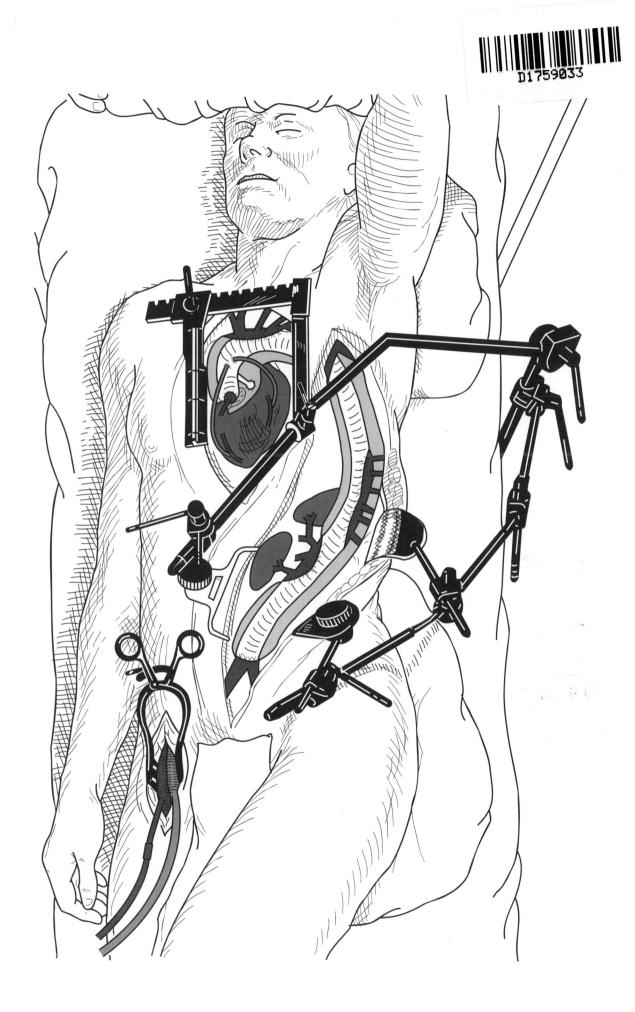

Cardiovascular and Vascular Disease of the Aorta

"For the life of all flesh is the blood thereof."
—Leviticus 17:14

"It profits one who is pondering on the movement, pulsation, performance, function, and services of the heart and arteries to read what his predecessors have written, and to note the general trend of opinion handed on by them. For by so doing he can confirm their correct statements, and through anatomical dissection, manifold experiments, and persistent careful observation emend their wrong ones. . . . and [with] much use of one's own eyes, to discern and investigate the truth."

—William Harvey, Introduction, *De Motu Cordis,* 1628
  (Latin translation by Kenneth J. Franklin)

Cardiovascular and Vascular Disease of the Aorta

Lars G. Svensson M.D., Ph.D.

F.R.C.S. (Edin), F.C.S. (S.A.), F.R.C.S. (C), F.A.C.C., F.A.C.S
Director, Center for Aortic Surgery and
Marfan Syndrome Clinic
Department of Cardiovascular and Thoracic Surgery
Lahey Clinic, Burlington, Massachusetts
Clinical Instructor in Surgery,
Harvard Medical School, Boston, Massachusetts
Formerly Assistant Professor of Surgery
Baylor College of Medicine
Attending Surgeon, Methodist Hospital
Chief of Cardiovascular Surgery, VAMC
Houston, Texas

E. Stanley Crawford M.D.

F.A.C.S., F.A.C.C., F.A.C.P
Late Professor of Surgery
Baylor College of Medicine
Attending Surgeon, Methodist Hospital
Houston, Texas

Illustrations by
Carol Pienta Larson B.S., A.M..I., and
Perrin Sparks Smith M.A., A.M.I.

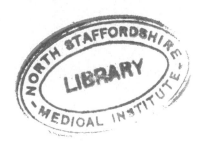

W. B. Saunders Company

A Division of Harcourt Brace & Company

Philadelphia London Toronto Montreal Sydney Tokyo

W.B. SAUNDERS COMPANY

A Division of Harcourt Brace & Company

The Curtis Center
Independence Square West
Philadelphia, Pennsylvania 19106

Library of Congress Cataloging-in-Publication Data

Svensson, Lars G.
    Cardiovascular and vascular disease of the aorta / Lars G.
Svensson, E. Stanley Crawford.
        p.   cm.
    ISBN 0-7216-5426-6
    1. Aorta—Diseases. 2. Aorta—Surgery. I. Crawford, E.
Stanley, 1924- . II. Title.
    [DNLM: 1. Aortic Diseases—surgery. WG 410 S968c 1997]
RC691.S92   1997
616.1'38—dc20
DNLM/DLC   96-18815

CARDIOVASCULAR AND VASCULAR DISEASE OF THE AORTA   ISBN 0-7216-5426-6

Printed in the United States of America

Last digit is the print number: 9   8   7   6   5   4   3   2   1

To Carolyn and Marion
without whose years of selfless sacrifice and loving
support this would not have been possible

and Geoffrey
who set the deadline

Preface

Dr. E. Stanley Crawford in his successful career of over 30 years operated on over 6,900 patients. I was privileged to have known and worked with him for six of those years. His modesty, tireless energy, enthusiasm for research and development of new techniques, keen mind, and surgical skill were extraordinary. At the inception of this writing, he and I discussed the need for a book that compiled our experience with aortic diseases. This book is a tribute to his achievements and also, I believe, a fulfillment of his wishes.

In this book, we have reviewed the available literature and also relied heavily on our own experience in managing aortic disease and, in particular, the wealth of experience of the senior author, E. Stanley Crawford. The recent exponential increase in knowledge relating to the subject of the aorta is compiled without losing sight of the pioneering work by the senior author previously published as a book and atlas. In medicine, the closest we can get to establishing scientific proof for the best method of management is the use of prospective randomized studies. For aortic diseases, however, there are few such prospective randomized studies and, certainly, none that have been blinded, and management of aortic disease is, therefore, based on prospective and retrospective studies, and many anecdotal reports. Thus principles of managing various aortic diseases are described. In addition, this book is a practical guide for those surgeons who wish to perform aortic operations and illustrates both the standard and modified operations in a step-by-step manner.

We also discuss the new developments in the field, in particular, the use of intraaortic stents and percutaneous methods which have become increasingly the favored approaches of choice under some circumstances. While there is great enthusiasm for some of these newer techniques, undoubtedly as the pitfalls are established, the pendulum will probably swing back again and the new techniques will find their indications in the spectrum of available options in the management of patients with aortic disease.

While many experts in the field could have written in great depth individual chapters for this book, we believe that there is virtue in describing a unified approach to the management of aortic disease based on our experience. Thus, we have presented a synthesis of the best techniques from our continued evaluation of our experience and observations to benefit the reader. We trust this book will be of value for both tyro and legerdemain. If the reader finds useful techniques in this manuscript on management and operative techniques for patients with aortic disease, this project will have been worthwhile.

We acknowledge with deep appreciation, our colleagues, who over the years have given valuable advice and have contributed to the development of aortic surgery, in particular, the residents and associates we have worked with; and, especially, Joseph S. Coselli, M.D., and Hazim J. Safi, M.D. Of particular note, is that without the pioneering work of surgeons at Baylor College of Medicine, during the 1950s and 1960s, the practice of aortic surgery would not have been established on such a firm footing as it was. Surgeons of note at Baylor who contributed to this expansion in aortic surgery included Michael E. DeBakey, M.D.; Denton A. Cooley, M.D.; George C. Morris, Jr., M.D.; and Gerald M. Lawrie, M.D. We also acknowledge the expert illustrations drawn mostly by Carol Pienta Larson, but also by Karen Perrin Park Smith at Baylor College of Medicine, and Francis E. Steckel and James Millerick at the Lahey Hitchcock Clinic, who took our rough drawings and made them into masterpieces of illustrative art, some of which have won prizes in national medical illustration competitions. Mark L. Silverman, M.D., Lahey Hitchcock Clinic, kindly provided the illustrative aortic histology slides. Jianping Sun, M.D., Ph.D., Dana Cardiovascular Research Fellow, diligently assisted in compiling Chapter 12 on the biochemistry of ischemia. We are also grateful to Marion Robinson, Ph.D., who edited and gave valuable advice concerning the book, and to Diane Carnevale who typed and obtained, with Carol Spencer, M.L.S., the references for the manuscript. I am also grateful to my colleagues Warren A. Williamson, M.D., Richard S. D'Agostino, M.D., and David M. Shahian, M.D., for their support and assistance during aortic operations and in the completion of this book. Lisette Bralow, Editor-in-Chief for Medical Books, from W.B. Saunders, encouraged the writing of the book and with Joan Sinclair, and Louise A. Gelinas, FSTM, efficiently produced it.

Lars G. Svensson, M.D., Ph.D.

Contents

1   Historical Aspects of Cardiovascular and Vascular Disease of the Aorta   1

2   Diagnosis and Evaluation of Aortic Disease   6

3   Degenerative Aortic Aneurysms   29

4   Aortic Dissection   42

5   Marfan Syndrome and Connective Tissue Diseases   84

6   Aortitis and Inflammatory Aneurysms   105

7   Aortic Infections   126

8   Congenital Abnormalities of the Aorta in Adults   153

9   Occlusive Disease of the Aorta   175

10   Traumatic Injuries of the Aorta   184

11   Primary Aortic Tumors   192

12   Ischemia, Reperfusion, and No-Reflow Phenomenon   194
With Jianping Sun, M.D., Ph.D.

13   Deep Hypothermia with Circulatory Arrest and Retrograde Brain Perfusion   219

14   Myocardial Protection   223

15   Pathophysiology of Aortic Cross-clamping and Influence of Spinal Cord Anatomy   226

16   Anesthesia and Perfusion Management   248

17   Techniques for Medial Degenerative Aneurysms of the Proximal Aorta   263

18   Techniques for Dissection Involving the Proximal Aorta   296

19   Techniques for Degenerative Disease of the Distal Aorta   335

20   Techniques for Dissection Involving the Distal Aorta   359

21 Procedures for Occlusive Disease of the Aorta   371

22 Repair of Aortic Fistulae   391

23 Aortic Aneurysms Associated with a Horseshoe Kidney   395

24 Replacement of the Entire Aorta   400

25 Complications of Proximal Aorta Operations   407

26 Complications of Distal Aorta Operations   414

27 Statistical Analyses of Operative Results   432

28 Late Follow-up and Management   456

    Index   460

Postscript

This book has attempted to concisely present the essential current knowledge concerning cardiovascular and vascular disease of the aorta based on that reported in the literature and our own experience, particularly that of my late mentor, E. Stanley Crawford, M.D., who was the motivator for this book. I have described in detail the operations we have found useful for operative repairs of the aorta. The factors that are important in reducing both the early and the late mortality rates and complication rates are presented as a compendium of our experience and that of other surgeons of a high caliber. New exciting and novel research is reviewed, particularly for neurological protection against ischemia and endovascular techniques, but will require observation over the ensuing years. This combination of world wide current expertise I hope will result in the synthesis of better or optimal patient care and further innovative research. If this is achieved in some small measure, my goal will have been attained.

Lars G. Svensson
December 24, 1995
Concord, Massachusetts

Historical Aspects of Cardiovascular and Vascular Disease of the Aorta

On the whole, disease of the aorta generally has not been of much interest except to a few inquiring persons. The reasons for this are many and include the utilitarian nature of the aorta, which may simply be regarded as a large pipe connecting various organs. The aorta does not capture the imagination as does the heart or brain, and it is not a distinctive organ like the lungs, liver, or kidneys with fascinating discrete and complex functions. Yet malfunction of the aorta is the thirteenth most common cause of death.[1] In more recent times, there has been a modest increase in public awareness of aortic disease as a result of some famous persons having succumbed to the condition. In 1989, despite emergency surgery, Lucille Ball died of acute aortic dissection involving the ascending aorta and aortic arch, and in 1993 Conway Twitty died of an infrarenal aortic rupture. Albert Einstein also died of a ruptured abdominal aortic aneurysm. He had previously had an abdominal aortic aneurysm wrapped with cellophane; Michael E. DeBakey, M.D., is said to have offered to repair the aneurysm for him, but Einstein refused another operation. Eventually, the aneurysm ruptured and was diagnosed initially as being due to acute cholelithiasis, hence the "Einstein sign."[2] Finally, and worthy of mention, is the sudden demise from aortic disease of a royal figure whose condition, one could argue, influenced the course of world events. On October 26, 1760, King George II suddenly died while moving his bowels.[3] Nichols, the King's physician, noted at autopsy that there was "intravasation of blood between (the) coats" of the aorta caused by aortic dissection. George II was succeeded by his unstable and stubborn grandson, George III, who imposed on the American colonies the taxes that led to the American War of Independence, and the rest is history.

EARLY DISCOVERIES CONCERNING THE AORTA

The early history of vascular surgery is illuminated by the creative genius of physicians such as Galen (c. AD 131–200), who based his anatomical knowledge on dissection of apes and other animals and stated, "When the arteries enlarged, the disease is called an aneurysm. If the aneurysm is injured, the blood gushes forth, and it is difficult to stanch it." Antyllus (second century AD) ligated arteries proximally and distally and evacuated the blood or clot. Ambrose Paré (1510–1590) repaired arterial war injuries by ligation of arteries. Andreas Vesalius (1514–1564) published *De Humani Corporis Fabrica* (*On the Fabric of the Human Body*) in 1543 and a description of an aneurysm in 1555.[4]

Although the aorta was known to anatomists, it was only when William Harvey wrote his momentous publication *Exercitatio Anatomica de Motu Cordis et Sanguinis in Animalibus* (*The Movement of the Heart and Blood in Animals*) in 1628 during the period known as the Enlightenment that the function of the aorta began to be understood. Harvey wrote in chapter 8 of his treatise

> when I meditated even further on the amount [i.e. of transmitted blood], and the very short time it took for its transfer, . . . having the veins, on the one hand, completely emptied and the arteries, on the other hand, brought to bursting through excessive inthrust of blood, unless the blood somehow flowed back again from the arteries into the veins and returned to the right ventricle of the heart; I then began to wonder whether it had a movement, as it were, in a circle. This I afterwards found to be true.

William Harvey proved that this connection had to exist when he conducted a simple yet ingenious experiment in which he used ligatures on the forearm and observed the direction of blood flow in the superficial veins.[5] He also observed that the aorta had a thicker wall because "the aorta sustains a stronger inthrust of blood from the left ventricle."

In 1732, three years after he graduated from Oxford University in England, Nichols published his compendium of lectures on cardiovascular physiology and disease. He had recognized aortic dissection in 1728, and he wrote extensively on the physiology of arteries, the innervation of arteries, and the autonomic nervous system, blood pressure control, and hypertension. His contributions to cardiovascular medicine have largely been overlooked and forgotten in the annals of history. His diagnosis of the cause of death of King George II has already been cited.[3] Also in 1728 came Lancisi's publication of *Motu Cordis et Aneurysmatibus* on the pathology and case reports of abdominal aneurysms.[6]

DEVELOPMENT OF AORTIC SURGERY

The first attempts at aortic operations were by John Hunter (1728–1793) and Cooper (1768–1841).[4] Nonetheless, it is only during the twentieth century that the successful operative repair of the aorta has been realized. The contributions of such men as Carrel[7] to basic operative techniques and experimental use of bypass grafts, Gibbon[8, 9] to the heart-lung machine, and Voorhees[4] and DeBakey[10] to graft prostheses will surely be landmarks in the historical annals of aortic surgery.[45] Other milestones are the development of operative techniques by Crafoord[11, 12] (coarctation), Dubost[13, 14] (infrarenal aorta repair), DeBakey[15-24] (ascending aorta and aortic arch repair, distal aortic arch, aortic dissection, and aortic surgery generally), Cooley and DeBakey[25] (ascending aorta), Morris[26, 31] (acute dissection, importance of profunda femoris artery in aortoiliac disease and aortofemoral bypass and renovascular surgery), and Crawford[32-44] (thoracoabdominal aneurysm, Marfan syndrome, and aortic dissection surgery).

For ease of reference, and because there have been so many important contributions to the field of aortic surgery, some of the particularly notable reports in the evolution of cardiovascular and vascular operations on the aorta are summarized below:

1817   Astley Cooper ligated an aortic bifurcation in a 38-year-old man with a ruptured external iliac aneurysm. This was done with the patient lying in his bed.[46]

1831   Alfred Velpeau inserted three pairs of sewing needles in an aneurysm to try to induce thrombosis.[4]

1922   Dshanelidze repaired a wound of the thoracic aorta.[47]

1923   Rudolph Matas used two cotton tapes in the first successful proximal ligation for a ruptured syphilitic aneurysm in a 28-year-old woman who died of tuberculosis 17 months later.[29] Matas also pioneered the technique of arteriorrhaphy for peripheral aneurysms.[48]

1932   Blalock repaired a stab wound of the ascending aorta caused by an ice pick in a patient with cardiac tamponade. On removal of the occluding clot, "bright red blood shot over the screen at the head of the table on the anesthetist." The use of only nitrous oxide and oxygen for the anesthetic may have contributed to Blalock's operative description.[47]

1944   Alexander and Byron excised an 8-cm thoracic aneurysm associated with coarctation and ligated the aorta both proximally and distally.[49]

1944   Clarence Crafoord performed two end-to-end repairs after resecting coarctations in a 12-year-old boy and a 27-year-old farmer.[11, 12]

1947   Shumacker reported the first excision of a post-coarctation saccular aneurysm and end-to-end repair in a 8½-year-old boy.[50]

1949   Swan repaired a 16-year-old boy's post coarctation aneurysm with a homograft.[51]

1950   Bigelow published the results of his experiments in dogs in which he used deep hypothermia with a view to its use for cardiovascular operations.[52, 53]

1950   (April) Lam and Aram reported the first successful repair of an aortic aneurysm not related to coarctation of the aorta.[54] They used a Hufnagel Lucite shunt within the replacement homograft during the repair. Postoperatively, the 56-year-old patient had paraparesis, particularly of the right leg. The patient had been treated for a luetic infection during World War I; he died of an empyema three months after surgery.

1950   (November 14) Jacques Oudot repaired a thrombosed aortic bifurcation in a 51-year-old woman; he used an extraperitoneal approach with an arterial homograft.[55]

1951   Charles Dubost repaired an infrarenal abdominal aortic aneurysm with a thoracic homograft, using an extraperitoneal approach through a thoracoabdominal incision in a 50-year-old man.[13, 14]

1952   DeBakey and Cooley inserted a bifurcated aortic homograft from below the renal arteries to the iliac arteries and reported a series of seven abdominal aortic aneurysm repairs with homografts.[15]

1952   Voorhees replaced an abdominal aortic aneurysm with plastic fiber, Vinyon-N.[4]

1952   Julian described the use of Dacron polyester prostheses.[56]

1953   Julian reported replacement of arteriosclerosis of the abdominal aorta with a homologous graft.[57]

1954   Gerbode reported the first repair of a ruptured infrarenal aneurysm with a homograft.[58]

1954   Etheredge reported the first successful thoracoabdominal aneurysm repair.[4]

1956   (August 18) Cooley and DeBakey replaced the ascending aorta with a homograft, using cardiac bypass.[25]

1956   Murray reported successful insertion of aortic valve homografts in the descending aorta to treat aortic and mitral valve insufficiency.[59]

1957   DeBakey and Cooley successfully repaired the aortic arch with a homograft.[20]

1958   DeBakey described the use of flexible knitted Dacron grafts.[21]

1958   DeBakey described treatment of thrombo-obliterative disease of the branches of the aortic arch, first performed in January, 1957.[10]

1959   Shumacker reported an ascending aorta–to–abdominal aorta bypass for a rupture of the descending thoracic aorta.[60]

1961 Crawford reported repair of saccular aortic aneurysms with patch grafts.[61]

1961 Bigelow and Heimbecker attempted insertion of an aortic homograft to replace the aortic valve, although the patient died of a myocardial infarct 24 hours after the operation.[62]

1961 Both Blaisdell (1961) and Stevenson (1961) independently reported thoracic aorta–to–femoral artery bypasses.[63, 64]

1961 Hufnagel and Conrad (1962) presented a series of seven patients in whom they repaired ascending aortic dissections; these repairs included the use of a tube graft and valve resuspension.[65]

1962 Wheat replaced the aortic valve, excised the aorta around the coronary ostia, and replaced the ascending aorta with a graft shaped to accommodate reattachment of the coronary ostia.[66]

1962 Ross reported successful insertion of an aortic valve homograft in an orthotopic subcoronary position.[67]

1963 Morris, Henley, and DeBakey reported repair of the ascending aorta for acute aortic dissection.[31] In 1992 their patient had a composite valve graft inserted by Lawrie.[68]

1963 Groves performed a separate aortic valve replacement and an ascending aortic replacement with a tubular graft in a 38-year-old patient with Marfan syndrome.[69]

1963 Barnard repaired the aortas of eight patients, including those with aortic dissection, using deep hypothermia and circulatory arrest or moderate hypothermia with atriofemoral bypass.[70]

1964 Borst reported direct suture repair of an arteriovenous fistula between the innominate vein and the aorta caused by shrapnel; he used deep hypothermia and circulatory arrest for 19 minutes.[71]

1965 Crawford replaced the thoracoabdominal aorta in a 55-year-old insurance salesman, who is still alive, using the inlay inclusion technique with bypasses to the renal arteries. The inclusion technique has become the principal method by which these aneurysms are repaired.[32-35, 38, 45]

1966 Waldhausen reported repair of coarctation of the aorta in three patients with a left subclavian artery flap bridging the coarctation.[72]

1967 Ross described replacement of the aortic root with a pulmonary autograft and repair of the pulmonary artery with a homograft.[73]

1968 Bentall and De Bono reported complete replacement of the ascending aorta with a composite valve graft in a 33-year-old man.[74]

1975 Griepp reported inversion of an aortic graft into the descending aorta for the distal anastomosis of aortic arch replacements with the use of deep hypothermia and circulatory arrest.[75]

1978 Goldstone characterized and elaborated on inflammatory aneurysms.[76]

1981 Cabrol reported composite valve graft insertion with reattachment of the coronary ostia with separate tube grafts.[77]

1983 Borst reported replacing the aortic arch and leaving a tube graft lying free in the descending aorta for a subsequent descending aortic repair, the so-called "elephant trunk" technique.[78]

1984 Crawford reported replacement of the entire aorta using multiple sequential operations.[37]

1986 Massimo reported extensive replacements of the aorta from and including the aortic arch to the celiac artery without replacement of the abdominal aorta with a tubular graft through predominantly a left thoracoabdominal incision.[79] The ascending aorta was not replaced.

1987 Coselli and Crawford reported insertion of an aortobifemoral graft to establish a cardiopulmonary bypass in conjunction with ascending aortic operations.[80]

1990 Svensson, Crawford, and colleagues reported their modification of the elephant trunk technique in which the graft was inserted into the descending aorta for the performance of the distal aortic anastomosis.[44, 81]

1990 Crawford and associates reported staged replacement of the entire aorta, using their modification of the "elephant trunk" technique.[42, 81]

1992 Svensson reported insertion of a composite valve graft with a tube graft to the left main coronary ostium and reattachment of the right coronary ostium as a free aortic button buttressed with a Teflon ring to reduce the risk of bleeding and postoperative formation of a false aneurysm.[82]

1993 (May 4) Svensson and colleagues successfully replaced the entire aorta from the aortic valve to the aortic bifurcation with a tubular graft during one operation, using deep hypothermia with circulatory arrest.[83]

1993 Massimo reported extensive replacements of the entire thoracic aorta during one operation and replacement of proximal segments of the abdominal aorta in some patients.[84]

1994 Svensson reported acute dissection repair with a composite valve graft and bypass from the composite valve graft to the supraceliac aorta in the abdomen for concurrent coarctation of the aorta.[85]

From 1955 to February 1991, Dr. Crawford performed 6900 aortic procedures. This included 1108 on the ascending aorta or aortic arch (or both), 887 on the descending thoracic aorta, 1679 on the thoracoabdominal aorta and on the infrarenal aorta, 1864 for aortic aneurysms, and 1362 for aortoiliac disease. This book is based on our experience and the operations pioneered by DeBakey and colleagues at Baylor College of Medicine.

REFERENCES

1. Majumber PP, St Jean PL, Ferrell RE, et al. On the inheritance of abdominal aortic aneurysm. Am J Hum Genet 1991;48:164-70.

2. Chandler JJ. The Einstein sign: the clinical picture of acute chole-cystitis caused by ruptured abdominal aortic aneurysm [letter]. N Engl J Med 1984;310:1538.

3. Nichols F. Observations concerning the body of his late majesty, October 26, 1760. Philos Trans R Soc Lond (Biol) 1761;52:265-74.

4. Slaney G. A history of aneurysm surgery. In: Greenhalgh RM, Mannick JA, Powell JT, eds: The Cause and Management of Aneurysms. London, England: WB Saunders, 1990:1-18.

5. Harvey W; Franklin KJ, trans. The circulation of the blood and other writings. London, England: JM Dent & Sons Ltd; 1963.

6. Lancisi GM; Wright WC, ed. Aneurysmatibus. New York, NY: Macmillan Publishing Co.: 1952:3, 24, 333.

7. Lawrie GM. The scientific contributions of Alexis Carrel. Clin Cardiol 1987;10:428-30.

8. Gibbon JH Jr. The maintenance of life during experimental occlusion of the pulmonary artery followed by survival. Surg Gynecol Obstet 1939;69:602.

9. Gibbon JH Jr. Application of a mechanical heart and lung apparatus to cardiac surgery. Minn Med 1954;37:171.

10. DeBakey ME, Cooley DA, Crawford ES, Morris GC Jr. Aneurysms of the thoracic aorta: analysis of 179 cases treated by resection. J Thorac Surg 1958;36:393.

11. Crafoord C, Nylin F. Congenital coarctation of aorta and its surgical treatment. J Thorac Surg 1945;14:347.

12. Crafoord C. Correction of aortic coarctation. Ann Thorac Surg 1980; 30:300.

13. Dubost C, Allanz M, Oeconomos N. Resection of an aneurysm of thoracoabdominal aorta: reestablishment of the continuity by a preserved human arterial graft, with results after five months. Arch Surg 1952;64:405.

14. Dubost C. The first successful resection of an aneurysm of the abdominal aorta followed by re-establishment of continuity using a preserved human arterial graft. Ann Vasc Surg 1986;1:147-9.

15. DeBakey ME, Cooley DA. Successful resection of aneurysm of thoracic aorta and replacement by graft. JAMA 1953;152:673.

16. DeBakey ME, Cooley DA. Successful resection of aneurysms of distal aortic arch and replacement of graft. JAMA 1954;155:1398-403.

17. DeBakey ME, Cooley DA, Creech O Jr. Surgical considerations of dissecting aneurysms of the aorta. Ann Surg 1955;142:586-92.

18. DeBakey ME, Creech O, Morris GC. Aneurysm of thoracoabdominal aorta involving the celiac, superior mesenteric, and renal arteries: report of four cases treated by resection and homograft replacement. Ann Surg 1956;144:549-73.

19. DeBakey ME, Crawford ES. Vascular prostheses. Transplant Bull 1957;4:2-4.

20. DeBakey ME, Cooley DA, Crawford ES, et al. Successful resection of fusiform aneurysm of aortic arch replacement by homograft. Surg Gynecol Obstet 1957;105:656-64.

21. DeBakey ME, Cooley DA, Crawford ES, et al. The clinical application of a new flexible knitted dacron arterial substitute. Arch Surg 1958;77:713-24.

22. DeBakey ME, Crawford ES. Surgical considerations of acquired disease of the aorta and major peripheral arteries. II. Dissecting aneurysms of the aorta. Mod Concepts Cardiovasc Dis 1959;28:563-5.

23. DeBakey ME, Henley WS, Cooley DA, et al. Surgical management of dissecting aneurysms of the aorta. J Thorac Cardiovasc Surg 1965;49:130-49.

24. DeBakey ME, McCollum CH, Crawford ES, et al. Dissection and dissecting aneurysms of the aorta: twenty-year follow-up of five hundred twenty-seven patients treated surgically. Surgery 1982;92:1118-34.

25. Cooley DA, DeBakey ME. Resection of the entire ascending aorta in fusiform aneurysm using cardiac bypass. JAMA 1956;162:1158.

26. Morris GC Jr, DeBakey ME, Cooley DA, et al. Surgical treatment of renal hypertension. Ann Surg 1960;151:854-5.

27. Lawrie GM, Morris GC Jr. Fifteen-year follow-up of emergency operation for acute dissecting aneurysm of the aorta with aortic insufficiency. JAMA 1978;239:724-5.

28. Lawrie GM, Morris GC Jr. Repair of aortic dissections. Ann Thorac Surg 1979;27:194.

29. Matas R. Aneurysm of the abdominal aorta at its bifurcation into the common iliac arteries. Ann Surg 1960;112:909.

30. Morris GC, DeBakey ME. Abdominal angina, diagnosis and surgical treatment. JAMA 1961;176:88.

31. Morris GC Jr, Henly WS, DeBakey ME. Correction of acute dissect-ing aneurysm of aorta with valvular insufficiency. JAMA 1963;184: 63.

32. Crawford ES, DeBakey ME. Hemodynamic alterations of circulation in patients submitted to reconstructive vascular operations. Bull Soc Int Chir 1960;85:13-23.

33. Crawford ES. Thoracoabdominal and abdominal aortic aneurysm involving renal, superior mesenteric, and celiac arteries. Ann Surg 1974;179:763-72.

34. Crawford ES, Snyder DM, Cho GC, et al. Progress in treatment of thoraco-abdominal and abdominal aortic aneurysms involving celi-ac, superior mesenteric, and renal arteries. Ann Surg 1978;188: 404-22.

35. Crawford ES, Palamara AE, Saleh SA, Roehm JOF. Aortic aneurysm: current status of surgical treatment. Surg Clin North Am 1979;59: 597-636.

36. Crawford ES, Walker HJ, Saleh SA, Normann NA. Graft replacement of aneurysm in descending thoracic aorta: results without bypass or shunting. Surgery 1981;89:73-85.

37. Crawford ES, Crawford JL, Stowe CL, et al. Total aortic replacement for chronic aortic dissection occurring in patients with and without Marfan's syndrome. Ann Surg 1984;199:358-62.

38. Crawford ES, Crawford JL. Diseases of the Aorta: including an Atlas of Angiographic Pathology and Surgical Technique. Baltimore, MD: Williams & Wilkins Co., 1984.

39. Crawford ES, Crawford JL, Safi HJ, et al. Thoracoabdominal aortic aneurysms: preoperative and intraoperative factors determining immediate and long-term results of operation in 605 patients. J Vasc Surg 1986;3:389-404.

40. Crawford ES, Svensson LG, Coselli JS, et al. Aortic dissection and dissecting aortic aneurysms. Ann Surg 1988;208:254-73.

41. Crawford ES, Svensson LG, Coselli JS, et al. Surgical treatment of aneurysm and/or dissection of the ascending aorta, transverse aortic arch, and ascending aorta and transverse aortic arch: factors influencing survival in 717 patients. J Thorac Cardiovasc Surg 1989;98: 659-73.

42. Crawford ES, Coselli JS, Svensson LG, et al. Diffuse aneurysmal disease (chronic aortic dissection, Marfan, and mega aorta syndromes) and multiple aneurysm: treatment by subtotal and total aortic replacement emphasizing the elephant trunk operation. Ann Surg 1990;211:521-37.

43. Svensson LG, Crawford ES, Coselli JS, et al. Impact of cardiovascular operation on survival in the Marfan patient. Circulation 1989;80(3 Pt 1):I233-42.

44. Svensson LG, Crawford ES, Hess KR, et al. Dissection of the aorta and dissecting aortic aneurysms: improving early and long-term surgical results. Circulation 1990;82(5 Supp):IV24-38.

45. Svensson LG, Crawford ES. Aortic dissection and aortic aneurysm surgery: clinical observations, experimental investigations and statistical analyses. Part I. Curr Probl Surg 1992;29:819-912.

46. Brock RC. The life and work of Sir Astley Cooper. Ann R Coll Surg Engl 1969;44:1.

47. Blalock A, Park EA. The surgical treatment of experimental coarctation (atresia) of the aorta. Ann Surg 1944;119:445.

48. Matas R. An operation for the radical cure of aneurysms based on arteriography. Ann Surg 1903;37:161.

49. Alexander J, Byron FX. Aortectomy for thoracic aneurysms. JAMA 1944;126:1139.

50. Shumacker HB Jr. Coarctation and aneurysm of the aorta: report of a case treated by excision and end-to-end suture of aorta. Ann Surg 1948;127:655.

51. Swan H, Maaske C, Johnson M, et al. Arterial homografts. II. Resection of thoracic aortic aneurysm using a stored human arterial transplant. Arch Surg 1950;61:732.

52. Bigelow WG, Callaghan JC, Hoops JA. General hypothermia for experimental intracardiac surgery. Ann Surg 1950;132:531-9.

53. Bigelow WG, McBirnie JE. Further experiences with hypothermia for intracardiac surgery in monkeys and groundhogs. Ann Surg 1953;137:361-8.

54. Lam CR, Aram HH. Resection of the descending thoracic aorta for aneurysm: a report of the use of a homograft in a case and an experimental study. Ann Surg 1951;134:743-52.

55. Oudot J, Beaconfield P. Thrombosis of the aortic bifurcation treated by resection and homograft replacement: report of five cases. Arch Surg 1959;66:365.

56. Julian OC, Dye WS, Olwin JH, et al. Direct surgery of arteriosclerosis. Ann Surg 1952;136:459.

57. Julian OC, Grove WJ, Dye WS, et al. Direct surgery of arteriosclerosis: resection of abdominal aorta with homologous aortic graft replacement. Ann Surg 1953;138:387.

58. Gerbode F. Ruptured aortic aneurysm: a surgical emergency. Surg Gynecol Obstet 1954;98:759.

59. Murray G. Homologous aortic valve segment transplants as surgical treatment for aortic and mitral insufficiency. Angiology 1956;7:466-71.

60. Shumacker HB, King H. Surgical management of rapidly expanding intrathoracic pulsating hematomas. Surg Gynecol Obstet 1959;109:155-64.

61. Crawford ES, DeBakey ME, Blaisdell FW. Simplified treatment of large, sacciform aortic aneurysms with patch grafts. J Thorac Surg 1961;41:479.

62. Gunning AJ. Ross' first homograft replacement of the aortic valve. Ann Thorac Surg 1992;54:809.

63. Blaisdell FW, DeMattei GA, Gauder PJ. Extraperitoneal thoracic aorta to femoral bypass graft as replacement for an infected aortic bifurcation prosthesis. Am J Surg 1961;102:583-5.

64. Stevenson JK, Sauvage LR, Harkins HN. A bypass homograft from thoracic aorta to femoral arteries for occlusive vascular disease. Am Surg 1961;27:632-7.

65. Hufnagel CA, Conrad PW. Dissecting aneurysms of the ascending aorta: direct approach to repair. Surgery 1962;51:84-9.

66. Wheat MN Jr, Wilson JR, Bartley TD. Successful replacement of the entire ascending aorta and aortic valve. JAMA 1964;188:717-9.

67. Ross DN. Homograft replacement of the aortic valve. Lancet 1962;2:287.

68. Svensson LG, Crawford ES. Aortic dissection and aortic aneurysm surgery: clinical observations, experimental investigations, and statistical analyses. Part II Curr Probl Surg 1992;29:915-1057.

69. Groves LK, Effler DB, Hawk WA, Guliti R. Aortic insufficiency secondary to aneurysmal changes in the ascending aorta: surgical management. J Thorac Cardiovasc Surg 1964;48:363-79.

70. Barnard CN, Schire V. The surgical treatment of acquired aneurysms of the thoracic aorta. Thorax 1963;18:101-5.

71. Borst HG, Schaudig A, Rudolph W. Arteriovenous fistula of the aortic arch: repair during deep hypothermia and circulatory arrest. J Thorac Cardiovasc Surg 1964;48:443-7.

72. Waldhausen JA, Nahrwold DL. Repair of coarctation of the aorta with a subclavian flap. J Thorac Cardiovasc Surg 1966;51:532-3.

73. Ross DN. Replacement of aortic and mitral valves with a pulmonary autograft. Lancet 1967;2:956-8.

74. Bentall H, DeBono A. A technique for complete replacement of the ascending aorta. Thorax 1968;23:338-9.

75. Griepp RB, Stinson EB, Hollingsworth JF, et al. Prosthetic replacement of the aortic arch. J Thorac Cardiovasc Surg 1975;70:1051-63.

76. Goldstone J, Malone JM, Moore WS. Inflammatory aneurysms of the abdominal aorta. Surgery 1978;83:425-30.

77. Cabrol C, Pavie A, Gandjbakhch I, et al. Complete replacement of the ascending aorta with reimplantation of the coronary arteries: new surgical approach. J Thorac Cardiovasc Surg 1981;81:309-15.

78. Borst HG, Walterbusch G, Schaps D. Extensive aortic replacement using "elephant trunk" prosthesis. Thorac Cardiovasc Surg 1983;31:37-40.

79. Massimo CG, Poma AG, Viligiardi RR, et al. Simultaneous total aortic replacement from arch to bifurcation: experience with six cases. Texas Heart Inst J 1986;13:147-51.

80. Coselli JS, Crawford ES. Femoral artery perfusion for cardiopulmonary bypass in patients with aortoiliac artery obstruction. Ann Thorac Surg 1987;43:437-9.

81. Svensson LG. Rationale and technique for replacement of the ascending aorta, arch, and distal aorta using a modified elephant trunk procedure. J Cardiac Surg 1992;7:301-12.

82. Svensson LG. Approach to the insertion of composite valve graft. Ann Thorac Surg 1992;54:376-8.

83. Svensson LG, Shahian DM, Davis FG, et al. Replacement of entire aorta from aortic valve to bifurcation during one operation. Ann Thorac Surg 1994;58:1164-6.

84. Massimo CG, Presenti LF, Favi PP, et al. Simultaneous total replacement from valve to bifurcation: experience with 21 cases. Ann Thorac Surg 1993;56:1110-6.

85. Svensson LG. Management of acute dissection with coarctation of the aorta in single operation. Ann Thorac Surg 1994;58:241-3.

2

Diagnosis and Evaluation
of Aortic Disease

Usually patients with aortic aneurysms, traumatic rupture of the aorta, aortitis, congenital lesions, or aortic dissection will require multiple tests to evaluate the aorta, followed by operative treatment in many cases. Factors that will weigh against the benefits of surgical treatment include aneurysms not large enough in diameter to warrant operation, medical conditions that make the risks excessively high, advanced age of the patient, minimal symptoms, and conditions (for example, dissection of the distal aorta) that are better managed initially by intensive medical therapy.

The diagnosis of aortic disease before an aortic catastrophe, such as rupture or dissection, is often missed or is made by chance. For example, asymptomatic disease of the thoracic aorta may be diagnosed from incidental findings on routine chest radiographs, computed tomography (CT) or magnetic resonance imaging (MRI) scans of the chest for other indications, or during cardiac catheterization for coronary artery or valvular disease. Similarly, abdominal aortic disease, particularly abdominal aortic aneurysms, may be fortuitously detected during routine physical examination of the abdomen, on ultrasound scans of the abdomen, or during radiography, CT, MRI, or angiography.

A patient's symptoms, particularly back pain or chest pain, may alert the physician to the need for further studies to identify the possible cause of the symptoms, thus leading to diagnosis of the aortic condition (Figs. 2-1 and 2-2).

On the basis of the diagnostic studies initially performed, the physician or surgeon will assess most patients for surgery, judging the risks versus the benefits in each patient and then presenting these findings, in addition to the recommended medical treatment, to the patient and the patient's family. The evaluation of the patient's condition is discussed later in this chapter. Subsequent chapters will deal in more detail with the evaluation of specific conditions (for example, aortic dissection, traumatic rupture of the aorta, congenital lesions, and aortitis).

The most important diagnostic tools for the detection and evaluation of the extent of aortic disease encompass CT with contrast, MRI, transesophageal echocardiography (TEE), and aortography. As with all innovations, there are inherent weaknesses in addition to the strengths of the various diagnostic methods. Therefore these will be covered in order of their overall importance and usefulness rather than in the order of their historical appearance.

COMPUTED TOMOGRAPHIC SCANS WITH CONTRAST

The principle of reconstructing images from projections was originally described by Radon in 1917, as discussed by Webb.[1] Later, in 1940, Gabriel Frank applied for a patent for an apparatus that could reconstruct an optical back-projection.[1] In the mid 1940's Takahashi built equipment that produced tomographic slices by back-projection. In 1957, in a remarkable development, Russian inventors in Kiev built a medical CT scanner, although this has only recently been discovered.[1] In 1963 Cormack reported building a CT scanner that was able to create images, but his research, published in an applied physics journal, generated little interest.[1] Similarly, there was scant enthusiasm when Kuhl, in May 1965, produced transmission CT scans of a patient's chest.[1] It was only later that Geoffrey Hounsfield, who collaborated with the EMI Company, produced his first images in October 1971. For his achievement he was knighted and, together with Alian Cormack, received the Nobel Prize in 1979.[1]

Indications and Advantages

When aortic disease is suspected on the evidence of clinical examination or routine radiographs, the most accurate and easily accessible method of noninvasively determining the diagnosis is to obtain a CT scan, with contrast, of the chest and abdomen. The reason for studying both the chest and the abdomen is that aneurysmal disease may be multisegmental according to our observation that, in up to 25% of patients with thoracic aneurysms and 10% of patients with abdominal aneurysms, more than one aortic aneurysm is present.[2] Furthermore, as the patient ages, the involvement of the thoracic aorta by aneurysmal disease is more frequently associated with infrarenal aneurysms. CT scanning, in our experience, is also the most accurate method of determining the external size of aneurysms and their extent, and CT can be speedily performed in patients suspected of having aortic dissection. In addition, CT is useful

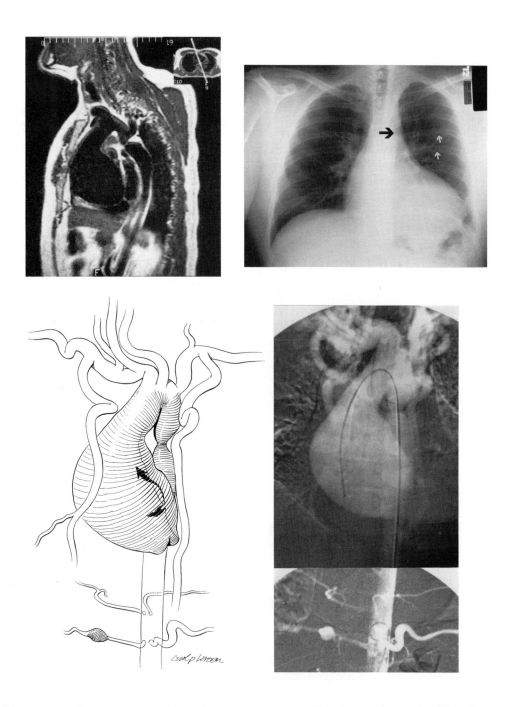

FIGURE 2–1 Diagnostic studies in a young male patient with shortness of breath and chest pain. Clinical examination revealed radiofemoral pulse delay with weak femoral pulses, distant heart sounds, and aortic valve regurgitation. Chest radiograph *(upper right window)* revealed a reversed "3" sign at the aortic knuckle *(black arrow)* suggesting aortic coarctation. This is further supported by the erosion of the ribs *(white arrows)*. Note that the heart shadow, particularly below the aortic knuckle, is globular in shape, suggesting a pericardial effusion. On chest radiographs of patients with ascending aortic aneurysms, the left heart shadow is often more prominent and the heart is displaced (pushed) downward and to the left, as in this patient. The reason for this is that an aneurysm not only increases in diameter but, particularly when the aneurysms reach larger diameters, also leads to lengthening of the aorta, thus causing downward and leftward displacement of the heart. Descending thoracic or thoracoabdominal aneurysms are seen as a bulge to the left of the descending aorta or as a shadow behind the heart. The MRI *(upper left window)* clearly shows coarctation of the aorta below the left subclavian artery, an ascending aortic aneurysm, and because the segment involving the sinus of Valsalva and the ascending aorta is continuous with a flask or wineskin bag appearance with loss of the sinotubular ridge, this is known as annuloaortic ectasia. There is severe displacement of the heart, with evidence of pericardial fluid. Cardiac catheterization, including aortogram *(lower right window)* revealed a posterior aortic tear, indicating aortic dissection, and confirmed the presence of the aortic coarctation with a 55 mm Hg gradient across it. The abdominal angiogram showed that there were small aneurysms of the intercostal arteries in keeping with late aortic coarctation. Note the enlarged internal mammary arteries. The left lower window is a composite diagram of the aortogram, with the arrow indicating the site of aortic dissection.

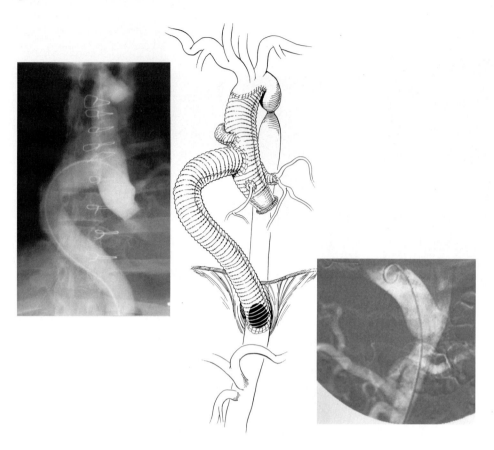

FIGURE 2–2 Postoperative repair aortogram showing, in the left window, the ascending aorta replacement with a composite valve graft, a tube interposition bypass to the left main coronary ostium, reattachment of the right coronary ostium as an aortic button, and a 25 mm tube graft from the ascending aorta to the infradiaphragmatic supraceliac aorta *(right lower window)*. The diagram shows the composite of the repair. The patient was extubated the morning after the operation with a hemoglobin level of 8.3 mg/dl, was discharged without any blood transfusion, and a year later is doing well without having had any problems. (Reprinted with permission from the Society of Thoracic Surgeons. From Svensson LG. Ann Thorac Surg 1994;58: 241–3.)

FIGURE 2–3 Windows **A, B,** and **C** show aortic dissection of the descending thoracic aorta on CT scan. Note the clear-cut septum in **A**. In **B** the two lumina can be seen, but there is partial thrombosis of the false lumen and evidence of calcification of the aortic wall *(white specules)*. **C** shows even more thrombosis of the false channel and no easily apparent septum; with the exception of the false channel indicated by the *arrow,* the appearance could be confused with a thrombus-lined aneurysm. The diagram shows the pathological changes. (From Svensson LG, Crawford ES. Curr Probl Surg 1992; 29:819–912.)

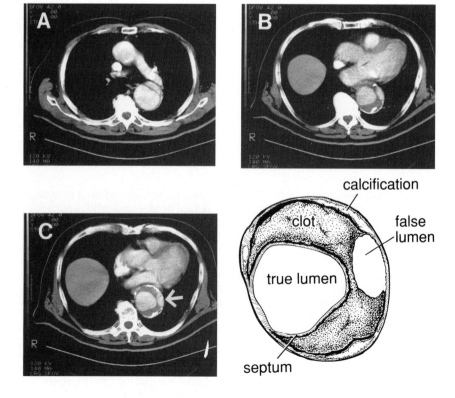

for the estimation of tissues surrounding the aorta, and the technique has a high specificity rate for ruling out aortic disease. The CT scan also reveals information concerning

- Cardiac ventricular wall thickness
- Coronary artery calcification and patency, as well as patency of bypass grafts
- Presence of pericardial disease or fluid, including cardiac tamponade
- Aortic wall dimensions and pathology
- Aortic contents, including thrombus or aortic dissection septum (Figs. 2–3 and 2–4)
- Patency of branch arteries
- Involvement of bony structures, particularly the sternum or vertebrae
- Extent in relation to repair required (Fig. 2–5)
- Position, involvement, and size of the greater vessels
- Relationship of an aneurysm to renal arteries, especially for juxtarenal aneurysms
- Size and thrombus in the iliac arteries
- Evidence of aortovenous fistulae as shown by simultaneous contrast in the aorta and inferior vena cava (Fig. 2–6).[3, 4]

Vertebral column erosion is not an infrequent observation in patients with descending thoracic aortic aneurysms and occurs in 6% of patients with abdominal aortic aneurysms, even though backache is considerably more common. Patients should be examined for evidence of malignant lesions because about 5% of patients have malignant tumors at the time of operation.[5] A patient whose operation is being deferred for various reasons (noncritical size, associated disease, age) can be conveniently followed up with regular CT scans. Hirose and colleagues[6] found in 171 patients with atherosclerotic aortic aneurysms, observed at 6-month intervals, that the average growth rate for thoracic aneurysms was 0.42 cm/y and for abdominal aneurysms

0.28 cm/y. Aortic arch aneurysms in particular grew rapidly at an average rate of 0.56 cm/y, even if corrected for initial size.

The time required for CT scanning has become considerably less in comparison with the original scans of the chest,[7, 8] and with the advances of ultrafast CT scanning it is likely that flow in even small arteries such as the coronary arteries will be imaged, allowing for evaluation of suspected coronary artery disease.[9] Furthermore, spatial resolution has improved to the extent that slices a couple of millimeters in size can be obtained. Thus diagnosis of a patient's problem can be quickly achieved and prompt institution of therapy commenced.[4]

A valuable new type of CT scanning is becoming available and will have an important impact on the preoperative evaluation of patients who require aortic operations.[10] Three-dimensional spiral CT angiography of the aorta results in a detailed picture of the inner lumen of the aorta and its branches. This image can be manipulated to view the aortic lumen in multiple projections or to produce a two-dimensional spatial image of the aorta analogous to a conventional angiogram. The sharp images allow for the diagnosis of stenoses in branches from the aorta and careful evaluation of the lumen. Thus it may, with time, supersede conventional angiography and become a more useful tool for evaluation of the aortic lumen (for example, with aortic dissection).

Disadvantages

One of the major disadvantages of CT scanning is that, either in the presence of renal disease or because of the need for subsequent arteriography, the patient may be given a large dose of contrast material that can then precipitate renal failure. When both a CT scan and an aortogram are required, an option is to obtain the aortogram first and the CT scan shortly thereafter. The circulating contrast material from the aortogram is usually sufficient to obtain good delineation of the aortic lumen. The inability of CT scanning to assess aortic valve insufficiency and detect

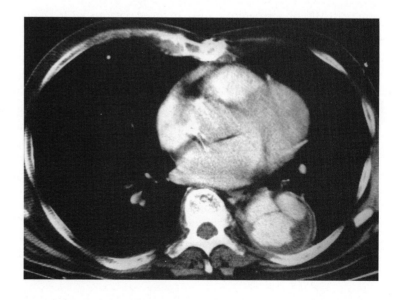

FIGURE 2–4 CT scan of the chest with contrast in a patient with Marfan syndrome. Note the unusual three lumina, two of them false, caused by repeated aortic dissection, a more common finding in patients with Marfan syndrome. There is also some thrombus formation in two of the lumina. Note the septa separating the lumina. (From Svensson LG, Crawford ES. Curr Probl Surg 1992; 29:819–912.)

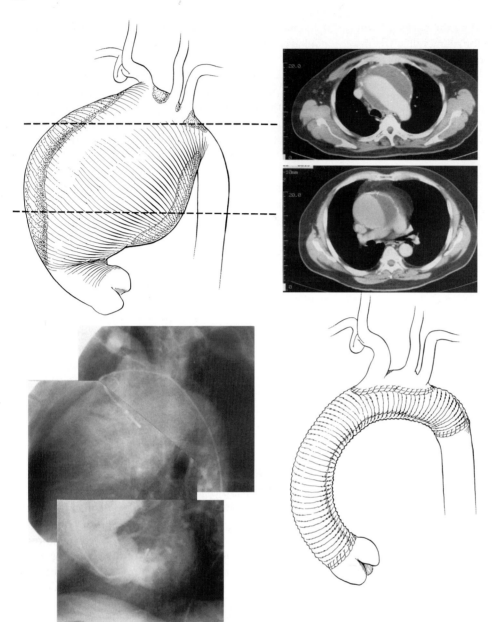

FIGURE 2–5 Right upper window shows the CT scans in an elderly patient with a thrombus-lined ascending and aortic arch aneurysm. Note that the inner lumen is clearly defined by the dye contrast in the blood. The aneurysm is interposed between the sternum and the vertebral column posteriorly, although there is no gross erosion of the bone cortex. It can be deduced from the scans that the aneurysm ends in the proximal descending aorta. The lower right aortogram, performed during cardiac catheterization, shows the inner lumen of the aneurysm. Note that thrombus within the aortic wall makes the aneurysm appear smaller than the true size seen on the CT scan. The lower diagram shows the postoperative repair performed with deep hypothermia, arterial circulatory arrest, and retrograde perfusion of the brain. The patient received no homologous blood or blood products for the operation and was discharged without any complications.

branch artery stenoses is a further disadvantage in comparison with MRI or aortography. Also, in those patients with aortic dissection, if the false lumen has completely thrombosed, then the septum between the true and false lumina often will not be detected by CT unless it is calcified. The aneurysm may therefore be diagnosed incorrectly as being caused by degenerative disease with thrombus rather than by aortic dissection (Fig. 2–3).[4]

AORTOGRAPHY

Arteriography, including cardiac catheterization, has evolved over a century to the present-day highly sophisticated techniques. Shortly after Roentgen's discovery of X-rays in 1895, a chalk solution was injected into a cadaver to image peripheral arteries.[11] Subsequently, in 1929, Reynaldo Dos Santos performed the first translumbar abdominal aortogram in a human patient.[12] In 1953 Seldinger[13] reported the technique for which he has become famous. This procedure involves the insertion of a needle, through which a guidewire is threaded, into the femoral artery. The needle is withdrawn, and a larger catheter can then be threaded over the guidewire. This is now the preferred technique for percutaneous transfemoral catheterization of the coronary arteries and the left ventricle and for general study of the aorta, irrespective of either the aortic disease or previous surgery. The technique of Sones,[14, 15] performed by means of a brachial artery cutdown, is used extensively by cardiologists for cardiac catheterization in patients with peripheral vascular disease.[4]

Indications

After the necessary diagnostic information has been obtained from the CT scan, the next step in planning the operation is usually an aortogram, especially for patients

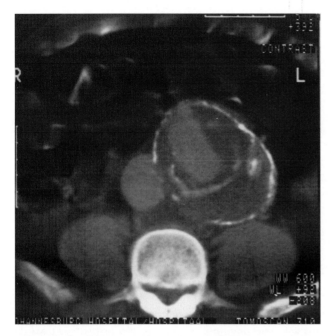

FIGURE 2–6   CT scan of the abdomen with contrast showing simultaneous contrast medium in the inferior vena cava and aorta. Note the thrombus-lined infrarenal aortic aneurysm with calcification of the outer wall. The ring of calcium is broken at the inferior vena cava with only some thrombus on this slice visible between the aortic lumen and the vena cava lumen. The patient, who had an aortocaval fistula with high-output cardiac failure, underwent successful repair. (From Svensson LG, Klepp P, Hinder AA. S Afr J Surg 1986;24:32–4.)

with thoracic or thoracoabdominal aneurysms (Figs. 2–7 to 2–9). Aortography is essential for the planning of complex operative procedures and avoiding unexpected intraoperative discovery of anatomic and pathologic conditions that may lead to life-threatening complications.

Standard Views of the Thoracic Aorta

For patients with extensive aortic disease, the standard views of the chest that should be obtained are anterior, left anterior oblique, and lateral views of the aorta, and the contrast medium should be injected with a catheter immediately above the aortic valve (Fig. 2–10). A separate injection of contrast may be needed to obtain a better view of the greater vessels; for this the catheter tip is placed immediately proximal to the innominate artery. In patients with suspected traumatic rupture of the proximal descending thoracic aorta, multiple views have to be obtained so that tangents to every part of the aortic circumference are imaged. The abdominal aorta is then studied on both anterior and lateral views, with the catheter tip positioned just above the diaphragm. If indicated, we request the radiologist to inject the left ventricle to check for mitral valve regurgitation and to obtain an estimate of the left ventricular ejection fraction. Injection of contrast immediately above the aortic valve enables the assessment of aortic valve regurgitation, and in the three thoracic views the coronary arteries are fairly well defined with high-speed injections

and newer equipment. Thus a good evaluation of the coronary arteries can be obtained; if evidence of coronary disease is noted, then selective cardiac catheterization can be performed at a later stage. The left anterior oblique view is most useful both for identifying the origins of the arch arteries and for detecting any stenoses. If clinical examination of the patient suggests the possibility of cerebrovascular disease, a flush aortic arch study should be performed; if evidence of carotid disease is found, then selective carotid artery studies should be undertaken. The lateral chest view is particularly important in the assessment of patients who are to undergo reoperation on the heart or ascending aorta, because this view gives an accurate measurement of the amount of space between the aorta and the sternum. However, care should be taken to check that a thrombus in the aorta does not falsely make the gap appear larger than it is. It should be noted that we prefer to use neither computerized digital subtraction angiography nor photographic subtraction angiography as the primary study for these chest views. The reason for this is that, with aortic dissections, the false lumen may be thrombosed or a large thrombus may be present in an aneurysm and the contrast in the lumen makes an aneurysm appear smaller than it actually is because the outer aortic wall is not shown. Aortic wall

FIGURE 2–7   Chest radiograph of a patient with a saccular aneurysm protruding from the aortic knuckle, not well seen in the reproduction. (From Svensson LG, Crawford ES. Curr Probl Surg 1992;29:819–912.)

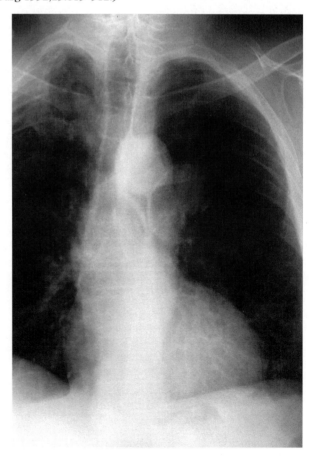

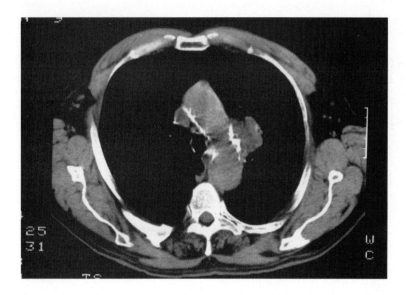

FIGURE 2–8 CT scan of the aortic arch confirming a saccular aneurysm from the aortic arch. (From Svensson LG, Crawford ES. Curr Probl Surg 1992;29:819–912.)

dilatations will thus often not be detected (Figs. 2-5 and 2-9). The implication of this is that a false aneurysm may be adjacent to or even eroding the posterior table of the sternum, and this would be missed by subtraction angiography. Thus when the surgeon opens the sternum, particularly during reoperations, the aorta is likely to be pierced, with potentially disastrous consequences. After conventional aortography, photographic positive subtraction angiograms of the aortic arch and carotid arteries can be obtained to better define arterial stenoses and small arteries. A positive mask of the chest, made before contrast injection, is overlaid on the negative film with the contrast injection study and then reexposed, resulting in the positive and negative cancellation of anatomical features other than the injected contrast. The injected contrast in the arteries is thus displayed as black instead of white, as in regular angiograms. Both the routine aortograms and the subtraction angiograms give a high-quality rendition of both the segmental intercostal arteries and the lumbar arteries arising from the aorta. The radicular arteries supplying the spinal cord, however, are usually not identified by this technique. Preoperative arteriographic studies of the spinal cord blood supply are not usually obtained because of the time and risks involved. On occasion we have performed postoperative highly selective spinal arteriographs using computerized digital subtraction angiograms (see spinal cord anatomy) to

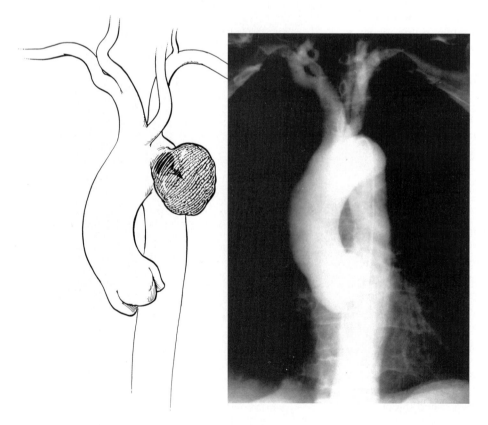

FIGURE 2–9 Aortogram showing that the saccular aneurysm does not fill with contrast, indicating that it is filled with thrombus. (From Svensson LG, Crawford ES. Curr Probl Surg 1992;29:819–912.)

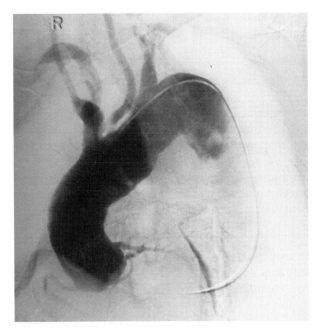

FIGURE 2–10 Left anterior oblique view of the ascending aorta and aortic arch with injection of contrast above the aortic valve. Note that the proximal right and left coronary arteries are visualized. The relationship of the greater vessels is also well seen in this view. The image was obtained by photographic subtraction to obtain better detail of the branch arteries. (Reprinted with permission from the Society of Thoracic Surgeons. From Svensson LG, Shahian DM, Davis FG, et al. Ann Thorac Surg 1994;58:1164–6.)

confirm intraoperative localization of the spinal cord blood supply.[4, 16]

Abdominal Aorta Views

Abdominal views of the aorta are obtained routinely for patients undergoing abdominal aortic surgery. If the thoracic aorta has not been imaged previously, particularly by CT scans, the radiologist is requested to examine the aorta by fluoroscopy; if there is evidence of aortic disease, then formal studies of the thoracic aorta should be performed. During fluoroscopy, the radiologist will usually inject contrast material to evaluate suspicious areas.

Anterior Abdominal View

The anterior view of the abdominal aorta is most useful for ascertaining the relationship of the renal arteries to the aortic aneurysm in order to identify juxtarenal aneurysms (Fig. 2–11). An argument that is sometimes raised against performing an anterior-view aortogram of the abdomen is that, with thrombus formation in the infrarenal aorta, the proximal limit of the aneurysm is difficult to define. Careful examination, however, usually shows a change in the luminal anatomy in the transition zone between the irregular atherosclerotic aortic wall and the smooth luminal thrombus, indicating where the aneurysm begins. Slow filling, or retrograde filling, of an unsuspected superior mesenteric artery occlusion is often detected. In this situation, the collateral flow from the inferior mesenteric artery is preserved

during surgery instead of being oversewn. A pelvic view that includes the common femoral arteries should also be obtained during evaluation of the abdominal aorta. Iliofemoral occlusive disease may considerably influence the type and placement of the distal anastomoses. Furthermore, when thoracic aortic surgery is contemplated, it is essential to ensure that blood flow will not be obstructed because of aortic dissection or atherosclerotic occlusive disease during femorofemoral bypass or atriofemoral bypass.[4]

Lateral Abdominal View

The lateral views of the abdominal aorta identify the anatomy of the celiac artery and the superior mesenteric and inferior mesenteric arteries and show whether any

FIGURE 2–11 Composite photographic image of the entire aorta. Note that the entire diameter of the aorta (indicated by the stippled line) is not visualized because the aneurysm is lined with thrombus. The arrow indicates where blood with contrast has tracked under the thrombus. The upper window is from the left anterior oblique views and the lower window from the anterior abdominal views. The entire aorta was replaced during one operation (see Chapter 24). (Reprinted with permission from the Society of Thoracic Surgeons. From Svensson LG, Shahian DM, Davis FG, et al. Ann Thorac Surg 1994;58:1164–6.)

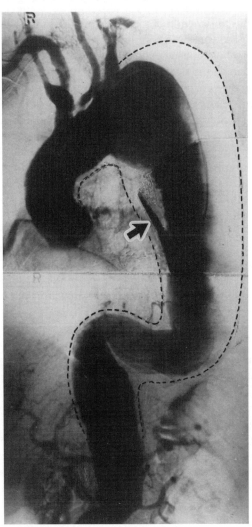

stenoses are present. A large juxtarenal aneurysm may be difficult to evaluate and delineate on the anterior view if the aneurysm overlaps and extends above the renal arteries. This is because the ectatic aorta of the dilated aneurysm sac may override the more proximal posterior aorta and be superimposed on it. On the lateral view, however, a juxtarenal aneurysm is clearly shown, provided that no thrombus is present. If a thrombus is present, then calcification in the aortic wall or displacement of the superior mesenteric artery and surrounding tissues may define the proximal limit. A CT or MRI scan transverse view at this level will also show whether the juxtarenal aneurysm has rolled over on top of the part of the aorta where the renal arteries arise.

Special Considerations

Of note, in those patients with horseshoe kidneys it is important to delineate the renal artery anatomy before surgery so that appropriate plans can be made for dealing with the kidney, its preservation, and reattachment of renal arteries if necessary.[17] Accessory renal arteries of some importance to renal blood supply are also frequently detected by aortography. The aortic and abdominal anatomy is well defined by aortography in most patients with aortic dissection. Aortocaval fistulae are clearly identified if there is a direct communication, although in some patients thrombus obstruction of the fistula prevents dye from crossing into the venous iliac or inferior vena cava circulation.[18] If a thrombus is obstructing the fistula, then the same problem exists in the detection of aortocaval fistulae by CT, in that the dye will not leak from the aorta into the vena cava. Mycotic aneurysms, which typically appear as bulging pseudoaneurysms posterior to the celiac and superior mesenteric arteries, are clearly seen on the lateral view, particularly since the aneurysms are seldom completely filled with thrombus. A digital subtraction angiogram may often miss mycotic aneurysms if they are filled with thrombus. Aortic rupture, infected aortic grafts, inflammatory aneurysms, and aortoduodenal fistulae are not always identified but may be suspected from characteristic luminal features such as pseudoaneurysms. We routinely obtain a nephrogram and a delayed ureterogram at a later phase after injection. The delayed ureterogram shows the relationship of the ureters to the aneurysm, which is particularly important in the case of inflammatory aneurysm repairs.[19]

Advantages

Aortography is still unsurpassed as a method of spatially mapping the entire aorta, particularly in representing three-dimensional (spatial) anatomy in a readily interpretable two-dimensional format. Furthermore, the technique of aortography sharply defines the anatomy of the aortic lumen, especially if multiple views are obtained, and also clearly identifies any stenoses or occlusions of branch vessels. The coronary arteries and the aortic valve can be evaluated. The presence of aortic tears, the true lumen tracking along the medial aspect of the aorta, reentry sites, and aortic rupture are clearly defined. Aortography is also indicated

for all patients with suspected traumatic rupture of the aorta.[4]

Disadvantages

The drawbacks of routine aortography are the potential complications associated with deleterious reactions to contrast material and catheter related problems. Contrast-related complications include renal failure, allergic reactions, and pain. Neurologic consequences include stroke, confusion, convulsions, cortical blindness, nausea, fever, pulmonary edema, and paraplegia or paraparesis. Hemodynamic alterations include vasodilatation or myocardial depression.[4, 16, 20-23]

RENAL FAILURE

In a study of 400 patients after angiography, 11.3% developed renal dysfunction, defined as a 50% increase in the serum creatinine or BUN levels. In patients with abnormal renal function, 41.7% developed renal dysfunction and 8.3% required dialysis.[24] To reduce the incidence of renal failure, patients should be well hydrated intravenously the night before elective aortography with 5% dextrose in water plus 0.25N saline with an ampule of mannitol and sodium bicarbonate added to each liter.[25] In particularly high-risk patients, dopamine at 3 μg/kg per minute should also be added. Those patients with a history of allergy or allergic reactions to contrast material are prophylactically premedicated with steroids, a histamine blocker, and an H2 blocker such as ranitidine before aortography. Nonetheless, these precautions do not always prevent an allergic reaction. Contrast-related renal failure is increased in patients with diabetes mellitus or proteinuria, the elderly, and patients with renal dysfunction, low blood flow states such as aortic dissection or ruptured aorta with shock, and dehydration.[20, 26] In such patients, nonionic agents, first developed by Almen,[20] may be safer, although the considerable cost of these contrast agents mitigates against their routine use.[4]

CATHETER-INDUCED COMPLICATIONS

Catheter-related complications include embolization of atherothrombotic material to branch arteries (including the brain, kidneys, and lower limbs), aortic dissection,[27] and puncture site complications such as hemorrhage, pseudoaneurysm formation, hematomas, arteriovenous fistulae, arterial thrombi, arterial stenoses, infection (including an increased operative infection rate[28]), and venous thrombosis.[29-31] Rarely, compartment syndromes with neuropraxia occur, particularly in the axilla with the brachial artery Sone's approach, commencing as a median nerve involvement followed by ulnar and radial nerve weakness.[22] It is recommended that any hematomas, particularly in the axilla, should be speedily evacuated to prevent later permanent neuropraxia or wound complications. Although translumbar arteriograms are rarely used now, they were associated with an increased risk of retroperitoneal hemorrhage,[21, 29, 30] aortic dissection and, more rarely, rupture of the aneurysms per se.[4]

Although there is a long list of potential complications after aortography, the risks are relatively small and, with expert radiologists, the risks are far outweighed by the benefits in planning of the operative procedure. The reported complication rate is 0.5% for transfemoral aortography, 0.6% for translumbar aortography, and 2% for the axillary approach.[31] The risk of stroke is reported to be less than 0.02%.[31] Controversy, however, remains over whether routine aortography is indicated for infrarenal abdominal aortic aneurysms.[4, 32, 33]

MAGNETIC RESONANCE IMAGING

History and Technique

Magnetic resonance imaging (MRI) has been a major advance in the accurate noninvasive evaluation of the aorta, its branches, and structures surrounding the aorta and the heart.[34-40] Because of the cost of MRI scans, the time required, and the fact that much of the information can be obtained from CT scans, MRI has not superseded CT scanning for most patients. With time, however, it may replace CT combined with aortography for aortic surgery.

The history of magnetism dates back to c. 1000 BC, when the shepherd Magnes, walking on Mount Ida in Turkey, noticed that the tacks in his sandals drew his feet to the earth. He dug into the earth and discovered magnetite, the magnetic oxide of iron, a mineral lodestone.[41] In 1924 Stern demonstrated that atoms had intrinsic magnetic moments, and in 1938 Rabi performed direct measurement of *nuclear magnetic resonance,* the term coined by Rabi.[41] For their research, Stern and Rabi received the Nobel Prizes in physics in 1943 and 1944, respectively. Bloch later introduced the terms for the "thermal" or "longitudinal" relaxation time (T1) and a "transversal" relaxation time (T2) in a 1946 paper. Both Bloch and Purcell performed early research on nuclear magnetic resonance, and in 1952 the Nobel Prize was awarded to them for their work on the measurement of magnetic fields in atomic nuclei.[41] This discovery showed that if atoms are placed in a strong magnetic field and radiofrequency energy is applied to them, when these atoms return to their unexcited state they emit a form of energy that can be measured with appropriate instruments. Of note, the method detects only atoms with odd-numbered protons. Thus the contrast between tissues is largely dependent on the hydrogen content; the contrast between water (H_2O)–containing tissues and muscle, for example, is sharp. The relationship of the image to hydrogen is more complex, however, than the mere presence of hydrogen. The image is dependent on the relaxation times of hydrogen, T1 and T2, which are the longitudinal and transverse relaxation times. The relaxation times are, in turn, determined by the chemical composition of the tissues.[4] Erik Odeblad of the Karolinska Institute in Stockholm performed extensive experiments on biological tissues. However, it was only when Lauterbur developed methods of mapping the quantities of relaxation times by encoding the spatial coordinates that the nuclear magnetic resonance scan, now known as MRI, became a practical apparatus.[41] Lauterbur's first paper on the subject was rejected, but it was later accepted by *Nature.*[41]

Indications

MRI is particularly advantageous for evaluating aortic dissection, fluid collections around previously placed aortic grafts, the aortic wall, and surrounding tissues. Also, MRI is used to accurately diagnose the presence of inflammatory aneurysms.

Studies by Nienaber and colleagues[42, 43] have shown that MRI is as sensitive as transesophageal echo (TEE) for detecting aortic dissection and is also more specific in accurately excluding the presence of aortic dissection. In 53 patients with suspected aortic dissection, both MRI and TEE were 100% sensitive in detecting aortic dissection. The specificity rate for MRI was 100%, although for TEE it was only 68.2% ($p < 0.01$).[42] The lower specificity rate for TEE was related to the difficulty of imaging the distal ascending aorta and because of artifacts mimicking aortic dissection. Of course, with experience these artifacts will be better recognized and a higher specificity rate will evolve. Appelbe and colleagues[44] found that linear artifacts in the ascending aorta noted in 44% of patients were due to external interference caused by reflection of ultrasound from the left atrium and were more common in patients with an enlarged aorta exceeding the left atrial diameter. In addition, mirror-image artifacts in the aortic arch and descending thoracic aorta resulted in the appearance of a septum. This appearance is due to the aorta–lung interface acting as a reflector and is seen in 80% of patients on both sagittal and transverse planes. For depiction of the septum in aortic dissection, however, MRI is one of the most accurate methods, even when the septum is very thin, because the contrast between blood and tissue is marked. Barbant and colleagues[45] have conveniently summarized the sensitivity, specificity, and predictive value of angiography, CT, MRI, and TEE reported in the literature for aortic dissections.[4]

Advantages

A great advantage of MRI is that it makes possible the determination of whether an area of fluid accumulation contains blood and, if the fluid is blood, whether the accumulation has occurred either acutely or chronically and whether it is a thrombus or hematoma or slow-flowing blood. This information is useful in the evaluation of aortic dissection and fluid collections around previously placed aortic grafts when graft infection is suspected. Furthermore, the assessment of blood flow and turbulence with appropriate techniques is advantageous. Gradient-echo imaging is also of importance for determining valve function, particularly that of the aortic valve. MRI is also useful for evaluating the aortic wall and surrounding tissues. For example, MRI accurately determines the presence of inflammatory aneurysms and, of interest, MRI scans of infrarenal

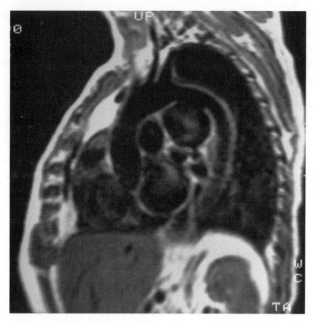

FIGURE 2–12   MRI scan of patient with a saccular aneurysm near the aortic isthmus on the distal lesser curve of the aortic arch and proximal descending aorta. Note turbulence within the aneurysm, as shown by blood within the aneurysm reflecting back the signal. The aorta and the greater vessel branches show no signal since the blood in these vessels passes through without reflecting any signals back in time to be detected. A saccular aneurysm at this site may be associated with a history of trauma, mycotic infections, or elderly debilitated patients. (From Svensson LG, Crawford ES. Curr Probl Surg 1992;29:819–912.)

inflammatory aneurysms have a laminated appearance even for specimens of explanted inflammatory aneurysms.[46]

MRI scanners do not need moving parts; therefore images can be visualized in any plane of the body. The ability to scan in any plane has a distinct advantage, particularly for obtaining three-dimensional (3D) information. Thus 3D images (for example, of the aorta and its branches, including stenosis of branch arteries) can be reconstructed. Even the coronary arteries can be imaged.[47] Movement of nuclei, however, affects the image. Thus, because of the relatively long scan times required, blood flowing at a high velocity in a vessel may not emit a signal and will appear as a void (Fig. 2–12). Newer techniques, however, are overcoming this problem of 3D imaging. To obtain images of flowing blood, the red cells have to be exposed to both 90 degree and 180 degree radiofrequency pulses. It should be noted, however, that if blood flow is more rapid than the sequence, then the red cells in the aortic lumen are not imaged. To obtain images of moving tissues, such as the heart, the image has to be gated with use of the patient's electrocardiogram. Therefore image acquisition in patients with cardiac arrhythmias, such as atrial fibrillation, can be a problem. Adipose tissue results in a strong spin-echo image, which helps delineate tissues surrounded by fat. Other techniques that allow the study of blood flow include gradient-recalled echoes that permit acquisition of images in a more rapid sequence.[4] With the continued evolution of MRI, static spin-echo allows for sharp depiction of the internal lumen and wall of the aorta. Dynamic MRI studies, cine gradient echo, and phase-velocity mapping techniques allow the assessment of physiological blood flow in relation to the vascular anatomy. The improvements in magnetic resonance angiography allow the depiction not only of the aorta and major vascular branches but also of the coronary anatomy.[48] Three-dimensional surface rendering of MRI scans allows the spatial depiction of vascular structures, such as the aorta, vena cava, and portal system, resulting in a better understanding of complex anatomical relationships.[49]

Thus the application of MRI enables the physician to obtain the same type of information as that provided by CT scanning, with some added advantages in evaluation of blood flow, 3D imaging, cardiac function, and aortic valve competence (Fig. 2–12). Furthermore, in addition to transverse images, coronal, sagittal, and oblique images can be obtained. Tennant and colleagues[50] compared ultrasonography, contrast-enhanced CT, and MRI in 79 patients with infrarenal aneurysms and found that MRI was the most accurate method of determining the level of the renal arteries, whether the aneurysm extended above the renal arteries, and whether it had the typical laminated appearance of inflammatory infrarenal aneurysms.[46] With time, MRI may become the primary method of diagnosing aortic disease and also of planning elective operative procedures.

Disadvantages

The drawbacks of MRI are that a patient may not enter the scanner if there are metal objects in proximity, including internal metal objects such as pacemakers and surgical clips made of material other than titanium. Special intravenous fluid pumps and respirators that can be safely placed in MRI scanners with the patient are becoming available. Another disadvantage is that long scan times are a problem in unstable patients. Also, the resolution of MRI is not as good as that of CT, but this will undoubtedly improve.[4, 43]

EVALUATION OF CORONARY ARTERY DISEASE

Abdominal Aortic Disease

The role of routine cardiac catheterization and thallium radioisotope scans before any abdominal aortic surgery is controversial.[31, 51-59] However, the information obtained with cardiac catheterization by Hertzer and his colleagues[55] at the Cleveland Clinic Foundation has been invaluable in defining the problem of concomitant coronary artery disease in patients with aortic disease and its influence on both early and late survival. In an autopsy study of 27 patients with abdominal aortic aneurysms more than 5 cm in diameter, Mautner and colleagues[60] from the National Institutes of Health confirmed the high incidence of coronary artery disease. Mautner and colleagues reported that 44% had symptoms of coronary artery disease, 37% died of myocardial ischemia, and 22% died of rupture. They concluded that "patients with AAA nearly always have diffuse and severe coronary atherosclerosis." Eagle and colleagues[53] used thallium scans to examine patients undergoing vascular operations on the basis of clinical parameters (age > 70 years, ECG Q waves, diabetes mellitus, and a history of ventricular arrhythmia or angina) and found that the risk of early cardiac complications was accurately predicted. McFalls and colleagues[61] found that not only redistribution of thallium on thallium-201 scintigraphy but also fixed defects are risk factors for predicting cardiac complications after vascular operations. McEnroe and associates[62] described similar results. Cutler and colleagues[63] have also shown the strong influence of coronary artery disease detected by thallium scans on the postoperative course of patients. They noted that the redistribution of thallium on scans was predictive of early postoperative events. This is not surprising since redistribution indicates areas of ischemia at risk of infarction during aortic operations. They also showed that areas of fixed defects were better predictors of long-term results. This would be consistent with the idea of fixed defects being due to areas of scarring caused by myocardial infarction and thus diminished muscle mass. A depressed left ventricular function is known to be one of the best predictors of long-term survival in patients after myocardial infarction and coronary bypass operations and in patients with malignant ventricular arrhythmias. Nevertheless, Mangano and colleagues[64] have reported that the test is not entirely accurate and have questioned the usefulness of thallium scans. Goldman and coauthors[65] have favored clinical examination of the patient and categorization of the patient into risk groups on the basis of a score developed from multivariate analysis of clinical findings. In contrast, Lalka and associates[66] have been enthusiastic about the use of dobutamine infusion and transthoracic echocardiography for the detection of coronary artery disease. The details of the reasoning for and against routine cardiac catheterization of patients undergoing infrarenal abdominal aortic surgery are discussed under Cardiac Complications in Chapters 16 and 26. Until recently, our approach has been not to perform cardiac catheterization or thallium radioisotope scans unless overt cardiac disease is present according to history, clinical examination, or electrocardiographic examination (including Holter monitoring), or echocardiography. (We routinely attempt to obtain the latter two before surgery.) Instead, we obtain information concerning the coronary artery vasculature from the aortogram, as discussed previously.

Thoracic Aortic Disease

If a patient has unstable angina, annuloaortic ectasia, or a proximal ascending aortic or arch aneurysm or chronic dissection, we forego initial aortography and request the cardiologist to examine the coronary arteries, the ascending aorta and arch vessels in particular, plus the remaining aorta by cinecatheterization (Fig. 2–1). The examination includes evaluation of the abdominal aorta and iliac arteries to ensure that cannulation of the femoral artery can be done safely for cardiopulmonary bypass. Increasingly, patients with descending thoracic or thoracoabdominal aortic aneurysms without symptoms or signs of coronary artery disease are undergoing selective coronary artery catheterization to identify coronary artery disease. If patients with coronary artery disease can undergo percutaneous transluminal coronary angioplasty (PTCA) before operation, this is advantageous. If, however, coronary artery bypass surgery is required, then there is the risk that the patient may die from the operation or that the aneurysm will rupture and need subsequent repair. The incidence of this is approximately 5% to 12%. Among the 263 patients examined by Suggs and colleagues[67] for selective screening of coronary artery disease, one of the 12 patients who had coronary artery surgery died of a ruptured aneurysm while awaiting abdominal aortic aneurysm repair. For this reason, we usually perform an infrarenal repair during the same hospital admission, and often 5 days after coronary bypass operation.

Whether cardiac catheterization is necessary before urgent thoracic aortic operations, such as for dissection or rupture, has not been clearly established. Kern and colleagues[57] were unable to show in 54 patients that knowledge of the coronary circulation under these circumstances was useful.

It should be emphasized that if a patient is to undergo a descending thoracic aortic or thoracoabdominal aortic operation involving the proximal descending aorta, the cardiac surgeon must be advised against using an in situ left internal mammary artery bypass graft. The reason for this is that the left subclavian artery will have to be clamped during repair of the aneurysm and thus the heart will be deprived of blood flow via the internal mammary artery. As an alternative approach, methods that we have used for coronary artery bypass are venous bypass grafts, right internal mammary artery bypass crossing the midline to the left anterior descending artery, or a free left internal mammary artery bypass. If perchance the patient has had a coronary artery bypass in the past and has patent internal mammary artery, deep hypothermia with circulatory arrest can be used for the proximal aortic anastomosis.

Prognostic Implications of Coronary Artery Disease

Hertzer and colleagues[54, 55, 68, 69] have stressed that knowledge of merely the incidence of immediate postoperative cardiac events in patients undergoing infrarenal aortic operations is not sufficient for determining whether preoperative tests are adequate to detect patients at high risk of perioperative death. A much broader consideration should be the patient's long-term prognosis. Hertzer and colleagues assert that physicians also need to examine the long-term impact of failing to search for coronary artery disease in those patients at high risk of ischemic cardiac disease. The reason for this is that repeated studies, including our own,[70-77] have shown that, irrespective of which segment of the aorta (ascending, aortic arch, descending, thoracoabdominal, and abdominal aorta) is operated on for degenerative aneurysms or aortic dissection, the 5-year survival is only approximately 60% in these patients after surgical repair, with most deaths being due to cardiac disease. Thus it is imperative that cardiac disease, whenever detected, be promptly treated to improve the long-term survival of patients after aortic surgery.

24-Hour Holter Electrocardiography

With the encouragement and medical advice of Corday,[78] Jeff Holter, a physicist, developed an apparatus that was able to monitor, collect, and store the ECG signals gathered from a patient and thus detect silent cardiac ischemia or arrhythmias.

Indications

One method of detecting silent myocardial ischemia is to perform single- or double-lead Holter monitoring.[79] Myocardial ischemia is silent in as many as 50% to 80% of patients; that is, no pain is experienced by these patients and therefore the ischemia remains unrecognized.[79, 80] This form of myocardial ischemia is deleterious to the heart and carries as high a risk of infarction as that observed for angina.[80] It has been shown that detection of silent myocardial ischemia, usually by ST segment changes, correlates with postoperative cardiac complications.[4, 79] In addition to the detection of silent ischemia, Holter monitoring is indicated for the detection of both atrial and ventricular arrhythmias, particularly in those patients with aortic valve regurgitation and Marfan syndrome. Of importance is the finding of ventricular tachycardia or a prolonged QT interval, which is associated with an increased risk of postoperative ventricular arrhythmias. The QT interval should be corrected for the patient's heart rate for a more accurate assessment of its significance.[4, 81]

Cardiac Catheterization

Cardiac catheterization has become one of the most common, sophisticated, and useful invasive radiographic techniques for evaluation of the heart. In 1929 Forssmann performed the first human catheterization on himself[82, 83] by devious means. After his superior refused to allow him to carry out his plan of passing a urethral type of catheter from his left forearm up into his heart, he tricked a nurse into allowing him access to surgical instruments. He then tied the nurse down on the operating table, inserted the catheter into himself, and proceeded to the basement, where he took x-ray photographs of himself with the catheter in his heart. In 1956 Forssmann, Cournand, and Richards were justly awarded the Nobel Prize in medicine.[84] Nevertheless, selective catheterization of the coronary arteries remained a problem, and it was not until 1958 that Sones and colleagues[14, 15] described a practical approach.

The Sones technique involved a brachial artery cutdown for insertion of the catheter. Subsequently, however, several investigators modified the Seldinger technique so that steerable preformed catheters could be inserted through a percutaneous femoral artery sheath; some of the most popular are still the Judkins catheters.[4, 85]

Advantages

The gold standard for determining the presence, extent, and course of treatment for coronary artery disease is cardiac selective catheterization. Although some physiological tests of coronary function, such as stress ECG, thallium scans, positron emission tomography (PET), and dobutamine echocardiography, can determine the physiological implications of coronary artery disease, the anatomical detail obtained from cardiac catheterization is currently unsurpassed.

Interpretation of Coronary Angiograms

Points to be borne in mind when one is interpreting coronary angiograms include the extent of disease in the artery, severity of stenoses, composition of the lesions, associated complications involving the lesion (e.g., thrombus, dissection, or ulceration),[86] the number and location of arteries involved, acuity of occlusion or development of collateral arteries that provide an alternative source of blood supply, age, and left ventricular function. Typically, collaterals develop only if a coronary artery is narrowed by more than 90%[87] and often will maintain good distal myocardial function if the stenosis forms gradually.[4]

Myocardial Function

Myocardial function is usually assessed by calculation of the ejection fraction from the left ventriculogram, despite the dependence of the calculated ejection fraction on preload, contractility, and afterload. The ejection fraction calculation is most often performed by comparing diastolic and systolic area–length determinations of volume with the basic assumption that the left ventricle is an ellipsoid. Such determinations, however, are prone to fairly high subjective variability by the observer and can vary by 10% or more between observers, particularly when determinations are made visually. Another method of assessing cardiac function is to examine segmental wall motion on ventriculography. Segmental wall motion is described as normal or hypokinetic (reduced contractility), akinetic (absence of contractility), or dyskinetic (paradoxical expansion with systolic contraction). The latter suggests formation of a left ventricular aneurysm. With continued improvements in cardiac surgery and myocardial preservation, the effect of decreased myocardial function (low ejection fraction or marked segmental abnormalities) has been reduced so that a poor ejection fraction no longer constitutes as great a risk factor for surgery as it used to. Paradoxically, long-term follow-up of patients treated either medically or surgically for ischemic heart disease has shown that those patients with decreased left ventricular function benefit more from coronary artery

bypass surgery than from medical therapy. The reasons are not entirely clear, but it is possible that patients treated medically who have normal ejection fractions maintain an adequate cardiac muscle reserve to tolerate many ischemic events, whereas those medically treated patients with low ejection fractions might be less able to tolerate ischemic events.[4]

Cardiac Valve Function

The status of cardiac valves and their function should be known before any cardiovascular operations on the aorta are undertaken. This may entail only listening to the patient's heart to assure that there are no murmurs. For patients undergoing operations on the descending thoracic or thoracoabdominal aorta, this knowledge is important because of the great afterload imposed on the valves. In particular, the aortic valve needs to be carefully evaluated if a murmur is present. This is conveniently done at the time of cardiac catheterization by obtaining pull-back pressures across the valve and injecting contrast medium above the aortic valve to judge the degree of aortic valve regurgitation. Aortic valve disease should also be actively investigated and treated in conjunction with ascending aortic operations because of the problems of reoperation in these patients for residual aortic valve disease. This approach reduces the rate of reoperation in these patients and thus lessens the attendant higher mortality rate. Thus valves with significant stenosis or regurgitation detected either by echocardiography or by cardiac catheterization will have to be replaced with prosthetic valves.[4]

Aortic conditions that should alert the physician to associated aortic valve disease include Marfan syndrome, Ehlers–Danlos syndrome, annuloaortic ectasia, sinus of Valsalva aneurysms, Erdheim's cystic medial necrosis, pseudoxanthoma elasticum, aortitis, Turner's syndrome, Noonan's syndrome, coarctation, syphilis, trauma, and aortic dissection.[4]

Percutaneous Cardiovascular Invasive Procedures

Increasingly, invasive procedures are being performed during cardiac catheterization and vascular imaging. Most of these are for occlusive disease, including coarctation of the aorta,[88] and use of stents,[89] and renovascular disease.[90] Percutaneous techniques have been described for the management of aortic dissection,[91, 92] aortic aneurysms,[93] and false aneurysms.[94] Although the most frequently used invasive technique is PTCA, restenosis continues to be a problem.[95] In these patients restenosis is associated with a significantly higher event rate, consisting of unstable angina, myocardial infarction, and the need for coronary artery bypass operations.[95] Furthermore, women and diabetics undergoing PTCA are at greater risk of dying after the procedure, possibly because of their smaller arteries associated with a smaller average body size.[96, 97] Nevertheless, PTCA is useful for tiding patients over aortic operations when coronary artery bypass is not an option.

Disadvantages

The additive contrast load of CT, aortography, and cine-cardiac catheterization in patients who have unstable angina and annuloaortic ectasia or a proximal ascending aortic aneurysm may be prohibitive and hence lead to renal complications. The routine examination of the coronary arteries by cardiac catheterization for patients undergoing elective aortic valve replacement or ascending aortic repair remains controversial.[98-100] Nevertheless, with the expanding numbers of elderly patients and the increased need for reoperation, we are placed in the position of having to perform many more preoperative coronary catheterizations and thus accumulate the risks of these multiple investigations. In patients undergoing urgent thoracic aortic surgery, preoperative cardiac catheterization has been reported to be of minimal benefit.[4, 57]

Fortunately, the risk of cardiac catheterization by itself is fairly small. In their reports on the respective incidences of complications, the Society of Cardiac Angiography[56] and the Collaborative Study of Coronary Artery Surgery (CASS)[101] have shown a death rate of 0.14% and 0.2%, an infarction rate of 0.07% and 0.25%, a stroke rate of 0.07% and 0.03%, and an incidence of vascular complications of 0.56% and 0.7%.[4]

Echocardiography and Doppler

Transthoracic echocardiography (TTE) is a noninvasive technique because it is performed by placing the probe on the chest wall, whereas transesophageal echocardiography (TEE) is considered invasive since the probe has to be inserted into the esophagus. Both methods have important advantages in the detection of cardiac and aortic disease.

Cardiac Functional Assessment

For cardiac and aortic evaluation, a synchronous electrocardiogram is used to average end-systolic and diastolic volumes for the calculation of ejection fraction. Assessment of segmental wall function, including that of the right ventricle, is accurately determined by both TTE and TEE. Furthermore, wall motion and contractility dysfunction on TTE and TEE have been closely correlated with regional ischemia, coronary stenoses, and blood flow.[102-105] Increasingly, dobutamine infusion with echocardiography is used for the detection of coronary artery disease on the basis of regional asynergy or new mitral valve regurgitation.[106] Eichelberger and associates[107] found that dobutamine echocardiography before vascular surgery was 100% sensitive in predicting which patients would not have cardiac complications. The specificity, however, was low, with no perioperative events in 69% of the patients with positive scans. Nevertheless, this would appear to be a useful physiological screening test for coronary disease; if the study is positive, then a further test, such as selective coronary artery catheterization, is warranted. Koolen and colleagues[108] have reported that TEE is more sensitive than surface ECG electrodes in detecting both myocardial ischemia and myocardial infarction resulting in enzyme leakage during and after abdominal aortic operations. Recent advances in the use of sonicated fluids or encapsulated microbubble contrast dyes have made possible the improved study and pathophysiological assessment of myocardial perfusion.[109] An important advancement to TTE and TEE has been the use of both continuous-wave and pulsed Doppler to determine flow on tomographic slices of the heart and vessels. By convention, flow directed toward the probe is colored red and that away from the probe is colored blue. The intensity of the color reflects velocity, and turbulent flow is indicated by a green hue. With echocardiography it is possible to determine the valve area, degree of regurgitation, velocity across the valve, and cardiac output.[110]

Assessment of Aortic Disease

Imaging of the aorta allows clear scans of aortic disease to be obtained. Thus patients can be screened for atherosclerotic disease of the ascending aorta, aortic dissection, and aneurysms, including rupture[111] and traumatic rupture.[112]

ATHEROMA AND ATHEROSCLEROSIS OF THE AORTA

Approximately 10% to 20% of patients with strokes are believed to have embolic strokes from the heart or ascending aorta. Ulcerated plaques in the aortic arch are also associated with stroke,[113] although the aortic arch cannot be entirely screened by TEE because of the trachea interposing between the transducer and the aortic arch. When patients with strokes are screened by TEE, a significant number are found to have atheroma in the ascending aorta as a possible source.[114] Whether the aorta should be operated on in these patients if there are no other indications for cardiovascular operations, however, is a problematic issue because of the high risks and questionable benefits, especially since anticoagulation may be all that is required.[115]

TEE is also being used for intraoperative examination of the aorta during cardiac operations.[116, 117] Alternatively, intraoperative epicardial and "epiaortic" echocardiography can be used to examine the aorta and to plan different methods of treating patients with evidence of severe ascending aortic atheroma. Kouchoukos and colleagues have used this technique and found that intimal thickening greater than 3 mm, indicating atheroma, is more frequent in elderly patients and in patients with diabetes; for 17% of the patients they had to change the operative procedure because of atheroma of the ascending aorta.[118] In some patients, the Kouchoukos group used circulatory arrest because of the atherosclerotic disease of the aorta (10/500, 2% of the patients).[119] Culliford and colleagues[120] have reported similar techniques and have performed endarterectomies of the ascending aorta and aortic arch for atherosclerosis of the aorta. In our limited experience with endarterectomy of the ascending aorta and aortic arch, our concern has been the risk of postoperative aortic dissec-

tion, although this has not occurred in our patients. Graft replacement may be a safer alternative.

AORTIC DISSECTION

Nienaber and colleagues[42, 43] recommend that TEE should be the primary procedure for the detection of aortic dissection, although it should be noted that artifacts can result in false diagnoses. Furthermore, rupture of the aorta has been reported to occur during TEE for the diagnosis of aortic dissection because of retching from the insertion of the probe.[121] The role of echocardiography in the evaluation of aortic dissection is discussed under the diagnostic evaluation of patients with suspected aortic dissection.[4]

CARDIAC TAMPONADE

In 1897 Starling[122] defined cardiac tamponade as compression of the heart by fluid within the pericardial sac that impairs diastolic filling of the ventricles. Patients with acute hemodynamic compromise associated with aortic dissection of the ascending aorta or after cardiovascular operations sometimes have cardiac tamponade. The severity of the cardiac tamponade is best evaluated by TEE. Beck's triad of hypotension, increased central venous pressure, and distant soft heart sounds may not be detected in patients with cardiac tamponade or may be absent, particularly if the patient is on a ventilator. Pulsus paradoxus may be absent with left ventricular dysfunction, localized right atrial tamponade, mechanical ventilation, atrial septal defect, pulmonary arterial obstruction, or severe aortic regurgitation.[123] TEE is useful for diagnosing subtle forms of tamponade when clinical signs are minimal. The echocardiographic features include right atrial collapse, right ventricular diastolic collapse, abnormal respiratory changes in ventricular dimensions or variation in flow across the tricuspid or mitral valves, a dilated inferior vena cava without collapse during inspiration, left atrial compression, left ventricular diastolic compression, and a swinging heart.[123] The patient's hemodynamic status and the cause of the tamponade will determine whether it should be drained and the urgency of drainage. For the patient who is not severely compromised by tamponade and who has acute aortic dissection, we recommend that it is better to take the patient to surgery without drainage, because drainage may precipitate fatal rupture of the dissected aorta.

Long-Term Follow-Up

TEE is particularly useful for the long-term follow-up of patients in whom composite valve grafts have been inserted. Before discharge from the hospital an image of the graft is obtained, usually by echocardiography or by angiography. This serves both as a baseline and to check that there are no problems with the repair. Evidence of false aneurysms, compression of the graft, and valve dysfunction can be detected. Similarly, Dent and Kaul[124] have reported the detection of postoperative endocarditis in patients who have had Cabrol repairs by means of TEE. Kouchoukos and colleagues[125] used TTE for the late follow-up of patients in whom the aortic valve had been replaced with a pulmonary autograft. TEE combined with CT has been used by Roudaut and colleagues[126] for the late follow-up of patients who have had ascending aortic repairs for aortic dissection. They found that there were no important differences in the accuracy of the two techniques. We have preferred to use CT because it provides a readily available hard copy that can easily be retrieved for later comparison of the diameters of the aorta on follow-up.

Duplex Scans

Ultrasonography combined with Dopper studies can be used as a duplex scanning technique for abdominal aortic and renal artery studies, including intraoperative determination of renal artery patency after surgical repairs.[4, 127, 128] O'Neil and colleagues[129] used renal duplex sonography to examine 21 patients with elevated serum creatinine levels above 2 mg/dl and found that the accuracy was 96% compared with conventional angiography in identifying stenoses.

DIAGNOSTIC AND PLANNING STRATEGIES

No single imaging technique offers the ideal solution for all patients undergoing aortic surgery. Furthermore, strategies will be dependent on the condition of the patient, the suspected diagnosis, the availability of the various methods in the hospital, and the expertise of the individual physician. A reasonable strategy is to evaluate all symptom-free candidates for elective surgery with potential aneurysms or chronic dissection with a CT scan of the abdomen and chest with contrast. This determines the diameter of the entire aorta, better delineates the cause and diagnosis, and focuses further attention on those studies appropriate for the segment involved. Thus, if the ascending aorta or aortic arch is involved by an aneurysm or by chronic aortic dissection, then cardiac catheterization with contrast studies of the coronary arteries, aortic valve, ascending aorta, aortic arch and flush aortography of the thoracoabdominal aorta, abdominal aorta, and iliofemoral arteries will suffice in most patients. This, however, requires careful coordination and discussion with the cardiologist performing the procedure. The importance of studying the iliofemoral arteries is to ensure that cardiopulmonary bypass can be safely established through the femoral arteries. If this study is inadequate for planning the operative procedure, an echocardiogram may be required for evaluation of the cardiac valves. Also, a total aortogram performed by a radiologist may be required, particularly if a thoracoabdominal aneurysm is also present, in which case careful evaluation of the visceral arteries is necessary. If CT findings indicate that the descending aorta or thoracoabdominal aorta is the aneurysmal or chronically dissected segment that requires repair, a total aortogram by a radiologist is preferable, with a flush aortic root study to

assess the aortic valve and proximal coronary artery segments. If, however, CT scanning shows that only the abdominal aorta is involved, then an abdominal aortogram is useful but not essential. In hemodynamically unstable patients and those with suspected acute dissection, the condition of the patient will determine which studies are chosen. If time permits, patients with suspected acute dissection should have either a TEE or an MRI, followed by an aortogram both for evaluation of branch arteries, particularly the iliofemoral arteries, and for planning the operation. If the TEE is inconclusive, MRI is more likely to be definitive. Some patients, however, will require operation immediately after the diagnosis is made by MRI, TEE, or aortography. In patients with suspected thoracic aortic rupture, a CT scan or aortography will support the diagnosis in most cases. For patients with suspected infrarenal rupture, the best course of action is usually immediate laparotomy and resuscitation in the operating room. Any delay will increase the risk of death or development of postoperative multiple organ dysfunction.

DETECTION OF OTHER COMORBID DISEASE

Carotid Artery Screening

With the increasing age at which patients are undergoing cardiovascular and vascular operations, the risk of stroke due to unrecognized carotid disease has increased. Hence, of late we have adopted a policy of performing noninvasive carotid studies with duplex ultrasonic Doppler scanners. When patients are found to have moderate or severe stenosis or occlusion of one carotid artery, then selective arteriograms are also obtained to better plan management and operative strategy. Carotid endarterectomy for symptomatic stenoses is warranted, although surgery for asymptomatic stenoses is more controversial. Gerraty and colleagues[130] studied 145 patients undergoing vascular operations and 213 undergoing cardiac operations. Of the 49 patients with a history of symptomatic cerebral ischemia, 10 had symptomatic stenoses of 50% or greater and 3 of these patients (30%) developed ipsilateral cerebral infarction, thus supporting the use of carotid endarterectomy before or during aortic operations. However, among the 53 patients with 50% or greater asymptomatic stenoses or occlusion, including 28 with 80% or greater stenoses or occlusion, none had an ipsilateral stroke. In a review[131] of our patients who had undergone coronary artery bypass operations, the risk of perioperative stroke was not increased in those in whom cerebrovascular disease was treated by carotid endarterectomy prior to coronary surgery. Similarly, in patients with strokes due to factors other than carotid artery disease, the risk of stroke was not increased. It is likely, however, that many, if not most, postoperative strokes are due to atheroembolic material. In the autopsy study by the Cleveland

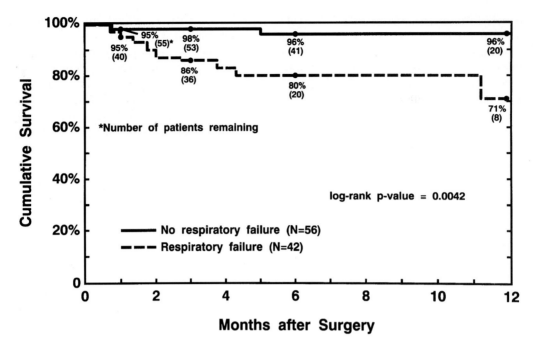

FIGURE 2–13   Influence of respiratory failure on long-term survival after Crawford type I or II thoracoabdominal aneurysm repairs. (From Svensson LG, Hess KR, Coselli JS, et al. J Vasc Surg 1991;14:271–82.)

Clinic Foundation,[132] 31.2% of the patients had evidence of embolism, including 16.3% to the brain.

Pulmonary Function Tests

Problem

A large proportion of patients with aortic disease have been smokers and thus have chronic pulmonary disease. For many of these patients undergoing thoracic, thoracoabdominal, or abdominal aortic operations, subsequent in-hospital and late deaths (Fig. 2–13) are associated with poor pulmonary function and associated complications.[133-142] Moreover, postoperative respiratory problems can be the cause of significant morbidity and dyspnea after operation.[4]

Patients who undergo either upper abdominal or thoracic surgery constitute the groups at highest risk of subsequent development of respiratory complications and even respiratory failure.[133, 134, 139, 143-146] Clearly, because both the upper abdomen and the thorax are operated on during thoracoabdominal aortic repairs, with division of the diaphragm and costal margin, these patients are particularly prone to respiratory problems. Since 1954, when pulmonary function tests were first introduced, several studies have tried to predict which patients would have postoperative pulmonary morbidity and those in whom the risks of surgery would be prohibitive.[4, 144-149] This has led to the subgrouping of patients undergoing abdominal and thoracic surgery into risk categories according to spirometric test results.[4, 135, 146-150] Calligaro and colleagues[151] retrospectively reviewed 181 patients who underwent elective abdominal aortic operations and found that postoperative respiratory

failure was associated with American Society of Anesthesiologists class IV, age greater than 70 years, body weight greater than 150% of ideal, calculated forced vital capacity of 80% or less, forced expiratory flow rate (25% to 75%) of 60% or less, crystalloid replacement greater than 6 L, and total operative time greater than 5 hours.

Indications

Most patients for whom aortic operations are planned should have pulmonary function tests unless they are undergoing emergency surgery. The tests should encompass spirometry and arterial blood gas analysis.[142] Patients also should have clinical and radiographic examinations for evidence of chronic pulmonary disease.

Determinants of Respiratory Failure

Although chronic pulmonary disease increases the risk of operations on the ascending aorta, the aortic arch, and the abdominal aorta, the patients at greatest risk of respiratory failure are those who undergo repairs of the descending thoracic or thoracoabdominal aorta. We therefore evaluated the factors associated with postoperative respiratory complications and respiratory failure in a prospective study of 98 patients undergoing thoracoabdominal aortic aneurysm repairs.[142] Respiratory failure was arbitrarily defined as the need for postoperative ventilation for longer than 48 hours. With this information, it was possible to assess the risk factors associated with respiratory failure and then to stratify patients into risk categories.[4]

The clinical diagnosis of chronic pulmonary disease and a history of smoking were the most significant independent predictors of the risk of respiratory failure, even when preoperative pulmonary function tests and operative variables were taken into account. This is in agreement with a previous retrospective report on patients undergoing cardiovascular surgery.[4, 134] Unfortunately, the incidence of chronic pulmonary disease (56%) and a history of smoking (82%) is high in those patients with thoracoabdominal aortic aneurysms, but it is lower for patients with aortic dissection or infrarenal aortic aneurysms.[142] Thus, if chronic pulmonary disease is present, further information is required to weigh the benefits versus the risks of surgery. Menzies and colleagues[137] reported that the independent predictors ($p <$ 0.05) of prolonged ventilation and death in nonsurgical patients with chronic obstructive pulmonary disease (COPD) in whom respiratory failure developed were premorbid activity, low FEV_1, decreased serum albumin, severe dyspnea, cor pulmonale, hypercarbia, and a history of left ventricular failure. Of the spirometric tests, we found the best independent predictor to be the $FEF_{25\%}$ in patients with chronic pulmonary disease. In the analysis of all patients, the following were predictive of postoperative respiratory failure on univariate analysis ($p < 0.05$): FEV_1; FEV_1 percentage of predicted; FVC; $FEF_{25\%}$; $FEF_{25\%}$ percentage of predicted; $FEF_{25\%-75\%}$; $FEF_{25\%-75\%}$ percentage of predicted; $PaCO_2$;

PaO_2; preoperative symptoms; smoking history; evidence of chronic pulmonary disease; cryoprecipitate volume infused; postoperative neuromuscular deficit; cardiac complications; reoperation because of bleeding; renal complications; stress ulceration; postoperative creatinine level; postoperative dialysis; and postoperative encephalopathy (Figs. 2–14 and 2–15).[4, 142]

Examination of the spirometric tests that were predictive on univariate analysis of respiratory failure in our analysis showed that the correlation of respiratory failure with spirometric tests (Figs. 2–14 and 2–15) was linear and not exponential, and thus it appears that there is no particular threshold value after which the risk of respiratory failure markedly increases in individual patients. Thus no single low value can be considered a contraindication to surgery. This linearity of risk versus pulmonary function tests has been extensively reported for both thoracic and abdominal operations.[143, 147, 152, 153] It is of interest that there was a close correlation between the various types of tests although, because of its common usage, the FEV_1 is probably the best measurement for routine screening.[4] It is generally accepted that the lower limit for adequate respiratory function without significant activity restriction is an FEV_1 of 0.6 L/s to 0.7 L/s.[143, 144, 153] When the FEV_1 is lower than this level, then

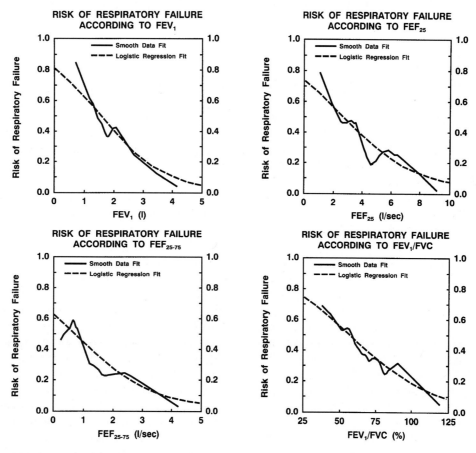

FIGURE 2–14 Risk of respiratory failure according to FEV_1, $FEF_{25\%}$, $FEF_{25\%-75\%}$, and FEV_1/FVC. Note the near linear relationship. (From Svensson LG, Hess KR, Coselli JS, et al. J Vasc Surg 1991;14:271–82.)

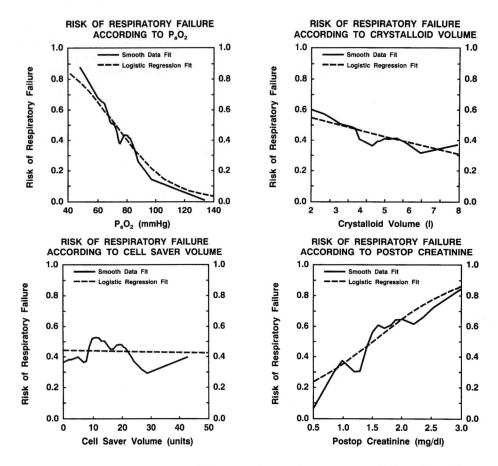

FIGURE 2–15 Risk of respiratory failure according to the preoperative PaO_2, volume of crystalloid administered during the operation, volume of cell-saver blood reinfused into the patients, and according to the postoperative serum creatinine level. (From Svensson LG, Hess KR, Coselli JS, et al. J Vasc Surg 1991;14:271–82.

CO_2 retention tends to occur, indicating failing respiratory reserves.[143, 144, 153] Furthermore, in patients with hypercarbia, the 5-year survival rate is less than 10%. For both coronary artery bypass surgery and thoracic pulmonary resections, the transient postoperative decrease in FEV_1 is at least 0.6 L/s.[133, 143, 152] The decrease in FEV_1 is similar in patients undergoing abdominal aortic aneurysm surgery.[136, 152, 154] Thus, by simply subtracting the minimal loss in function of 0.6 L/s from a preoperative value of 1.2 L/s, one could calculate a patient's postoperative FEV_1 to be 0.6 L/s. This low value would indicate either that transient respiratory failure is likely to occur or that the respiratory reserve is severely limited with no allowance for unforeseen pulmonary complications. Furthermore, CO_2 retention may occur.[4]

Several variables that are difficult to evaluate and predict in the individual patient influence the risk of respiratory failure. These include respiratory complications, retained secretions, the way the diaphragm is managed for thoracoabdominal aneurysms, the size of the aneurysm that may be compressing the lung, and prior leaks from the aneurysm resulting in fluid collections or scarring, which restricts normal lung expansion. Statistically, we found that those patients who were below the lowest quartile for FEV_1 (< 1.4 L) had

the highest incidence of respiratory failure. This is in keeping with at least a 0.6 L transient loss in postoperative FEV_1, some of which is recovered with time and even exceeded if lung compression was present preoperatively.[4]

There was noted to be an inverse linear correlation between either $FEF_{25\%-75\%}$ or $FEF_{25\%}$ and the risk of postoperative respiratory failure. This has also been reported for other surgical procedures.[134, 147, 153] These tests appear to correlate with the postoperative strength of a patient's cough. This is particularly important in patients who have preoperative bronchitis associated with COPD or who stop smoking immediately before surgery and thus are likely to produce excessive amounts of secretions[144, 147, 148] that have to be expectorated.[4]

Although preoperative variables were found to be important predictors of respiratory failure, particularly chronic pulmonary disease, smoking history, and $FEF_{25\%}$, when operative and postoperative variables were entered into our statistical model, renal and cardiac complications became additional independent predictors of respiratory failure. Nevertheless, encephalopathy and paralysis were also important univariate predictors of respiratory failure. Both of these factors compromise central respiratory drive and strength of respiratory muscles.[145, 155] However, as in patients with encephalopathy, we[74, 156] have reported that about two thirds of patients with paraparesis and some with paraplegia recover from their deficits with subsequent improvement of their respiratory function, and these patients can then be extubated. This has also been confirmed in patients who sustain traumatic injuries of the spinal cord.[155] Our research suggests that the risks of postoperative neuromuscular deficits can be reduced, thus decreasing the risk of respiratory failure in these patients.[16, 76, 77, 156] Furthermore, aside from the cardiac benefits,[157] fluid loading may reduce the risk of renal failure or postoperative hypotension resulting in paralysis.[142, 156] Stress ulceration, which often occurs after cardiac and aortic surgery,[140, 158] was also associated with respiratory failure. The association between respiratory complications, including pulmonary edema, with unclamping of the aorta and reperfusion of ischemic tissues has been reported.[4, 159]

Of interest, a study of 481 of our patients with chronic pulmonary disease who underwent thoracoabdominal aortic aneurysm surgery revealed that the risk of death increased slightly with the time spent on the ventilator up to the eighth postoperative day, and thereafter the risk increased markedly. This is in keeping with the development of multiple organ failure and nosocomial pneumonias in patients with prolonged ventilation. The prevention and management of patients with respiratory failure will be discussed later.[4]

Since no single variable correlated with a prohibitive risk of thoracoabdominal aortic surgery because of respiratory failure, on the basis of the univariate and multivariate analysis, then the following should be deemed as particularly high risks: $CO_2 > 45$ mm Hg; $FEV_1 < 1.2$ L; $FEF_{25\%} < 2.0$ L/s; $FEF_{25\%-75\%} < 0.5$ L/s; $PaO_2 < 55$ mm Hg; and renal occlusive disease or a serum creatinine value > 2 mg/dl.[4]

Patients undergoing thoracoabdominal repairs undoubtedly have the greatest risk of respiratory failure. Those patients who have thoracoabdominal incisions combined with midline chest incisions for extensive aortic operations are even more at risk.[160] Patients undergoing ascending aorta or aortic arch surgery, or both, from a respiratory standpoint, tolerate extensive operations remarkably well if the transfusion of blood is kept to a minimum and if aggressive diuresis is established after operation. Thus in these patients preoperative chronic pulmonary disease and a depressed FEV_1, even as low as 0.8 to 1.0 L, is not considered to be prohibitive for operation, particularly in smaller patients, such as females. Similarly, in view of the risk–benefit ratio and the high likelihood that an unresected abdominal aortic aneurysm will rupture, patients with abdominal aortic aneurysms are not turned down for surgery solely on the basis of poor preoperative pulmonary function tests. Nevertheless, both in our experience[142] with high-risk thoracoabdominal aortic aneurysm repairs and in the experience of Kispert and colleagues[161] with patients undergoing vascular surgery, including abdominal aortic repairs, patients with diminished pulmonary function have a decreased long-term

survival rate. The management of patients with depressed pulmonary function, chronic pulmonary disease, and respiratory complications is discussed in Chapters 16 and 26.

CONCLUSIONS

For safe aortic operations with minimal morbidity, elective surgery requires careful evaluation of the aorta, the cause of the aortic disease, and associated factors that will increase the risk of the operation. On the basis of the preoperative evaluation, the condition of the patient undergoing an elective operation should be optimized for the operation, not only to reduce the immediate risks of the operation but also to improve the patient's long-term survival.

REFERENCES

1. Webb S. Historical experiments predating commercially available computed tomography. Br J Radiol 1992;65:835-7.
2. Crawford ES, Cohen ES. Aortic aneurysm: a multifocal disease. Arch Surg 1982;117:1393-400.
3. Svensson LG, Klepp P, Hinder RA. Spinal cord anatomy of the baboon: comparison with man and implications on spinal cord blood flow during thoracic aortic cross-clamping. S Afr J Surg 1986;24:32-4.
4. Svensson LG, Crawford ES. Aortic dissection and aortic aneurysm surgery: clinical observations, experimental investigations and statistical analyses. Part I. Curr Probl Surg 1992;29:819-912.
5. Henry LG, Doust B, Korns ME. Abdominal aortic aneurysm and retroperitoneal fibrosis. Arch Surg 1978;113:1456.
6. Hirose Y, Hamada S, Takamiya M, et al. Aortic aneurysms: growth rates measured with CT. Radiology 1992;185:249-52.
7. Alfid RJ, Haaga J, Meaney TF, et al. Computed tomography of the thorax and abdomen: a preliminary report. Radiology 1975;117:257.
8. Anderson MW, Higgins CB. Should the patient with suspected acute dissection of the aorta have MRI, CAT scan, or aortography as the definitive study. Cardiovasc Clin 1990;21:293-304.
9. Bateman TM. X-ray computed tomography of the cardiovascular system. Curr Probl Cardiol 1991;16:765-829.
10. Rubin GD, Walker PJ, Dake MD, et al. Three-dimensional spiral computed tomographic angiography: an alternative imaging modality for the abdominal aorta and its branches. J Vasc Surg 1993;18:656-65.
11. Haschek E, Lindelthal OT. A contribution to the practical use of the photography according to Rontgen. Wien klin Wochenschr 1896;9:63.
12. Dos Santos R, Lamas AC, Pereira-Caldas J. L'arteriographie des membres de l'aorte et de ses branches abdominales. Bull Mem Soc Natl Chir 1929;55:587.
13. Seldinger SI. Catheter replacement of needle in percutaneous arteriography: new technique. Acta Radiol 1953;39:368-76.
14. Sones FM Jr, Shivey EK, Proudfit WL, et al. Cinecoronary arteriography (abstract). Circulation 1959;20:773.
15. Sones FM, Shirey EK. Cine coronary arteriography. Mod Concepts Cardiovasc Dis 1962;31:735.
16. Svensson LG, Patel V, Coselli JS, Crawford ES. Preliminary report of localization of spinal cord blood supply by hydrogen during aortic operations. Ann Thorac Surg 1990;49:528-35.
17. Crawford ES, Mizrahi EM, Hess KR, et al. The impact of distal aortic perfusion and somatosensory evoked potential monitoring on prevention of paraplegia after aortic aneurysm operation. J Thorac Cardiovasc Surg 1988;95:357-67. (Published erratum appears in J Thorac Cardiovasc Surg 1989;97:665.)
18. Svensson LG, Gaylis H, Barlow JB. Presentation and management of aorto-caval fistula. S Afr Med J 1987;72:876-7.
19. Svensson LG, Crawford ES. Aortic dissection and aortic aneurysm surgery: clinical observations, experimental investigations, and statistical analyses. Part II. Curr Probl Surg 1992;29:915-1057.
20. Almen T. Contrast agent design: some aspects on the synthesis of

water soluble agents of low osmolality. J Theor Biol 1969;24: 216-26.

21. Bergman T, Neiman HL. Computed tomography in the detection of retroperitoneal hemorrhage after translumbar aortography. AJR 1978;131:831-3.

22. Dudrick S, Masland W, Mishkin M. Brachial plexus injury following axillary artery puncture: further comments on management. Radiology 1967;88:271-3.

23. Svensson LG, Coselli JS, Safi HJ, et al. Appraisal of adjuncts to prevent acute renal failure after surgery on the thoracic or thoracoabdominal aorta. J Vasc Med 1989;10:230-9.

24. Martin-Paredero V, Dixon SM, Baker JD, et al. Risk of renal failure after major angiography. Arch Surg 1983;118:1417.

25. Morris GC, Crawford ES, Beall AC Jr, et al. Hyperhydration: a method of decreasing the nephrotoxic effects of urokon as employed in aortography. Surg Forum 1957;7:319-22.

26. Svensson LG, Coselli JS, Safi HJ, et al. Appraisal of adjuncts to prevent acute renal failure after surgery on the thoracic or thoracoabdominal aorta. J Vasc Surg 1989;10:230-9.

27. Gaylis H, Laws JW. Dissection of the aorta as a complication of translumbar aortography. Br Med J 1956;2:1141.

28. Landnenau MD, Raju S. Infections after bypass surgery for lower limb ischemia: the influence of preoperative transcutaneous aortography. Surgery 1981;90:956-61.

29. Beall AC Jr, Crawford ES, Couves CM, et al. Complications of aortography, factors influencing renal function following aortography with 70 per cent urokon. Surgery 1958;43:364-80.

30. Beall AC Jr, Morris GC Jr., Crawford ES, et al. Translumbar aortography: re-evaluation. Surgery 1961;49:772-8.

31. Hessel SJ, Adams DF, Abrams HL. Complications of angiography. Radiology 1981;138:273-81.

32. Couch NP, O'Mahony J, McIrvine A, et al. The place of abdominal aortography in abdominal aortic aneurysm resection. Arch Surg 1983;118:1029-34.

33. Gaspar MR. Role of arteriography in the evaluation of aortic aneurysms: the case against. In: Bergan JJ, Yao JST, eds. Aneurysms—Diagnosis and Treatment. New York: Grune & Stratton; 1982: 233-41.

34. Amparo EG, Higgins CB, Hricak H, et al. Aortic dissection: magnetic resonance imaging. Radiology 1985;155:399-406.

35. Dinsmore RE, Liberthson RR, Wismer GL, et al. Magnetic resonance imaging of thoracic aortic aneurysms: comparison with the other imaging methods. AJR 1986;146:309-14.

36. Grenier P, Pernes JM, Desbleds MT, et al. Magnetic resonance imaging of aneurysms and chronic dissections of the thoracic aorta. Ann Vasc Surg 1987;9:531-41.

37. Higgins CB. MR of the heart: anatomy, physiology, and metabolism. AJR 1988;151:239.

38. Johnston DL, Liu P. Evaluation of myocardial ischemia and infarction by nuclear magnetic resonance techniques. Can J Cardiol 1988;4: 116.

39. Lotan CS, Cranney GB, Doyle M, et al. Fat-shift artifact simulating aortic dissection on MR images. AJR 1989;152:385-6.

40. Schaefer S, Peshock RM, Malloy CR, et al. Nuclear magnetic resonance imaging in Marfan's syndrome. J Am Coll Cardiol 1987;9:70.

41. Mourino MR. From Thales to Lauterbur, or from the lodestone to MR imaging: magnetism and medicine. Radiology 1991;180:593-612.

42. Nienaber CA, Spielmann RP, von KY, et al. Diagnosis of thoracic aortic dissection: magnetic resonance imaging versus transesophageal echocardiography. Circulation 1992;85:434-47.

43. Nienaber CA, von Kodolitsch Y, Nicolas V, et al. The diagnosis of thoracic aortic dissection by noninvasive imaging procedures. N Engl J Med 1993;328:1-9.

44. Appelbe AF, Walker PG, Yeoh JK, et al. Clinical significance and origin of artifacts in transesophageal echocardiography of the thoracic aorta. J Am Coll Cardiol 1993;21:754-60.

45. Barbant SD, Eisenberg MJ, Schiller NB. The diagnostic value of imaging techniques for aortic dissection. Am Heart J 1992;124:541-3.

46. Tennant WG, Hartnell GG, Baird RN, Horrocks M. Inflammatory aortic aneurysms: characteristic appearance on magnetic resonance imaging. Eur J Vasc Surg 1992;6:399-402.

47. Manning WJ, Li W, Edelman RR. A preliminary report comparing magnetic resonance coronary angiography with conventional angiography. N Engl J Med 1993;328:828-32.

48. Link KM, Loehr SP, Baker DM, Lesko NM. Magnetic resonance imaging of the thoracic aorta. Semin Ultrasound CT MR 1993;14:91-105.

49. Kandarpa K, Sandor T, Tieman J, et al. Rapid three-dimensional surface reconstruction of magnetic resonance images of large arteries and veins: a preliminary evaluation of clinical utility. Cardiovasc Intervent Radiol 1993;16:25-9.

50. Tennant WG, Hartnell GG, Baird RN, Horrocks M. Radiologic investigation of abdominal aortic aneurysm disease: comparison of three modalities in staging and the detection of inflammatory change. J Vasc Surg 1993;17:703-9.

51. Boucher CA, Brewster DC, Darling RC, et al. Determination of cardiac risk by dipyridamole-thallium imaging before peripheral vascular surgery. N Engl J Med 1985;312:389.

52. Cutler BS, Leppo JA. Dipyridamole thallium 201 scintigraphy to detect coronary artery disease before abdominal aortic surgery. J Vasc Surg 1987;5:91-100.

53. Eagle KA, Coley CM, Newell JB, et al. Combining clinical and thallium data optimizes preoperative assessment of cardiac risk before major vascular surgery. Ann Intern Med 1989;110:859-66.

54. Hertzer NR, Young JR, Kramer JR, et al. Routine coronary angiography prior to elective aortic resection. Arch Surg 1979;114:1336.

55. Hertzer NR, Beven EG, Young JR, et al. Coronary artery disease in peripheral vascular patients: a classification of 1000 coronary angiograms and results of surgical management. Ann Surg 1984; 199:223-33.

56. Kennedy JW. Complication associated with cardiac catheterization and angiography. Cathet Cardiovasc Diag 1982;8:13.

57. Kern MJ, Serota H, Callicoat P, et al. Use of coronary arteriography in the preoperative management of patients undergoing urgent repair of the thoracic aorta. Am Heart J 1990;119:143-8.

58. McCann RL, Clements FM. Silent myocardial ischemia in patients undergoing peripheral vascular surgery: incidence and association with perioperative cardiac morbidity and mortality. J Vasc Surg 1989;9:583-7.

59. Pasternack PF, Imparato AM, Riles TS, et al. The value of the radionuclide angiogram in the prediction of perioperative myocardial infarction in patients undergoing lower extremity revascularization procedures. Circulation 1985;72:11.

60. Mautner GC, Berezowski K, Mautner SL, Roberts WC. Degrees of coronary arterial narrowing at necropsy in men with large fusiform abdominal aortic aneurysm. Am J Cardiol 1992;70:1143-6.

61. McFalls EO, Doliszny KM, Grund F, et al. Angina and persistent exercise thallium defects: independent risk factors in elective vascular surgery. J Am Coll Cardiol 1993;21:1347-52.

62. McEnroe CS, O'Donnell TF Jr, Yeager A, et al. Comparison of ejection fraction and Goldman risk factor analysis to dipyridamole-thallium 201 studies in the evaluation of cardiac morbidity after aortic aneurysm surgery 'see comments'. J Vasc Surg 1990;11:497-504.

63. Cutler BS, Hendel RC, Leppo JA. Dipyridamole-thallium scintigraphy predicts perioperative and long-term survival after major vascular surgery. J Vasc Surg 1992;15:972-81.

64. Mangano DT, London MJ, Tubau JF, et al. Dipyridamole-thallium 201 scintigraphy as a preoperative test: a re-examination of its predictive potential. Circulation 1991;84:493-502.

65. Goldman L, Caldera DL, Southwick FS, et al. Cardiac risk factors and complications in non-cardiac surgery. Medicine 1978;57:357.

66. Lalka SG, Sawada SG, Dalsing MC, et al. Dobutamine stress echocardiography as a predictor of cardiac events associated with aortic surgery. J Vasc Surg 1992;15:831-42.

67. Suggs WD, Smith RB III, Weintraub WS, et al. Selective screening for coronary artery disease in patients undergoing elective repair of abdominal aortic aneurysms. J Vasc Surg 1993;18:349-57.

68. Hertzer NR, Young JR, Beven EG, et al. Late results of coronary bypass in patients with infrarenal aortic aneurysms: the Cleveland Clinic Study. Ann Surg 1987;205:360-7.

69. Hertzer NR. Basic data concerning associated coronary disease in peripheral vascular patients. Ann Vasc Surg 1987;1:616-20.

70. Crawford ES, Saleh SA, Babb JW, et al. Infrarenal abdominal aortic aneurysm: factors influencing survival after operation performed over a 25-year period. Ann Surg 1981;193:699-709.

71. Crawford ES, Bomberger RA, Glaeser DH, et al. Aortoiliac occlusive disease: factors influencing survival and function following reconstructive operation over a twenty-five year period. Surgery 1981; 90:1555-67.

72. Crawford ES, Crawford JL, Safi HJ, et al. Thoracoabdominal aortic

aneurysms: preoperative and intraoperative factors determining immediate and long-term results of operation in 605 patients. J Vasc Surg 1986;3:389–404.

73. Crawford ES, Svensson LG, Coselli JS, et al. Surgical treatment aneurysm and/or dissection of the ascending aorta, transverse aortic arch, and ascending aorta and transverse aortic arch: factors influencing survival in 717 patients. J Thorac Cardiovasc Surg 1989;98:659–74.

74. Svensson LG, Crawford ES, Hess KR, et al. Dissection of the aorta and dissecting aortic aneurysms: improving early and long-term surgical results. Circulation 1990;82(5 Supp):iV24–38.

75. Svensson LG, Crawford ES. Aneurysms involving the descending and upper abdominal aorta. Chest Clin North Am 1992;2:311–28.

76. Svensson LG, Crawford ES, Hess KR, et al. Variables predictive of outcome in 832 patients undergoing repairs of the descending thoracic aorta. Chest 1993;104:1248–53.

77. Svensson LG, Crawford ES, Hess KR, et al. Experience with 1509 patients undergoing thoracoabdominal aortic operations. J Vasc Surg 1993;17:357–70.

78. Corday E. Historical vignette celebrating the 30th anniversary of diagnostic ambulatory electrocardiographic monitoring and data reduction systems. J Am Coll Cardiol 1991;17:286–92.

79. Mangano DT, Hollenberg M, Fegert G, et al. Perioperative myocardial ischemia in patients undergoing noncardiac surgery. I. incidence and severity during the four day perioperative period. J Am Coll Cardiol 1991;17:843–50.

80. Fu LX, Hjalmarson A. An update to silent myocardial ischemia: pathophysiological, diagnostic, and therapeutic approaches. Clin Cardiol 1990;13:452–6.

81. Statters DJ, Ward DW, Camm AJ. Units for QTc. Lancet 1993;341:629.

82. Forssmann W. Experiments on myself: memoirs of a surgeon in Germany. New York: Saint Martin's Press 1974:75–8, 84–5.

83. Warren JV. Fifty years of invasive cardiology. Werner Forssman (1904–1979). Am J Med 1980;60:10.

84. Cournand A. Cardiac catheterization: development of the technique, its contribution to experimental medicine, and its initial application in man. Acta Med Scand 1978;7(Supp):S79.

85. Judkins MP. Selective coronary arteriography. Radiology 1967;89:815.

86. Glagov S, Zarins CV. Quantitating atherosclerosis: problems of definition. In: Bond MA, Insull W, Glagov S, et al. (eds). Clinical Diagnosis of Artherosclerosis: Quantitative Methods of Evaluation. New York: Springer-Verlag 1982:11–35.

87. Levin DC. Pathways and functional significance of the coronary collateral circulation. Circulation 1974;50:831.

88. Waldman JD, Karp RB. How should we treat coarctation of the aorta? Circulation 1993;87:1043–5.

89. Grifka RG, Vick GW III, O'Laughlin MP, et al. Balloon expandable intravascular stents: aortic implantation and late further dilation in growing minipigs. Am Heart J 1993;126:979–84.

90. Meier GH, Sumpio B, Setaro JF, et al. Captopril renal scintigraphy: a new standard for predicting outcome after renal revascularization. J Vasc Surg 1993;17:280–7.

91. Lacombe P, Mulot R, Labedan F, et al. Percutaneous recanalization of a renal artery in aortic dissection. Radiology 1992;185:829–31.

92. Saito S, Arai H, Kim K, et al. Percutaneous fenestration of dissecting intima with a transseptal needle: a new therapeutic technique for visceral ischemia complicatign acute aortic dissection. Cathet Cardiovasc Diagn 1992;26:130–5.

93. Chuter T, Green RM, Ouriel K, et al. Transfemoral endovascular aortic graft replacement. J Vasc Surg 1993;18:185–97.

94. Sorrell KA, Feinberg RL, Wheeler JR, et al. Color-flow duplex-directed manual occlusion of femoral false aneurysms. J Vasc Surg 1993;17:571–7.

95. Weintraub WS, Ghazzal ZMB, Douglas JS Jr, et al. Long-term follow-up in patients with angiographic restudy after successful angioplasty. Circulation 1993;87:831–40.

96. Greenberg MA, Mueller HS. Why the excess mortality in women after PTCA? Circulation 1993;87:1030–2.

97. Kelsey SF, James M, Holubkov AL, et al. Results of percutaneous transluminal coronary angioplasty in women: 1985–1986 National Heart, Lung, and Blood Institute's Coronary Angioplasty Registry. Circulation 1993;87:720–7.

98. Rahimtoola SH. The need for cardiac catheterization and angiography in valvular heart disease is not disproven. Ann Intern Med 1982;97:433.

99. Roberts WC. Reasons for cardiac catheterization before cardiac valve replacement. N Engl J Med 1982;306:1291.

100. St. John SMG, St. John SM, Oldershaw P, et al. Valve replacement without preoperative cardiac catheterization. N Engl J Med 1981;305:1233.

101. Davis K, Kennedy JW, Kemp HG, et al. Complications of coronary arteriography from the Collaorative Study of Coronary Artery Surgery (CASS). Circulation 1979;59:1105.

102. Armstrong WF, Odonnel J, Ryan T, et al. Effect of prior myocardial infarction and extent and location of coronary disease on accuracy of exercise echocardiography. J Am Coll Cardiol 1987;10:531.

103. Buda AJ, Zotz RJ, Gallagher KP. Characterization of the functional border zone around regionally ischemic myocardium using circumferential flow-function maps. J Am Coll Cardiol 1986;8:150.

104. Meltzer RS, Woythaler JN, Buda AJ, et al. Two-dimensional echocardiographic quantification of infarct size alteration by pharmacologic agents. Am J Cardiol 1979;44:257.

105. Wyatt HL, Meerbaum S, Heng MK, et al. Experimental evaluation of the extent of myocardial dysynergy and infarct size by two-dimensional echocardiography. Circulation 1981;63:607.

106. Mazeika PK, Nadazdin A, Oakley CM. Dobutamine stress echocardiography for detection and assessment of coronary artery disease. J Am Coll Cardiol 1992;19:1203.

107. Eichelberger JP, Schwarz KQ, Black ER, et al. Predictive value of dobutamine echocardiography just before noncardiac vascular surgery. Am J Cardiol 1993;72:602–7.

108. Koolen JJ, Visser CA, Reichert SLA, et al. Improved monitoring of myocardial ischaemia during major vascular surgery using transoesophageal echocardiography. Eur Heart J 1992;13:1028–33.

109. Feinstein SB, Lang RM, Dick C, et al. Contrast echocardiographic perfusion studies in humans. Am J Cardiac Imaging 1986;1:29.

110. Gorlin R, Gorlin G. Hydraulic formula for calculation of area of stenotic mitral valve, other cardiac valves and central circulatory shunts. Am Heart J 1951;41:1.

111. Hust MH, Metzler B, Bickel W, et al. Transmural rupture of a nondissecting aortic aneurysm diagnosed by transesophageal echocardiography. Am Heart J 1993;125:1778–80.

112. Galvin IF, Black IW, Lee CL, Horton DA. Transesophageal echocardiography in acute aortic transection. Ann Thorac Surg 1991;51:310.

113. Amarenco P, Duyckaerts C, Tzourio C, et al. The prevalence of ulcerated plaques in the aortic arch in patients with stroke. N Engl J Med 1992;326:221–5.

114. Rubin DC, Plotnick GD, Hawke MW. Intraaortic debris as a potential source of embolic stroke. Am J Cardiol 1992;69:819–20.

115. Tunick PA, Lackner H, Katz ES, et al. Multiple emboli from a large aortic arch thrombus in a patient with thrombotic diathesis. Am Heart J 1992;124:239–41.

116. Katz ES, Tunick PA, Rusinek H, et al. Protruding aortic atheromas predict stroke in elderly patients undergoing cardiopulmonary bypass: experience with intraoperative transesophageal echocardiography. J Am Coll Cardiol 1992;20:70–7.

117. Ribakove GH, Katz ES, Galloway AC, et al. Surgical implications of transesophageal echocardiography to grade the atheromatous aortic arch. Ann Thorac Surg 1992;53:758–63.

118. Davila-Roman VG, Barzilai B, Wareing TH, et al. Intraoperative ultrasonographic evaluation of the ascending aorta in 100 consecutive patients undergoing cardiac surgery. Circulation 1991;84(supp III):III-47–III-53.

119. Wareing TH, Davila-Roman VG, Barzilai B, et al. Management of the severely atherosclerotic ascending aorta during cardiac operations: a strategy for detection and treatment. J Thorac Cardiovasc Surg 1992;103:453–62.

120. Culliford AT, Colvin SB, Rohrer K, et al. The atherosclerotic ascending aorta and transverse arch: a new technique to prevent cerebral injury during bypass: experience with 13 patients. Ann Thorac Surg 1986;41:27–35.

121. Silvey SV, Stoughton TL, Pearl W, et al. Rupture of the outer partition of aortic dissection during transesophageal echocardiography. Am J Cardiol 1991;68:286–7.

122. Starling EH. Some points in the pathology of heart disease. Lancet 1897;1:652–5.

123. Fowler NO. Cardiac tamonade: a clinical or an echocardiographic diagnosis? Circulation 1993;87:1738–41.

124. Dent J, Kaul S. Utility of transesophageal echocardiography in the diagnosis of aortic conduit endocarditis in patients who have undergone the Cabrol procedure. J Am Soc Echocardiogr 1992;5:434-6.

125. Kouchoukos NT, Davila-Roman VG, Spray TL, et al. Replacement of the aortic root with a pulmonary autograft in children and young adults with aortic-valve disease. N Engl J Med 1994;330:1-6.

126. Roudaut RP, Marcaggi XL, Deville C, et al. Value of transesophageal echocardiography combined with computed tomography for assessing repaired Type A aortic dissection. Am J Cardiol 1992;70: 1468-76.

127. Okuhn SP, Reilly LM, Bennett JB, et al. Intraoperative assessment of renal and visceral artery reconstruction: the role of duplex scanning and spectral analysis. J Vasc Surg 1987;5:137-47.

128. Taylor DC, Kettler MD, Moneta GL, et al. Duplex ultrasound scanning in the diagnosis of renal artery stenosis: a prospective evaluation. J Vasc Surg 1988;7:395-9.

129. O'Neil EA, Hansen KJ, Canzanello VJ, et al. Prevalence of ischemic nephropathy in patients with renal insufficiency. Am Surg 1992; 58:485-90.

130. Gerraty RP, Gates PC, Doyle JC. Carotid stenosis and perioperative stroke risk in symptomatic and asymptomatic patients undergoing vascular or coronary surgery. Stroke 1993;24:1115-8.

131. Beall ACJ, Jones JW, Guinn GA, et al. Cardiopulmonary bypass in patients with previous completed stroke. Ann Thorac Surg 1993; 55:1383-5.

132. Blauth CI, Cosgrove DM, Webb BW, et al. Atheroembolism from the ascending aorta: an emerging problem in cardiac surgery. J Thorac Cardiovasc Surg 1992;103:1104-12.

133. Berrizbeitia LD, Tessler S, Jacobwitz IJ, et al. Effect of sternotomy and coronary bypass surgery on postoperative pulmonary mechanics. Chest 1989;96:873-6.

134. Cain HD, Stevens PM, Adaniya R. Preoperative pulmonary function and complications after cardiovascular surgery. Chest 1979;76: 130-5.

135. Cosio M, Ghezzo H, Hogg JC, et al. The relations between structural changes in small airways and pulmonary function tests. N Engl J med 1977;298:1277-81.

136. Diehl JT, Cali RF, Hertzer NR, et al. Complications of abdominal aortic reconstruction: an analysis of perioperative risk factors in 557 patients. Ann Surg 1983;97:49-56.

137. Menzies R, Gibbons W, Goldberg P. Determinants of weaning and survival among patients with COPD who require mechanical ventilation for acute respiratory failure. Chest 1989;95:398-405.

138. Robison JG, Beckett WC Jr, Mills JL, et al. Aortic reconstruction in high-risk pulmonary patients. Ann Surg 1989;210:112-7.

139. Sabanathan S. Alterations in respiratory mechanics following thoracotomy. J R Coll Surg Edinb 1990;35:144-50.

140. Svensson LG, Decker G, Kinsley R. A prospective study of hyperamylasemia and pancreatitis after cardiopulmonary bypass. Ann Thorac Surg 1985;39:409-11.

141. Svensson LG, Loop FD. Prevention of spinal cord ischemia in aortic surgery.In:Bergan JJ, Yao JST, eds. Arterial surgery: new diagnostic and operative techniques. New York: Grune & Stratton. 1988; 273-85.

142. Svensson LG, Hess KR, Coselli JS, et al. A prospective study of respiratory failure after high-risk surgery on the thoracoabdominal aorta. J Vasc Surg 1991;14:271-82.

143. Gass GD, Olsen GN. Preoperative pulmonary function testing to predict postoperative morbidity and mortality. Chest 1986;89: 127-35.

144. Milledge JS, Nunn JF. Criteria of fitness for anesthesia in patients with chronic obstructive lung disease. Br Med J 1975;3:670-3.

145. Tisi GM. Preoperative evaluation of pulmonary function: validity, indications, and benefits. Am Rev Respir Dis 1979;119:293-310.

146. Williams CD, Brenowitz JB. "Prohibitive" lung function and major surgical procedures. Am J Surg 1976;132:763-6.

147. Gracey DR, Divertie MB, Didier EP. Preoperative pulmonary preparation of patients with chronic obstructive pulmonary disease: a prospective study. Chest 1979;76:123-9.

148. Lazar HL, Plehn J. Intraoperative echocardiography. Ann Thorac Surg 1990;50:1010-18.

149. Miller WF, Wu N, Johnson RL Jr, et al. Convenient method of evaluating pulmonary ventilatory function with a single breath test. Anesthesiology 1956;17:480-93.

150. Hodgkin JE, Dines DE, Didier EP. Preoperative evaluation of the patient with pulmonary disease. Mayo Clin Proc 1973;48:114-8.

151. Calligaro KD, Azurin DJ, Dougherty MJ, et al. Pulmonary risk factors of elective abdominal aortic surgery. J Vasc Surg 1993;18:914-21.

152. Latimer RG, Dickman M, Day WC, et al. Ventilatory patterns and pulmonary complications after upper abdominal surgery determined by preoperative and postoperative computerized spirometry and blood gas analysis. Am J Surg 1971;122:622-32.

153. Stein M, Cassara EL. Preoperative pulmonary evaluation and therapy for surgery patients. JAMA 1970;211:787-90.

154. Smith PK, Fuchs JCA, Sabiston DJ Jr. Surgical management of aortic abdominal aneurysms in patients with severe pulmonary insufficiency. Gynecol Obstet 1980;151:407-11.

155. Huldgren AC, Fugl-Meyer AR, Jonasson E, et al. Ventilatory dysfunction and respiratory rehabilitation in post-traumatic quadriplegia. Eur J Respir Dis 1980;61:347-56.

156. Crawford ES, Svensson LG, Hess KR, et al. A prospective randomized study of cerebrospinal fluid drainage to prevent paraplegia after high-risk surgery on the thoracoabdominal aorta. J Vasc Surg 1991;13:36-45.

157. Whittmore AD, Clowes AW, Hectman HB, et al. Aortic aneurysm repair: reduced operation mortality associated with maintenance of optimal cardiac performance. Ann Surg 1980;193:414-21.

158. Svensson LG, Von Ritter C, Oosthuizen MM, et al. Prevention of gastric mucosal lesions following aortic cross-clamping. Br J Surg 1987;74:282-5.

159. Klausner JM, Paterson IS, Mannick JA, et al. Reperfusion pulmonary edema. JAMA 1989;261:1030-5.

160. Svensson LG, Shahian DM, Davis FG, et al. Replacement of entire aorta from aortic valve to bifurcation during one operation. Ann Thorac Surg 1994;58:1164-6.

161. Kispert JF, Kazmers A, Roitman L. Preoperative spirometry predicts perioperative pulmonary complications after major vascular surgery. Am Surg 1992;58:491-5.

Degenerative Aortic Aneurysms

CLASSIFICATION OF ANEURYSMS

An aneurysm is an irreversible dilatation of the aorta exceeding the normal diameter for age and height of the patient. As a rule of thumb, we define an aneurysm as being present when the aortic transverse diameter exceeds twice the normal aortic diameter. It should also be noted that not only is the diameter enlarged, but also the aorta is lengthened in the aneurysmal segment.

True aortic aneurysms can be broadly classified as those associated with degeneration of the aortic media (medial degenerative aneurysms), aortic dissection, disorders of connective tissue, blunt trauma, aortitis, primary mycotic infections, previous graft insertion, and congenital abnormalities. We prefer the term *aneurysmal medial degenerative disease* rather than *atherosclerotic aneurysms* to describe the aneurysms that typically occur in the elderly. The reason for this distinction is that atherosclerosis is not always present and, when it is, the atherosclerosis is most commonly located in the media of the aorta (Fig. 3–1), in contrast to the smaller arteries where it usually involves the intima. Furthermore, the infiltration of the aortic media by atheroma, fibrosis, and scar tissue is the result of degeneration rather than the primary event.

Aneurysms that are not lined with the intima of the aortic wall are known as false or pseudoaneurysms. False aneurysms tend to occur in the following situations: at sites of previous aortic anastomoses such as those with prosthetic material, end-to-end repairs, patch repairs for coarctation of the aorta, burrowing of infections through the aortic wall by mycotic aneurysms, and posttraumatic aneurysms, including from penetrating injuries of the aorta. In contrast to those fusiform true aneurysms that involve the entire circumference of the aorta, false aneurysms often have a saccular appearance, mimicking saccular aneurysms. Figures illustrating the different types of aneurysms are shown in the relevant chapters.

For ease of reference, the aorta is divided into various aortic segments. The segment above the cusp of the aortic valve extending to the sinotubular ridge is known as the sinus of Valsalva. The sinotubular ridge is the narrowing, sometimes "shelflike," transition from the sinuses of Valsalva to the ascending aorta proper. The ascending aorta proper extends from the sinotubular ridge to a line drawn at a right angle to the origin of the innominate artery. When an aneurysm involves the sinus segment but the sinotubular ridge is also lost because of dilatation, this type of aneurysm is known as having *annuloaortic ectasia,* a term coined by Cooley.[1] This "flasklike," "hourglass," or "wine-skin-like" deformity is typically associated with Marfan syndrome. The aortic arch extends from the line drawn at a right angle proximal to the innominate artery origin to a line drawn at a right angle distal to the origin of the left subclavian artery. The descending thoracic aorta extends from the left subclavian artery to the aortic hiatus in the diaphragm. The abdominal aorta extends from the aortic hiatus to the bifurcation of the aorta. The abdominal aorta is further divided into subsegments. The supraceliac segment lies between the diaphragm and the celiac artery and is essentially wrapped by the crura of the diaphragm. The suprarenal aorta lies above the level of the renal arteries, and the infrarenal aorta extends from distal to the renal arteries to the bifurcation. The term *juxtarenal* is sometimes used to describe aneurysms that extend to the immediate origin of the renal arteries with no space for placing a clamp below the renal arteries.[2] The term *thoracoabdominal aneurysm* implies involvement of varying extents of the descending thoracic and abdominal aorta.

These thoracoabdominal aneurysms have been subclassified by us.[3–6] Figure 3–2 illustrates the Crawford classification of thoracoabdominal aortic aneurysms. Type I involves the proximal half of the descending aorta to the renal arteries; type II extends from the proximal half of the descending thoracic aorta to below the renal arteries; type III extends from the distal half of the descending thoracic aorta into varying extents of the abdominal aorta; type IV involves most of the abdominal aorta. More recently, we examined the influence on postoperative neurologic deficits of subdividing type I aneurysms into those ending at the celiac artery (A) and those with a bevel extending behind the celiac artery but ending above the renal arteries (B). The incidence of postoperative paraplegia or paraparesis was increased in the subgroup B when compared with subgroup A.[7]

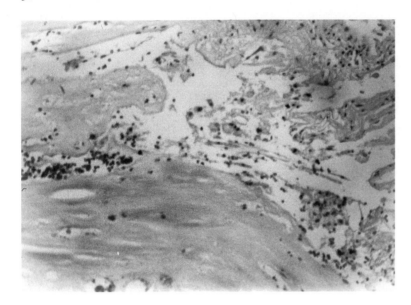

FIGURE 3–1   Medial degenerative aneurysm showing medial friable atheromatous debris (*central*) and surrounding hyalinized component (*lower left*). H&E stain 100×.

AORTIC HISTOLOGY

Normal Histology

The normal aorta in the human adult consists of five distinctive layers. The tunica intima is composed of an endothelial layer of cells on a basement membrane with minimal ground substance and connective tissue. Bordering the tunica intima and the tunica media is the fenestrated sheet of elastic fibers known as the internal elastic lamina. The tunica media consists of elastic tissue arranged concentrically

and forms the bulk of the aortic wall. It also contains smooth muscle cells and ground substance consisting of proteoglycans. The outer third of the tunica media is supplied by the nutrient vasa vasorum and a variable number of lymphatics and nerves. The outermost layer is the external elastic lamina bordering the adventitia. The tunica adventitia consists of a strong, tough layer of collagen and elastic fibers.

There is no universally accepted classification for aortic micropathology. In fact, pathologists differ quite markedly in their opinions about how best to identify aortic medial

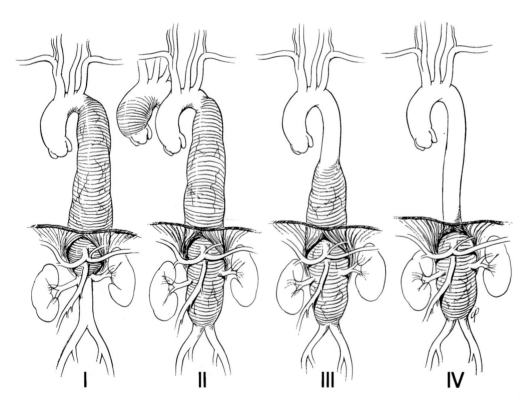

FIGURE 3–2   Crawford classification of thoracoabdominal aortic aneurysms. Type I originates in the proximal descending thoracic aorta and ends above the renal arteries. Type II begins in the proximal descending thoracic aorta and terminates below the renal arteries. Type III originates in the distal descending aorta, below approximately thoracic vertebra T6, conveniently identified by being below the level of the thoracic incision in the sixth intercostal space. Type IV involves most of the abdominal aorta (8).

I   II   III   IV

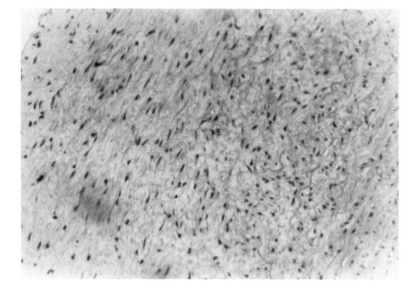

FIGURE 3–3   Medial degeneration of media with diffuse fibrosis and splaying and filling of the spaces. H&E stain 100×.

disease. As a result of these problems, the histologic classification we have used[8] is based on the presence of elastic fibers, smooth muscle cells, atherosclerosis, and inflammatory cells. Thus aortic histology is based on the observation of loss of elastic fibers (medial degenerative disease), loss of smooth muscle cells (medial necrosis), the presence of atherosclerosis (atherosclerosis usually superimposed on medial degenerative disease), and evidence of chronic inflammatory cell infiltration (inflammatory disease).

Medial Degeneration

In most patients microscopic analysis of the aorta with special staining techniques often reveals loss and disruption of the elastic fibers (Figs. 3-3 and 3-4), particularly when there is chronic hypertension or Marfan syndrome or when the patient is elderly. The exact cause remains unknown. There-

fore these patients are referred to as having medial degenerative disease.

Medial Necrosis

With more advanced medial degeneration, for example in Marfan patients, smooth muscle cells appear to be lost, and this form is referred to as showing medial necrosis (Fig. 3-5). Controversy still exists as to whether medial necrosis antedates or follows acute aortic dissection.[8] It has been our observation that in a few patients with aortic infections or those patients with aortic dissection at a remote and different site, an apparently uninvolved segment of aorta can easily be separated into two layers. Histological examination of the seemingly uninvolved aorta has revealed medial necrosis. With chronic dissection the tear and false lumen may become lined by endothelial cells (Fig. 3-6).

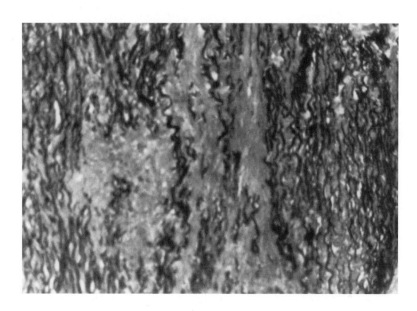

FIGURE 3–4   Advanced fragmentation of elastic laminae of media. Elastic stain 100×.

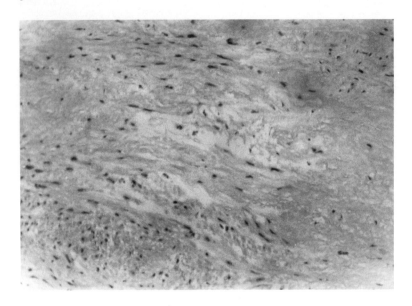

FIGURE 3–5   Medial necrosis, sometimes referred to as cystic medial necrosis in advanced forms, often associated with Marfan syndrome, characterized by loss of smooth muscle cells and pools of mucopolysaccharide (*center*). H&E stain 100×.

Atherosclerosis

Atherosclerosis can be associated with any type of medial disease and is more commonly seen in elderly patients with chronic aneurysms (Fig. 3–1).[9] Indeed, the farther distal from the aortic valve the aorta is examined, the greater the probability of finding atherosclerosis, including atheroma and calcification, in the aortic wall.[8] Dense aortic calcification is often associated with inactive chronic aortitis that has been present for a long time.

Inflammatory Aneurysm (Aortitis), Including Infection of the Aorta

The microscopic presence of chronic inflammatory cells, particularly lymphocytes, histiocytes, and plasma cells, in association with intimal fibrosis, medial degeneration, and adventitial fibrosis, is suggestive of aortitis (Fig. 3–7). These findings should be assessed in conjunction with the macroscopic clinical observations of a thickened white or pearl gray aortic wall. Of importance is whether the patient has undergone a previous operation on or in the vicinity of the aorta and whether the aorta is possibly infected. Classically, the findings of syphilitic aortitis are characteristic. Plasma cells and lymphocytes occur in the adventitia, particularly surrounding the vasa vasorum. Perivascular inflammation and endarteritis of the vasa vasorum are typical. On histologic examination, a gumma may be identified but it is extremely unusual to identify *Treponema palladum* organisms, and some pathologists believe bacteria are never found. In patients with evidence of an inflammatory etiology, intimal hyperplasia is frequently noted.

More rarely, chronic tuberculous infiltration of the aorta can cause a type of aortitis that is often difficult to differentiate from other forms of aortitis.[10] Giant cells are observed, as in certain forms of aortitis; in addition, caseation may be

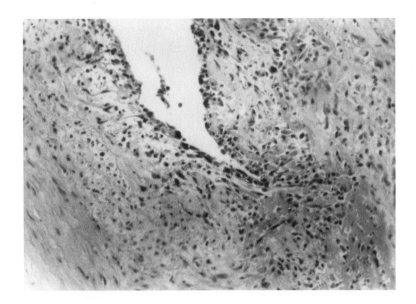

FIGURE 3–6   Aortic dissection showing false channel lined by endothelium. Scattered nonspecific inflammatory cells suggest an organizing lesion. H&E stain 100×.

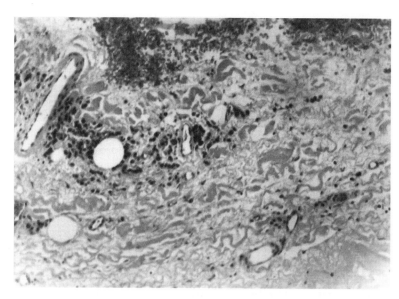

FIGURE 3–7 Aortitis with dense inflammation of the adventitial layer. Note inflammation centered near vasa vasorum. Tissue planes appear obliterated. H&E stain 100×.

found. The tuberculous bacillus or a cell-mediated hypersensitivity to the antigen may play a role. When there is invasion of the aortic wall by tuberculous bacilli, acid-fast bacilli in association with the Langhans giant cells may be detected. Evidence of old or active tuberculosis should be sought on the chest radiograph. A strongly positive Mantoux skin test is characteristic. An elevated erythrocyte sedimentation rate is further evidence of a tuberculous infection.[10] In endemic areas, this form of inflammatory aneurysm is often seen in the descending thoracic or abdominal aorta and tends to be characterized by a particularly thick-walled aorta, but often without evidence of a tuberculous bacterial infection. Spread to the aorta can be directly from surrounding structures such as the lungs or vertebrae (Pott's disease of the spine). Nonetheless, for most patients the seeding either appears to be hematogenous or there is no evidence of bacterial infection. Clearly demarcated areas of involvement of the aorta are common. Periaortic fibrosis and inflammation occurs at the involved segments. Macroscopically, granulomas of the aorta with caseation may also be present.[11]

Noninflammatory Fibroplasia

Noninflammatory arterial fibroplasia, which is more commonly associated with aortic branch artery stenoses rather than with aortic aneurysms, has been classified into four subgroups by Stanley and colleagues.[12] These include intimal fibroplasia, medial fibroplasia, medial hyperplasia, and perimedial dysplasia.

ETIOLOGY

The etiology of degenerative aneurysms is multifactorial, and a few studies have identified those factors that are associated with the development of degenerative aneurysms in certain groups of patients. Nevertheless, for the majority of

cases, the cause remains unknown. Some of the clinical parameters that are statistically associated with aneurysm formation include genetic inheritance such as Marfan syndrome, infectious agents, hypertension, increasing age, and smoking history. Cocaine abuse has also been associated with the cause of both aneurysm formation and aortic dissection.[13, 14]

Genetic Inheritance

Familial clustering of aortic dissection was noted in 1951 by Griffiths and colleagues,[15] although it was not until 1977 that Clifton[16] reported on the family grouping of degenerative aneurysms of the abdominal aorta. A strong family history has been reported in 11% to 15% of patients with abdominal aortic aneurysms.[17, 18] Furthermore, 15% of patients have first-degree relatives with abdominal aortic aneurysms.[19] Familial clustering has been documented by several authors.[16, 17, 20-25] One report demonstrated that identical (monozygotic) twins were particularly prone to both being affected.[20] Adoki and Stoodley[26] reported a familial syndrome of glaucoma, deafness, or both associated with the development of abdominal aortic aneurysms. In their study of 10 siblings from the same kindred, five had confirmed development of abdominal aortic aneurysms. Also, autoimmune or collagen vascular diseases such as rheumatoid arthritis have been implicated in formation of aortic aneurysm and thus may occur in some family pedigrees. Calcification of the ascending aorta has also been reported to develop in families in association with abnormal levels of globulins and T lymphocyte ratios.[27]

Tilson and Seashore[24] have suggested an autosomal dominant or X-linked pattern of inheritance for aneurysm formation in certain families they studied. From the analysis of 91 families, Majumber and colleagues[18] concluded that the mode of inheritance was determined by a recessive gene at an autosomal diallelic major locus. Powell and Greenhalgh,[23] using a multifactorial model, estimated the heritability of aneurysms to be 70%. An abnormal type III procollagen

(COL3A1) has been found in some patients with familial aortic aneurysms associated with a single base mutation in the gene for type III procollagen.[28] Abnormalities of type III collagen in familial aneurysm have also been reported by Greenhalgh's group.[29, 11]

In conclusion, it appears that several gene defects are associated with the formation of aortic aneurysms. Marfan syndrome, for example, is caused by a defective mutation in the fibrillin gene on chromosome 15 and has a dominant inheritance. Other defective genes are possibly X-linked, whereas others are autosomal recessives.

Biochemical Factors

The biochemical etiology of aneurysmal disease has been extensively studied by Tilson,[30] Zairns and associates,[31-33] and Greenhalgh and Powell.[34-36] From their thorough research and that of other investigators, it would appear that central to the causative mechanism of aneurysm formation is the excessive presence of elastase, an enzyme possibly released from activated white cells but more likely produced from other sources.[37] It is now further accepted that elastase results in the destruction of the elastic fiber lamellae in the aorta.[38] This, in turn, results in a nonelastic and noncompliant aorta that dilates. To further support the theory that destruction of elastin, either by abnormal elastase activity or by other causes, is central to the development of many aneurysms, much research has been conducted. Baxter and colleagues[38] compared the elastin content of the abdominal aorta in patients with and without abdominal aneurysms. They found that the amount of insoluble elastin was markedly decreased in patients with aneurysms (1.3% versus 12%, $p < 0.001$). They did not, however, find that cross-linking was deficient or that elastin mRNA was lowered: this suggests that gene expression is retained in aneurysms and that the loss of elastin is due to other factors. This same group of investigators have reported that although mRNA is not altered, there is enhanced COL I gene expression that may account for the increased levels of collagen.[39] A marked accumulation of a high polar amino acid that was not elastin was measured and was apparently of a composition consistent with a microfibrillar protein.[38] Experiments in rats have shown that perfusion of the aorta with elastase or activated macrophages or plasmin chemically induces aneurysms by destroying elastin.[11, 40] Interestingly, increased levels of serum elastase continue to be present in patients after abdominal aortic aneurysm repairs, in contrast to patients with aortic occlusive disease.[41] Abnormal elastin synthesis, fibers, and destruction are well known in Marfan syndrome and will be discussed in Chapter 5. Other than the role of an elastase, Busuttil and associates[42] have noted that in infrarenal aneurysms there are decreased levels of collagen in the aortic wall, whereas levels of collagenase are increased. Levels of collagenase appear to be particularly increased in patients with ruptured aneurysms.[29] Rizzo and colleagues,[43] however, did not find reduced levels of type III collagen in patients with aneurysms,

although ruptured aneurysms exhibited a higher level of collagenase activity.

Minion and colleagues[44] examined the influence of an extract of aortic aneurysms on smooth muscle cells in culture. They hypothesized that, because procollagen gene expression and synthesis are increased in abdominal aortic aneurysms, there may be a factor that modulates gene function. Of the six types of collagen present in the abdominal aorta, most are type 1. Type 1 collagen is made up of a triple helix with two 1δ (I) procollagen units. Both collagen and the procollagen levels are increased in abdominal aortic aneurysms, including gene expression for 1δ (I) procollagen, suggesting that the gene and collagen are possible factors in the causation of aneurysms.[38, 39] The structural collagen proteins are synthesized by smooth muscle cells in the media and are regulated by transforming growth factor β (TGF-β1).[38, 39, 44] In addition, inflammatory cell cytokines from the aorta can modulate smooth muscle cell synthesis.[38, 39, 44] Minion and colleagues[44] tested whether aortic wall extract could modulate cultured smooth muscle activity. By analyzing mRNA and 1δ (I) procollagen levels, they found that factors from the abdominal aortic aneurysms but not from atherosclerotic diseased aortas increased smooth muscle gene expression and synthesis.

The proposed sequence of events appears to be that the elastase destroys the elastin fibers, collagen replaces elastin during the formation of aneurysms, and collagenase weakens the collagenase fibers prior to aortic rupture. The source of the proteases (elastase and collagenase) is unclear.

Other factors have been postulated. Cannon and Read[45] have reported increased serum levels of elastolytic activity and decreased antiproteolytic activity, which may be related to decreased levels of alpha-$_1$-antitrypsin.[46] Cell-mediated immunity, especially in inflammatory aneurysms[47] and immunoglobins, may play a role.[48] Of interest, according to a study of dog aortas, farther away from the aortic valve elastin content appears to be less and the fenestrations observed in the internal elastic laminae are larger.[11, 49]

The evidence that bacterial infections may trigger the onset of medial degeneration and atherosclerosis of the aorta, resulting in aneurysmal formation, is still tenuous, although it is well documented that certain chronic bacterial infections such as syphilis and tuberculosis can result in aneurysms of the inflammatory aortitis type. More recently, however, a high correlation has been reported between increasing levels of the circulating autoantibody to hsp65 and the development of carotid artery plaques.[50] The hsp65 protein is one of the heat-shock proteins produced by injury due to heat, oxygen free radicals, and cytokines. It is not unique to humans and, of interest, it is also produced by bacteria. In fact, in tests for hsp65 antibodies, *Mycobacterium tuberculosis* is used for the synthesis of the reagent. Antibodies to hsp65 have been found in autoimmune and inflammatory diseases such as rheumatoid arthritis, systemic lupus erythematosus, diabetes, and atherosclerosis, all of which are also associated with aneurysm formation. It may be that after exposure to bacterial antigens, antibodies cross-react with human homologues, resulting in atherosclerosis and aneurysm formation. Of further interest is the finding that Kawasaki disease is associated with the toxic shock syndrome *Staphylococcus aureus* bacterium, and the subsequent development of coronary artery aneurysms and, rarely, aortic aneurysms.[51]

Clinical Syndromes and Diseases Associated with Aneurysms

Syndromes associated with aneurysmal disease but not with an inflammatory process (aortitis) include Marfan syndrome, Ehlers-Danlos syndrome, pseudoxanthoma elasticum (autosomal recessive elastin defect), homocystinuria, Erdheim's syndrome (annuloaortic ectasia), Noonan's syndrome, Klippel-Feil syndrome, fragile X syndrome, familial hemorrhagic telangiectasia, hereditary polycystic kidney disease, and Turner's syndrome. We have had a few patients with both osteogenesis imperfecta and cardiovascular disease, but this may be coincidental.

We have also seen patients in whom aortitis is related to either the collagen vascular or autoimmune type of diseases. Those conditions that are considered to be associated with aortic aneurysm formation include Takayasu's disease (nonspecific aortoarteritis), giant cell arteritis (Horton's disease), temporal arteritis, Behçet's disease, relapsing polychondritis, thromboangiitis obliterans, periarteritis nodosa, systemic lupus erythematosus, scleroderma, Kawasaki's disease, rheumatoid arthritis, juvenile rheumatoid arthritis, Reiter's syndrome, Sjögren's syndrome, polymyalgia rheumatica, ankylosing spondylitis, Paget's disease, osteoarthritis of unknown origin, ulcerative colitis, and autoimmune disease of the thyroid such as Reidel's struma and Hashimoto's thyroiditis. Although some of these associations may be incidental, it is of interest that the aortic tissue in these patients usually shows evidence of chronic inflammation.[11]

INCIDENCE OF AORTIC ANEURYSMS

Mortality

Aortic aneurysms are the thirteenth most common cause of death in the United States.[18] In Great Britain, ruptured abdominal aortic aneurysms account for 1.3% of all deaths (not including aortic dissection).[52] Approximately 0.6% of all women and 1.2% of all men die of aortic aneurysms (National Center for Health Statistics, 1987). In older age groups, rupture of aneurysms becomes a more common cause of death. Of the patients who die of ruptured abdominal aortic aneurysms, 83% are over the age of 65 years.[53] Infrarenal aneurysm rupture is the most common cause of death among patients with aneurysms. In about 80% of patients who die of an abdominal or thoracic aneurysm, death has been attributed to aortic rupture.[54]

It should be recognized, however, that aortic dissection is considered by others and ourselves to be a more common cause of death than infrarenal aneurysm rupture.[8] The reason is discussed below. This observation is further supported by Waller and colleagues.[55] In their study of forensic autopsies after sudden deaths, they found that 22.3% of the deaths were due to cardiac disease and 0.45% were due to aortic disease, with the ratio of aortic dissection to ruptured aortic aneurysm being 8:1. Nevertheless, abdominal aortic ruptures may have been less likely than aortic dissection to cause sudden death. From the analysis by Lilienfeld and colleagues[54] of deaths reported in the United States, using the international classification of diseases, the incidence of death in white males for abdominal aortic aneurysms for 1981 was 5/100,000 per year; unspecified aneurysms, 2/100,000 per year; dissecting aneurysms, 1.5/100,000 per year (a figure that does not necessarily include all patients with aortic dissection); and thoracic aneurysms, 0.7/100,000 per year, for a total of 9.2/100,000 per year. As many as 35% of deaths due to aortic dissection are not diagnosed before death but are discovered only at the time of autopsy, which may account for some of the apparent discrepancies reported with regard to the incidence of deaths due to aortic dissection.[56] Similarly, it is our impression that more cases of aortic dissection are increasingly being diagnosed by the newer imaging techniques (CT, MRI, TEE) and thus are being successfully treated surgically, with the result that fewer patients are dying of aortic dissection. This could account for the apparent decline in reported deaths due to aortic dissection as documented by Lilienfeld and colleagues.[54] A further factor may be that because hypertension is being diagnosed earlier and treated more aggressively, the risk of hypertension causing aortic dissection has declined. In contrast, the incidence of thoracic aortic aneurysms not due to aortic dissection has not lessened, suggesting that hypertension is not likely to be a major causative factor in the formation of thoracic aneurysms, which would parallel our clinical impressions.[54]

In addition to deaths caused by rupture of aortic aneurysms and aortic dissection, another large group of deaths due to aortic disease involve blunt trauma. In an autopsy study of 530 persons killed in motor vehicle accidents, 90 of the injuries were associated with rupture of the aorta (17%).[57] The incidence of death from other causes, such as congenital coarctation of the aorta, infections, and penetrating trauma, is less but is not known.

Incidence of Thoracic Aortic Aneurysms

Very little is known about the true extent of occurrence of thoracic aortic aneurysms in any particular population. It is clear that these aneurysms occur more commonly in older population groups in Western countries, but how frequently is difficult to determine. Bickerstaff and colleagues[58] found the prevalence of thoracic aortic aneurysms in Rochester, Minnesota, to be 5.9/100,000 per year on the basis of the 72 residents who were found to have aneurysms. Thirty-seven (51%) involved the ascending aorta, 8 (11%) the aortic arch, and 27 (38%) the descending thoracic aorta. The cause was aortic dissection in 53%; "atherosclerosis" (medial degenerative disease) in 29%; aortitis in 8%; "cystic medial necrosis" (medial necrosis) in 6%; and syphilis in 4%. Twenty-five percent of the patients had a concomitant infrarenal abdominal aortic aneurysm, an incidence similar to the 28% noted by Pressler and McNamara.[59] In a review of 1510 patients with aortic aneurysms, Crawford and Cohen[60] found that 12.6% had multisegmental aortic disease. The most common combination consisted of descending thoracic and associated infrarenal aneurysms (44%). This finding led to the recommendation that the entire aorta should be evaluated by aortography or computerized tomography.[11]

Bickerstaff and colleagues[58] reported an equal gender distribution of thoracic aortic aneurysms. Their report is in marked contrast to that by DeBakey and Noon,[61] who found among patients referred for surgery that males with thoracic aortic aneurysms were nine times as frequent. In our own series of patients with repairs of the ascending aorta or aortic arch or both,[62] aortic dissection,[5] and descending thoracic or thoracoabdominal aneurysms, males outnumbered females by approximately 2:1.[6, 11, 63]

Prevalence of Abdominal Aortic Aneurysms

Bickerstaff and associates[64] found the incidence of abdominal aortic aneurysms in Rochester, Minnesota, to be 21/100,000 people per year. For the period from 1971 to 1980, the occurrence was 36.5/100,000 people per year. Seventy-eight percent of the patients had asymptomatic aneurysms that were found incidentally or had minimal symptoms, whereas 12% had ruptured aneurysms. Likewise, the increasing incidence of infrarenal aneurysms would also suggest that hypertension is not a major etiological factor;[54] this, coupled with the apparent increase in younger patients dying of infrarenal abdominal aortic aneurysms, makes it interesting to speculate whether a new etiological factor has recently evolved in the formation of abdominal aneurysms. The prevalence of infrarenal aneurysms appears to be increasing in both the United States and the United Kingdom[54, 65] concurrent with the increasing age of the populations. Furthermore, there may be an increasing incidence of younger patients with aneurysms.

Operative Procedures

Although it appears that the ratio of thoracic aneurysms to abdominal aortic aneurysms is approximately 1:3, the number of persons with thoracic aneurysms who undergo operative repair is probably considerably less and more likely is 1:10.[54, 66] The exact number of aortic operations performed each year is not known, but it approximates 80,000 to 100,000. This estimate is based on 35,000 infrarenal aortic aneurysm resections performed annually, 35,000 aortobifemoral bypasses for occlusive disease,[66] and about 10,000 thoracic operations. In addition, repairs are performed for other conditions such as traumatic injuries and the coarctation of the aorta. Coarctation of the aorta occurs in 50/100,000 live births; of these, 40 are isolated coarctations of the aorta, and most are repaired during infancy by either dilatation or operation.

ULTRASOUND DIAGNOSIS

Abdominal Aneurysm

Ultrasound screening for abdominal aortic aneurysms has become usual, particularly in Europe, but the question of when an aneurysm is present remains to be fully answered. When one is dealing with normal parameters for the human body, it is generally accepted that a measurement beyond the range of plus or minus 2 standard deviations (2 SD) is abnormal.

Problems with ultrasound screening are the interobserver variation in the estimation of size, magnification errors and inaccurate size estimation if a different plane is used, and even the finding of an aneurysm that is apparently getting smaller because of an overestimation of size on initial examinations.[67, 68] Nevertheless, patients with "aneurysms" of 3.5 to 3.9 cm are reported to have growth rates of about 0.29 cm per year and 6-month screenings by ultrasound appear to be safe.[69]

To determine the normal range of the diameter of the infrarenal aorta, Lucarotti and colleagues[52] used ultrasonography to examine 1748 men over the age of 65 years. They found that the aortic diameters were less than 2.5 cm in 88% of the population, between 2.6 and 4 cm in 10%, and greater than 4 cm in 1.5% of the population. The mean aortic diameter was 2.1 cm with an SD of 0.55 cm. Thus, on average, 97.5% (2 SD) of men older than 65 years will have an aorta less than 3.3 cm in diameter, whereas those with aortas larger than 3.3 cm should be suspected of having aortic aneurysms. In a study of younger patients with peripheral vascular disease, Pedersen and colleagues[70] found the mean size to be 1.69 cm for men and 1.5 cm for women aged 50 years to 89 years, with respective 2 SD sizes of 2.66 cm and 2.36 cm. They found aortic size correlated with age and gender on multivariate analysis but not with body weight and height. Aortic expansion with systole also decreased with increasing age. Of interest, as systolic expansion decreases with age in the ascending aorta the velocity of blood flow increases.[71]

Infrarenal Aortic Aneurysms

While the population ages further, the incidence of infrarenal aneurysms has increased to the extent that aneurysms are expected to develop in approximately 3% of patients older than 50 years of age.[72-74] Several authors[68, 74-77] have advocated ultrasound screening as being cost-effective in patients at risk. Among elderly men, 83% of the patients who suffer ruptured abdominal aortic aneurysms are over

65 years of age;[53] patients with peripheral vascular disease or those with hypertension are particularly likely to have abdominal aortic aneurysms.[68, 73, 75-77] Hypercholesterolemia may also be a factor in the development of aortic disease of the aorta.[78] In the Oxford study, 426 men between the ages of 65 and 75 years were screened by ultrasound and 23 (5%) were found to have abdominal aortic aneurysms; of these, 10 had aneurysms larger than 4 cm.[11, 76] It should be noted, however, that 50% of patients with abdominal aortic aneurysms are not in the high-risk group of patients who have hypertension or have been smokers.[52, 79]

ULTRASOUND MONITORING, EXPANSION RATE, AND SURVIVAL

Imakita and colleagues[80] found that the expansion rate for abdominal aortic aneurysms was 0.28 cm/y. A similar growth rate for abdominal aortic aneurysms was confirmed in a study by Bengtsson and colleagues,[81] who found that the expansion rate was 0.08 cm/y for aneurysms less than 4 cm and 0.33 cm/y for those larger than 4 cm. They concluded that aneurysms less than 4 cm in diameter have a low risk of rupture, inasmuch as none of their patients with small aneurysms died of rupture, although the mortality rate in this group of patients was higher than in the normal population because of concurrent disease, particularly coronary artery disease. Only 60% of patients were 5-year survivors. This finding is similar to our own results with infrarenal aneurysm repairs[82] and also with other segment repairs.[1-3, 6, 62, 63, 83-85] The normal rate of increase in size of the aorta with age has been reported to be 0.005 to 0.008 cm/y.[70]

Nevitt and colleagues[68] claimed that in their population-based study aneurysms less than 5 cm in diameter did not rupture. It is apparent from their study, however, that one fourth of their patients underwent operations, suggesting that at least some of the aneurysms became symptomatic and required operation. In a study of 8944 ultrasound-scanned patients in West Sussex, England, Scott and colleagues[86] detected that 4% of the population had aneurysms defined as 3 cm or greater. They followed up all patients with aneurysms smaller than 6 cm with regular scanning, and if the aorta either grew greater than 6 cm, expanded more than 1 cm a year, or became symptomatic, the patients were scheduled for operation. Most patients (43.7%) were observed for up to 3 years, and 13.3% were observed for 5 years. Of the 232 patients with aneurysms that did not meet the criteria for operation, 0.4% died of rupture. It should be noted that during a 10-year period, 14% of the patients who underwent surgery for aortic rupture had aneurysms less than 6 cm. Of interest, Cronenwett and colleagues[87] were unable to show a correlation between expansion rate and rupture, possibly because growth rates may vary from year to year or even be quiescent, but they did find that 15% of aneurysms less than 6 cm eventually ruptured.[88] Bernstein and colleagues[89, 90] reported an expansion rate of 0.5 cm/y

as a useful criterion for operation. Moreover, Geroulakis and Nicolaides[91] have calculated that the risk of rupture for aneurysms greater than 5 cm is 8%/y and 25% to 49% for a patient's lifetime. Although small aneurysms can be safely watched from the standpoint of rupture, Hallett and colleagues[92] in Minnesota examined the outcome of patients with small aneurysms less than 5 cm in size. One third of the patients underwent surgery because of the aneurysms' being present (49%), expansion on follow-up (28%), symptoms (18%), and patient anxiety in 5%, with an operative mortality rate of 2.6%. As is the case in many reported series of patients, including our own, operated on for aneurysms irrespective of site,[1-3, 6, 62, 63, 83-85] the survival rate in this study was only 62% at 5 years, the same as in Bengtsson's series of patients treated nonoperatively by follow-up. Similarly, most of the deaths were due to coronary artery disease. Hallett and colleagues therefore question whether early operation for small abdominal aortic aneurysms will enhance survival.

Currently, at least three prospective randomized studies are in progress, treating patients either surgically or with close follow-up for small aneurysms. Even if these studies should show no difference in survival according to whether or not small aneurysms are operated on, there are two caveats that should be borne in mind. First, aneurysms tend to increase in size over time and, even if there is no difference in early survival at 5 years, there may well be at 10 or 20 years, because the older the patient is at the time of operation, the greater the risk of death. Second, because an aneurysm should be considered a marker of coronary artery disease and because patients are screened more carefully before operations for coronary artery disease, a greater number of such patients will probably be treated for their coronary artery disease. This will result in an improved long-term survival, not only because of the reduced risk of abdominal aortic rupture but also because of a reduced risk of death due to myocardial infarction from coronary artery disease. Hertzer and colleagues[93-96] noted that the survival rate improved from 72% to 78% at 5 years with revascularization, although this is still lower than the 84% survival rate for patients with no coronary artery disease.

The low cost of the ultrasound examination allows regular screenings of at-risk patient populations and permits the follow-up of patients with small aneurysms. The patients probably should also be tested for coronary artery disease to justify conservative management, since coronary artery disease is a more likely cause of death than aneurysm rupture in this group of patients.[11]

MONITORING OF THE THORACIC AORTA

Although the abdominal aorta can be studied with ultrasound, the thoracic aorta cannot be easily and cheaply screened for aneurysms. For accurate screening, either CT, TEE, or MRI is required, although chest radiographs will show aneurysmal disease. In one of the few studies we are aware of concerning thoracic aneurysms,[80] the growth rate was reported to be 0.42 cm/y; for aortic arch aneurysms, it was 0.56 cm/y, even when growth rate was corrected for initial size of the aorta. This latter study suggests that thoracic aneurysms may be at greater risk of rupture because of the greater growth rate.

RISK OF ANEURYSM RUPTURE AND WHEN TO OPERATE

Modern aortic operations are mostly prophylactic; sometimes they are therapeutic, and they should rarely be palliative. The reason for the prophylactic operations is that they may prevent rupture of aneurysms that cause death. As Darling and associates[97] succinctly stated, "The natural history of an abdominal aortic aneurysm terminates in its rupture unless the host dies from other causes." To this statement may be added that rupture is the course for all types of aneurysm, regardless of aortic site or cause. The decision as to when a patient should undergo prophylactic operation to prevent rupture is dependent on the risk of rupture causing death versus the risk of other comorbid conditions. If the patient has symptoms or signs related to the aneurysm, then surgery is justified on the basis that it is therapeutic, especially since the risk of rupture (if it has not already occurred) is high. Palliative operations, such as aneurysm exclusion with bypass, have few indications in the modern era.

Thus it is of paramount importance to know the risk of rupture according to size, cause, and segment involved. Unfortunately, the assessment of this risk must be made with reference to the limited number of historical studies in which patients did not benefit from aortic operations or cardiovascular medications such as beta-blockers. A prospective randomized study cannot be justified on ethical grounds, with the possible exception of small infrarenal aneurysms in elderly patients without symptoms.

ABDOMINAL ANEURYSMS AND THE RISK OF DEATH

In 1950, Estes[98] reviewed the course of 102 patients with abdominal aortic aneurysms seen at the Mayo Clinic. Of the patients, 97 had atherosclerotic aneurysms and the remainder had either syphilis ($n = 4$), or a history of trauma ($n = 1$), or both. In one patient the aneurysm was wrapped with cellophane, and one underwent an attempted ligation of the neck with fascia lata. The survival rate was 50% at 3 years, 19% at 5 years, and 10% at 8 years. None of the patients survived as long as 10 years. Rupture of the aortic aneurysm was the cause of death in 63% of the patients.

Darling and associates[97] found, in an autopsy study of deceased patients with abdominal aortic aneurysms, that 29.4% had died of rupture of the aneurysm. In patients with untreated infrarenal aneurysm, the incidence of death due to rupture of the aneurysm has been reported to be between 30% and 63%.[97, 98] Szilagyi and colleagues[99] published an actuarial survival rate of 19% for untreated infrarenal abdominal aortic aneurysms, with the most common cause of death being rupture. Darling and associates[97] studied 473 patients who apparently had died with intact infrarenal abdominal aortic aneurysms. In the group of aneurysms measuring 4 to 7 cm, 25% had ruptured and caused death (4 to 5 cm, 23.4%; 5 to 7 cm, 25.3%). Among patients with aneurysms between 7 and 10 cm, 45.6% died of aneurysm rupture; among those with aneurysms larger than 10 cm, 60.5% had died of rupture. Of interest, of the patients who had aneurysms measuring 4 cm or less, 9.5% had died of rupture, confirming that even small aneurysms can rupture but at a lower rate. Among the 102 patients with rupture, the majority of the ruptures occurred posterolaterally into the retroperitoneum (65%, 66/102) with a total of 84 (82%) being retroperitoneal. Of the 52 patients who were known to have aneurysms before death, the majority died of aortic rupture. Of interest, in 12% of our patients with thoracic aortic rupture associated with aortic dissection who survived long enough to have an operation, the aorta was less than 5 cm in diameter.[5] In a population-based study of thoracic aneurysms, Pressler and McNamara[100] found that the aorta ruptured in 44% of patients with "atherosclerotic" aneurysms.[11]

THORACIC AND THORACOABDOMINAL ANEURYSMS AND RISK OF DEATH

Bickerstaff and colleagues[58] reported that rupture occurred in 74% of patients with thoracic aneurysms (95% for aortic dissection, 51% for nondissecting aneurysms), of whom 94% died of aortic rupture. Eleven percent of their patients underwent surgery with a 40% mortality rate.[58] The overall 5-year survival after diagnosis was 13% (7% for patients with aortic dissection, 19.2% for patients without dissection) compared with a matched expected survival rate of 75%. Those patients who did not have elective surgery had a 3-year survival rate of 25.7%.

In 94 patients who did not undergo thoracoabdominal aortic aneurysm repairs because of associated disease, age, small size of aneurysm, more urgent procedures, or refusal to have surgery, Crawford and DeNatale[101] found, by Kaplan–Meier analysis, that only 24% were 2-year survivors. Half of the deaths occurred because of rupture.

CLINICAL PRESENTATION

Approximately 75% of aneurysms are asymptomatic and are detected incidentally by physicians, either during routine physical examination or on chest radiographs or ultrasonography. In the past, when aneurysms were not as aggressively searched for, the incidence of asymptomatic aneurysms was 30%.[97] In the patients with symptomatic aneurysms, there are certain signs and symptoms that should alert the physician. In patients with medial degenerative aneurysms of the ascending aorta or aortic arch, manifestations may include heart failure, myocardial infarction, rupture, cardiac tamponade, right-sided heart failure, superior vena cava syndrome, arrhythmias, murmurs, fever, brain ischemia or neurological events, seizures, stroke, vertebrobasilar symptoms, nonischemic atypical chest pain, backache, shortness of breath, wheezing, dysphagia, hoarseness, aspiration, hemoptysis, chest fullness, palpitations, neck fullness, and less frequent signs such as erosion of the sternum with presentation as a pulsatile chest mass similar to that observed in classic syphilis. In addition to any of these indications, those patients with descending thoracic aortic aneurysms may show other signs that include right or left chest pain, pleuritic chest pain, paraplegia or paraparesis, renal failure, and shoulder pain, the latter probably arising from irritation of the diaphragm. Abdominal aneurysms typically cause symptoms related to tenderness or backache. Pain may also occur in the flank, abdomen, shoulder, or groin. Less frequent manifestations are an abdominal mass, nausea, vomiting, gastric retention, weight loss, hematemesis, melena, jaundice associated with fever in patients with chronic rupture, renal failure, abdominal angina, urinary frequency, leg weakness, leg pain, inferior vena cava obstruction, and abdominal distention. Distal embolization of aneurysmal thrombus is not uncommon, nor is the presentation of "blue toes" as a result of distal embolization. A ruptured aneurysm may have manifestations typical of acute cholecystitis, as in the case of Einstein (Einstein sign).[102] The symptoms, particularly those observed with rupture, may also be similar to those observed with a ureteric stone. Flank pain due to ureteric obstruction with resultant hydronephrosis or nephritis may also occur with inflammatory aneurysms.

Points to remember on clinical examination include placement of the patient in a relaxed position on a flat surface and palpation of the aorta between the tips of the fingers with both hands; one should also remember that displacement of the aortic impulse to below the umbilicus suggests downward displacement of the aortic bifurcation by an aortic aneurysm. However, palpation of the lateral expansile sides of the aneurysm is dependent on the patients' habitus and should be taken into account during examination for a suspected aneurysm. The examiner should listen for abdominal thrills and bruits.

The manifestations of aneurysms can be variable; therefore we grade symptoms into groups according to severity. This grading also has an important value in predicting the risks of postoperative death, paraplegia, and renal failure in patients with thoracic aortic aneurysms.[4, 5, 62, 103] Thus patients with no symptoms are designated grade I; those with mild symptoms, grade II; patients with severe pain are classified as grade III; and those patients in extremis with one or more life-threatening signs such as shock, renal failure, paraplegia, strokes, rupture, and acute dissection are in grade IV.[11]

INDICATIONS FOR SURGERY

Controversy exists concerning when aortic surgery is appropriate in patients who have no symptoms.

Thoracic Aneurysms

Among patients with thoracic aneurysms, we advise that repair should be considered in healthy symptom-free young patients with aortic dilation exceeding twice the size of a normal aorta or with aneurysms greater than 5 cm in diameter. This is based on the lower mortality rate we have observed in patients with asymptomatic aneurysms exceeding 5 cm who undergo thoracic aorta repairs (less than 2% mortality)[104] and on the incidence of rupture in patients with aneurysms exceeding 5 cm.[5, 105] Nonetheless, 12% of our patients with rupture of the thoracic aorta, including dissection, have had aortic aneurysms less than 5 cm.[4, 5] Thus in patients with Marfan syndrome an asymptomatic aneurysm of more than 4.7 to 5 cm is considered appropriate for surgery.[103] In Marfan patients operative survival is currently 99% or better.[105]

Abdominal Aneurysms

We recommend that patients who have asymptomatic abdominal aortic aneurysms twice the normal size or aneurysms exceeding 4 cm also should undergo operative repair if they are otherwise healthy.[106, 107] Treiman and colleagues[108] reported that in 73 patients with abdominal aortic aneurysms, 37% of aneurysms less than 4 cm required elective resection and 2% ruptured. In the 30 patients with aneurysms measuring 4 to 4.9 cm, 40% of the aneurysms were resected and 10% ruptured within 3 to 6.5 years. Treiman and colleagues advised that all asymptomatic aneurysms larger than 4 cm should be surgically repaired, which is in agreement with guidelines published by the Society for Vascular Surgery and the North American Chapter of the International Society for Cardiovascular Surgery.[109] Accepted indications include size twice that of the normal aorta, size greater than 4 cm if the patients are young and fit, associated symptoms, documented increase in size, pressure or erosion into surrounding structures, infection, inflammation, distal embolization, occlusion, and saccular shape. The decision of whether to carefully observe patients with small aneurysms between 4 and 5 cm or to operate on them may be better defined by the prospective randomized studies being conducted.

Preoperative Evaluation

Studies performed before aortic surgery include blood tests (complete blood count, electrolytes, blood urea nitrogen, creatinine, liver function, total protein and albumin, glucose, clotting profile [platelets, prothrombin time, partial thromboplastin time, fibrinogen, erythrocyte sedimentation rate]), urinalysis, ECG, posteroanterior and lateral chest radiographs, noninvasive carotid studies, and cardiac function tests when deemed appropriate (thallium scans, echocardiograms, Holter monitoring, and cardiac catheterization). These latter tests are discussed elsewhere.

REFERENCES

1. Svensson LG, Crawford ES, Hess KR, et al. Composite valve graft replacement of the proximal aorta: comparison of techniques in 348 patients. Ann Thorac Surg 1992;54:427-39.
2. Crawford ES, Beckett WC, Greer MS. Juxtarenal infrarenal abdominal aortic aneurysm: special diagnostic and therapeutic considerations. Ann Surg 1986;203:661-70.
3. Crawford ES, Crawford JL, Safi HJ, et al. Thoracoabdominal aortic aneurysms: preoperative and intraoperative factors determining immediate and long-term results of operation in 605 patients. J Vasc Surg 1986;3:389-404.
4. Crawford ES, Svensson LG, Hess KR, et al. A prospective randomized study of cerebrospinal fluid drainage to prevent paraplegia after high-risk surgery on the thoracoabdominal aorta. J Vasc Surg 1991;13:36-45.
5. Svensson LG, Crawford ES, Hess KR, et al. Dissection of the aorta and dissecting aortic aneurysms: improving early and long-term surgical results. Circulation 1990;82(5 Supp):IV 24-38.
6. Svensson LG, Crawford ES, Hess KR, et al. Experience with 1509 patients undergoing thoracoabdominal aortic operations. J Vasc Surg 1993;17:357-70.
7. Svensson LG, Hess KR, Coselli JS, Safi HR. Influence of segmental arteries, extent, and atrio-femoral bypass on postoperative paraplegia after thoracoabdominal aortic aneurysm repairs. J Vasc Surg 1994: 20:255-62.
8. Svensson LG, Crawford ES. Aortic dissection and aortic aneurysm surgery: clinical observations, experimental investigations, and statistical analyses. Part II. Curr Probl Surg 1992;29:915-1057.
9. Trotter SE, Olsen EG. Marfan's disease and Erdheim's cystic medionecrosis: a study of their pathology. Eur Heart J 1991;12:83-7.
10. Costa M, Robbs JV. Abdominal aneurysms in a black population: clinico-pathological study. Br J Surg 1986;73:554-8.
11. Svensson LG, Crawford ES. Aortic dissection and aortic aneurysm surgery: clinical observations, experimental investigations, and statistical analyses. Part III. Curr Probl Surg 1993;30:1-172.
12. Stanley JC, Gewertz BC, Bove EL, et al. Arterial fibroplasia: histopathologic character and current etiologic concepts. Arch Surg 1975;110:561.
13. Bacharach JM, Colville DS, Lie JT. Accelerated atherosclerosis, aneurysmal disease, and aortitis: possible pathogenetic association with cocaine abuse. Int Angiol 1992;11:83-6.
14. Gadaleta D, Hall M-H, Nelson RL. Cocaine-induced acute aortic dissection. Chest 1989;96:1203-5.
15. Griffiths AJ, Hayhurst AP, Whitehead R. Dissecting aneurysm of the aorta in mother and child. Br Heart J 1951;13:364-8.
16. Clifton MA. Familial abdominal aortic aneurysm. Br J Surg 1977;64: 765-6.
17. Bengtsson H, Norrgard O, Angquist KA, et al. Ultrasonographic screening of the abdominal aorta among siblings of patients with abdominal aortic aneurysms. Br J Surg 1989;76:589-91.
18. Majumber PP, St Jean PL, Ferrell RE, et al. On the inheritance of abdominal aortic aneurysm. Am J Hum Genet 1991;48:164-70.
19. Webster MS, St Jean PL, Steed DL, et al. Abdominal aortic aneurysm: results of a family study. J Vasc Surg 1991;13:366-72.
20. Borkett JHJ, Stewart G, Chilvers AS. Abdominal aortic aneurysms in identical twins. J R Soc Med 1988;81:471-2.
21. Cole CW, Barber CG, Bouchard AG, et al. Abdominal aortic aneurysm: consequences of a positive family history. Can J Surg 1989;32:117-20.
22. Loosemore TM, Child AH, Dormandy JA. Familial abdominal aortic aneurysms. J R Soc Med 1988;81:472-3.
23. Powell JT, Greenhalgh RM. Multifactorial inheritance of abdominal aortic aneurysm. Eur J Vasc Surg 1987;1:29-31.
24. Tilson MD, Seashore MR. Fifty families with abdominal aortic aneurysms in two or more first-order relatives. Am J Surg 1984;147: 551-3.
25. Tilson MD, Roberts MP. Molecular diversity in the abdominal aortic aneurysm phenotype. Arch Surg 1988;123:1202-6.
26. Adoki II, Stoodley BJ. Abdominal aortic aneurysm, glaucoma and deafness: a new familial syndrome. Br J Surg 1992;79:637-8.
27. Tentolouris C, Kontozoglou T, Toutouzas P. Familial calcification of aorta and calcific aortic valve disease associated with immunologic abnormalities. Am Heart J 1993;126:904-9.
28. Kontusaari S, Tromp G, Kuivaniemi H, et al. A mutation in the gene for type III procollagen (COL3A1) in a family with aortic aneurysms. J Clin Invest 1990;86:1465-73.
29. Menashi S, Campa JS, Greenhalgh RM, Powell JT. Collagen in abdominal aortic aneurysm: typing, content, and degradation. J Vasc Surg 1987;6:578-82.
30. Tilson MD. Histochemistry of aortic elastin in patients with nonspecific abdominal aortic aneurysmal disease. Arch Surg 1988;123: 503-5.
31. Zarins CK, Zatina MA, Giddens DP, et al. Shear stress regulation of artery lumen diameter in experimental atherogenesis. J Vasc Surg 1987;5:413-20.
32. Zarins CK, Glagov S, Vesselinovitch D, Wissler RW. Aneurysm formation in experimental atherosclerosis: relationship to plaque evolution. J Vasc Surg 1990;12:246-56.
33. Zarins CK, Xu CP, Glagov S. Aneurysmal enlargement of the aorta during regression of experimental atherosclerosis. J Vasc Surg 1992; 15:90-8.
34. Powell JT, Muller BR, Greenhalgh RM. Acute phase proteins in patients with abdominal aortic aneurysms. J Cardiovasc Surg (Torino) 1987;28:528-30.
35. Powell JT, Greenhalgh RM. Cellular, enzymatic, and genetic factors in the pathogenesis of abdominal aortic aneurysms. J Vasc Surg 1989;9:297-304.
36. Powell JT, Adamson J, MacSweeney ST, et al. Genetic variants of collagen III and abdominal aortic aneurysm. Eur J Vasc Surg 1991;5:1458.
37. Campa JS, Greenhalgh RM, Powell JT. Elastin degradation in abdominal aortic aneurysms. Atherosclerosis 1987;65:13-21.
38. Baxter BT, McGee GS, Shively VP, et al. Elastin content, cross-links, and mRNA in normal and aneurysmal human aorta. J Vasc Surg 1992;16:192-200.
39. Mesh CL, Baxter BT, Pearce WH, et al. Collagen and elastin gene expression in aortic aneurysms. Surgery 1992;112:256-61.
40. Anidjar S, Salzmann JL, Gentric D, et al. Elastase-induced experimental aneurysms in rats. Circulation 1990;82:973-81.
41. Cohen JR, Faust G, Tenenbaum N, et al. The calcium messenger system and the kinetics of elastase release from human neutrophils in patients with abdominal aortic aneurysms. Ann Vasc Surg 1990; 4:570-4.
42. Busuttil RW, Cardenas A. Collagenase activity of the human aorta. Arch Surg 1980;115:1373-8.
43. Rizzo RJ, McCarthy WJ, Dixit SN, et al. Collagen types and matrix protein content in human abdominal aortic aneurysms. J Vasc Surg 1989;10:35-73.
44. Minion DJ, Wang Y, Lynch TG, et al. Soluble factors modulate changes in collagen gene expression in abdominal aortic aneurysms. Surgery 1993;114:252-7.
45. Cannon DJ, Read RC. Blood elastolytic activity in patients with aortic aneurysms. Ann Thorac Surg 1982;34:10-15.
46. Cohen JR, Mandell C, Margolis I, et al. Altered aortic protease and antiprotease activity in patients with ruptured abdominal aortic aneurysms. Surg Gynecol Obstet 1987;164:355-8.
47. Stella A, Gargiulo M, Pasquinelli G, et al. The cellular component in the parietal infiltrate of inflammatory abdominal aortic aneurysms (IAAA). Eur J Vasc Surg 1991;5:65-70.
48. Brophy CM, Reilly JM, Smith GJ, Tilson MD. The role of inflammation in nonspecific abdominal aortic aneurysm disease. Ann Vasc Surg 1991;5:229-33.
49. Song SH, Roach MR. Comparison of fenestrations in internal elastic laminae of canine thoracic and abdominal aortas. Blood Vessels 1984;21:90-7.
50. Hansson GK. Atherosclerosis: immunological markers of atherosclerosis. Lancet 1993;341:278-9.
51. Leung DYM, Meissner HC, Fulton DR, et al. Toxic shock syndrome toxin-secreting Staphyloccus aureus in Kawasaki syndrome. Lancet 1993;342:1385-8.
52. Lucarotti ME, Shaw E, Heather BP. Distribution of aortic diameter in a screened male population. Br J Surg 1992;79:641-2.
53. Amundsen S, Trippestad A, Viste A, Soreide O. Abdominal aortic aneurysms—a national multicenter study. Eur J Vasc Surg 1987;1: 239-43.
54. Lilienfeld DE, Gunderson PD, Sprafka JM, Vargas C. Epidemiology of

aortic aneurysms. I. Mortality trends in the United States, 1951 to 1981. Arteriosclerosis 1987;7:637–43.

55. Waller BF, Clark MA, et al. Cardiac pathology in 2007 consecutive forensic autopsies. Clin Cardiol 1992;15:760–5.

56. Jamieson WRE, Munro AI, Miyagishima RT, et al. Aortic dissections: early diagnosis and surgical management are the keys to survival. Can J Surg 1982;25:145–9.

57. Williams JS, Graff JA, Uku JM, Steinig JP. Aortic injury in vehicular trauma. Ann Thorac Surg 1994;57:726–30.

58. Bickerstaff LK, Pairolero PC, Hollier LH, et al. Thoracic aortic aneurysms: a population-based study. Surgery 1982;92:1103–9.

59. Pressler V, McNamara JJ. Aneurysm of the thoracic aorta: review of 260 cases. J Thorac Cardiovasc Surg 1985;89:50–4.

60. Crawford ES, Cohen ES. Aortic aneurysm: a multifocal disease. Arch Surg 1982;117:1393–400.

61. DeBakey M, Noon G. Aneurysms of the thoracic aorta. Mod Concepts Cardiovasc Dis 1975;44:53–8.

62. Crawford ES, Svensson LG, Coselli JS, et al. Surgical treatment of aneurysm and/or dissection of the ascending aorta, transverse aortic arch, and ascending aorta and transverse aortic arch: factors influencing survival in 717 patients. J Thorac Cardiovasc Surg 1989;98:659–73.

63. Svensson LG, Crawford ES, Hess KR, et al. Thoracoabdominal aortic aneurysms associated with celiac, superior mesenteric and renal artery occlusive disease: methods and analysis of results in 271 patients. J Vasc Surg 1992;16:378–90.

64. Bickerstaff LK, Hollier LH, Van Peenen H. et al. Abdominal aortic aneurysms: the changing natural history. J Vasc Surg 1984;1:6–12.

65. Fowkes FG, Macintyre CC, Ruckley CV. Increasing incidence of aortic aneurysms in England and Wales. BMJ 1989;298:33–5.

66. Rutkow IM, Ernst CB. An analysis of vascular surgical manpower requirements and vascular surgical rates in the United States. J Vasc Surg 1986;3:74.

67. Lederle FA. Management of small abdominal aortic aneurysms [editorial]. Ann Intern Med 1990;113:731–2.

68. Nevitt MP, Ballard DJ, Hallet JW Jr. Prognosis of abdominal aortic aneurysm: a population-based study. N Engl J Med 1989;321:1009–14.

69. Collin J, Heather B, Walton J. Growth rates of subclinical abdominal aortic aneurysms—implications for review and rescreening programmes. Eur J Vasc Surg 1991;5:141–4.

70. Pedersen OM, Aslaksen A, Vik-Mo H. Ultrasound measurement of the luminal diameter of the abdominal aorta and iliac arteries in patients without vascular disease. J Vasc Surg 1993;17:596–601.

71. Mohiaddin RH, Firmin DN, Longmore DB. Age-related changes of human aortic flow wave velocity measured noninvasively by magnetic resonance imaging. J Applied Physiol 199;74:492–7.

72. Allen PI. Screening for abdominal aortic aneurysm. Biomed Pharmacother 1988;42:451–4.

73. Bengtsson H, Ekberg O, Aspelin P, et al. Ultrasound screening of the abdominal aorta in patients with intermittent claudication. Eur J Vasc Surg 1989;3:497–502.

74. Bengtsson H, Bergqvist D, Ekberg O, Janzon L. A population based screening of abdominal aortic aneurysms (AAA). Eur J Vasc Surg 1991;5:53–7.

75. Cheatle TR, Scurr JH. Abdominal aortic aneurysms: a review of current problems. Br J Surg 1989;76:826–9.

76. Collin J, Araujo L, Walton J, Lindsell D. Oxford screening programme for abdominal aortic aneurysm in men aged 65 to 74 years. Lancet 1988;2:613–5.

77. Collin J, Araujo L, Walton J. A community detection program for abdominal aortic aneurysm. Angiology 1990;41:53–8.

78. Matsuzaki M, Ono S, Tomochika Y, et al. Advances in transesophageal echocardiography for the evaluation of atherosclerotic lesions in thoracic aorta—the effects of hypertension, hypercholesterolemia, and again on atherosclerotic lesions. Jpn Circ J 1992;56:592–602.

79. OKelly TJ, Heather BP. General practice-based population screening for abdominal aortic aneurysms: a pilot study. Br J Surg 1989;76:479–80.

80. Imakita S. Naito H, Nishimura T. Aortic aneurysms: growth rates measured with CT. Radiology 1992;185:249–52.

81. Bengtsson H, Nilsson P, Bergqvist D. Natural history of abdominal aortic aneurysm detected by screening. Br J Surg 1993;80:718–20.

82. Crawford ES, Saleh SA, Babb JW, et al. Infrarenal abdominal aortic aneurysm: factors influencing survival after operation performed over a 25-year period. Ann Surg 1981;193:699–709.

83. Crawford ES, Bomberger RA, Glaeser DH, et al. Aortoiliac occlusive disease: factors influencing survival and function following reconstructive operation over a twenty-five year period. Surgery 1981;90:1555–67.

84. Svensson LG, Crawford ES, Hess KR, et al. Deep hypothermia with circulatory arrest: determinants of stroke and early mortality in 656 patients. J Thorac Cardiovasc Surg 1992;106:19–31.

85. Svensson LG, Crawford ES, Hess KR, et al. Variables predictive of outcome in 832 patients undergoing repairs of the descending thoracic aorta. Chest 1993;104:1248–53.

86. Scott RAP, Wilson NM, Ashton HA, Kay DN. Is surgery necessary for abdominal aortic aneurysm less than 6 cm in diameter? Lancet 1993;342:1395–6.

87. Cronenwett JL, Sargent SK, Wall MH, et al. Variables that affect the expansion rate and outcome of small abdominal aortic aneurysms. J Vasc Surg 1990;11:260–8.

88. Cronenwett JL, Murphy TF, Zelenock GB, et al. Actuarial analysis of variables associated with rupture of small abdominal aortic aneurysms. Surgery 1985;98:472–83.

89. Bernstein EF, Dilley RB, Goldberger LE, et al. Growth rates of small abdominal aortic aneurysms. Surgery 1976;80:765–73.

90. Bernstein EF, Chan EL. Abdominal aortic aneurysm in high-risk patients: outcome of selective management based on size and expansion rate. Ann Surg 1984;200:255–63.

91. Geroulakis G, Nicolaides A. Infrarenal abdominal aortic aneurysms less than five centimeters in diameter: the surgeon's dilemma. Eur J Vasc Surg 1992;6:616–22.

92. Hallett JW Jr, Naessens JM, Ballard DJ. Early and late outcome of surgical repair for small abdominal aortic aneurysms: a population-based analysis. J Vasc Surg 1993;18:684–91.

93. Hertzer NR, Young JR, Beven EG, et al. Late results of coronary bypass in patients with infrarenal aortic aneurysms: The Cleveland Clinic Study. Ann Surg 1987;205:360–7.

94. Hertzer NR, Beven EG, Young JR, et al. Coronary artery disease in peripheral vascular patients: a classification of 1000 coronary angiograms and results of surgical management. Ann Surg 1984;199:223–33.

95. Hertzer NR, Young JR, Karmer JR, et al. Routine coronary angiography prior to elective aortic resection, Arch Surg 1979;114:1336–44.

96. Hertzer NR. Basic data concerning associated coronary disease in peripheral vascular patients. Ann Vasc Surg 1987;1;616–20.

97. Darling RC, Messina CR, Brewster DC, Ottinger LW. Autopsy study of unoperated abdominal aortic aneurysms: the case for early resection. Circulation 1976;56(2 Supp):161.

98. Estes JR Jr. Abdominal aortic aneurysm: a study of one hundred and two cases. Circulation 1950;2:258–64.

99. Szilagyi DE, Elliot JP, Smith RF. Clinical fate of the patient with asymptomatic abdominal aortic aneurysm and unfit for surgical treatment. Arch Surg 1972;104:600–6.

100. Pressler V, McNamara JJ. Thoracic aortic aneurysm: natural history and treatment. J Thorac Cardiovasc Surg 1980;79:489–98.

101. Crawford ES, DeNatale RW. Thoracoabdominal aortic aneurysm: observations regarding the natural course of the disease. J Vasc Surg 1986;3:578–82.

102. Chandler JJ. The Einstein sigh: the clinical picture of acute cholecystitis caused by ruptured abdominal aortic aneurysm [letter]. N Engl J Med 1984;310:1538.

103. Svensson LG, Crawford ES, Coselli JS, et al. Impact of cardiovascular operation on survival in the Marfan patient. Circulation 1989;80(3 Pt 1):i233–42.

104. Svensson LG, Sun J, Nadolony E, Kimmel WA. Prospective evaluation of minimal blood use for ascending aorta and aortic arch operations. Ann Thorac Surg 1995;59:1501–8.

105. Crawford ES, Hess KR, Cohen ES, et al. Ruptured aneurysm of the descending thoracic and thoracoabdominal aorta: analysis according to size and treatment. Ann Surg 1991;213:417–25.

106. Crawford ES, Hess KR, Abdominal aortic aneurysm. N Engl J Med 1989;321:1040–2.

107. Crawford ES. Ruptured abdominal aortic aneurysm [editorial]. J Vasc Surg 1991;13:348–50.

108. Treiman RL, Hartunian SL, Cossman DV, et al. Late results of small untreated abdominal aortic aneurysms. Ann Vasc Surg 1991;5:359–62.

109. Hollier LH, Taylor LM, Ochsner J. Recommended indications for operative treatment of abdominal aortic aneurysms. J Vasc Surg 1992;15:1046–56.

4

Aortic Dissection

HISTORICAL NOTE

Aortic dissection was first described in the second century, at the time of Galen and Antyllus. Vesalius made mention of aortic dissection in 1557,[1] and of particular historical interest is the comprehensive compendium of lectures published by Nicholls in Oxford, England, in 1732. Nicholls noted the process of aortic dissection in 1728 and also described the nervous innervation of arteries, the effect of small arteries on blood pressure, and hypertension.[2] Later, in 1761, Morgagni[3] described in detail the pathologic features of a patient whose aorta had ruptured into his pericardium. The term *dissection* arose when, in 1819, Laennec[4] coined the phrase *aneurysme dissequant.* This latter term is something of a misnomer, because dissection may be present without aneurysmal formation. A landmark contribution to the knowledge concerning the clinical and pathological findings of aortic dissection was the treatise published by Shennan in 1934.[1, 5] However, the successful management of aortic dissection was achieved only in the latter half of this century by DeBakey and colleagues.[6] Since then, the understanding of the pathogenesis and management of aortic dissection has rapidly evolved.[5]

The first attempts to treat aortic dissection surgically by fenestration were made by Gurin and colleagues[7] in 1935, but their patient died of renal failure. Similarly, in 1955 Shaw[8] reported another attempt at treating a DeBakey type III dissection by fenestration, and this patient also died of renal failure. Only in 1955 did DeBakey, Cooley, and Creech[6] first report a successful repair of aortic dissection. Later, in 1963, Morris and colleagues[9] described the successful repair of acute aortic dissection involving the ascending aorta. The patient subsequently underwent an aortic valve replacement in 1977 and then had a composite valve graft inserted successfully in 1990.[10, 11]

DEFINITIONS

Aortic dissection is best defined as a splitting of the aortic tunica media with extraluminal blood in the aortic wall. In most patients, a tear is present in the aortic intima, resulting in an abnormal communication between the true aortic lumen and the split aortic media. Thus the media, split by the process of aortic dissection, forms an abnormal extraluminal channel, known as the false lumen. The amount of splitting and, accordingly, the amount of blood in the aortic wall may vary greatly. The splitting of the aortic wall may be less than 1 mm thick, or it may involve the entire diameter of the aorta, resulting in total occlusion of the true lumen by the false lumen. Sometimes the tearing is completely circumferential, creating an inner tube of intima and inner aortic wall surrounded by blood with an outer tube that consists of the outer aortic wall. The extent of the dissection may be localized with minimal tracking along the aorta, such as observed in DeBakey type II dissections, or it may involve the entire length of the aorta and extend into the interventricular septum and to beyond the aortic bifurcation. The inner lining of the aorta intima and usually the inner third of the media that is dissected from the outer wall is referred to as the septum, since it separates the blood flow between the true and false lumina. This is the classic form of aortic dissection. When the false lumen is clotted and no tear is found for communication between the two lumina by imaging studies (13% of patients), particularly transesophageal echocardiography, or by autopsy (4% of patients), the dissection is known as an intramural hematoma. More rarely (6% of our 151 patients with Marfan syndrome) only a luminal intimal tear is seen exposing the media without extensive undermining of the intimal layer. Some authors refer to the septum as a "flap." In fact, rarely is there an actual true free "flap" in the aorta, and we do not use this somewhat misleading term *flap* in reference to the septum. Rather, the term is better applied to the commotion created by the finding of an aortic dissection septum.[11]

CLASSIFICATION

The time of onset of an aortic dissection determines the classification of the dissection as either acute or chronic. Thus an onset less than 2 weeks in duration is arbitrarily defined as acute. This definition is generally appropriate because it has been found that, in untreated patients, 74% of deaths occur within this 2-week period.[12] Furthermore, this is the stage when the aorta is most friable from the dissection and when inflammation is maximal.

Classifications have been proposed to describe the extent of aortic dissection, the site of the tear, and whether the false lumen is thrombosed. Currently, surgical literature, including our own reported findings,[13] indicates that the site of the aortic tear and thrombosis or lack of thrombosis of the false lumen do not influence either early or late operative results. Of greater importance are the extent of the aortic dissection and the diameter of the aorta, because these determine the operative approach, the extent of resection, and the long-term prognosis, including the late risk of rupture.[13] The most widely used terminology is that of DeBakey[14-16] (Fig. 4–1). In the DeBakey classification, type I dissection is defined as extending from the ascending aorta, through the transverse aortic arch, and into the descending aorta for a variable extent. Type II involves only the ascending aorta and is often association with Marfan syndrome.[17] Type III extends from the region of the left subclavian artery to the diaphragm (IIIa) or into the abdomen (IIIb). Figure 4–1 shows the classification graphically. The uncommon type of dissection that begins in the aortic arch, without involvement of the ascending aorta, and extends into the descending thoracic aorta is not included as a separate subgroup in this classification, although DeBakey would classify this as a type I dissection (personal communication). This is appropriate because we

concur with Miller of the Stanford group[18, 19] in recommending immediate operative repair of these dissections.

The original Stanford classification described by Daily and colleagues[20] grouped aortic dissection into two types, with type A involving the ascending aorta and type B involving all other extents beyond the left subclavian artery. It should be noted, though, that aortic arch dissections without involvement of the ascending aorta are now currently classified as type B whereas in the original system these patients were classified as type A.[20] This latter point has an important bearing on treatment of patients and will be discussed later.

Classification Used in This Text

We prefer to classify aortic dissections as either proximal or distal, acute or chronic and, when necessary, to describe other attributes of importance, such as aortic regurgitation, widest aortic diameter, area involved, tear site, and thrombosis of the lumen. Inclusion of these latter descriptive details within a classification code would make a classification unnecessarily complicated and cumbersome. Furthermore, unless one is using a database with multidimensional array capabilities (hierarchical), for example, MUMPS, the data string of the classification would have to be subdivided for most relational databases to allow for convenient analysis.

Influence of Classification on Management

The crux of surgical therapy is determined by whether the aorta, either proximal or distal to the left subclavian artery, is involved by aortic dissection.[13] Thus all patients with aortic dissection involving only the ascending aorta and aortic arch, irrespective of the extent of involvement beyond the left subclavian artery, are considered by us to have *proximal* dissection.[11, 13] Those patients with aortic dissection beyond the left subclavian artery and without involvement of the proximal aorta are classified as having *distal* dissection. The great significance of this classification is that the initial course of therapy is determined by whether proximal or distal dissection is present.[13, 21, 22] Therefore, a patient with acute proximal dissection will undergo immediate repair of the ascending aorta, the aortic arch, or both, even if more distal segments of the aorta are involved, because most deaths are caused by rupture of the ascending aorta into the pericardium. Chronic proximal dissections should also be repaired as soon as possible. In contrast, those patients with acute distal dissection are best treated initially by medical means. If this approach fails, then all dilated segments of the descending thoracic or thoracoabdominal aorta will be repaired. Chronic distal dissections are treated according to symptoms and size. A fusiform aneurysm may be present if the outer aortic wall has dilated or if an aneurysm was present before the dissection. Thoracoabdominal aneurysms are divided into four groups as shown in Figure 4-2.[11, 23]

FIGURE 4–1 DeBakey classification of aortic dissection. Type I extends from the ascending aorta down into the descending aorta and usually to the aortic bifurcation. Type II involves only the proximal aorta. Type III originates in the descending aorta and ends in either the descending aorta (IIIa) or the abdominal aorta (IIIb). (From Svensson LG, Crawford ES. Curr Probl Surg 1992;29:915-1057.)

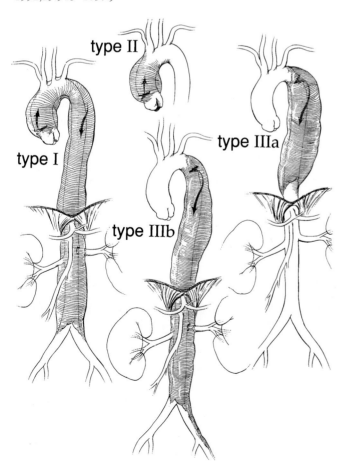

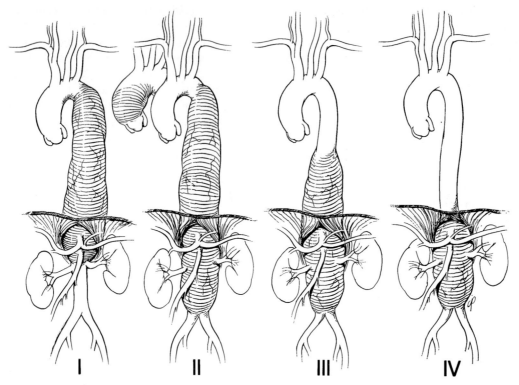

I II III IV

FIGURE 4–2 Crawford classification of thoracoabdominal aortic aneurysms. Type I originates in the proximal descending thoracic aorta and ends above the renal arteries. Type II begins in the proximal descending thoracic aorta and terminates below the renal arteries. Type III originates in the distal descending aorta, below approximately thoracic vertebrae T6, conveniently identified by being below the level of the thoracic incision in the sixth intercostal space. Type IV involves most of the abdominal aorta. (From Svensson LG, Crawford ES. Curr Probl Surg 1992;29:915–1057.)

INCIDENCE

In the United States, aortic dissection is diagnosed in approximately 2000 patients annually, although the exact incidence is not known.[24] On the basis of the number of aortic dissections diagnosed, the listed causes of death, and the known ratios of aortic dissection to ruptured abdominal aortic aneurysms, we estimate that the rate of occurrence is probably 10 per 100,000 of the population per annum, with the incidence increasing in older population groups.[11] In the United States, 2 deaths per 100,00 males and 0.8 death per 100,000 females are classified annually as being due to aortic dissection, although we surmise that this is probably a significant underestimate because many cases of aortic dissection are not diagnosed before death.[25] Jamieson and colleagues[26] noted that, of those patients who died of aortic dissection in hospitals, 35% had aortic dissection that was not detected before death. Furthermore, only one third of fatal aortic dissections originating in the aortic arch are diagnosed before death.[27] Thus, on the basis of these figures, the incidence of aortic dissection is probably about 10 per 100,000 per annum. There is general agreement in the literature that aortic dissection is the most common aortic disaster and appears to surpass the incidence of rupture in the infrarenal aorta, although more living patients with

the latter condition are seen by surgeons.[11] In one of the few community-based studies, Ponraj and Pepper[28] found that in a borough of London aortic dissection was the most common aortic catastrophe, outnumbering rupture of abdominal aortic aneurysms by a ration of 2:1. Furthermore, during a 3-year period, 4.2% of all sudden deaths in men were attributed to aortic dissection. Unfortunately, many patients with aortic dissection do not survive long enough to undergo operation.

PREDISPOSING FACTORS

Hereditary and Congenital Factors

Certain familial syndromes, particularly those with abnormal connective tissue, are associated with aortic dissection: Marfan (autosomal dominant, chromosome 15), Turner's (45, XO), Noonan's (XY, 5%XO), and Ehlers–Danlos (arterial type IV, either autosomal dominant or, occasionally, recessive).[11] In our series of 151 patients with Marfan syndrome,[29] three fourths had aortic dissection, with most of the dissections occurring in antecedent fusiform aneurysms.

The incidence of aortic dissection in families who are prone to the disease is high; in fact, aside from patients known to have a described syndrome, such as Marfan syndrome, familial aortic dissection appears to be inherited as an autosomal dominant trait.[30, 31] Furthermore, Kontusaari and colleagues[32] have shown that in these families aortic dissection may be due to a mutation in the gene for type III procollagen, namely, COL3A1.

Pregnancy

Pregnancy is also a predisposing factor.[11] In women under the age of 40 years, 50% of all aortic dissections occur during pregnancy.[33, 34] The highest incidence is in the third trimester, and is probably related to the hemodynamic and hormonal alterations that take place during pregnancy, particularly the increased levels of relaxin.[11]

Congenital Aortic Valve Defects

Congenital defects such as those of the bicuspid and stenotic aortic valves and coarctation of the aorta also appear to predispose a patient to aortic dissection. In 186 autopsies on patients who died of aortic dissection, Roberts and Roberts[35] found that the aortic valve was tricuspid in 91.4%, bicuspid in 7.5%, and unicuspid in 1.1%. Thus the aortic valve was five times more likely to be congenitally malformed in adults who died of aortic dissection. It is of interest that in the 16 patients with congenitally malformed valves (bicuspid or unicuspid), the entry site was always in the ascending aorta (compared with 68% in patients without congenital malformation); in the 11 patients who did not undergo operation, rupture of the false channel into the pericardium resulted in death within 24 hours of aortic dissection. Although six of the 16 patients had aortic stenosis, it was not reported whether there was poststenotic dilatation or whether any of the patients had a dilated aorta.

Coarctation of the Aorta

In 1928, Abbott[36] found that dissection occurred eight times more frequently in the segment of aorta proximal to aortic coarctation. The reason for this is probably that both proximal hypertension and medial degenerative disease are present in this segment. Also, it appears that aortic dissection arising in the ascending aorta does not progress beyond the coarctation site. The management of patients with simultaneous acute aortic dissection and coarctation of the aorta can be difficult. We have reported inserting a composite valve graft for the ascending aortic repair and also placing a tube graft from the ascending aorta to the supraceliac aorta.[37] The preoperative studies and postoperative results are illustrated in Figure 2-1.

Fusiform Aortic Aneurysms

We have observed that fusiform aneurysms of the aorta often antedate or precede aortic dissections, particularly in patients with Marfan syndrome.[29] In an extensive retrospec-

tive review of preoperative studies and operative notes, we noted that in all but two of 102 patients who had Marfan syndrome with aortic dissection there was evidence of some aortic dilatation. It should be cautioned that some families with Marfan syndrome are more prone to aortic dissection with minimal aortic dilatation.

It is well recognized that patients who undergo aortic valve replacement are at greater risk of intraoperative or postoperative aortic dissection.[38, 39] It has not been clearly determined whether this is because the aorta is abnormal or because of associated aortic dilatation, including poststenotic dilatation. Pieters and colleagues[38] performed a meta-analysis to examine the risk of aortic dissection after aortic valve replacement. They reported that, of 31 patients in whom aortic dissection developed after valve replacement, 68% had hypertension, 88% had dilation of the ascending aorta at the time of operation, and 55% had pure aortic regurgitation. The average interval between valve replacement and the development of aortic dissection was 4.3 years (range, 0.1 to 15 years), and 55% of the patients died of dissection. Of the patients seen with aortic dissection after valve replacement at their own institution, the size of the aorta before dissection varied between 5.3 and 6 cm. In addition, in 18 of 330 preoperative echocardiograms of patients undergoing aortic valve replacement at their own institution, the ascending aorta was noted to be larger than 5 cm. On late follow-up, four of these 18 patients were found to have developed postoperative dissection after valve replacement. In most of the patients in whom aortic dissection developed, monodisk valves had been inserted. These valves may entail a greater risk of dissection because they direct the ejecting jet of blood against the aortic wall, increasing the risk that dissection will occur. Left ventricular function had no correlation. Furthermore, three of the remaining 14 patients required reoperation to replace the ascending aorta. None of the patients with aortas less than 5 cm in diameter had dissection after valve replacement. Thus, in view of the 22% risk of aortic dissection occurring and also the subsequent need for surgery in 21% of the other patients, Pieters and associates recommended that the ascending aorta should be replaced at the time of aortic valve replacement.

Inflammatory Diseases, Infections, and Hormonal Abnormalities

Giant cell arthritis, systemic lupus erythematosus, relapsing polychondritis, juvenile nephropathic cystinosis, polycystic kidneys, pheochromocytoma, and Cushing's syndrome are associated with dissection, perhaps because of the hypertension that develops in these patients.[11] Cocaine may also precipitate aortic dissection.[40] Occasionally even mild trauma may cause dissection, although this is controversial. Infections may also induce aortic dissection. On one occasion in our experience,[11] while an aortic valve was being replaced because of bacterial endocarditis associated with an annular abscess, aortic dissection occurred during cardioplegia administration. This was repaired without mishap, although the undissected, more distal aortic wall could easily be peeled into two layers along a plane in the media. Aortic tissue histology revealed medial necrosis.[11] Paradoxically, it should be noted that syphilitic aortitis is believed to protect against the occurrence of dissection. This is because the cellular infiltrate (lymphocytes and plasma cells), scarring and periadventitial fibrosis of the aorta result in obliteration of the aortic wall planes.[11, 12]

ETIOLOGY AND HISTOLOGY

The two clinical variables most frequently associated with aortic dissection are medial degenerative disease of the aorta and hypertension The causes of medial degenerative disease and hypertension remain largely unknown.[11]

Medial Degenerative Disease

The intimal layer of the aorta consists of a thin connective tissue layer of collagenous tissue with myofibroblasts, elastic fibers, and smooth muscle with a covering of endothelial cells. The tunica media lies adjacent to the intima and consists of concentrically arranged fenestrated layers of elastic lamellae with a delicate layer of elastin microfibrils and interwoven collagen and smooth muscle cells. From a surgical point of view, the adventitia is the strongest and toughest layer for holding sutures. It consists of irregularly arranged collagenous tissue, come incorporated circumferential elastic fibers, and the vasa vasorum, which branch in between the outer and middle layers of the media. Gsell,[41] in 1928, noted necrosis of small muscle cells and the degeneration of the elastic and collagen fibers on histological examination of the aortas from eight patients with aortic dissection. Shortly thereafter, in 1929, Erdheim[42] described the cystic lesions of mucoid ground substance between the degenerated fibers in two patients without aortic dissection but with ascending aneurysms, and coined the phrase *medionecrosis aortae idiopathica cystica.* Contrary to Erdheim's[42] postulate, it appears that the loss of smooth muscle cells and elastic fibers precedes the accumulation of ground substance. Moreover, the accumulated ground substance in the aorta is not truly contained within cysts. Nevertheless, medial degeneration is present in most patients with aortic dissection, although there is a wide difference of opinion as to both the presence and the significance of medial degeneration.[43, 11]

In most of our patients, evidence of aortic disease is found on histologic examination.[21] Histologic specimens were obtained in 818 patients with proximal aortic dissection, ascending or aortic arch aneurysms, or both.[11] In patients with Marfan syndrome, medial necrosis was present in 33% ($N = 9$) of those with acute proximal dissection versus 31% of patients with acute dissection but without Marfan syn-

drome ($N = 72$). The incidence of atherosclerosis or medial degeneration alone was similar in both groups. Medial necrosis was more common (35%, $N = 158$) in patients with aortic dissection who required aortic arch replacement than in those who required only ascending aortic replacement (20%, $N = 149$). In other words, medial degeneration alone was more frequent in patients who required only ascending aortic repairs. Medial necrosis was present in 31% of patients with acute dissection ($N = 83$) and in 24% of patients with chronic dissection ($N = 231$). In patients with proximal aortic aneurysms without aortic dissection ($N = 511$), only 11% had medial necrosis and 51% had associated atherosclerosis. Atherosclerosis was found in 37% ($N = 307$) of patients with aortic dissection. Aortitis was found in 1.6% ($N = 307$) of patients with aortic dissection and in 4.3% ($N = 511$) of patients without dissection. In patients ($N = 220$) with distal aortic dissection, 21% had medial necrosis, 65% had atherosclerosis, and 48% had medial degeneration alone. There was no variation in incidence for patients with Marfan syndrome, acute dissections, or chronic dissections. It is of interest that the incidence of atherosclerosis and medial necrosis was, respectively, higher and lower in patients with distal aortic dissection than in patients with proximal dissection. Aortitis was present in 1.3%.[11]

There has been speculation as to whether medial necrosis precipitates aortic dissection or is produced by the dissection per se.[44] Medial necrosis is more frequently observed in patients with Marfan syndrome and, as pointed out previously, aortic dissection is present in two thirds of the patients who require surgery. It is likely that some patients have medial necrosis, perhaps caused by severe hypertension, that results in aortic dissection. Nevertheless, medial necrosis cannot be the sole factor.[12, 45] Of interest is the finding that aortic dissection can occur spontaneously in fish that have no vasa vasorum and that do not have hypertension, atherosclerosis, or aortic enlargement but do have medionecrosis of the aortic wall.[11, 46]

Healing of Dissection

After acute dissection, intense inflammation of the aortic wall occurs and thus, over time, as with chronic dissection, parts of the septum seem to disappear. This partial disappearance of the septum may occur because the areas with medial necrosis are reabsorbed during healing and later new endothelial cells line the false channel to create a new pseudointima. Occasionally true healing will occur if the false lumen is small and thrombosed and if the lumen is obliterated.[11]

Atherosclerosis

In accordance with our findings,[11] atherosclerosis has previously been reported to be more frequently found in the media from patients with distal aortic dissection.[12] This could be explained by the fact that these are older patients.

There is some controversy as to whether atherosclerosis causes aortic dissection.[12, 45] We believe that it does not, because atherosclerosis may limit dissection, atherosclerosis is more common in the abdominal aorta or descending thoracic aorta and yet dissection most often arises in the ascending aorta, and atherosclerosis of the aorta does not always involve the intima. We have noted that the dissection process often stops at sites of gross atherosclerosis, perhaps because the surrounding fibrosis limits extension of the dissection. That atherosclerosis is not an important factor is further supported by the finding that aortic dissection is more frequent in the ascending aorta where atherosclerosis less common. There has been some debate as to whether ulcerated atherosclerotic plaque typically seen in the descending aorta precipitates aortic dissection. In affected patients, the extent of dissection, if present at all, is very limited and hardly ever extends to the left subclavian artery, unlike DeBakey type III dissections. Ulcerated plaques occur infrequently in the ascending aorta.[11] Sariola and colleagues,[47] however, believe that penetrating ulcers with defects in type IV collagen and the basement membrane may be etiologic factors in aortic dissection. The latter type of dissection related to penetrating ulcers tends to be in the plane between the media and adventitia and to be more limited without involving the entire aorta or even the entire descending thoracic aorta. Furthermore, these latter patients more often have frank aortic rupture into the mediastinum (see also Chapter 9).

Hypertension

The role of hypertension in the development of aortic dissection is unclear, although it is frequently associated with aortic dissection. In our patients,[48] the incidence of hypertension was 75%. Others[15] have reported an incidence of up to 90%. In an experimental study Prokop and colleagues[49] found that the pulsatile component of hypertension is an important indicator for the progression of dissection. They observed that nonpulsatile hypertension at 400 mm Hg did not result in dissection, whereas pulsatile flow at 120 mm Hg resulted in dissection. It is of interest that, while aortic dissection may occur on total cardiopulmonary bypass for cardiac surgery, dissection is more likely to occur with an ejecting heart.[50] The higher the dP/dt_{max}, the more rapid the progression of the dissection.[51] Turbulence in the ascending aorta may also precipitate dissection.[11, 52]

Iatrogenic and Traumatic Factors

Aortic dissection can be precipitated by invasive procedures that damage the aorta, particularly the intima. These iatrogenic factors include cardiac catheterization, aortography, arterial and aortic cannulation for cardiopulmonary bypass, coronary artery bypass surgery, aortic valve replacement, intraaortic balloon pumps, and simple aortic cross-clamping for aneurysm repairs.[11, 12, 39, 53, 54] More recently one

of us (L.G.S.) performed emergency repairs in two patients with acute type II aortic dissection of the ascending aorta and coronary artery dissection caused by percutaneous coronary angioplasty (PTCA) (Fig. 4–3). Rarely, retrograde dissection from the abdominal aorta may follow repair of an infrarenal aortic aneurysm.[55] Patients placed on a regimen of steroids, particularly for organ transplants, are also prone to develop aortic dissection.[11]

Of concern during cardiac surgery is the risk or iatrogenic aortic dissection.[39, 50, 56, 57] Still and colleagues[50] reported their experience with 24 patients (0.16% of patients undergoing cardiac operations). The origin of the intraoperative dissections included the aortic cannulation site in 10, the cross-clamp site in eight, and the site of application of the partial occluding clamp in seven. The high incidence reported in this study may have been due to the proximal vein graft anastomoses and the aortic cannulations being performed with a partial occluding clamp while the heart was ejecting prior to cardiopulmonary bypass. This would lead to a greater risk of dissection because of the greater dP/dt_{max} of an ejecting heart as opposed to the heart on bypass. Boruchow and colleagues[58] have implicated partial occlusion clamps in the development of aortic dissection after cardiac operations. Lam and colleagues[56] performed autopsy studies on 50 patients who died after cardiac surgery and found that seven (14%) died of aortic dissection. None had any obvious predisposing factors such as hypertension or medial degenerative disease, but all seven patients had undergone cannulation of the femoral arteries. It is noteworthy that trauma during surgical cannulation, particularly in the femoral arteries, was considered to be a factor in five of the seven patients. In six of seven patients the

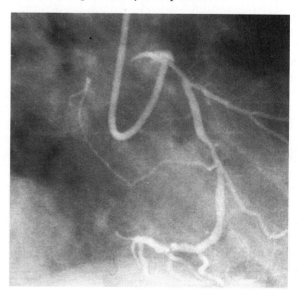

FIGURE 4–3 Aberrant right coronary artery arising from the left coronary sinus of Valsalva with dissection of the ascending aorta at catheter tip caused by attempted PTCA.

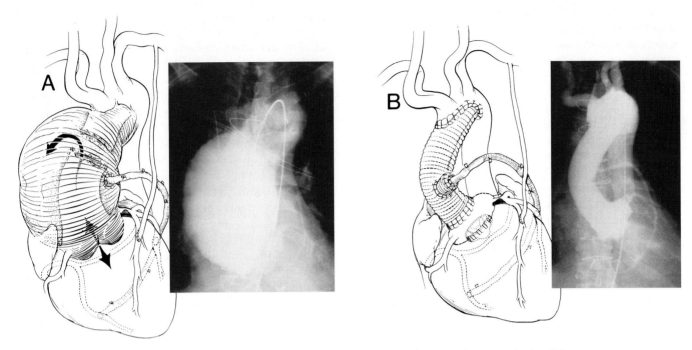

FIGURE 4–4 **A,** Patient with proximal aortic dissection and aortic valve regurgitation follow-ing coronary artery bypass graft operation. **B,** Postoperative result after hemiarch replacement, insertion of aortic valve, and reattachment of saphenous graft to the ascending aorta with an interposition tube graft.

dissection was DeBakey type I, and it was type II in the other patient. This report should serve as a warning against excessive use of the femoral arteries for cannulation in patients with severe atherosclerosis of the ascending aorta and aortic arch. For most patients, however, cannulation of the ascending aorta is the safest procedure to follow, as dis-cussed in the review by Taylor and colleagues.[59] They found that, of 9000 patients operated on with ascending aortic cannulation, only two developed aortic dissection; one of these was fatal. Orszulak and colleagues[60] reported late operations on six patients in whom aortic dissection had developed as a result of cardiac surgery. Of the seven patients who had a dilated ascending aorta at the time of the initial cardiac operation, three subsequently developed aortic dissection. Figures 4–4 to 4–9 illustrate various aortic dissection problems in patients.

Experimental Precipitation of Dissection in Animals

In animals aortic dissection has been produced by epinephrine, vitamin D, electrocautery, sweet-pea feeds (*Lathyrus odoratus,* the active ingredient of which is B-aminopropionitrile), copper-deficient diet, special breeding such as cattle with aortas of the marfanoid type, and hyper-tension.[11, 12, 61] The broad-breasted bronze variety of turkeys is reported to be prone to aortic dissection. Rather than aortic dissection, a transmural aortic rupture occurs. These tur-keys are particularly prone to hypertension, with blood

pressures reaching 400 mm Hg, the highest values observed in any species.[11]

PATHOPHYSIOLOGY

Aortic dissection originates at a tear in the aortic intima in more than 95% of patients.[12, 62] On occasion no obvious site of an intimal tear communicating with the false lumen is found, and a split may not be identified on postmortem examination in as many as 4% of patients.[12] These rare excep-tions give credence to the theory that aortic dissection may also originate from the vasa vasorum[63] or that it may arise from an area of medial necrosis. Usually the tear is trans-verse and involves more than half the circumference. In 65% of patients the tear is 1 to 3 cm distal to the coronary arteries, in 20% of patients the tear is in the upper descend-ing thoracic aorta, in 10% it is in the aortic arch, and in fewer than 5% it is in the abdominal aorta.[12, 18, 22, 62, 64] How-ever, it should be noted that, once dissection occurs, the dissection process can extend either proximally or (more often) distally. Dissection of the distal aorta may occasionally extend proximally.[29] In 65% to 85% of autopsies, the ascend-ing aorta is found to be involved by acute dissection.[65, 66] In 70%, cardiac tamponade is the cause of death.[11, 12]

The sequence of events appears to evolve with blood being forcefully pumped through the tear into the aortic wall, creating a second or false channel, which rapidly pro-gresses, often within a matter of seconds, distally to the

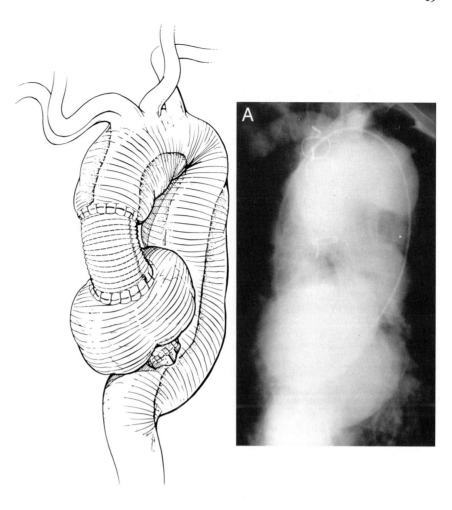

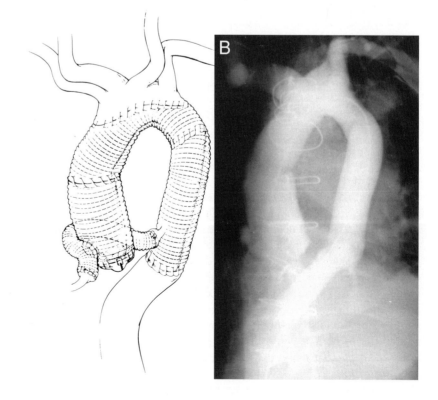

FIGURE 4–5 **A,** Patient with Marfan syndrome who presented with aortic dissection beyond previous attempted repair done elsewhere for aortic valve regurgitation and annuloaortic ectasia. Note large sinus of Valsalva aneurysm. **B,** Postoperative repair after insertion of composite valve graft by the Cabrol technique, replacement of the aortic arch by our modification of the elephant trunk technique, and subsequent repair of the descending aorta. The descending aorta second-stage elephant trunk operation was performed a few weeks after the initial operation. (From Svensson LG, Crawford ES. Curr Probl Surg 1992;29:915–1057.)

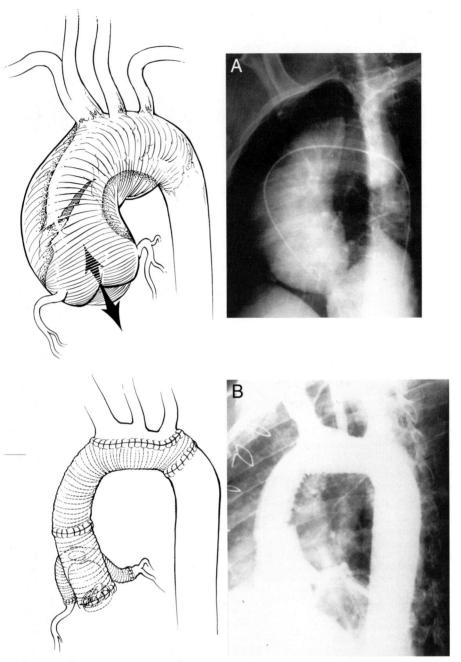

FIGURE 4–6 **A,** Patient with Marfan syndrome with proximal aortic dissection and aortic regurgitation. **B,** Postoperative result after replacement of the aortic arch and insertion of a composite valve graft by the Cabrol method. (From Svensson LG, Crawford ES. Curr Probl Surg 1992;29:915–1057.)

outer part of the media. The dissection may be arrested anywhere along the course of the aorta, but most often the dissection ends either in the iliac arteries on in an arterial side branch. The false channel characteristically spirals from the right outer curve of the ascending aorta, then to the anterior or left lateral side of the arch, and then down the left side of the aorta (Fig. 4-10). In most patients, more than half the circumference of the aorta is involved. We have observed in approximately 80% of patients that the left iliac artery is supplied by the false channel, whereas in Hirst's autopsy study[12] the incidence was found to be equal. The importance of this is that when the femoral arteries need to be cannulated for cardiopulmonary bypass, the true lumen should also be cannulated. Distal to the point of entry into

the aortic wall, the dissection false channel can either terminate as a blind pocket or reenter the true aortic lumen, often with multiple fenestrations, or tear through the adventitia, resulting in rupture, exsanguination, and subsequent death of most patients.[11]

In either the acute stage or the chronic stage, the false lumen may compress or obstruct the true lumen. During the chronic stage, the true lumen often shrinks in size and becomes redundant.[12, 13, 62] When the aorta is occluded by the false lumen, distal perfusion of the aorta, including the branches, is dependent on reentry tears occurring into the true lumen to reestablish perfusion of critical arteries. If this does not happen during the acute phase, the complications such as bowel ischemia, renal failure, and lower limb gangrene may occur. Occlusion of aortic branches is observed in about 30% of patients.[67] The mechanisms for arterial occlusion include a true flap obstructing the lumen, compression of the artery by an external hematoma, the dissection extending into the proximal artery, or shearing of the arteries off the true lumen. When the arteries are sheared off the true lumen, they are usually perfused by the false lumen. This is typically seen with the left renal artery. However, obstructed arteries may thrombose, contributing to end-organ ischemia.[11]

Proximal ascending aortic dissections often extend into the coronary sinuses, resulting in aortic valve prolapse or coronary artery occlusion; they may even extend retrograde into the ventricular septum, resulting in heart block or atri-

oventricular valve incompetence. Usually the dissecting false channel burrows outside the noncoronary cusp, between the anterior commissure and the right posterior lateral commissure, and then into the left ventricle. The entire annular circumference from the right coronary artery around to the left main coronary artery may also be dissection free. Aortic valve regurgitation is particularly severe when this occurs and may lead to fatal heart failure. The right coronary artery ostium, because of its location, is more frequently involved by the aortic dissection. As a consequence, it may be either compressed, dissected, torn off the true lumen, or interrupted by a flap of the septum, resulting in acute myocardial ischemia. Retrograde dissection from the distal aorta into the proximal aorta is rare but

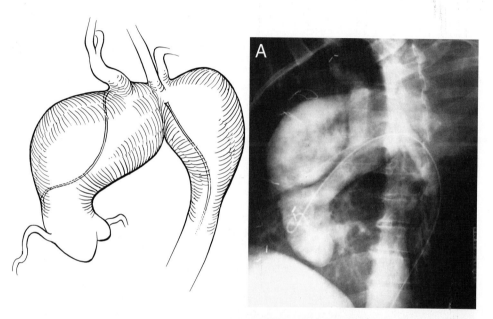

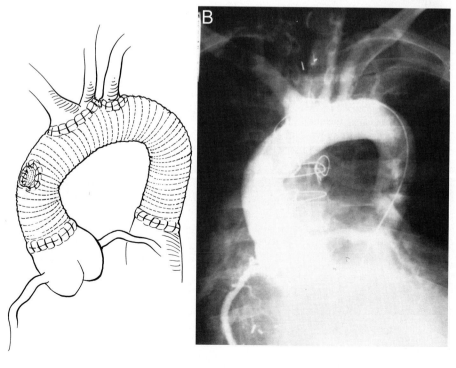

FIGURE 4–7   A, Patient with a DeBakey type I aortic dissection following previous cardiac surgery. **B,** Postoperative result after replacement of the aortic arch with separate reimplantation of the left subclavian artery.

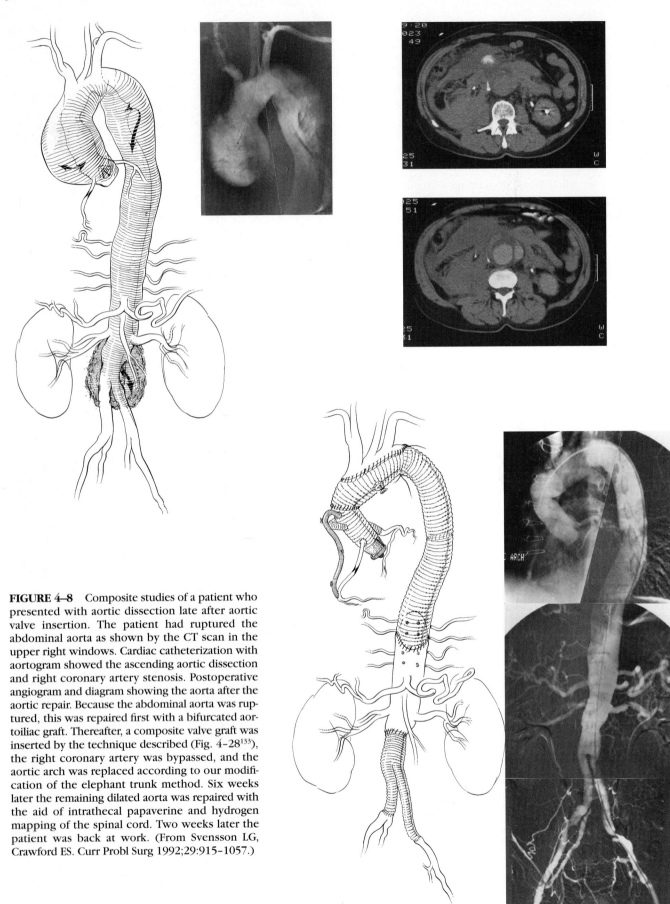

FIGURE 4–8 Composite studies of a patient who presented with aortic dissection late after aortic valve insertion. The patient had ruptured the abdominal aorta as shown by the CT scan in the upper right windows. Cardiac catheterization with aortogram showed the ascending aortic dissection and right coronary artery stenosis. Postoperative angiogram and diagram showing the aorta after the aortic repair. Because the abdominal aorta was ruptured, this was repaired first with a bifurcated aortoiliac graft. Thereafter, a composite valve graft was inserted by the technique described (Fig. 4–28[133]), the right coronary artery was bypassed, and the aortic arch was replaced according to our modification of the elephant trunk method. Six weeks later the remaining dilated aorta was repaired with the aid of intrathecal papaverine and hydrogen mapping of the spinal cord. Two weeks later the patient was back at work. (From Svensson LG, Crawford ES. Curr Probl Surg 1992;29:915–1057.)

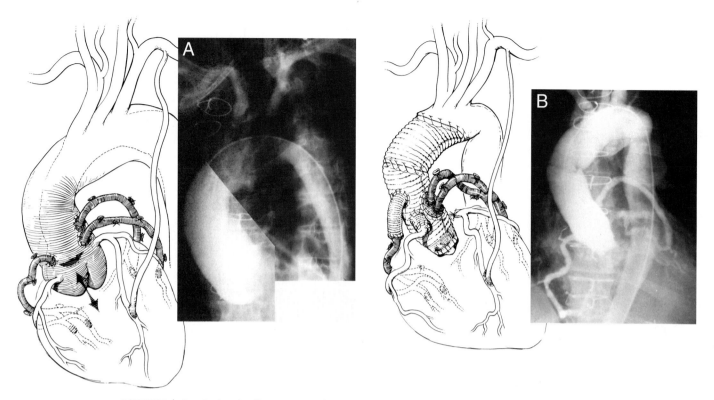

FIGURE 4–9   **A,** Aortic dissection and aortic valve regurgitation following coronary artery bypass with three veins and internal mammary artery done elsewhere. **B,** Aortogram following repair of the proximal aortic arch using deep hypothermia with circulatory arrest, insertion of composite valve graft, reattachment of the right coronary artery with an interposition tube graft, oversewing of the left main coronary artery ostium, and reattachment of the saphenous vein grafts. (From Svensson LG, Crawford ES. Curr Probl Surg 1992;29:915–1057.)

has been reported, including in our patients with Marfan syndrome.[29] Rarely, intussusception of the intima can occur with resultant obstruction of the aorta (Fig. 4–11).[11, 29, 68]

AORTIC RUPTURE CAUSED BY DISSECTION

Early Rupture

Death from acute proximal aortic dissections is frequently due either to aortic rupture or to a leak of fluid, often by transudation, into the pericardial cavity. The accumulation of blood and fluid in the pericardial cavity leads to cardiac tamponade or occlusion of the coronary arteries. Acute right-sided heart failure may develop because of rupture into or compression of the pulmonary artery. Both proximal and distal dissections can rupture into the mediastinum, pleural cavities, or abdomen with exsanguination. Roberts[62] has documented that the most common site of rupture in the acute stage is at the site of the mural tear in the aorta. Necrosis of the outer layer of the aortic wall at the site of the tear weakens the wall, allowing for rupture. Thus, for dissections arising in the ascending aorta, rupture within the closed confines of the pericardial cavity can cause cardiac tamponade. Rupture of the aorta in patients with dis-

section arising just beyond the left subclavian artery (DeBakey type III) results in a usually fatal exsanguination into the left side of the chest from the upper portion of the descending thoracic aorta. Rupture, however, may occur at a more distal site, often in the abdomen. Because proximal dissections have more potential causes of death, it is not surprising that the 1-year survival in untreated patients with proximal dissections is a mere 10% compared with 40% for untreated patients with distal aortic dissection. With both types of dissection, death usually occurs within the first 30 days.[12, 62, 66, 69–71]

During the early period after acute dissection, survival depends on minimal progression of the dissection as in DeBakey type II dissections, reentry of the dissection false lumen into the aortic true lumen, or the severity of end-organ ischemia because of occlusion of the branch arteries. In addition to the acute complications related to branch artery occlusions and aortic valve regurgitation, chronic complications include the development of fusiform aneurysms, new dissections, aortic rupture, and complications of older surgical techniques.[11, 13, 29, 48, 61, 72-74]

Late Rupture

Late rupture of aneurysmal segments of the aorta has been reported to be the cause of death in as many as 30% of

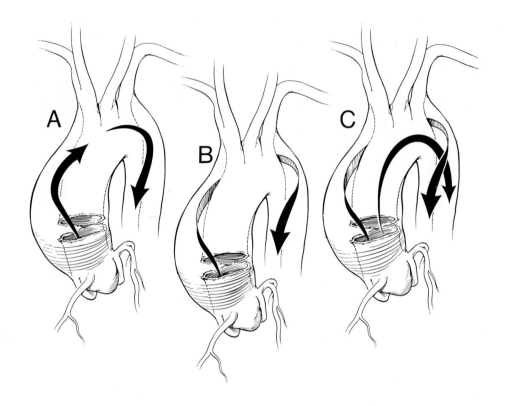

FIGURE 4–10 Possible courses taken by the false lumen after aortic dissection. **A,** Anterior to the arch. **B,** Posterior course. **C,** Combined anterior and posterior course with complete circumferential dissection of the aorta, leaving an inner tube of the intima with the inner layers of the media. Note how in most patients the false lumen follows the outer curve of the distal aortic arch and proximal descending aorta and then extends down the posterolateral aspect of the aorta on the left side. (From Svensson LG, Crawford ES. Curr Probl Surg 1992;29:915–1057.)

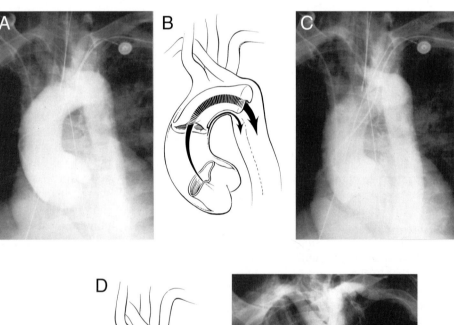

FIGURE 4–11 A, Aortogram of patient with intussusception of inner dissection tube (intimal layer and inner media layer) into the distal aortic arch and proximal descending aorta. **B,** Diagram of intimal prolapse. **C,** Aortogram with a later phase of injection. **D,** Diagram of repair and postoperative result on aortography.

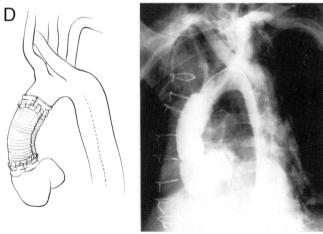

our patients.[15] In our earlier experience, about 20% of our patients died of late rupture (that is, rupture occurring 30 days or more postoperatively),[21] but this has been reduced to 10% with more aggressive resections for all aneurysmal disease.[13] DeBakey and colleagues[15] have reported that late rupture appears to be associated with the presence of uncontrolled hypertension. Rupture occurred in 46% of patients with hypertension and in 17% of those without hypertension.[15] We have observed that the risk of rupture is also directly dependent on aneurysm size, so that 88% of patients with aortic rupture have aneurysms less than 10 cm in diameter whereas 23% have ruptured aneurysms of less than 6 cm.[13] This has also been supported by the work of Glower and colleagues[75] and by Japanese studies.[76] These latter studies showed that when the aorta exceeded a diameter of 5 cm, the risk of rupture increased markedly.[11] Therefore, operative repair should be considered in all patients with dissected segments of the aorta exceeding 5 cm in diameter.

CLINICAL MANIFESTATIONS

Acute Aortic Dissection

During the acute phase of aortic dissection the most frequent complications are aortic rupture, aortic valve regurgitation, aortic obstruction, obstruction of the aortic branches, rarely rupture into an aortic chamber, or obstruction or rupture into the pulmonary artery. These complications of acute dissection influence the clinical findings in patients.[11]

Symptoms

In most patients, the onset of the excruciating pain associated with aortic dissection is sudden and intense. It is often described as a tearing or ripping sensation. The initial locality of the pain suggests where the dissection has occurred. Thus proximal dissection commences with severe anterior chest pain that usually progresses down the length of the back. The patient will often describe the migration of pain as progressing along the course of the aorta and even into the upper thighs. Radiation of pain may extend to the neck, jaw, or both arms. The precipitation of the pain may be reported to follow vigorous and sudden movements, such as chopping wood with an axe, weight-lifting, swinging a golf club, or playing basketball or baseball. Other activities may have been coughing, straining, or defecation. Occasionally, minor trauma may precede the event. Descriptions of the pain include "ripping," "burning," "splitting," "cutting," or "a hit in the chest." In contrast to myocardial ischemia, nausea and vomiting are infrequent. Patients are often restless, agitated, and apprehensive and can precisely recount the time of onset of the pain. In contrast, with myocardial ischemia, the pain tends to rise to a crescendo. Either because of the severe pain or because of the dissection transiently occluding the origin of the head vessels of interfering with the aortic arch baroreceptors, syncope or loss of consciousness is often associated with the onset of pain. Distal dissection characteristically results in pain commencing in the upper back, and then the pain appears to migrate down into the abdomen. For either proximal or distal dissection, the severe pain first experienced with aortic dissection may then subside over a couple of hours, to be replaced by a deep ache. Later, the pain may recur or be noted to migrate with further dissection. A cautionary note is that during the interval of diminished pain experienced by some patients the physician may be lulled into a false belief that the cause of the pain has disappeared. For this reason, it is imperative to perform an imaging study of the aorta in patients in whom myocardial ischemia has been ruled out as the cause of pain. Other potential causes of the chest pain, such as pulmonary embolic disease, should also be borne in mind and excluded by appropriate tests.[11]

Although most patients have chest pain, a few patients, particularly those with Marfan syndrome or those who are taking steroid medication, may have no pain associated with the dissection. Transient syncope, or giving way or collapsing of the legs may be the only presenting symptom as the dissection process shears the intercostal arteries off the aortic lumen.[11] Some patients will be seen in shock and in extremis. The shock is usually due to rupture into the pericardial space, resulting in cardiac tamponade. Less often, the cause is hypovolemia due to rupture of the aorta in the abdomen or, occasionally, into the left side of the chest. Shock may also be cardiogenic because of dissection of the coronary arteries, resulting in frank myocardial infarction.

Narrowing or occlusion of arteries arising from the aorta occurs in 30% of patients. Thus, in 3% of patients, narrowing of the coronary arteries results in characteristic myocardial ischemic chest pain. In 7% of patients involvement of the aortic arch arteries leads to transient strokes or in the patients being mentally obtunded. Leg weakness or paralysis develops in 2.5% of patients; this is possibly related to intercostal artery dissection. Limb ischemia occurs in 13% because of iliac and femoral artery involvement, and abdominal angina occurs in 1.5% as a result of visceral ischemia. Aortic valve incompetence is present in two thirds of patients, and severe aortic valve incompetence, present in 55% of patients, can result in acute onset of dyspnea and heart failure.[48]

Signs

Paradoxically, the patient, despite being hypertensive, may appear shocked, cold, and clammy, with poor peripheral perfusion. The hypertension is probably the result of involvement of the aortic arch baroreceptors, release of catecholamines, and possible activation of the renin-angiotensin system.[11] The release of the latter hormones may be due to renal artery obstruction causing renal ischemia, particularly in the left kidney. Hypertension may not always be present with acute dissection. Cardiac tamponade from proximal dissection or rupture into the left side of the chest or abdomen may result in hypotension. Tachycardia, however, is almost universally present. On auscultation, aortic regurgitation is detected in about 50% of patients[77] and is often the first clue to the presence of aortic dissection. Aortic regurgitation is due to either a single commissure being dissected loose with prolapse of the cusp, a tear of the leaflet, preexistent regurgitation, particularly if associated with annuloaortic ectasia, or prolapse of the entire valve.[11] Aortic regurgitation may disappear, however, as the dissection spreads proximally into the annulus and leaflet coaptation once again occurs. Sometimes auscultation also reveals a pericardial rub or distant heart sounds suggesting cardiac tamponade, particularly if this is associated with a raised central venous pressure and a pulsus paradoxus. Cardiac tamponade or pericardial effusion can be confirmed by radiography of the chest, electrocardiography (ECG), and echocardiography. Cardiac tamponade is acute in onset either from frank rupture of the aorta, usually from the anterior aorta in close proximity to the right coronary artery, or from transudation of fluid from the acutely inflamed exudative and very thin ascending aorta. The aorta may be so translucent that blood flowing in it can be observed through the adventitia at the time of operation. Distal rupture or leakage is suggested by the accumulation of fluid in the left hemithorax with the classic findings of a pleural effusion on auscultation. Rupture can also occur into the esophagus, trachea, or a bronchus. Very rarely, a systolic murmur may be heard over the back between the scapulae.[11] This is due to a thrombosed false lumen narrowing the true lumen, creating a type of long coarctation of the aorta.[11]

Obstruction of arteries arising from the aorta, either transiently or permanently, results in ischemia of the tissues supplied by the artery. The ischemia may be transient or incomplete. Thus strokes are often transient and may be fully reversible with surgery.[13, 18, 19, 67] If the innominate artery or a common carotid artery is obstructed at its origin, collateral blood flow from the other carotid artery probably maintains brain viability. Similarly, collateral blood may prevent renal dysfunction and bowel necrosis, and ischemia is sometimes reversible with a prompt operation. Renal ischemia often results in reduced urine output and elevation of the serum creatinine level. Unfortunately, bowel necrosis is usually detected a few days after an operative repair, and by then it is too late to prevent gangrene. It is interesting that some patients who have chronic iliac artery occlusion from dissection describe claudication in the region of their thighs. In contrast, claudication in the calf muscles is more indicative of atherosclerotic iliofemoral disease. If, by error, a femoral embolectomy is performed for acute limb ischemia due to dissection, then the catheter will be found both to easily pass proximally and to withdraw without difficulty, but no clot will be extracted and flow will not be reestablished. The diagnosis of aortic dissection is also suggested by a hematoma in the femoral artery wall; this has a bluish discoloration from the stagnant deoxygenated blood or thrombus.[11]

On occasion, patients with aortic dissection have unusual presenting symptoms, such as superior vena cava obstruction, right atrial obstruction, lower neck pulsation, hemoptysis, hematemesis, gastrointestinal bleeding, fistulae into the right side of the heart, unexplained fever with or without weight loss, mild jaundice (particularly associated with elevated levels of LDH from reabsorption of the dissection hematoma), and abdominal cramps. Rarely, the aorta will rupture into another cardiac chamber, including the right atrium, right ventricle, and left atrium, as documented by Lindsay.[78] This can manifest suddenly after previous cardiac operations, and then the patient will have acute heart failure. By contrast, after chronic dissections, the complication of rupture into a chamber will result in a more chronic or subacute heart failure. A continuous murmur is almost always heard. Because of the presence of postoperative adhesions, previous operations tend to lead to the development of fistula formation rather than free rupture. There is danger that a false diagnosis of endocarditis may be made, particularly if fever is observed a few days after dissection or if the false lumen has marked thrombus formation.[11]

The vagaries of aortic dissection may be illustrated by one of our patients who had been treated with streptokinase for chest pain of probable myocardial origin. When the pain failed to subside, the cardiologist noted a murmur on auscultation of the chest. A transthoracic echo then detected the acute ascending aortic dissection. Aortography confirmed the diagnosis, and the patient underwent an operation. Thus it is important that the possibility of aortic dissection should always be considered in patients with chest pain. Furthermore, the three most common features of acute aortic dissection that should alert the physician are a history or presence of hypertension, sudden onset of pain, and subsequent caudal migration of the pain.[11, 79]

Chronic Aortic Dissection

In one fourth of the patients an aneurysm develops within 5 years of aortic dissection.[15] The clinical signs of chronic dissection are frequently related to an enlarging aortic aneurysm. Chronic dissecting aneurysm may rupture or dissect again, with manifestations similar to those for acute aortic dissection.

The severity of the patient's symptoms at the time of presentation with aortic dissection,[13] Marfan syndrome,[29] and ascending and/or aortic arch aneurysms[80] significantly influence the risk mortality rate and often also the long-term prognosis after aortic operation. Therefore patients are classified at presentation as follows: patients with no symptoms or pain are classified as grade I; those with mild pain, occasional discomfort or symptoms, such as a chronic dry cough, hoarseness, dysphagia, or Horner's syndrome, are classified as grade II; patients with severe, continuous pain not related to aortic dissection are classified as grade III; and those with aortic dissection or dissection associated with complications such as cardiac tamponade, myocardial infarct, renal shutdown, paresis/paraplegia, shock, or rupture are classified as grade IV.[11, 80, 81] Figure 4–12 shows the influence of aneurysm symptom grade on survival after surgery.

It is noteworthy that the clinical signs of a chronic dissection may be minimal or absent. Most often they are related to expansion of the aorta, resulting in findings such as pulsation at the base of the neck, wheezing from tracheal or bronchial compression, or a pulsatile abdominal mass. Of interest, marked depression of left ventricular function may be present with minimal evidence of coronary artery disease or valve dysfunction. This may be related to compression of the heart by the aneurysms and to lateral displacement of the heart. If aortic valve regurgitation is present, signs of aortic incompetence may be found; these include Duroziez's sign (femoral murmurs), Quinke's sign (capillary pulsation), de Musset's sign (head nodding), Traube's sign (pistol shot femorals), Corrigan's pulse (water hammer pulse), and Branham's sign (increased swinging movement of the upper leg when a patient sits with his legs crossed). Interestingly, it has been speculated from the photographs of Abraham Lincoln, which show blurring of movement in the region of his crossed leg, that this effect might have arisen because of excessive motion caused by an incompetent valve associated with his probable Marfan syndrome.[11]

DIAGNOSIS OF ACUTE DISSECTION

A high index of suspicion is the most important reason for investigating aortic dissection.[11] Radiographic or echocardiographic techniques are crucial to the diagnosis of aortic dissection.

Chest Radiographs

A posteroanterior (PA) chest radiograph has an accuracy of 85%[68] and, indeed, may be the only test that shows aortic dissection. Typically, the aortic knob is enlarged on the anterior or PA chest film. Of particular diagnostic value is the presence of calcification in the aortic arch. If present, the outer border of the aorta can be seen to be displaced by more than 0.75 cm from the inner border. Other suggestive findings include a widened mediastinum, downward displacement of the left bronchus, upward displacement of the right bronchus, and deviation of the esophagus to the right as indicated by a nasogastric tube.[11] A chest radiograph will not show the septum between the true and false lumina unless it is calcified. The presence of a left pleural effusion is also indicative of aortic dissection. It should be recalled that chest radiographs of supine patients or of larger patients may be misleading in falsely indicating a widened mediastinum.[11]

On one occasion, we saw a patient in the emergency room with chest pain and an enlarged aortic knuckle that was observed on a radiograph of the chest. Two aortograms, a computed tomography (CT) scan, and a magnetic resonance imaging (MRI) scan, however, were all falsely negative. Although transesophageal echocardiography (TEE) was not used, it undoubtedly would also have been negative according to the operative findings. On the basis of the chest radiograph and aspiration of a bloody effusion from the left side of the chest, the patient was taken to the operating room, where a distal aortic dissection was found and repaired. The intramural hematoma in the aorta was only 2 mm wide and therefore the preoperative tests were unable to detect the aortic dissection.[11]

CT Scans

The diagnosis of aortic dissection is made by searching for a septum between the true and false aortic lumina by the use of CT scans, particularly when contrast is used. Differences in the opacification of the two aortic lumina by contrast may be detectable because of different blood flow velocities. Sometimes a thickened aortic wall will also be suggestive, even if a septum is not demonstrated (Fig. 4–13). When the false lumen is thrombosed, a septum is not seen unless it is calcified (see Chapter 2.) Care should

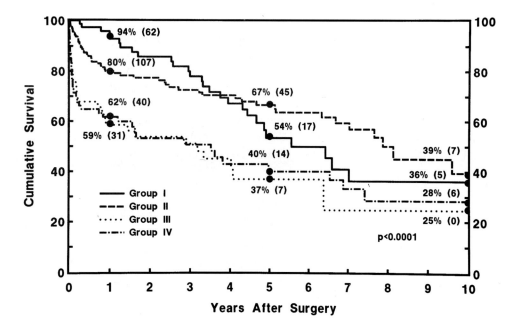

FIGURE 4–12 Long-term survival for patients who underwent distal aortic operations according to the preoperative symptom grading (includes operative in-hospital deaths). (From Svensson LG, Crawford ES, Hess KR, et al. Circulation 1990;82(5 Supp):IV 24–38.)

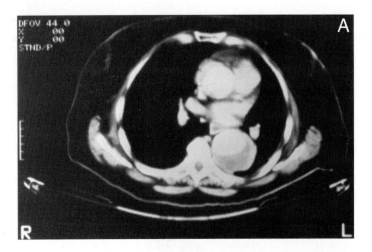

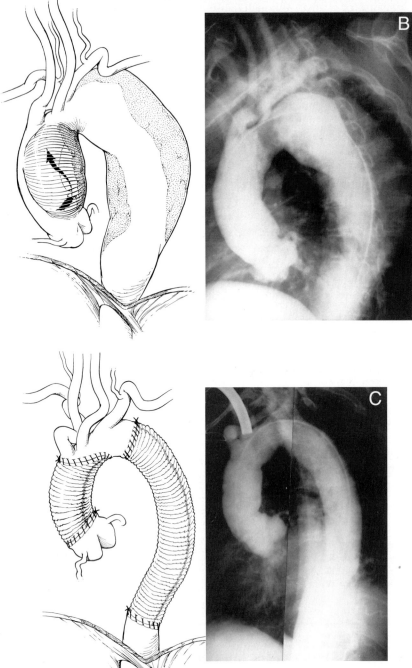

FIGURE 4–13   **A,** CT scan of patient with thrombus formation in a descending aortic aneurysm. The patient, however, was complaining of anterior chest pain and, on careful examination of the ascending aorta, an area of intramural dissection was noted on the CT scan. **B,** Left anterior oblique view of the thoracic aorta. Note the area of dissection immediately above the origin of the left main coronary artery. Note also how the thrombus in the descending thoracic aorta results in an irregular appearance of the aortic lumen. **C,** Postoperative appearance after first replacing the ascending aorta by means of deep hypothermia with circulatory arrest and then turning the patient on her side and repairing the descending aorta. (From Svensson LG, Crawford ES. Curr Probl Surg 1992; 29:915–1057.)

be taken to ensure that a streak artifact, often caused by the vertebral bodies, does not create a false appearance of a septum. A septum will tend to have a slight curvature, whereas a streak artifact is usually a straight line that can be traced back to the vertebral body. CT is very accurate in detecting calcification, and thus displacement of aortic calcium from the outer border is highly suggestive. Typically, in aneurysms of the degenerative type with thrombus formation in the aortic wall, calcium is located in the outer circumference of the aorta.[15, 48] Determination of the outer aortic diameter is important in the decision as to further management of both acute and chronic dissection.[11] Occasionally, when a patient is seen with a recurrent aortic dissection, more than one lumen may be noted on CT scans, as shown in Figure 4–13.

As discussed in Chapter 2, CT scanning has several advantages. CT scans are readily available in most institutions, the size of the aorta is accurately delimited, the true and false lumina are usually clearly seen unless the false lumen is thrombosed, the aortic wall can be assessed, and surrounding structures can be evaluated. Among the disadvantages are the fact that imaging is performed only in an axial plane (although with spiral CT this is not the case), contrast material is injected and sometimes leads to complications, the origin of branch arteries from the aorta can be difficult to determine, thrombosis of the false lumen may confuse the diagnosis, aortic valve regurgitation and cardiac function cannot be assessed, metal clips or wires may make it impossible to clearly evaluate the scan, movement of the patient will interfere with the quality of the scan, and streak artifacts (particularly from the vertebral bodies) may result in a false diagnosis. The site of the tear is usually not seen on CT, although this is of little consequence from a surgical point of view (see discussion on TEE). With the improvement in spiral CT angiography, this technique may become the preferable method in many institutions.

MRI Scans

On MRI scans, the septum appears as a linear structure of medium intensity, separating the two flow voids of the true and false lumina. If the false lumen is clotted, the false channel will not appear as a void since protons will reflect signals without exiting the imaging plane and may appear similar to thrombi in a degenerative aneurysm. Blood flow at a rate of less than 10 cm/s in the false channel will appear as an intraluminal signal. Imaging in multiple planes can be useful in detecting occlusion of arteries arising from the aorta. The presence of aortic valve regurgitation, pericardial effusion, and flow in the false lumen can also be detected. False-positive findings have been reported in 64% of MRI scans,[82] although more recent studies have found higher specificity rates.[83-85] The specificity was better than that of TEE.[83-85] Most problems that arise in diagnosing aortic dissection occur in the patient with acute dissection. As these patients are often unstable, requiring careful monitoring and blood pressure control with infusion of hypotensive agents, MRI is usually not a suitable investigative method.

The reasons for this are the prolonged scanning times required and the problems associated with metallic monitoring devices and infusion pumps within the magnetic field.[11]

TTE and TEE

The combination of transthoracic echocardiography (TTE) and transesophageal echocardiography (TEE) is reported to be very sensitive and specific in the diagnosis of aortic dissection.[83, 84, 86-90] Findings on TTE that are associated with aortic dissection include the presence of an aortic septum, a dilated aorta, widening or thickening of the aortic wall, compression of the left atrium, aortic regurgitation, and pericardial or pleural fluid.[91] TTE has a reported sensitivity of 59% and a specificity rate of 83%.[84] TEE and TTE detect associated cardiovascular complications such as pericardial effusions, cardiac tamponade, aortic valve regurgitation, localized myocardial segmental abnormalities, and aortic arch vessel occlusions. Figure 4–14 illustrates findings on TEE in a patient with ascending aortic dissection. TEE or TTE and the recognition of cardiac tamponade is discussed in Chapter 2.

TEE is reported to have a sensitivity rate of 95% to 100%.[83, 84, 87, 92] The specificity, however, is not as good as that for MRI.[83, 84] Specificity rates of 68% and 76.9% have been reported by Nienaber and associates[83, 84]; with knowledge of the false-positives, the specificity rate can be improved. Erbel and colleagues[87] assessed TEE scans in 164 patients and found the sensitivity rate for TEE to be 99% and the specificity rate 98%, with a positive predictive value of 98%. Ballal and colleagues[92] reported similar results in 34 patients, with a sensitivity of 97% and a specificity of 100%. They also reported that they were able to diagnose coronary artery involvement in 21% of patients. Goldstein and colleagues[91] have listed the criteria for diagnosing a septum.

FIGURE 4–14   CT scan showing dissection of the descending thoracic aorta. Note the three separate lumina caused by repeat dissection in a patient with Marfan syndrome.(From Svensson LG, Crawford ES. Curr Probl Surg 1992;29:915–1057.)

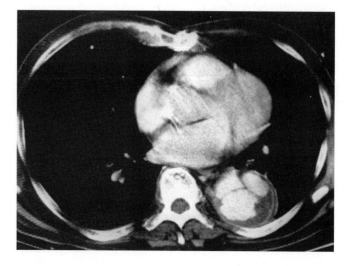

These include oscillation of the septum independent of aortic movement; visualization in more than one plane; and clear distinction from a calcified aortic annulus, aortic wall, atherosclerotic plaque, pulmonary catheters, dilatation of the sinus of Valsalva, or pericardial fluid. The addition of spectral Doppler is useful in that turbulence characteristically occurs at entry and reentry sites across the septum. Furthermore, jets typically flow from the true lumen to the false lumen during systole and from the false lumen to the true lumen during diastole. It should be noted, however, that small (approximately 2 mm wide) jets in the descending aorta are not entry or reentry sites but, rather, sites where the intercostal arteries have been sheared off, leaving small holes in the aortic septum. We have also confirmed this at the time of operation.[93] Flow rate detected by Doppler is usually slower in the false lumen. Typically, as confirmed at the time of surgery, the false lumen, particularly in the descending aorta, is larger than the true lumen. Compression of the false lumen during systole and the reverse during diastole may be seen. Swirling echodensities of spontaneous echocontrast material or thrombus may be seen in the false lumen.

From a surgical standpoint, the essential information that can be obtained from TEE is whether the ascending aorta, the arch, or both are involved by aortic dissection. TEE also shows whether aortic valve regurgitation is present and the severity of the regurgitation. Although echocardiographers place much emphasis on detecting the site of the tear, this evidence is not of primary importance to the surgeon. If an ascending aortic repair is being performed, this is usually achieved by the use of deep hypothermia with circulatory arrest, therefore, if the tear is not in the ascending aorta, it is usually visualized in the arch. Should a decision be made not to use deep hypothermia with circulatory arrest but to use moderate hypothermia instead, the aorta can be unclamped and the arch can be briefly inspected with circulatory arrest; if a tear is found in the arch or if the arch vessels are compromised, then the aorta can be reclamped. Next, the patient is further cooled down for deep hypothermia and circulatory arrest for a longer period. In those patients with type III or distal dissections, the tear site is usually observed at the left subclavian artery. If retrograde dissection is present, with involvement of the aortic arch or the ascending aorta, then the surgeon will operate on both the ascending aorta and the arch.

More recently, we have routinely used intraoperative TEE for surgical patients with aortic dissection. The advantages include ensuring that arterial perfusion through the femoral artery does not produce hemodynamic problems during bypass (for example, occlusion by the septum, functioning like a flutter valve, so that perfusion of vital organs is not maintained); detection of possible loose thrombi or atheromatous debris; and checking the repair after completion of the operation. For those patients in whom an elephant trunk type of procedure is performed, ensuring that the elephant trunk graft perfuses both the true and false lumina is of vital importance to the preservation of bowel and renal function.

Kyo and colleagues[94] found that in 13.5% of patients problems from arterial perfusion developed during type I repairs and that intraoperative TEE detected these problems and was also useful for cardiopulmonary bypass management. In two of the five patients, problems with cardiopulmonary bypass perfusion occurred with aortic cross-clamping; in three patients problems occurred with unclamping. However, the cause or site of the problem could not always be ascertained. We have noted that the malperfusion problems can be related to iliofemoral occlusive disease, the dissection septum or flap acting as a valve, or the only communication between the true and false lumina being in the ascending aorta. In the latter situation, if a clamp is applied, only one lumen or neither may be adequately perfused, resulting in organ ischemia, particularly of the brain, loss of the radial arterial line pressures, or both. Similarly, if circulatory arrest is used, which lessens the risk of the latter problem, when the pump is restarted, it will sometimes be noted that the intimal flap that has been sutured back to the outer wall bulges from perfusion of the obliterated false lumen. Should this happen, the arterial perfusion is best switched to the aortic arch via an end-to-side graft.

PROBLEMS WITH TEE

Most of the difficulties with TEE are related to imaging the distal ascending aorta. When the diagnosis is not certain, MRI can be used to exclude false-positives. The disadvantages include the learning curve required to become skilled interpreter of TEE, the difficulty in detecting fresh thrombus, the fact that TEE is invasive, and the fact that the aortic arch is poorly visualized because of the trachea.[90] Moreover, during TEE, retching by the patient is frequent and therefore tachycardia with hypertension can occur, potentially precipitating the onset of aortic rupture, as has been reported by Silvey and colleagues[95] and Nienaber and colleagues.[84] Geibel and colleagues[96] noted that in 77% of patients an increase in systolic blood pressure developed during TEE. Atrial and ventricular arrhythmias, hypotension, heart block, and arterial oxygen desaturation may also occur. Furthermore, the use of TEE cannot accurately detect the distal extent of aortic dissection in the abdominal aorta, including disease of the iliofemoral arteries. The reason for this is the problem of maintaining good contact between the probe and the gastric mucosa and also the interposing intestinal gas. Nor can dissection be diagnosed if the aorta is to the right side of the vertebral bodies. The blind spot in the distal ascending aorta and the proximal aortic arch is better visualized with the newer biplane and multiplane probes.[91]

False-positive findings and causes of artifacts include pulmonary artery catheters, echoes from the anterior wall of the left atrium, or calcium or other surrounding structures. These artifacts typically appear to traverse the wall of the aorta, or the distance between the apparent septum and the probe is twice the distance between the structure (for example, the anterior atrium) and the probe.[93] Figures 4-15 to 4-19 illustrate false-positive TEE scans. Appelbe and

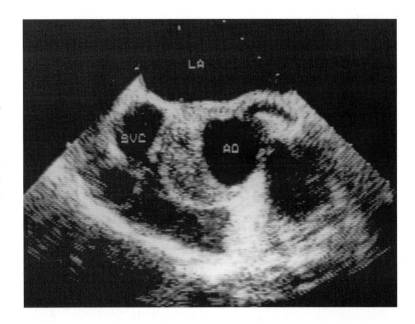

FIGURE 4–15 Transesophageal echocardiogram of the ascending aorta showing a septum separating the false lumen with thrombus in it (between *AO* and *SVC*) and the true lumen *(AO)*. *LA*, Left atrium; *SVC*, superior vena cava; *AO*, aorta. Note the left main coronary artery arising from the aorta without any evidence of dissection in the coronary artery. (From Svensson LG, Labib S. Curr Opinion Cardiol 1994;9: 191–9.)

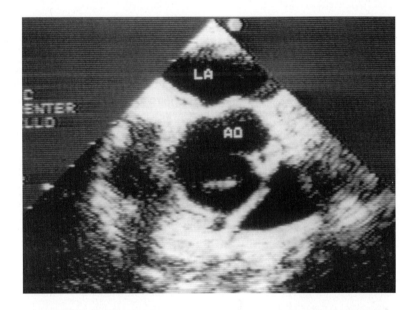

FIGURE 4–16 Transesophageal echocardiogram showing artifact in the aorta *(AO)* due to the posterior wall of the left atrium *(LA)*. Note that the distance of the false septum is twice the distance from the probe and does not extend across the entire width of the aorta. (From Svensson LG, Labib S. Curr Opinion Cardiol 1994;9:191–9.)

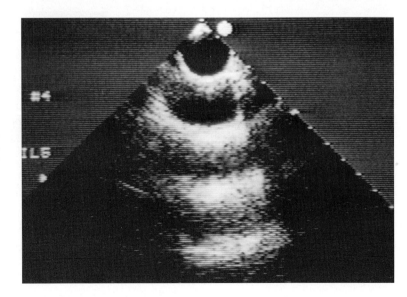

FIGURE 4–17 Transesophageal echocardiogram showing multiple mirror images of the posterior wall of the aorta. Note the regular intervals. (From Svensson LG, Labib S. Curr Opinion Cardiol 1994;9:191–9.)

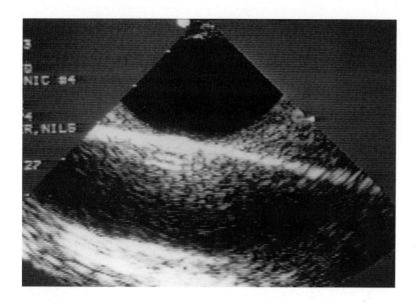

FIGURE 4–18 Transesophageal echocardiogram showing linear artifact extending across the aorta, probably due to the aorta lung interface.

colleagues[97] found that, of 36 patients with aortic disease, 44% had linear artifacts in the ascending aorta. Interestingly, these artifacts were more common in patients with aortic diameters that exceeded the left atrial diameter ($p < 0.001$). The aorta-lung interface resulted in the appearance of a double-barrel aorta in the aortic arch and the descending aorta. These mirror-image artifacts were seen in 80% of patients. Clearly, TEE alone should not be relied on if the patient is hemodynamically stable. Of concern, we are aware of cases in which patients were taken to surgery for repair of the ascending aorta on the basis of TEE findings alone but no dissection was found when the aorta was opened.

False-positive diagnoses are also associated with hiatal hernias, atelectatic lung, and simple mural thrombus.[11, 88, 89, 98] Although uncommon, false-negative images may occur with TEE. We recently encountered a patient with Marfan syndrome who had myocardial infarction and a suspected acute ascending aortic dissection that was missed on TEE but was found during cardiac catheterization and contrast study of the aorta. The presence of acute dissection was con-firmed at the time of operation and was repaired with insertion of a composite valve graft. Failure of TEE to identify a type II aortic dissection involving the distal ascending aortic blind spot has also been reported by Dacosta and colleagues.[99] Similarly, Aoyagi and colleagues[100] found that both echocardiography and angiography failed to detect an ascending aortic dissection that caused the patient's death. Thus, if there is a strong suspicion of aortic dissection, even after CT, MRI, or TEE, another imaging technique may be required to detect aortic dissection. If the patient has pain, an ascending aortic aneurysm, and aortic valve disease, the patient should undergo surgery. Of 125 patients we have operated upon recently (L.G.S.), 5 for aneurysms with pain were found to have intimal tears that had been missed by imaging studies. Intraaortic ultrasonography is also being evaluated for the diagnosis of aortic dissection.[101]

Aortography

When a patient is hemodynamically unstable, the issue arises as to which study should be done to confirm suspected

FIGURE 4–19 Transesophageal echocardiogram of the descending aorta with calcification of the aorta. Note the poor image beyond the calcium and the appearance of two layers of the aortic wall, which could be mistaken for aortic dissection.

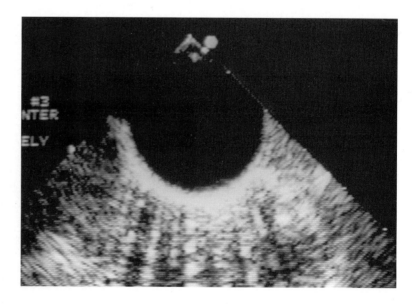

aortic dissection before one proceeds to immediate operation. Our practice has been to obtain an aortogram immediately. The diagnosis of aortic dissection by aortography is dependent on the finding of one or more of the following: an intimal tear, a nonopacified outer aortic wall more than 0.75 cm thick (particularly in the ascending aorta and aortic knuckle), a compressed true aortic lumen, an unusual catheter course (especially if it crosses over from one lumen into the other), aortic regurgitation (particularly if severe), and characteristic occlusion of branch arteries. The most sensitive of these signs is the finding that the outer aortic wall has been displaced from the opacified lumen. Care should be taken to compare this finding with the CT scan, particularly below the mid-descending thoracic aorta and further distally, where a thrombus lining an aortic aneurysm may have the same appearance. Because the outer aortic wall needs to be seen on the radiographs, subtraction angiograms frequently miss the diagnosis of aortic dissection. Thus a digital subtraction angiogram alone is not indicated. Although we are in general agreement with the radiological literature concerning the diagnosis of aortic dissection (namely, that the preferable *diagnostic* techniques are CT, MRI, or TEE), we firmly maintain that aortography is essential both for the appropriate management of patients and for the *planning* of operative procedures, unless the patients are in extremis.[11] None of the other studies, such as TEE, CT, and MRI, are currently as accurate as aortography in showing occlusion of branch arteries and compromise of blood supply to vital organs, such as the kidneys and intestines. Furthermore, if there is severe occlusive disease or dissection of the iliac or femoral arteries, cardiopulmonary bypass may not be possible through the femoral arteries. This will usually not be detected by the other studies. Figure 4–20 shows a patient with an ascending aortic dissection that had to be repaired but in whom the abdominal aorta also had to be bypassed because of occlusive disease so that the patient could be perfused with the heart lung machine. If only TEE, CT, or MRI had been obtained, the patient might not have survived the operation.

Although for most patients we use standard aortography, supplemented with either photographic or digital subtraction techniques for planning the operation, in selected patients we have recently been performing aortography at the time they undergo cardiac catheterization. Figure 4–21 shows an example of a patient in whom cardiac catheterization was used to evaluate both the aorta and the coronary arteries in planning for the operation. The question of whether the coronary arteries should be evaluated in hemodynamically stable patients before cardiovascular operations on the ascending aorta is difficult to answer. Our previous studies have shown that coronary artery disease and the need for coronary artery bypass are associated with a higher 30-day and long-term mortality rate[13, 102] (Fig. 4–22). Similar results were found by the Stanford group, although they do not believe coronary catheterization is indicated.[103] Kouchoukos and colleagues found that coronary artery bypass was necessary in 45% (23 of 51) of their patients who were operated on for acute dissection (38% because of coronary artery disease). On late follow-up, we found that patients who underwent coronary artery bypass for coronary artery disease had a better long-term survival.[13] Kern and colleagues[105] examined this problem. Of 27 patients with aortic dissection involving the ascending aorta that required urgent repair, 16 had symptoms or signs suggestive of coronary artery disease. In none of the patients who were catheterized (5 of 16 and 6 of 11, respectively) was coronary artery bypass surgery necessary. One patient with a history of coronary disease who was not catheterized had a postoperative infarct. Of 27 other patients who had distal aortic dissections, 10 had a history of coronary disease, only one of these underwent catheterization, for which the patient required coronary artery bypass surgery. In the other 17 patients, two were catheterized with no evidence of coronary artery disease. In this group also, catheterization before surgery did not appear to influence the outcome. It should be noted, however, that this study evaluated only postoperative outcome and not long-term outcome.

The studies used preoperatively for chronic aortic dissection other than those discussed here are reviewed in Chapter 2.

Summary

Barbant and colleagues[106] used Bayes' theorem to calculate predictive values and accuracies of the various diagnostic tests for the detection of acute aortic dissection based on previous reports. They found that the accuracy was influenced by the prevalence of aortic dissection in the population under study. When the prevalence was high (50%), then the positive predictive values were 86% for angiography, 99% for CT, 100% for MRI, and 99% for TEE. The negative predictive values were 94% for angiography, 85% for CT, 100% for MRI, and 98% for TEE. This resulted in an accuracy rate of 90% for angiography, 90% for CT, 100% for MRI, and 98% for TEE. If the prevalence of aortic dissection was only 10% in the group of patients under study, then Barbant's group found that angiography had only a 15% positive predictive value. They reported the positive predictive value to be 45% for CT and 50% for TEE. MRI, however, had a 100% positive predictive value even in this low-risk group of patients. The negative predictive value for this population was 100% for all the tests.[106]

Thus it appears that only MRI continues to have a 100% accuracy rate in a low-risk population, although we have seen patients in whom intimal tears have been missed by MRI. Since CT scanning is safe, generally available, and easy to interpret under most circumstances, it is currently recommended as the primary diagnostic technique. The use of CT has resulted in the earlier detection of aortic dissection and the more prompt referral of patients for operation in recent years.[13, 48] Spiral CT may further improve the accuracy of CT. Nonetheless, the increasing availability of and improvements in TEE with the use of Doppler flow probes make this the preferred method of diagnosis in some institutions.[87, 107] Cigarroa and colleagues[85] reviewed the various methods and concluded that the technique of choice should depend on the tests that are available in any particular institution and on expertise in interpreting the findings. This applies particularly to TEE. At the Lahey Clinic we use both CT and TEE, depending on which is available first, which is usually TEE. The new technology of intraaortic ultrasound examination may also become a useful adjunctive technique. At present, for planning the operative procedure, aortography is the preferred method of determining the extent of dissection, the condition of branch arteries, and evaluating aortic valve regurgitation. Furthermore, the use of aortography enables the surgeon to determine the involvement of the iliofemoral arteries by dissection or atherosclerosis or the presence of coronary artery stenoses, and hence to modify the operative strategies.[11]

For a surgeon who is considering repair of an acutely dissected aorta, the essential information required is whether the ascending aortic arch segment or only the segment beyond the left subclavian artery is involved by aortic dissection. If the ascending aortic arch is involved, clearly an anterior mediastinal approach is indicated; if only the distal aorta beyond the left subclavian artery is involved, the patient is initially treated conservatively. It is also essential to know whether the aortofemoral arteries on the side of arterial cannulation are patent. (If occluded or severely stenosed, an alternative arterial cannulation site, such as the axillary artery, subclavian artery, ascending aorta, or the ascending aorta through the left ventricle, is required, or the infrarenal aorta has to be bypassed or replaced. Other important information is whether aortic valve incompetence is present (aortic valve prolapse requires commissure resuspension or aortic valve replacement) and whether significant cardiac tamponade is present (cardiac tamponade with severe hemodynamic instability or hypotension requires immediate drain-

FIGURE 4–20   Patient with aortic dissection and severe occlusive disease of the iliac artery. An aorto-bi-iliac bypass was performed first and then the ascending aorta was repaired with the use of one of the aorto-bi-iliac graft limbs for arterial blood infusion from the heart lung machine.

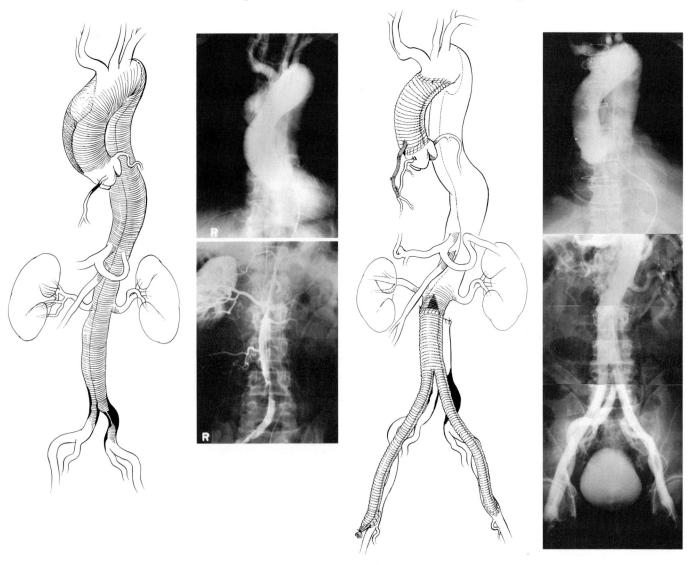

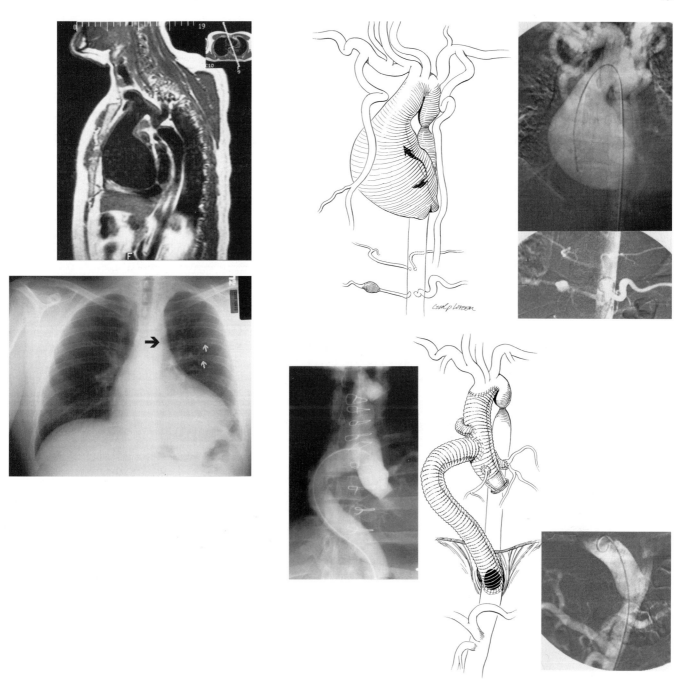

FIGURE 4–21 Diagnostic studies in a young male patient with shortness of breath and chest pain. Clinical examination revealed radiofemoral pulse delay with weak femoral pulses, distant heart sounds, and aortic valve regurgitation. Chest radiograph *(above)* revealed a reversed 3 sign at the aortic knuckle *(black arrow)* suggesting aortic coarctation. This is further supported by erosion of the ribs *(white arrows)*. Note that the heart shadow, particularly below the aortic knuckle, is globular in shape, suggesting a pericardial effusion. On chest radiographs in patients with ascending aortic aneurysms, the left heart shadow is often more prominent and the heart is displaced (pushed) downward and to the left, as in this patient. The reason for this is that an aneurysm not only increases in diameter but, particularly when the aneurysm reaches larger diameters, also lengthens the aorta, thus causing displacement of the heart downward and to the left. Descending thoracic or thoracoabdominal aneurysms are seen as a bulge to the left of the descending aorta or as a shadow behind the heart. The MRI *(upper left window)* clearly shows coarctation of the aorta below the left subclavian artery and an ascending aortic aneurysm. Because the segment involving the sinus of Valsalva and ascending aorta is continuous with a flask or a wine-skin appearance, with loss of the sinotubular ridge, this is known as annuloaortic ectasia. There is severe displacement of the heart, with evidence of pericardial fluid. Cardiac catheterization, including aortogram *(upper right window)*, revealed a posterior aortic tear indicating aortic dissection and confirmed the presence of the aortic coarctation with a 55 mm Hg gradient across it. The abdominal angiogram showed that there were small aneurysms of the intercostal arteries in keeping with late aortic coarctation. Note the enlarged internal mammary arteries. The *left lower window* is a composite diagram of the aortogram, with the *arrow* indicating the site of aortic dissection. (Reprinted with permission from the Society of Thoracic Surgeons. From Svensson LG. Ann Thorac Surg 1994;58:241–3.)

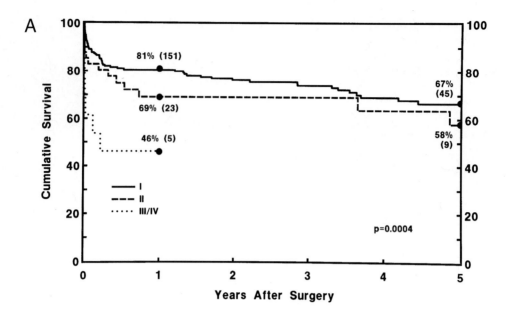

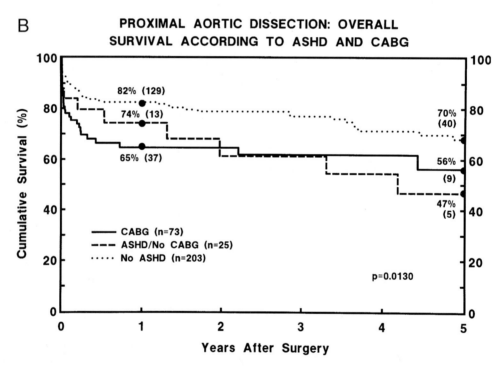

FIGURE 4–22 Influence of coronary artery disease on early survival after operation and on long-term survival as measured by preoperative New York Heart Association angina grading (**A**) and any preoperative evidence (history, symptoms, ECG, cardiac catheterization) of coronary artery disease (**B**) *ASHD,* Atherosclerotic heart disease; *CABG,* coronary artery bypass grafting. Note that patients who had atherosclerotic heart disease and underwent coronary artery bypasses had a higher initial mortality rate but a better long-term survival rate than patients without bypass operations. (From Svensson LG, Crawford ES, Hess KR, et al. Circulation 1990;82(5 Supp):IV24–38.)

age). It should be noted that, except for cardiac tamponade, aortography can provide all this required information, which is not possible with the newer techniques such as MRI with magnetic resonance angiography. Other useful but not essential information is the myocardial function, the site of the aortic tear, whether the aortic arch is aneurysmal or has ruptured, whether any of the arch vessels are occluded, which lumen supplies the kidneys (usually the false lumen supplies the left kidney), and whether intimal prolapse is present. The nonessential information should not change the operative strategy. Furthermore, much of this information is obtained intraoperatively, including inspection of the inside of the aortic arch during deep hypothermia with circulatory arrest. Thus whether or not the aortic arch requires replacement is dependent on the operative findings (see Surgical Techniques).[11]

Occasionally the patient's condition is so severe that time is not available for diagnostic studies. In these circumstances, on the basis of a high clinical index of suspicion, exploratory left thoracotomy or median sternotomy should be undertaken with intraoperative TEE.[11]

PROGNOSIS OF UNTREATED ACUTE AND CHRONIC DISSECTION

In 1934 Shennan[1] found that 40% of patients with proximal dissection died immediately, 70% within 24 hours (1% to 3% per hour), 94% within 1 week, and 100% within 5 weeks. Similarly, in 1967 Lindsay and Hurst[66] found that one third of their patients died within 24 hours, 50% within 48 hours, 80% within 1 week, and 95% in the first month. Three fourths of the deaths were due to rupture of the aorta into the pericardium, mediastinum, and pleural cavity. In patients with chronic dissection, the 5-year survival was found to be approximately 10% to 15%. In patients with distal dissection, 75% survived more than 1 month.[66] In a collected series of 963 patients reported in 1972, Anagnostopoulos and colleagues[69] reported that 70% of patients with dissection died within 1 week and 90% died within 3 months: by 3 years after dissection, only 8% of patients were alive.[11] Clearly, both aggressive medical therapy and surgery are required to improve survival rates after aortic dissection.[11]

INITIAL MANAGEMENT OF ACUTE DISSECTION

All patients suspected of having aortic dissection on the basis of clinical criteria should immediately be started on medical therapy with beta-blockers combined with vasodilators to control heart rate and blood pressure. A central line has to be placed for the administration of nitroprusside and intravenous beta-blockers. At the same time, a right radial arterial line should be inserted for pressure monitoring, and the patient should be attached to a portable ECG monitor. An indwelling urinary catheter should be inserted for urine output monitoring. Pain is usually controlled by reducing the heart rate and blood pressure, but if this fails morphine is added to any other medications that have been given for pain. Oxygen is administered by nasal cannulae and adjusted according to arterial blood gases. Administration of large volumes of fluid should be avoided, as this may dangerously raise the blood pressure with the risk of rupture, result in coagulation problems, and possibly result in respiratory complications. If large volumes are required or if the hematocrit decreases, rupture or leakage of the aorta, particularly in the abdomen, should be suspected.[11]

Beta-Blockers

Since nitroprusside will tend to increase the heart rate and also increase the force of left ventricular contraction by decreasing *afterload while increasing the dP/dt of the pulse wave,* a beta-blocker such as propranolol (Inderal) should be started prior to the commencement of nitroprusside.[13, 16, 48, 61, 71, 108] Inderal is best administered intravenously in 1 mg increments every 5 minutes until the heart rate is between 60 and 70 beats per minute. This is the most effective agent in patients with severe resistant hypertension associated with aortic dissection. With milder forms of hypertension, metoprolol (Lopressor), labetalol, or esmolol will often be effective. The advantages of using the latter two beta-blockers are that they have fewer respiratory side effects and can be administered as continuous infusions. Also, the half-life of esmolol is approximately 9 minutes, which is desirable if the effect needs to be rapidly reversed. Labetalol also has postsynaptic alpha I-receptor blockade effects, which is of value in lowering the blood pressure. Once the heart rate has been controlled, the use of metoprolol, 50 to 10 mg intravenously every 6 hours, is usually effective in maintaining blood pressure and controlling heart rate. If the patient has distal dissection and operation is not indicated, the intravenous administration should be replaced by oral administration once the patient is hemodynamically stable.[11]

Vasodilators

Nitroprusside is mixed in a concentration of 50 to 100 mg in 250 ml of 5% dextrose water and is infused at whatever rate is necessary to reduce the systolic blood pressure to below 100 mm Hg. If extremely high doses are required, then other vasodilators can be added, provided the heart rate is being controlled with beta-blockers. The effect of nitroprusside is to act directly on the arterial smooth muscle, resulting in mostly arterial vasodilatation and, less so, venous dilatation. The mechanism of action of nitroprusside is apparently independent of both the sympathetic nervous control and the renin-angiotensin system via nitric oxide. Restlessness, nausea, and somnolence are not uncommon effects of nitroprusside infusion, although far more serious are the side effects of cyanide and thiocyanate toxicity. Toxicity is indicated by vomiting, headaches, psychosis, altered mental state, confusion, restlessness, and loss of consciousness. Toxicity is confirmed by checking serum cyanide levels. Evidence of thiocyanate toxicity includes metabolic acidosis, methemoglobinemia, and hypoxia, which can be reversed by the administration of hydroxycobalamin.[16] The ganglion blocking agent, trimetaphan camsylate (Arfonad), is rarely required as a primary agent unless the blood pressure does not respond to other hypotensive agents, although good results with the use of Arfonad have been reported by Wheat.[61] The drug is prepared by mixing 500 mg in 500 ml of 5% dextrose water and infusing it at a rate 0.5 to 4 mg/min. Arfonad does, however, have significant side effects, including cholinergic effects and those of the sympathetic blockade (blurred vision, pupillary dilation, constipation, ileus, and urinary retention).[11]

Medical therapy to treat hypertension as outlined should be instituted while arrangements are being made for the diagnosis of aortic dissection. In most facilities, the latter will usually be by CT scan or TEE. Once the diagnosis has been established, we recommend aortography to plan further management if the patient is hemodynamically stable. Conversely, if aortography has been performed before referral and shows distal aortic dissection (type III), then CT scans should be obtained to confirm both the extent of dissection and the aortic diameters of involved segments. Patients with proximal dissections will require immediate operation without CT or TEE.[11]

INDICATIONS FOR SURGERY

Proximal Dissection

Acute Dissection

Most medical and surgical experts agree that acute proximal dissection should be managed with immediate operation, because fatal rupture or cardiac tamponade may occur at any time. The appropriate analogy is that of a ruptured infrarenal aortic aneurysm. In addition, in patients with evidence of severe cardiac tamponade and hypotension, a subxiphoid incision of the pericardium may be required immediately under local anesthetic to resuscitate the patient while an operating room is being prepared. However, this may result in free rupture when the blood pressure increases, and it should be done with discretion. Stroke should not be considered a contraindication to operation, since many patients will recover without a neurological deficit.[11, 13, 67]

Chronic Dissection

All patients with chronic proximal aortic dissection, irrespective of size or symptoms related to aneurysmal disease, and patients with complications of previous dissection or operations should undergo surgical repair. Similarly, if aortic valve regurgitation is moderate to severe, both surgical repair and aortic valve replacement should be performed. In patients with Marfan syndrome, a more aggressive approach is required to prevent rupture or aortic dissection. When the nondissected aorta exceeds twice the normal size, or approximately 4.7 cm in diameter, operation is indicated.[29] Similarly, if the aorta is growing at a rate of more than 1 cm per year, it should probably be repaired. It should be noted that the number of reoperations we have performed on the ascending aorta, the aortic arch, or both has increased from 29% *prior* to 1985 to 52% of patients after 1985.[11] These figures reflect the fact that initial acute proximal dissections were often done elsewhere and subsequent repairs were

needed because of aortic dissection progression, further aortic dilatation, or complications. Reoperation should be considered in those patients with previous repairs who have dissection beyond the tube graft and in whom the aorta exceeds 6 cm in diameter, either in the aortic arch or in the descending thoracic or thoracoabdominal aorta.[11]

Distal Dissection

Acute Dissection

In patients with acute distal dissection, surgery is advised if medical therapy fails to adequately control both blood pressure and pain. Moreover, surgery is recommended if pain recurs or if complications related to branch artery obstruction arise. Thus frequent indications include pain, diameter greater than 5 cm, renal failure, paresis/paraplegia, leg ischemia, bowel ischemia, bloody pleural effusion, frank rupture, and respiratory compromise. Operative repair for distal dissections, either acute or chronic, must include repair of the aorta at the origin of the dissection, usually at the left subclavian artery, irrespective of the aortic size.[11]

Peripheral Vascular Operations

The lesser abdominal aortic or peripheral vascular procedures, such as femorofemoral bypass, renal artery bypass, or aortic fenestration, are usually inadequate for aortic dissection because these procedures do not repair the origin of the acute aortic dissection and do not have a lower morbidity or mortality rate. Repair of the origin of the aortic dissection with a tube graft will, however, result in reperfusion of the true lumen, reverse more distal ischemic complications in most patients, and lower the risk of late aortic rupture.[13, 48, 67, 109] Thus, for most patients, peripheral vascular operations are not indicated, furthermore, such procedures do not reduce the risk of subsequent rupture from the aorta because residual areas of dissection and aneurysms are left behind.[13] Sometimes, however, emergency procedures are needed, as illustrated in Figure 4–8 where the patient required emergency insertion of an aortoiliac bypass to repair a rupture of the dissection in the abdomen before the rest of the aorta could be repaired,

Chronic Dissection

Operative repair should be considered in patients with distal chronic dissection associated with symptoms or with an aneurysm exceeding 5 cm in diameter in low-risk patients. It should also be considered if the annual growth rate exceeds 1 cm per year, particularly in young patients. In those patients who are a higher risk because of associated medical conditions, operation is advised on the basis of potential benefit to the individual patient versus the risk of aortic rupture.[13] If both the proximal and distal parts of the aorta are aneurysmal, the most symptomatic and life-threatening portion is treated first and the other is repaired 6 to 12 weeks later. Occasionally, if both segments are symptomatic and enlarged, then both segments have to be repaired during the same operation (see Chapter 24).[11, 13, 110]

MEDICAL MANAGEMENT OF DISTAL AORTIC DISSECTION

Once the diagnosis of acute distal aortic dissection has been established, medical therapy is continued unless indications for surgery develop. The signs are continued uncontrolled hypertension, ongoing pain, aorta diameter greater than 5 cm, evidence of leakage, and arterial branch occlusion, including renal failure. The aim of early and long-term medical treatment is to control both the blood pressure and the forceful ejection of blood from the heart by lowering *dP/dt* with beta-blockers and thus prevent aortic dilatation or rupture.

Initially beta-blocker therapy is intravenous, but this is converted to per os medication as soon as the patient is stable and can take oral medications. Propranolol in increasing intravenous doses is still the preferred initial agent, followed by metoprolol. Metoprolol can be given intravenously before it is switched to per os administration. Furthermore, metoprolol has been shown in prospective randomized studies to prevent late death associated with hypertension and myocardial infarction, and there is also some evidence that the drug increases the cross-linking of collagen fibers in the aorta.[11, 111]

Chronic obstructive pulmonary disease is common in patients with acute distal dissection, and in conjunction with the administration of Inderal, nitroprusside, morphine, sedatives, oxygen, or bedrest respiratory complications such as atelectasis and pneumonia may develop. Treatment with bronchodilators and incentive spirometry, therefore, is usually needed when distal aortic dissection is diagnosed. Not infrequently, an antibiotic and intravenous theophylline have to be added despite the drugs' side effects of increasing both myocardial contractility and heart rate.[11]

Patients with acute distal dissection should be monitored in an intensive care unit until pain and hypertension have been controlled with oral medications. Despite control of blood pressure, an occasional patient will experience rupture of the aorta 3 to 5 days after dissection when the aortic inflammatory response and repair processes are maximal. Excessive fluid requirements and a decreasing hematocrit may indicate leakage or rupture of the aorta. Repeat studies to rule out rupture or periaortic hematoma, particularly in the abdomen, may be required. In addition, urine output has to be carefully monitored, particularly in patients with chronic hypertension, since renal failure may develop. Blood pressure should be lowered as much as possible, provided that the urine output exceeds 0.5 ml/kg per hour. We recommend that systolic blood pressure be maintained at less than 100 mm/Hg. Should serum creatinine levels rise that can lead to renal dysfunction, the possible causes that should be considered include obstruction of the renal arteries by the dissection septum, excessive lowering of blood pressure, ACE blockers such as enalapril and captopril, and administration of high doses of radiographic contrast medium. If pain has been controlled, then the blood pressure may have to be allowed to rise slightly. If renal artery obstruction is

not the cause of the rise in the creatinine level, this will usually result in a decrease in the serum creatinine level. A renal radioisotope scan will usually differentiate renal artery occlusion from the other causes. Once the patient is taking a regular diet and blood pressure is controlled after some 10 days to 2 weeks, the aorta should be imaged to determine whether the aorta is aneurysmal and to establish a baseline aortic diameter. The patient can thereafter be discharged from the hospital but will have to be followed up regularly.[11]

In 1988 we reviewed our experience with the medical management of 25 patients with acute distal dissection.[21] Medical therapy failed in two patients, who then underwent successful operations. Because of their advanced age and other prohibitive risk factors, six patients were treated medically despite having aneurysmal aortas and ongoing pain. Three of these latter patients' aneurysms ruptured in the hospital, and one patient underwent surgery and required a ventilator for more than a year because of respiratory failure related to chronic pulmonary disease. The other two patients died later of untreated ruptures in nursing homes. A total of 47 patients with chronic dissection were not treated initially by surgery because one died of rupture before an operation could be performed, 31 did not require operation on the basis of size or symptoms, and in 15 the risks of surgery were considered to be too high. In 12 of the 31 (41%) in whom surgery initially was not indicated, indications for surgery subsequently developed. Eight of the 15 in whom surgery was considered too risky and was not recommended subsequently died of rupture.[11]

Kazui and Komatsu[112] examined the long-term outcome of their patients treated for acute aortic dissection. Of 83 patients with proximal aortic dissection, 47 were operated on immediately, 26 were operated on in the chronic phase, and 10 had no operations. The 10-year survival rate for surgically treated patients was 62%, which was significantly better than for those patients who did not have surgery. For the 77 patients with distal aortic dissections, 27 were operated on in the acute phase and 22 in the chronic phase, whereas 28 were treated nonoperatively. The 10-year survival rate for surgically treated patients was 64%, which was no different from medically treated patients. Neya and colleagues[113] examined the outcome of 58 patients with acute type III aortic dissection. Thirteen were treated by emergency operation, with a 69% mortality rate. Of the remaining 45 patients who were treated medically, 8% died within 2 weeks and 19% died in the chronic phase. Of the total of 42 patients treated medically, 12% died of aortic rupture although none of the 11 patients who survived surgery subsequently died of either rupture or any other cause. Of interest, of the discharged patients treated either surgically or medically, the survival rate was 83% at 5 years. If hypertension was uncontrolled, however, the survival rate was 61% compared with 96% when the blood pressure was normal. Koide and colleagues[114] examined the outcome of 74 patients with DeBakey type III dissections. Before 1987, their mortality rate was 40% for 21 patients treated with various approaches. They then chose to administer antihypertensives in treating all patients who had thrombosed false channels and they operated on patients with blood flow in the false channel. Of the 51 patients treated medically because of thrombosed false lumina, one patient died (2%) of respiratory failure. Of the 23 surgically treated patients who had a patent nonthrombosed false channel, four (17%) died of multiple organ failure. This approach resulted in an improved hospital survival rate of 92%, including both the medically and surgically treated patients. The unanswered question from this study is whether more of the surgically treated patients could have been treated medically in view of the higher mortality rate and since complete thrombosis of the false channel was noted in 69% of the patients.

Clearly, many patients with acute distal aortic dissection can be treated medically, provided that they do not have indications for surgery as described previously. It should be noted that we do not use lack of false channel thrombosis as a prerequisite for surgery. Medically treated patients must be observed closely in the chronic phase for expansion of the aorta that will require an elective operation. With the improving results of descending aortic operations,[115] an argument may be made for performing elective operations in these patients earlier rather than later.

INTERVENTIONAL CARDIOVASCULAR PROCEDURES

Various percutaneous procedures have been used to reestablish blood flow in patients who have acute dissection with malperfusion of critical arteries to organs, particularly the renal arteries and those to the lower limbs. These procedures are more appropriate for distal aortic dissections because these dissections are initially treated medically. Lacombe and colleagues[116] reported percutaneous insertion of a stent to open an occluded left renal artery. Saito and colleagues[117] reported fenestration of the intimal septum in two patients; they used a transeptal type of needle and peripheral angioplasty balloon catheters to reestablish visceral blood flow and lower limb perfusion. We have had experience with this technique in one high-risk patient with severe coronary artery disease and angina. Intraaortic ultrasound has also been used in combination with TEE to diagnose and evaluate aortic dissections.[101, 118]

SURGICAL TECHNIQUES

Principles

In their classic report, DeBakey, Cooley, and Creech[6] first reported the successful repair of aortic dissections in four of six attempts. Certain principles that they proposed in the management of aortic dissection are still relevant some four decades later.

1. Blood flow must be directed distally into the true lumen if possible.
2. The proximal extent of the descending aortic dissection should be resected. Subsequently, this was also espoused for ascending aortic dissections.[15]
3. The acutely dissected septum should be tacked to the outer wall by either a running stitch or interrupted sutures.
4. Patients with acute descending dissections who develop complications should be operated on as soon as possible.
5. Both preoperative and postoperative hypertension must be controlled.
6. Hypothermia may protect the spinal cord.
7. Patients should be closely observed postoperatively.
8. Abdominal or peripheral fenestration is not applicable for the reestablishment of branch artery occlusions.

DeBakey and colleagues[16, 15] noted that, with few exceptions, dissection commences in the ascending aorta in 75% of patients and at the left subclavian artery in most of the others and that successful surgery was dependent on excision of the proximal origin of the tear. From these seminal concepts have evolved the current methods of aortic repair.[11]

To prevent later rupture or the development of fusiform aortic aneurysms, the entire proximal part of the dissection and all distal dilated segments of aorta should be replaced by a tubular graft.[11, 13, 80] Thus, for proximal dissections, the entire ascending aorta should be replaced usually with deep hypothermia plus circulatory arrest; for distal dissections, at least the proximal half of the descending aorta (including the tear and the distal aorta dilated more than 4 cm in diameter) will have to be replaced. For both proximal and distal dissections, the aorta is transected circumferentially and the intimal septum is sutured to the outer adventitial layers so that the true lumen is reperfused and the false channel is obliterated. Galloway and colleagues[119] reported using the inclusion technique alone without transection combined with circulatory arrest. However, some of their patients were noted on postoperative studies to either have false aneurysms or blood flow outside the graft.[120]

We believe that insertion of an aortic prosthesis by direct suture is the safest technique and involves the lowest risk of recurrence or problems. Ablaza and colleagues, Lemole and colleagues, and Dureau and colleagues have reported the use of intraluminal grafts although in our experience many of these patients have required reoperation because of the formation of false aneurysms, stenosis, hemolysis, migration, and rupture.[13, 80, 121] Figures 4-23 to 4-25 illustrate postoperative problems that we have encountered after insertion of intraluminal grafts.

In summary, operations for acute dissections are therapeutic and life-saving; for chronic dissection, operations are prophylactic against later rupture; and for DeBakey type II dissections, operation can often be curative.

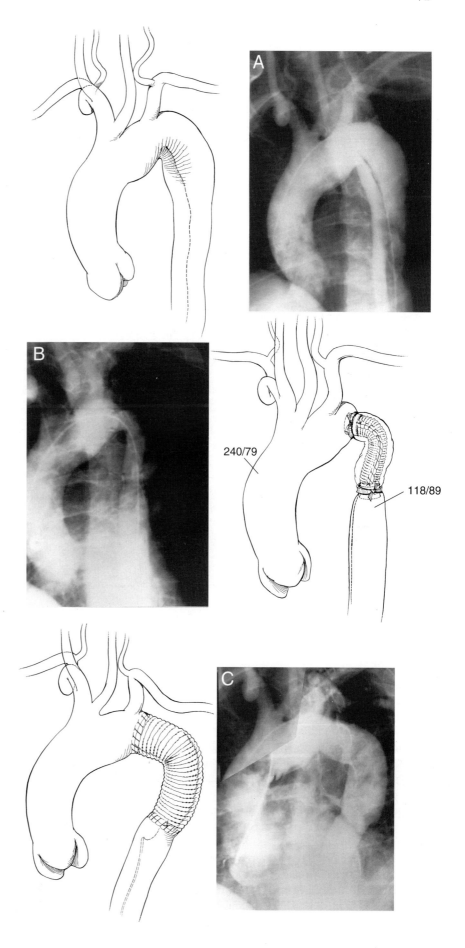

FIGURE 4–23   A, Type III aortic dissection seen at another institution and treated by insertion of an intraluminal graft. **B,** Aortogram showing the pressure gradients across the graft. The proximal pressure was 240/79, and the distal pressure was 118/89. **C,** Diagram and postoperative aortogram after reoperation and repair.

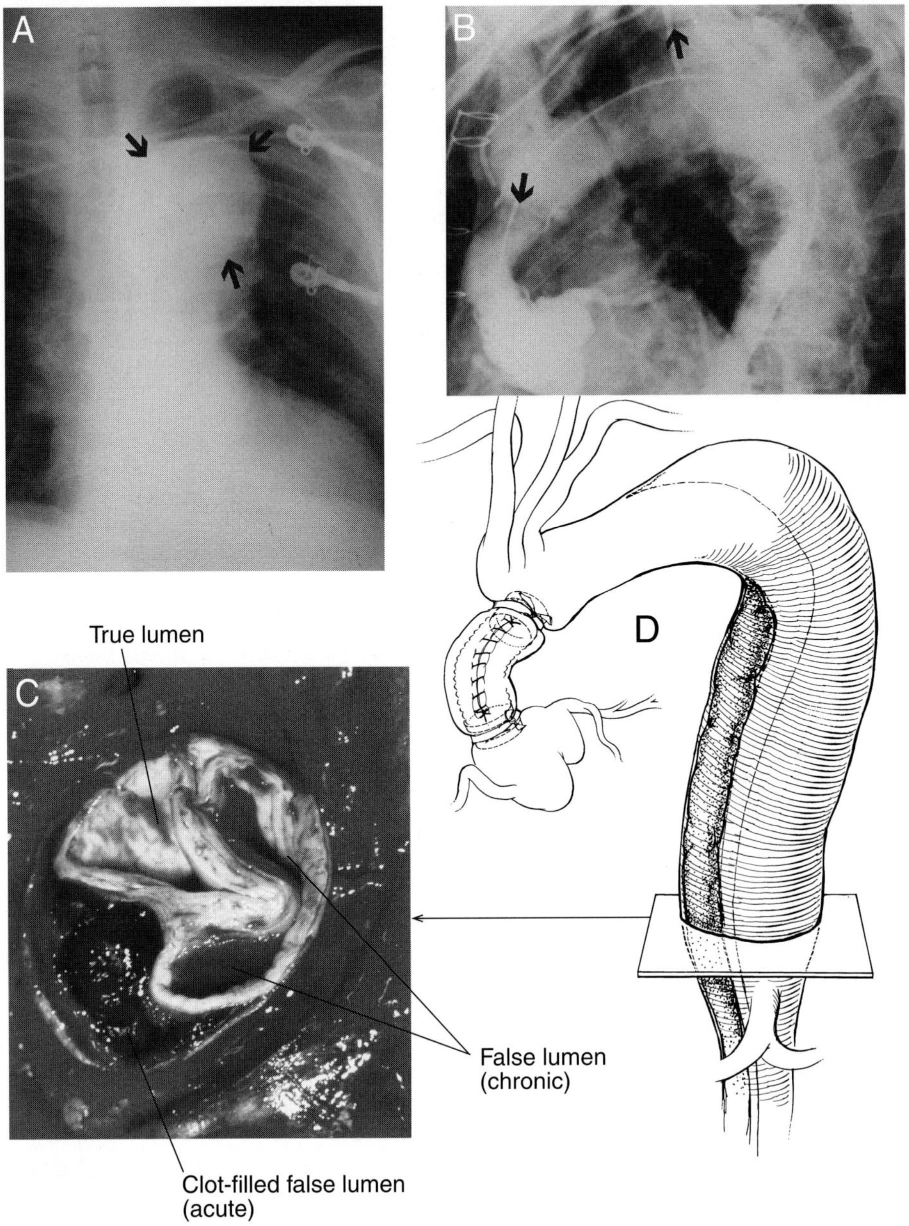

FIGURE 4–24 **A** and **B,** Aortogram after aortic dissection repair with intraluminal graft performed elsewhere. *Arrows* indicate false lumen of the outer wall of the aorta. **C,** Intraoperative photograph of operative specimen showing three separate lumina. **D,** Diagram of aorta and level of section of the specimen.

Repair of the Aortic Arch for Acute Dissection

In patients with either intimal tears or rupture of dissected aneurysms in the aortic arch, the distal extent of the repair should be extended well into the lesser curve of the aortic arch so that a complete repair can be performed. Tears of the intima in the aortic arch resulting in aortic dissection are uncommon; in our series of 82 acute dissections, we found that this type accounted for 10%.[102] Tears in the arch are not necessarily an indication for total arch replacement because a tear can sometimes be repaired with pledgeted sutures if it is small. Occasionally, the entire arch may have to be replaced by a technique that we have described.[13] On the basis of 82 patients with proximal acute dissection,[102] we believe that the indications for replacement of the entire arch are a large aneurysm in the arch, transmural rupture of the aorta, and an extensive intimal tear that cannot be repaired by pledgeted sutures. In collating the data for this study, we reviewed every operation note to identify the reason the entire aortic arch was replaced. The indications were those listed above. The overall 30-day survival rate was 83% for patients in whom only the ascending aorta was repaired, usually by the open technique with the distal anastomosis in the proximal aortic arch with a slight bevel. When the entire arch had to be repaired, however, the mortality rate increased to 31% (8 of 26). Clearly, the increased mortality rate in this latter group of patients occurred not only because of the more extensive procedure but also because repair of the dissection was a more complicated operation. Thus there were two important risk factors for the patients who had arch replacement,

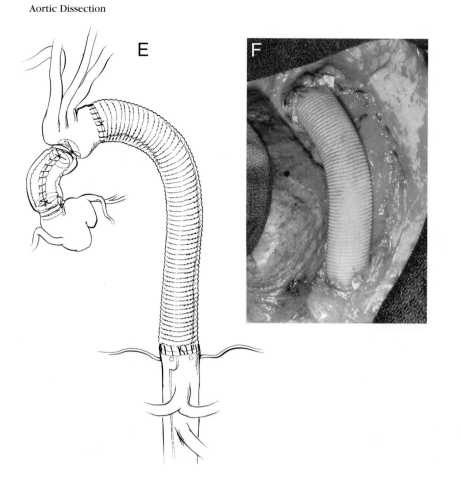

FIGURE 4–24 *Continued* **E,** Diagram of repair. **F,** Intraoperative photograph of operative repair.

namely, the more exacting surgery and the more severe antecedent problem in these patients. Therefore clinical judgment should be used to decide whether the arch needs replacement on the basis of the indications listed. If only an intimal tear in the aortic arch is present without and aneurysm or if other indications for replacement exist, then whether or not the total arch should be resected is open to debate. If possible, we repair the tear in the arch with pledgeted sutures, using the open aorta technique (see Surgical Technique).[102] By following these principles, we achieved a survival rate of 79%.

Miller[122] found no advantage to resecting intimal tears in the arch. In the combined Stanford and Duke University series, Yun and colleagues[123] reported a series of 33 patients, of whom 26 had Stanford type A and 7 had Stanford type B. Whether the arch was included or not made no difference in survival or long-term follow-up, although 9% of type A patients required a subsequent arch repair. Carrel and associates[124] prospectively evaluated 61 patients with ascending aortic dissection and found that in 80% the tear was in the ascending aorta and in 20% the tear was in the arch. The mortality rate for repairs of the ascending aorta alone using moderate hypothermia was 10% (5 of 48) compared with 20% (2 of 10) for arch repairs that were performed with deep hypothermia with circulatory arrest. Although the site of the tear was a risk factor for death ($p < 0.01$), resection of the intimal tear did not influence early mortality. Tabayashi

and colleagues[125] reported a series of 20 patients in whom they described replacement of the aortic arch for tears originating in the "ascending to arch" (nine patients), arch (nine patients), and "arch to descending" aorta (two patients). The mortality rate was 1 in 14 for partial arch repairs and 2 in 6 for complete arch replacements. The partial arch type of replacements that they performed are our standard operation for most patients with acute aortic dissections; therefore this operation cannot be used as an argument for aortic arch replacement. Their high mortality rate for total arch replacements to treat acute dissection adds support to our view that the total arch should not be routinely replaced unless, on the basis of sound clinical judgment and the factors listed above, there is an indication for replacement of the entire arch. Bachet et al.[126, 127] reported that in 10 of their patients who required reoperation to replace the aortic arch, the original tear in the arch had not been resected. Laas and colleagues[107] and Heinemann and colleagues[128] reported the use of resorcinol formol glue for the arch repair but cautioned against the toxicity of the formol glue. In our experience with 27 patients, we have found that the time required to tan the aorta adds unnecessary time to the period of circulatory arrest. Massimo and colleagues[129] advocate an even more radical approach. In 14 patients, one of whom died postoperatively (7%), they resected the entire aortic arch and performed the distal anastomosis in the descending aorta. Kirklin and Kouchoukos[130] advocated that

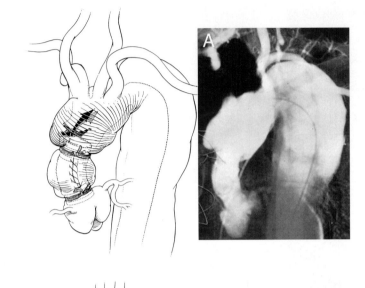

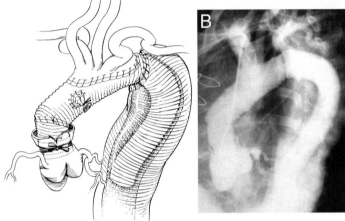

FIGURE 4–25 **A,** Attempted repair of acute dissection of the ascending aorta with an intraluminal ring. Note the stenosis caused in the ascending aorta by the prosthesis, which resulted in a significant gradient across the prosthesis and associated hemolysis. **B,** Aortogram after repair, including insertion of "elephant trunk" into the descending aorta. **C,** The patient subsequently underwent a second-stage elephant trunk procedure without incident. (From Svensson LG, Crawford ES. Curr Probl Surg 1992;29:915–1057.)

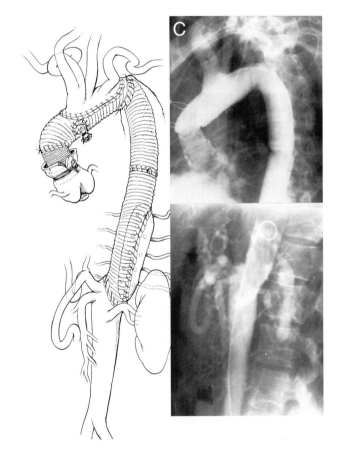

the arch should be included in the repair when the tear is in the arch, rupture of the arch has occurred, the false channel wall is tenuous, or the septum is fragmented.[11] The methods of operative repair are discussed in the relevant chapters dealing with the surgical technique.

Surgical Management of Proximal Aorta

In patients who have proximal dissection without significant involvement of the sinuses of Valsalva, the anastomosis is performed to the transected aorta immediately above the left and right coronary artery ostia. Sometimes the intima has to be tacked to the outer adventitia so that it will be easier to perform the anastomosis. When the aortic valve commissures are dissected off the aorta and the valve prolapses, the result is aortic regurgitation. The commissures are resuspended if this can easily be done in patients with acute dissection. In either patients with chronic dissection or those in whom acutely dissected valves cannot be resuspended, the valve is replaced by a prosthetic valve with preservation of the coronary ostia according to the Wheat technique.[131] We avoid the use of biologic valves because they tend to degenerate and have to be replaced, and thus the patient may be subjected to a particularly high-risk reoperation. St. Jude's composite valve aortic tubular grafts are inserted if the proximal aorta is ruptured, destroyed, or too fragile to suture or if annuloaortic ectasia exists. Coronary arteries are reattached either by mobilizing a button of the aorta with the coronary ostia or by using our modification of the Cabrol technique.[132] The latter method involves the interposing of an 8 mm Dacron tube graft between the composite graft and the coronary ostia. Figures 4–26 and 4–27 illustrate methods of operative repair with composite valve grafts. Alternatively, only the left main ostium is reattached by an interposition graft and the right coronary ostium is implanted as a button (Fig. 4–28) as described by one of us.[133] This technique is particularly useful in patients undergoing reoperation or to prevent blood loss. When the coronary arteries are involved and cannot be reattached, the ostia are oversewn and reversed autogenous saphenous vein or internal mammary artery bypasses are performed to the circumflex, left anterior descending, and right coronary arteries.[11]

Sometimes perfusion cannot be established by the femoral arteries for cardiopulmonary bypass because of either aortic dissection of atherosclerotic aortoiliac disease. Under these circumstances, we have inserted an infrarenal aortic bifurcated graft and used one limb of the graft for arterial inflow.[134] Other options include bilateral axillary artery cannulation; subclavian artery cannulation; cannulation through the apex of the heart into the ascending aorta,[135] or transection of the ascending aorta and excision of a wedge of the septum with reclamping of the aorta.[13] Gelatin-resorcin-formol glue has not been found to be particularly advantageous, although Guilmet and Bachet and colleagues reported its use and have reported a series of 105 patients with a 23% operative mortality rate and a 9% reoperation rate.[136, 137] The Cabrol fistula technique is also rarely used because the aorta is circumferentially transected as advocated by Kouchoukos and colleagues.[104, 138] This reduces the risk of late false aneurysm formation and reoperation.[121, 139] The technical aspects of surgical repairs are discussed in greater detail in subsequent chapters.

Follow-up

After operative repair, patients require careful follow-up, both to control blood pressure and to check for further aneurysmal formation. DeBakey and colleagues[15] reported that the risk of aneurysm development in the remaining aorta was 45.5% if the blood pressure was uncontrolled and 17% if the patients were normotensive postoperatively. This result was confirmed by Neya and colleagues,[113] who reported a rupture-free survival rate of 96% at 5 years for normotensive patients and a 61% survival rate for patients with uncontrolled blood pressure ($p < 0.05$). We prefer to use beta-blockers for blood pressure control to reduce both the dP/dt_{max} of cardiac contraction and the risk of further dissection requiring a repeat operation. Although we did not perform a prospective randomized study and there were undoubtedly selection factors, it is interesting how postoperative medications were associated with long-term survival (Fig. 4–29).

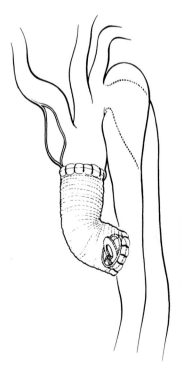 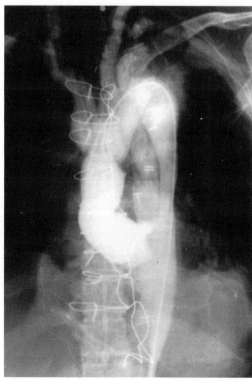

FIGURE 4–26 Postoperative angiogram revealing residual false lumen extending into the innominate artery and into the descending aorta after insertion of composite valve graft by the classic Bentall operation with wrapping of the graft. This technique is no longer used.

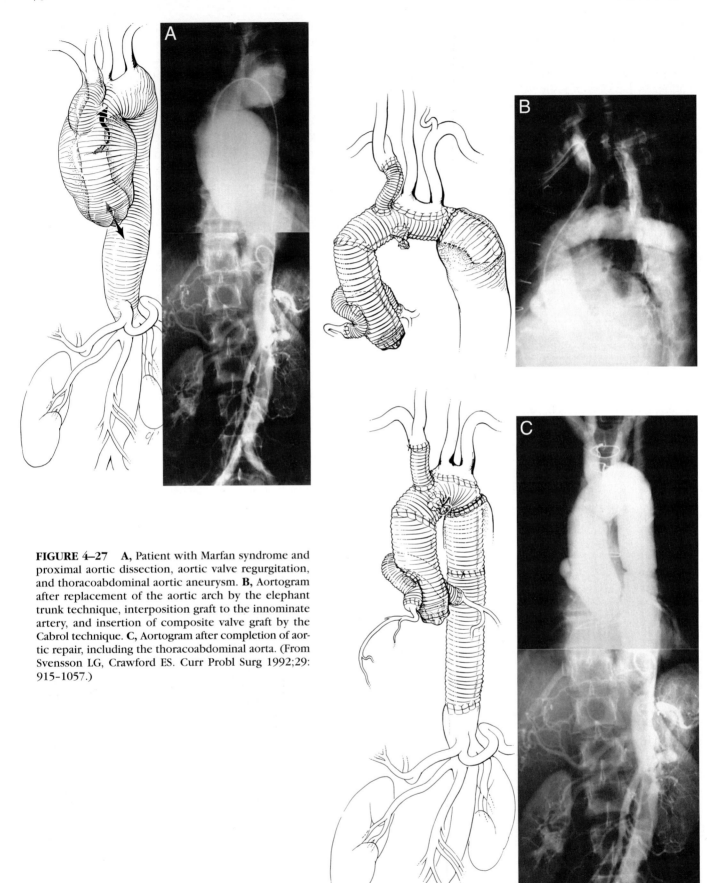

FIGURE 4–27 **A,** Patient with Marfan syndrome and proximal aortic dissection, aortic valve regurgitation, and thoracoabdominal aortic aneurysm. **B,** Aortogram after replacement of the aortic arch by the elephant trunk technique, interposition graft to the innominate artery, and insertion of composite valve graft by the Cabrol technique. **C,** Aortogram after completion of aortic repair, including the thoracoabdominal aorta. (From Svensson LG, Crawford ES. Curr Probl Surg 1992;29: 915-1057.)

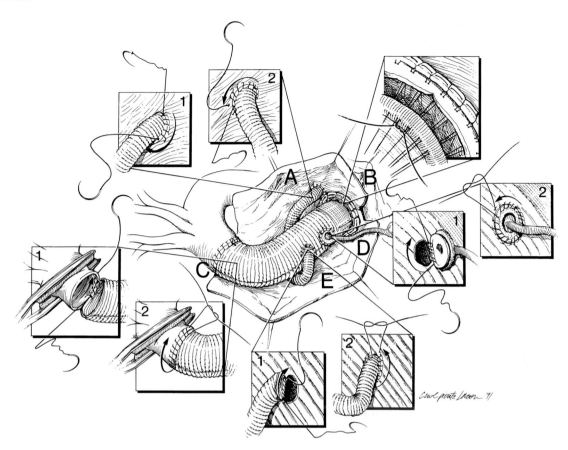

FIGURE 4–28   Currently preferred method (L.G.S.) for inserting a composite valve graft to avoid the risks of graft occlusion, false aneurysm formation, and blood transfusion. (Reprinted with permission from the Society of Thoracic Surgeons. From Svensson LG. Ann Thorac Surg 1992;54:376–8.)

FIGURE 4–29   Kaplan-Meier curve showing long-term survival according to postoperative medications in hospital survivors of aortic dissection operations. Patients either received the medications (Yes) or not (No). Medications: beta-blockers; calcium channel blockers; aspirin; coumadin.

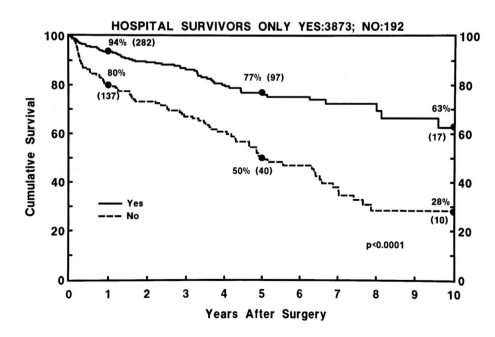

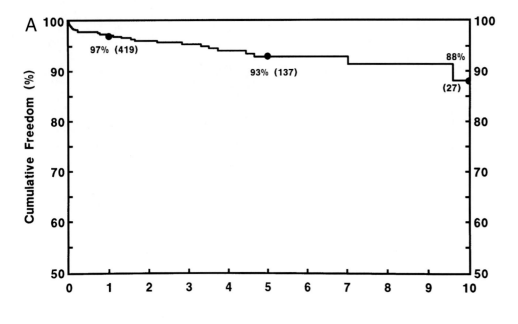

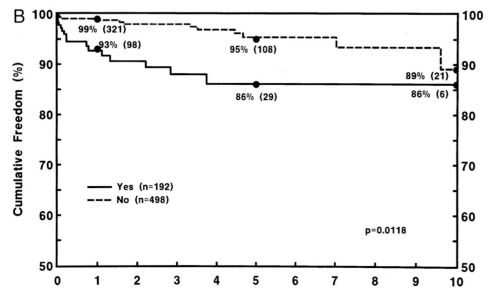

FIGURE 4–30 **A,** Kaplan-Meier curve of overall freedom from aortic rupture in all patients ($N = 432$) discharged from hospital. **B,** Overall freedom from rupture according to whether the residual aorta after the repair was dilated and aneurysmal in all patients ($N = 690$, including in-hospital deaths). **C,** Influence of residual aneurysm on survival for all patients with proximal aortic dissection and for patients recently operated on **(D).** **E,** Overall freedom from reoperation for all patients on long-term follow-up.

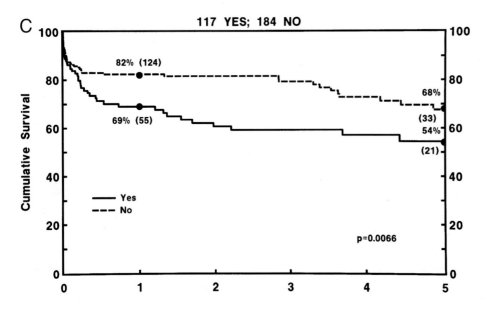

FIGURE 4–30 *Continued*

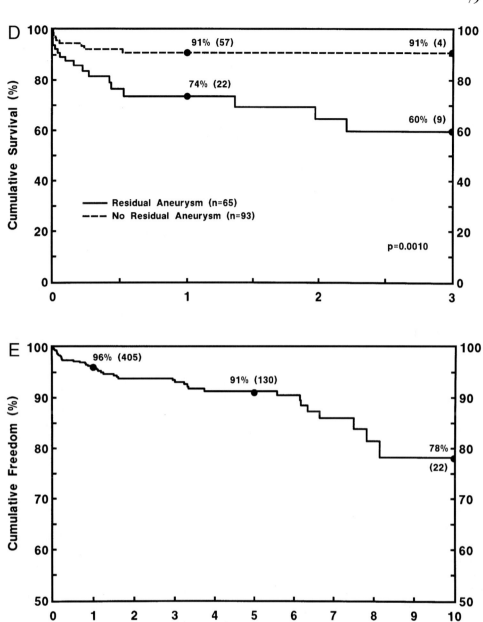

We found that if there was residual dilatation of the aorta after either ascending or ascending plus arch or descending aortic repairs, then on long-term follow-up the dilatation was a significant risk factor for aortic rupture and death (Fig. 4-30). Clearly, patients with dilated aortas after aortic dissection repair still have double lumina, usually without thrombosis. Our data, however, did not show that the risk of rupture was greater when a double lumen was present and the aorta was not dilated or aneurysmal. Thus it would appear to us that the risk of subsequent rupture is mostly influenced by the diameter of the residual aorta and probably a growth rate of more than 0.5 cm to 1 cm per year rather than the presence of a double lumen. Erbel and colleagues[140] performed a multicenter prospective study of 168 patients who had undergone operation and observed them with TEE. On follow-up after operation, 80% of type I patients had some thrombosis of the false lumen, with only 6.6%

showing complete thrombosis. Thus 93% of the patients had a residual patent false lumen; for type II repairs, 11% had a residual lumen. After medical therapy for type III dissections, 81% of type III dissection repairs showed evidence of some thrombosis in the false lumen. However, after operation for type III dissection, only 17% (2 of 12) had complete thrombosis of the false lumen. For both type II and type III dissections, 4% healed spontaneously. These data emphasize that after either medical or surgical treatment complete obliteration of the remaining dissected aorta is rare, which warrants meticulous follow-up of the aorta for possible aneurysm formation. The risk of reoperation or rupture may be higher for patients with communication between the true and false lumina or with no thrombus formation in the false lumen.[141] However, with their careful follow-up, Erbel and colleagues[140] were unable to conclusively prove that this was the case. Dinsmore and colleagues[142] also have argued that the long-term results are better if the false channel is thrombosed. It is not known whether either the size of the aorta or the presence of thrombus is the critical factor because the two factors are directly interrelated. Parenthetically, the history of vascular surgery is replete with early reports of inducing thrombosis in aneurysms that later ruptured despite the thrombus formation. Roudaut and colleagues[143] used CT, TTE, or TEE to follow-up 32 patients who had ascending aortic (25 patients) or ascending aorta plus arch (7 patients) repair for type A proximal aortic dissection. Dilatation of the ascending aorta developed in 31% of the patients. Persistence of flow in the distal false lumen was significantly ($p < 0.05$) more frequent in patients with a dilated (> 4 cm) distal aorta (7 of 9, 77%) than in those with non-dilated aortas (3 of 21, 14%), There was no apparent difference whether or not the aortic arch was repaired, although the numbers were small. Both CT and TEE were found to be consistent in size calculations, but TEE consistently underestimated the size of the aortic root (0.6 cm), ascending aorta (0.6 cm), aortic arch (1.1 cm), upper descending aorta (0.5 cm), and the lower descending aorta (0.3 cm). However, it is not clear from the study whether the internal diameter of the aorta was measured by TEE, whereas usually with CT the external diameter is measured. Of interest, in the 6 (19%) patients in whom late false aneurysms developed at the suture lines, all had been operated upon with the use of glue to reapproximate the layers of the aorta. By contrast, in none of those in whom glue was not used for repairs, some of which included Teflon when needed, did false aneurysms develop. With the Bentall technique, development of false aneurysms is not uncommon,[139] particularly in patients with Marfan syndrome.[29] We have found that false aneurysms can be detected by echocardiography.[144] Currently, our (L.G.S.) patients routinely undergo TEE after insertion of a composite valve graft. No false aneurysms have been detected at any of the anastomoses in those patients in whom the left main ostium was reanastomosed by a separate tube graft and in whom the right coronary artery was reattached as an aortic button with a Teflon doughnut.[133] We perform TEE in all patients who have had a tube graft replacement of the ascending aorta and/or arch. Rofsky and colleagues[120] examined the aorta with MRI or CT after repair by the graft inclusion technique for either aortic dissection or aneurysms of the ascending aorta. The two methods were equivalent in detecting flow outside the graft (15% versus 17%), mass effect on the graft (12% and 13%), and persistence of the false lumen after dissection repair (50% and 40%). For late follow-up, we tend to favor CT because of its greater accuracy in measuring aortic diameter and the possibility that CT is also better for detecting false aneurysms.[143] Furthermore, evidence of calcification of the aortic neointima and aortic wall may indicate a lower risk of rupture. For patients who have had ascending aorta or aortic arch repairs with prosthetic tube grafts only, we prescribe aspirin to reduce the risk of cardiac events and of stroke. Late results of aortic dissection are discussed in greater detail in Chapters 27 and 28.

In conclusion, the results of managing patients with both acute and chronic aortic dissection have improved markedly because of both earlier diagnosis and improved treatment of aortic dissection. Further improvements will depend on even earlier operation on patients with proximal aortic dissection and better determination of when patients with distal dissections need to be operated on.

REFERENCES

1. Shennan T. Dissecting aneurysms. Medical Research Clinical Special Report Series No. 193. London: His Majesty's Stationery Office, 1934.
2. Nichols F. Observations concerning the body of his late majesty, October 26, 1760. Philos Trans R Soc Lond (Biol) 1761;52:265–74.
3. Morgagni GB. De sedibus et causis morborum per anatomen indagatis libri quinque, Venice, Ex Typog. Remondiana, 1761, ep. 26 (1761). Translated from Latin by Alexander B. London: A. Miller & T. Cadele. 1769. Cited by Sailer S. Dissecting aneurysm of the aorta. Arch Pathol 1942;33:704. Reprinted with introduction by Klemperer P, 1960.
4. Laennec RTH. De l'auscultations mediate, ou traité du diagnostic des maladies des poumons et du coeur, fondé principalement sur ce nouveau moyen d'exploration. Paris: JA Brosson & JS Chaude 1819;2:411.
5. Svensson LG, Crawford ES. Aortic dissection and aortic aneurysm surgery: clinical observations, experimental investigations, and statistical analyses. Part III. Curr Probl Surg 1993;30:1–172.
6. DeBakey ME, Cooley DA, Creech O Jr. Surgical considerations of dissecting aneurysms of the aorta. Ann Surg 1955;142:586–92.
7. Gurin D, Bulmer JW, Derby R. Dissecting aneurysm of aorta: diagnosis and operative relief of acute arterial obstruction due to this cause. New York State J Med 1935;35:1200–2.
8. Shaw RS. Acute dissecting aortic aneurysm: treatment by fenestration of the internal wall of the aneurysm. N Engl J Med 1955;253:331–3.
9. Morris GC Jr, Henly WS, DeBakey ME. Correction of acute dissecting aneurysm of aorta with valvular insufficiency. JAMA 1963;184:63–4.
10. Lawrie GM, Morris GC Jr. Fifteen-year follow-up of emergency operation for acute dissecting aneurysm of the aorta with aortic insufficiency. JAMA 1978;239:724–5.
11. Svensson LG, Crawford ES. Aortic dissection and aortic aneurysm surgery: clinical observations, experimental investigations, and statistical analyses. Part II. Curr Probl Surg 1992;29:915–1057.
12. Hirst AE Jr, Johns VJ Jr, Klime SW Sr. Dissecting aneurysm of the aorta: a review of 505 cases. Medicine (Baltimore) 1958;37:217–79.
13. Svensson LG, Crawford ES, Hess KR, et al. Dissection of the aorta and dissecting aortic aneurysms: Improving early and long-term surgical results. Circulation 1990;82(5 Supp):IV 24–38.
14. DeBakey ME, Henley WS, Cooley DA, et al. Surgical management of dissecting aneurysms of the aorta. J Thorac Cardiovasc Surg 1965;49:130–49.
15. DeBakey ME, McCollum CH, Crawford ES, et al. Dissection and dissecting aneurysms of the aorta: twenty-year follow-up of five hundred twenty-seven patients treated surgically. Surgery 1982;92:1118–34.
16. Eagle KA, DeSanctis RW. Aortic dissection. Curr Probl Cardiol 1989;14:225–78.
17. Svensson LG, Coselli JS, Safi HJ, et al. Appraisal of adjuncts to prevent acute renal failure after surgery on the thoracic or thoracoabdominal aorta. J Vasc Surg 1989;10:230–9.
18. Miller DC. Surgical management of aortic dissections: indications, perioperative management, and long-term results. In: Doroghazi RM, Slater EE, eds. Aortic Dissection. New York: McGraw-Hill, 1983;193–243.
19. Miller DC, Mitchell RS, Oyer PE, et al. Independent determinants of operative mortality for patients with aortic dissections. Circulation 1984;70(Supp I):I-153–I-164.
20. Daily PO, Trueblood W, Stinson EB, et al. Management of acute aortic dissections. Ann Thorac Surg 1970;10:237–47.
21. Crawford ES, Svensson LG, Coselli JS, et al. Aortic dissection and dissecting aortic aneurysms. Ann Surg 1988;108:254–73.

22. Crawford ES. The diagnosis and management of aortic dissection. JAMA 1990;264:2537–41.

23. Crawford ES, Crawford JL, Safi HJ, et al. Thoracoabdominal aortic aneurysms: preoperative and intraoperative factors determining immediate and long-term results of operation in 605 patients. J Vasc Surg 1986;3:389–404.

24. Demos TC, Posniak HV, Marsan RE. CT of aortic dissection (review). Semin Roentgenol 1989;24:22–37.

25. Lilienfeld DE, Gunderson PD, Sprafka JM, Vargas C. Epidemiology of aortic aneurysms. I. Mortality trends in the United States, 1951 to 1981. Arteriosclerosis 1987;7:637–43.

26. Jamieson WRE, Munro AI, Miyagishima RT, et al. Aortic dissections: early diagnosis and surgical management are the keys to survival. Can J Surg 1982;25:145–9.

27. Roberts CS, Roberts WC. Aortic dissection with the entrance tear in transverse aorta: analysis of twelve autopsy patients. Ann Thorac Surg 1990;50:762–6.

28. Ponraj P, Pepper J. Aortic dissection. Br J Clin Pract 1992;46:127–31.

29. Svensson LG, Crawford ES, Coselli JS, et al. Impact of cardiovascular operation on survival in the Marfan patient. Circulation 1989;80(3 Pt 1):i233–42.

30. Nicod P, Bloor C, Godfrey M, et al. Familial aortic dissection aneurysm. J Am Coll Cardiol 1989;13:811–19.

31. Toyama M, Amano A, Kameda, T. Familial aortic dissection: a report of rare family cluster. Br Heart J 1989;61:204–7.

32. Kontusaari S, Tromp G, Kuivaniemi H, et al. A mutation in the gene for type III procollagen (COL3A1) in a family with aortic aneurysms. J Clin Invest 1990;86:1465–73.

33. Schnitker MA, Bayer CA. Dissecting aneurysm of the aorta in young individuals, particularly in association with pregnancy: with report of a case. Ann Intern Med 1944;20:486–511.

34. Pedowitz P, Perrell A. Aneurysms complicated by pregnancy. I. Aneurysms of the aorta and its major branches. Am J Obstet Gynecol 1957;73:720–35.

35. Roberts C, Roberts W. Dissection of the aorta associated with congenital malformation of the aortic valve. J Am Coll Cardio 1991; 17:712–6.

36. Abbott ME. Coarctation of the aorta of the adult type II. Am Heart J 1928;3:574–618.

37. Svensson LG. Management of acute dissection with coarctation of the aorta in single operation. Ann Thorac Surg 1994;58:241–3.

38. Pieters F, Widdershoven J, Gerardy A, et al. Risk of aortic dissection after aortic valve replacement. Am J Cardiol 1993;72:1043–7.

39. Murphy DA, Craver JM, Jones EL, et al. Recognition and management of ascending aortic dissecting complicating cardiac surgical operations. J Thorac Cardiovasc Surg 1983;85:247–56.

40. Gadaleta D, Hall M-H, Nelson RL. Cocaine-induced acute aortic dissection. Chest 1989;96:1203–5.

41. Gsell O. Wandnekrosen der Aorta als selbstandig Erkrankung und ihre Beziehung für spontan Ruptur. Virchows Arch A Pathol Anat Histopathol 1928;270:1–36.

42. Erdheim J. Medionecrosis aortae idiopathica cystica. Virchows Arch A Pathol Anat Histopathol 1930;276:187–229.

43. Schlatmann TJM, Becker AE. Histologic changes in the normal aging aorta: implications for dissecting aortic aneurysm. Am J Cardiol 1977;39:13–20.

44. Hartman JD, Eftychiadis AS. Medial smooth-muscle cell lesions and muscular arteries. Arch Pathol Lab Med 1990;114:50–61.

45. Nakashima Y, Kurozami T, Sueishi K, et al. Dissecting aneurysm: a clinicopathologic and histopathololgic study of 111 autopsied cases. Hum Pathol 1990;21:291–6.

46. Benjamin M. A dissecting aneurysm in the bulbus arteriosus of a brook stickleback, Culaea inconstans. J Comp Pathol 1985;95: 37–43.

47. Sariola H, Viljanen T, Luosto R. Histological pattern and changes in extracellular matrix in aortic dissections. J Clin Pathol 1986;39: 1074–81.

48. Crawford ES, Svensson LG, Coselli JS, et al. Aortic dissection and dissecting aortic aneurysms. Ann Surg 1988;208:254–73.

49. Prokop EK, Palmer RF, Wheat MW Jr. Hydrodynamic forces in dissecting aneurysms: in-vitro studies in a Tygon model and in dog aortas. Circ Res 1970;27:121–7.

50. Still RJ, Hilgenberg AD, Akins CW, et al. Intraoperative aortic dissection. Ann Thorac Surg 1992;53:374–9.

51. Svensson LG, Crawford ES, Hess KR, et al. Thoracoabdominal aortic aneurysms associated with celiac, superior mesenteric and renal artery occlusive disease: methods and analysis of results in 271 patients. J Vasc Surg 1992;16:378–90.

52. Peacock JA. An in vitro study of the onset of turbulence in the sinus of Valsalva. Circ Res 1990;67:448–60.

53. Gaylis H, Laws JW. Dissection of the aorta as a complication of translumbar aortography. Br Med J 1956;2:1141–6.

54. Muna WF, Spray TL, Morrow AG, et al. Aortic dissecting after aortic valve replacement in patients with valvular aortic stenosis. J Thorac Cardiovasc Surg 1977;74:65–9.

55. Stricharty SD, Gelabert HA, Moore WS. Retrograde aortic dissection with bilateral renal artery occlusion after repair of infrarenal aortic aneurysm. J Vasc Surg 1990;12:41–4.

56. Lam R, Robinson MJ, Morales AR. Aortic dissection complicating aortocoronary saphenous vein bypass. Am J Clin Pathol 1977;68: 729–35.

57. Nicholson WJ, Crawley IS, Logue RB, et al. Aortic root dissection complicating coronary bypass surgery. Am J Cardiol 1978;41:103–7.

58. Boruchow I, Iyengar R, Jude J. Injury to ascending aorta by partial-occlusion clamp during aorta-coronary bypass. J Thorac Cardiovasc Surg 1977;73:303–5.

59. Taylor P, Groves L, Loop F, Effler ID. Cannulation of the ascending aorta for cardiopulmonary bypass: experience with 9,000 cases. J Thorac Cardiovasc Surg 1976;71:255–8.

60. Orszulak T, Pluth J, Schaff H, et al. Results of surgical treatment of ascending aortic dissections occurring late after cardiac operation. J Thorac Cardiovasc Surg 1982;83:538–45.

61. Wheat MW Jr. Intensive drug therapy. In: Doroghazi RM, Slater EE, eds. Aortic Dissection. New York: McGraw-Hill, 1983:165–92.

62. Roberts WC. Aortic dissection: anatomy, consequences, and causes. Am Heart J 1981;101:195–214.

63. Wilson SK, Hutchins GM. Aortic dissecting aneurysms: causative factors in 204 cases. Arch Pathol Lab Med 1982;106:175–80.

64. Becquemin JP, Deleuze P, Watelet J, et al. Acute and chronic dissections of the abdominal aorta: clinical features and treatment. J Vasc Surg 1990;11:397–402.

65. Larson EW, Edwards WD. Risk factors for aortic dissection: a necropsy study of 161 cases. Am J Cardiol 1984;53:849–55.

66. Lindsay J Jr, Hurst JW. Clinical features and prognosis in dissecting aneurysms of the aorta: a re-appraisal. Circulation 1967;35:880–8.

67. Sarris GE, Miller DC. Peripheral vascular manifestations of acute aortic dissection. In: Rutherford RB, ed. Vascular Surgery. ed 3. Philadelphia: WB Saunders, 1989:942–51.

68. Kastan DJ, Sharma RP, Keith F, et al. Intimo-intimal intussusception: an unusual presentation of aortic dissection. AJR 1988;151:603–4.

69. Anagnostopoulos CE, Prabhakar MJS, Vittle CF. Aortic dissections and dissecting aneurysms. Am J Cardiol 1972;30:263–73.

70. Applebaum A, Karp RB, Kirklin JW. Ascending vs. descending aortic dissections. Ann Surg 1976;183:296–300.

71. Doroghazi RM, Slater EE, DeSanctis RW, et al. Long-term survival of patients with treated aortic dissection. J Am Coll Cardiol 1984;3: 1026–34.

72. Crawford ES, Saleh SA. Transverse aortic arch aneurysm: improved results of treatment employing new modifications of aortic reconstruction and hypothermic cerebral circulatory arrest. Ann Surg 1981;194:180–8.

73. Crawford ES, Walker HJ, Saleh SA, Normann NA. Graft replacement of aneurysm in descending thoracic aorta: results without bypass or shunting. Surgery 1981;89:73–85.

74. Crawford ES, Crawford JL. Diseases of the aorta including an atlas of angiographic pathology and surgical technique. Baltimore: Williams & Wilkins: 1984.

75. Glower DD, Fann FJI, Speier RH, et al. Comparison of medical and surgical therapy for uncomplicated descending aortic dissection (abstract). Circulation 1990;80(Supp IV):IV-39–46.

76. Watanabe S, Inagaki Y, Masuda Y, et al. Prognosis of dissecting aneurysms of the aorta by medical treatment. In: Strano A, Novo S, eds. Advances in Vascular Pathology. Amsterdam: Elsevier Science Publishing Co, Inc: 1989:1331–5.

77. Alexander J, Byron FX. Aortectomy for thoracic aneurysms. JAMA 1944;126:1139–45.

78. Lindsay J Jr. Aortocameral fistula: a rare complication of aortic dissection. Am Heart J 1993;126:441–3.

79. Eagle KA, Quertermous T, Kritzer GA, et al. Spectrum of conditions initially suggesting acute aortic dissection but with negative aortograms. Am J Cardiol 1986;57:322–6.

80. Crawford ES, Svensson LG, Coselli JS, et al. Surgical treatment of aneurysm and/or dissection of the ascending aorta, transverse aortic arch, and ascending aorta and transverse aortic arch: factors influencing survival in 717 patients. J Thorac Cardiovasc Surg 1989; 98:659–73.

81. Svensson LG, Crawford ES. Aortic dissection and aortic aneurysm surgery: clinical observations, experimental investigations and statistical analyses. Part I. Curr Probl Surg 1992;29:819–912.

82. Solomon SL, Brown JJ, Gazer HS, et al. Thoracic aortic dissection: pitfalls and artifacts in MR imaging. Radiology 1990;177:223–8.

83. Nienaber CA, Spielmann RP, von Kodolitsch Y, et al. Diagnosis of thoracic aortic dissection: magnetic resonance imaging versus transesophageal echocardiography. Circulation 1992;85:434–47.

84. Nienaber CA, von Kodolitsch Y, Nicolas V, et al. The diagnosis of thoracic aortic dissection by noninvasive imaging procedures. N Engl J Med 1993;328:1–9.

85. Cigarroa JE, Isselbacher EM, DeSanctis RW, Eagle KA. Diagnostic imaging in the evaluation of suspected aortic dissection. N Engl J Med 1993;328:35–43.

86. Erbel R, Mohr-Kahaly S, Visser C, et al. Diagnosis of aortic dissection: the value of transesophageal echocardiography. Thorac Cardiovasc Surg 1987;35:126–33.

87. Erbel R, Engberding R, Daniel W, et al. Echocardiography in diagnosis of aortic dissection. Lancet 1989;1:457–61.

88. Freedberg RS, Weinreb J, Gluck M, et al. Paraesophageal hernia may prevent cardiac imaging by transesophageal echocardiography. J Am Soc Echocardiogr 1989;2:202–3.

89. Kronzon I, Demopoulos L, Schrem SS, et al. Pitfalls in the diagnosis of thoracic aortic aneurysm by transesophageal echocardiography. J Am Soc Echocardiogr 1990;3:145–8.

90. Sasaki S, Matsui Y, Youda T, et al. The value and limitation of two-dimensional transesophageal echocardiography in diagnosis of dissecting aortic aneurysm. Nippon Kyobu Geka Zasshi 1989;37:2495–501.

91. Goldstein S, Mintz G, Lindsay J Jr. Aorta: comprehensive evaluation by echocardiography and transesophageal echocardiography. J Am Soc Echocardiogr 1993;6:634–59.

92. Ballal RS, Nanda NC, Gatewood R, et al. Usefulness of transesophageal echocardiography in assessment of aortic dissection. Circulation 1991;84:1903–14.

93. Svensson LG, Labib S. Aortic dissection and aneurysm surgery. Curr Opinion Cardiol (in press) 1994;.*

94. Kyo S, Takamoto S, Omoto R, et al. Intraoperative echocardiography for diagnosis and treatment of aortic dissection. Herz 1992;17:377–89.

95. Silvey SV, Stoughton TL, Pearl W, et al. Rupture of the outer partition of aortic dissection during transesophageal echocardiography. Am J Cardiol 1991;68:286–7.

96. Geibel A, Kasper W, Behroz A, et al. Risk of transesophageal echocardiography in awake patients with cardiac diseases. Am J Cardiol 1988;62:337–9.

97. Appelbe AF, Walker PG, Yeoh JK, et al. Clinical significance and origin of artifacts in transesophageal echocardiography of the thoracic aorta. J Am Coll Cardiol 1993;21:754–60.

98. Chandrasekaran K, Currie PJ. Transesophageal echocardiography in aortic dissection. J Invasive Cardiol 1989;1:6.

99. Dacosta A, Guy JM, Lamaud M, et al. Localized Type 2 dissection unrecognized by transesophageal echography: a propos of a case. Ann Cardiol Angeiol (Paris) 1992;42:35–8.

100. Aoyagi S, Akashi H, Fujino T, et al. Spontaneous rupture of the ascending aorta. Eur J Cardiothorac Surg 1991;5:660–2.

101. Weintraub AR, Schwartz SL, Pandian NG, et al. Evaluation of acute aortic dissection by intravascular ultrasonography. N Engl J Med 1990;323:1566–7.

102. Crawford ES, Kirklin JW, Naftel DC, et al. Surgery for acute dissection of ascending aorta: Should the arch be included? (See comments.) J Thorac Cardiovasc Surg 1992;104:46–59.

103. Haverich A, Miller DC, Scott WC, et al. Acute and chronic aortic dissections: determinants of long-term outcome for operative survivors. Circulation 1985;72(Supp II):II-22–II-34.

104. Kouchoukos NT, Marshall WG Jr, Wedige STA. Eleven-year experience with composite graft replacement of the ascending aorta and aortic valve. J Thorac Cardiovasc Surg 1986;92:691–705.

105. Kern MJ, Serota H, Callicoat P, et al. Use of coronary arteriography in the preoperative management of patients undergoing urgent repair of the thoracic aorta. Am Heart J 1990;119:143–8.

106. Barbant SD, Eisenberg MJ, Schiller NB. The diagnostic value of imaging techniques for aortic dissection. Am Heart J 1992;124:541–3.

107. Laas J, Jurmann MJ, Heinemann M, Borst HG. Advances in aortic arch surgery. Ann Thorac Surg 1992;53:227–32.

108. DeSanctis RW, Doroghazi RM, Austen WG, et al. Aortic dissection. N Engl J Med 1987;317:1060–7.

109. Lawrie GM. In discussion of vascular complications associated with spontaneous aortic dissection. J Vasc Surg 1988;7:207–8.

110. Svensson LG, Shahian DM, Davis FG, et al. Replacement of entire aorta from aortic valve to bifurcation during one operation. Ann Thorac Surg 1994;58:1164–6.

111. Yusuf S, Wittes J, Friedman L. Overview of results of randomized clinical trials in heart disease. I. Treatments following myocardial infarction. JAMA 1988;260:2088–93.

112. Kazui T, Komatsu S. Comparison of long-term results of surgical and nonsurgical therapy in acute aortic dissection. Nippon Geka Gakkai Zasshi 1992;93:1028–31.

113. Neya K, Omoto R, Kyo S, et al. Outcome of Stanford Type B acute aortic dissection. Circulation 1992;86(Supp II):II-1–II-7.

114. Koide S, Kanabuchi K, Inamura S, et al. Combined medical and surgical treatment of 74 cases of acute Type III aortic dissection. Nippon Geka Gakkai Zasshi 1992;93:1032–5.

115. Svensson LG, Crawford ES, Hess KR, et al. Variables predictive of outcome in 832 patients undergoing repairs of the descending thoracic aorta. Chest 1993;104:1248–53.

116. Lacombe P, Mulot R, Labedan F, et al. Percutaneous recanalization of a renal artery in aortic dissection. Radiology 1992;185:829–31.

117. Saito Y, Hirota K, Ito I, et al. Clinical and pathological studies of five autopsied cases of aortitis syndrome. Part I. Findings of the aorta and its branches, peripheral arteries and pulmonary arteries. Jpn Heart J 1992;13:20–33.

118. Iliceto S, Carella L, Chiddo A, et al. Integrated ultrasound evaluation of dissecting aneurysm of the aorta by the combined use of transesophageal echocardiography and intravascular ultrasound. Cardiologia 1992;37:555–9.

119. Galloway AC, Colvin SB, Grossi EA, et al. Surgical repair of type A aortic dissection by the circulatory arrest-graft inclusion technique in sixty-six patients. J Thorac Cardiovasc Surg 1993;105:781–90.

120. Rofsky NM, Weinreb JC, Grossi EA, et al. Aortic aneurysm and dissection: normal MR imaging and CT findings after surgical repair with the Continuous-Suture Graft-Inclusion Technique. Radiology 1993;186:195–201.

121. Crawford ES, Svensson LG, Coselli JS, et al. Surgical treatment aneurysm and/or dissection of the ascending aorta, transverse aortic arch, and ascending aorta and transverse aortic arch: factors influencing survival in 717 patients. J Thorac Cardiovasc Surg 1989;98:659–74.

122. Miller DC. Replacement of the transverse aortic arch during emergency operations for type-A aortic dissection (letter). J Thorac Cardiovasc Surg 1989;98:310–13.

123. Yun KL, Glower DD, Miller DC, et al. Aortic dissection resulting from tear of transverse arch: is concomitant arch repair warranted? J Thorac Cardiovasc Surg 1991;102:355–68.

124. Carrel T, Pasic M, Vogt P, et al. Retrograde ascending aortic dissection: a diagnostic and therapeutic challenge. Eur J Cardiothorac Surg 1993;7:146–52.

125. Tabayashi K, Niibori K, Iguchi A, et al. Replacement of the transverse aortic arch for Type A acute aortic dissection. Ann Thorac Surg 1993;55:864–7.

126. Bachet J, Teodori G, Goudot B, et al. Replacement of the transverse aortic arch during emergency operations for type A acute aortic dissection: report of 26 cases. J Thorac Cardiovasc Surg 1988;96:878–86.

127. Bachet J, Goudot B, Teodori G, et al. Surgery of type A acute aortic dissection with gelatine-resorcine-formol biological glue: a twelve-year experience. J Cardiovasc Surg (Torino) 1990;31:263–73.

128. Heinemann M, Laas J, Jurmann M, et al. Surgery extended into the aortic arch in acute type A dissection: indications, techniques, and results. Circulation 1991;84(5 Supp):iII25–30.

129. Massimo CE, Presenti LE, Favi PP, et al. Excision of the aortic wall in the surgical treatment of acute type-A aortic dissection. Ann Thorac Surg 1990;50:274–6.

130. Kirklin JW, Kouchoukos NT. When and how to include arch repair in patients with acute dissections involving the ascending aorta. Semin Thorac Cardiovasc Surg 1993;5:27–32.

131. Wheat MW Jr, Harris PD, Malm JR, et al. Acute dissecting aneurysms

of the aorta: treatment and results in 64 patients. J Thorac Cardiovasc Surg 1969;58:344-51.

132. Coselli JS. Treatment of acute aortic dissection involving the right coronary artery and aortic valve. J Cardiovasc Surg (Torino) 1990; 31:305-9.

133. Svensson LG. Approach to the insertion of composite valve graft. Ann Thorac Surg 1992;54:376-8.

134. Coselli JS, Crawford ES. Femoral artery perfusion for cardiopulmonary bypass in patients with aortoiliac artery obstruction. Ann Thorac Surg 1987;43:437-9.

135. Robicsek F, Guarino RL. Compression of the true lumen by retrograde perfusion during repair of aortic dissection. J Cardiovasc Surg (Torino) 1985;26:36-40.

136. Guilmet D, Bachet J, Goudot B, et al. Use of biological glue in acute aortic dissection: preliminary clinical results with a new surgical technique. J Thorac Cardiovasc Surg 1979;77:516-21.

137. Rahimtoola SH. The need for cardiac catheterization and angiography in valvular heart disease is not disproven. Ann Intern Med 1982;97:433-*.

138. Kouchoukos NT. Inclusion (aneurysm wrap) technique for composite graft replacement of the ascending aorta and aortic valve (letter). J Thorac Cardiovasc Surg 1988;96:967-*.

139. Svensson LG, Crawford ES, Hess KR, Coselli JS, Safi HJ. Composite valve graft replacement of the proximal aorta: comparison of techniques in 348 patients. Ann Thorac Surg 1992;54:427-39.

140. Erbel R, Oelert H, Meyer J, et al. Effect of medical and surgical therapy on aortic dissection evaluated by transesophageal echocardiography: implications for prognosis and therapy. Circulation 1993; 87:1604-15.

141. Khandheria B. Aortic dissection: the last frontier. Circulation 1993; 87:1765-8.

142. Dinsmore RE, Rourke JA, DeSanctis RD, et al. Angiographic findings in dissecting aortic aneurysm. N Engl J Med 1966;275:1152-7.

143. Roudaut RP, Marcaggi XL, Deville C, et al. Value of transesophageal echocardiography combined with computed tomography for assessing repaired Type A aortic dissection. Am J Cardiol 1992;70: 1468-76.

144. Barbetseas J, Crawford S, Safi HJ, et al. Doppler echocardiographic evaluation of pseudoaneurysms complicating composite grafts of the ascending aorta. Circulation 1992;85:212-22.

5

Marfan Syndrome and Connective Tissue Diseases

$\mathbf{M}$arfan syndrome and connective tissue diseases have a strong genetic component and are characterized by the development of catastrophic vascular complications, such as aortic dissection and rupture that, until recently, often resulted in death by the third decade of life. McKusick and his team[1] found that the most commonly encountered inherited connective tissue disorder is Marfan syndrome; the other two less frequently inherited syndromes are Ehlers-Danlos syndrome and pseudoxanthoma elasticum. More rarely, other disorders, such as osteogenesis imperfecta, polycystic kidney disease, Menkes' syndrome, alkaptonuria, homocystinuria, mucopolysaccharidoses, Noonan's syndrome, Klippel-Feil syndrome, fragile X syndrome, Turner's syndrome, familial mitral valve prolapse, and dwarfism, may have involvement of the aorta.

MARFAN SYNDROME

Marfan syndrome is an inherited disorder of the connective tissues that often evolves over time to cause heart failure and blood vessel dilatation, particularly a deterioration and eventual rupture or dissection of the aorta. Marfan syndrome is usually diagnosed in young patients, often young parents. This is unfortunate because the syndrome is inherited as an autosomal dominant trait and thus half of the progeny of an affected person will inherit the defective gene. More uncommonly, elderly patients are seen with Marfan syndrome, as we have noted in two patients in their 70s, both with a strong family history of Marfan syndrome. More rarely, neonatal Marfan syndrome may occur and is usually fatal soon after birth. In the latter patients, elastic tissue in the aorta is absent, resulting in early death, and the genetic mutation has not been characterized.

It is increasingly clear that a multidisciplinary approach to the treatment of Marfan syndrome is a prerequisite. As will be revealed in this chapter, an early knowledge of whether a child of an affected family has inherited the disorder is important for the optimal management of the disease. Evidence shows that early medical and surgical intervention for certain patients with Marfan syndrome is the best course of action. Thus a detailed knowledge of the patient's family history, particular gene mutation, and pathologic findings in the connective tissue and careful monitoring of the progression of the disease over time are of great importance.

History

In 1896 the skeletal and ocular manifestations of Marfan syndrome were described by a Parisian pediatrician.[1-4] In 1943 Etter and Glover[5] and later Baer, Taussig, and Oppenheimer[6] reported the cardiovascular manifestations of the disorder.[7] In a classic article published in 1955, McKusick[1] detailed the syndrome and the manifestations. Pyeritz and McKusick established the criteria for diagnosing Marfan syndrome in 1979[2,3] and 1980.[4]

HISTORY OF OPERATIONS

Muller and colleagues[8] first reported the direct surgical treatment of cardiovascular complications in patients with Marfan syndrome in 1960, using the techniques of aortoplasty, graft replacement, and aortic valve valvuloplasty. The successful development and application of the prosthetic valve described by Starr[9,10] for the mitral and aortic valve positions led to Groves and associates[11] reporting the use of the valves and separate tubular graft replacement of the aorta in patients with Marfan syndrome. Groves, in the discussion of their paper, commented that replacement of the entire ascending aorta with reimplantation of the coronary arteries would be needed to replace the dilated segment of the aorta between the valve and the aortic tubular prosthesis.[11] In 1964 Wheat and coauthors[12] described near total replacement of the ascending aorta in a patient with syphilis, although this technique still left some remaining aorta that could dilate. The method that Bentall and DeBono[13] introduced in 1968, involving insertion of a composite valve graft for replacement of the aortic valve and the entire ascending aorta with reimplantation of the coronary artery ostia was used by Crosby and associates[14] in 1973 in patients with Marfan syndrome. The main problems with the classic Bentall technique are the formation of false aneurysms at the aortic annulus and at the coronary artery ostia, particularly in patients with Marfan syndrome.[15-17] Excision of aortic buttons for the right and left coronary arteries and the reattachment of these buttons to the ascending aorta has been found to be a safe method, both in our experience and that of Gott[18] and Kouchoukos[19, 20] in patients with Marfan syndrome. However, control of bleeding from the left anastomoses can be difficult to achieve. Cabrol and colleagues[21] described a technique of interposing prosthetic material between the coronary ostia and the ascending graft, which allowed for easier control of intraoperative bleeding. The graft to the right coronary artery ostium, however, sometimes occluded and resulted in right ventricular dysfunction.[17] To overcome the problems with the Cabrol technique and the right coronary artery, Svensson[16] described an approach of interposing graft material to the left main coronary artery but not to the right coronary artery whereby the right coronary artery is attached as a separate aortic button buttressed with Teflon. This procedure, combined with a transaortic annulus replacement of the mitral valve without the need for any intraoperative homologous blood transfusion, was successfully performed in a patient with Marfan syndrome in August 1992.

In 1964 Dietzmann and colleagues[22] first described replacement of the mitral valve with a Starr-Edward valve in a patient with Marfan syndrome. Subsequently, in 1994, Gillinov and colleagues[23] reported mitral valve repair in 29 patients with Marfan syndrome, of whom 88% were free, by actuarial analysis, from recurrent regurgitation 5 years after surgery. Repair of the descending or thoracoabdominal aorta for either aneurysms or dissection in patients with Marfan syndrome was described, respectively, by DeBakey and associates[24, 25] in 1958 and 1965. In 1974 Crawford and colleagues[26-30] repaired the thoracoabdominal aorta by the inclusion technique and direct reattachment of the branch arteries.

Genetic Findings

Marfan syndrome is inherited as an autosomal dominant disease. Of the patients who first present with clinical manifestations of the disorder, about 70% to 85% (74% in one study of 564 Chinese patients[31]) have a family history of the disorder, with the remainder being either the result of new spontaneous mutations or, possibly, heterogeneous disease (that is, phenotypically similar manifestations that have a different genetic origin).[15] It is noteworthy that there is a higher incidence of spontaneous mutations in the progeny of an elderly father.

The gene for Marfan syndrome was first isolated to a locus on chromosome 15 (D10S45) by Kainulainen and colleagues[32] in 1990. This is the same gene (FBN1) that codes for fibrillin, the major protein of microfibrils that make up elastin fibers.[33] Fibrillin genes have been found on chromosome 15 (classic Marfan syndrome) and chromosome 5 (Marfanlike congenital contractual arachnodactyly). Elastin fibers consist of elastin protein and 10 to 20 mm fibrils. The parallel fibrils are made up of a microfibril scaffolding on which elastin is deposited. The microfibrils consist of glycoproteins, of which the most important is fibrillin.

Many unique missense, nonsense, and deletion mutations in FBN1 (the gene that codes for fibrillin) have been reported in patients with Marfan syndrome, suggesting that involvement of this gene is primarily responsible for the manifestations of Marfan syndrome.[34] Apparently, various stages of fibrillin production and incorporation into the extracellular matrix may be affected. McGookey-Milewicz and associates[35] showed that approximately one fourth of patients synthesized inadequate amounts of fibrillin, one fourth secreted fibrillin inefficiently, one fourth incorporated the fibrillin poorly into the extracellular matrix, and in the remaining patients the fibrillin defect was not defined.

The gene on chromosome 15 encoding fibrillin, a 350-kDa glycoprotein, is characterized by different missense gene mutations within the epidermal growth factor–like repeats of the gene in patients with Marfan syndrome.[36] The missense gene mutations appear to be cysteine residue substitutions within the gene[36] and, furthermore, family members within a kindred affected with Marfan syndrome exhibit the same fibrillin mutations. These observations provide further evidence of the pivotal role of the mutated glycoprotein in expression of the Marfan phenotype.

Reports reveal that fibrillin is important in determining the structural integrity of tissues by helping the organization of tropoelastin molecules into maturing elastic fibers.[37] Aoyama and colleagues[34] studied cysteine-labeled fibrillin in fibroblasts from skin samples in 55 patients with Marfan syndrome and 10 normal controls. They noted five groups of defects, which included reduced synthesis of normal-sized fibrillin, reduced deposition of fibrillin, abnormal fibrillin, and a combination of these defects. The groups were defined as follows:

I. Decreased synthesis and normal fibrillin deposition.

II. Decreased synthesis and impaired fibrillin deposition with a large percentage of abnormal fibrillin.

III. Normal synthesis of fibrillin and mildly impaired fibrillin deposition.

IV. Normal synthesis and severely impaired deposition of fibrillin with drastically reduced amounts of normal fibrillin.

V. Normal synthesis secretion and deposition of fibrillin with no noted difference between the four patients with sporadic-onset Marfan syndrome and control patients.

Curiously, the phenotypic finding of Marfan syndrome in this group of four patients without apparent fibrillin problems is not further discussed. Aoyama and colleagues[34] postulated that the disease in their patients was due to either reduction in microfibrils or an altered fibrillin product synthesized in low amounts. In 51 of the 55 patients (93%), differences in fibrillin synthesis, matrix deposition, or both were found, with 50% of the patients having group I or II defects. This high incidence of abnormal fibrillin defects may be useful for screening indeterminate patients for Marfan syndrome. Furthermore, these findings would account for the different types of fibrillin problems and the phenotypic grouping of certain clinical characteristics in affected family members, but they do not entirely explain interfamily phenotypic variation.

Thus, studies have shown that the fibrillin gene (FBN1) mutation on chromosome 15 that encodes the glycoprotein abnormality in extracellular microfibril is central to the causation of Marfan syndrome. This is further confirmed by the finding that linkage between FBN1 and classic phenotype Marfan syndrome has been observed in all families tested, suggesting that mutation in the FBN1 gene is probably the sole cause of classic Marfan syndrome. It is noteworthy, however, that the mutation in the fibrillin gene (FBN1) appears to be unique in each family and more than 50 have been found.[37] Although hopes were initially high that RFLP linkage analysis of the FBN1 gene would be useful in genetic counseling and follow-up of patients and their families, the great variability in the mutations in the FBN1 gene and thus the difficulty of finding the escort mutation in a particular family have precluded the widespread use of RFLP linkage analysis for clinical management and treatment.

Pereira and colleagues,[37] however, have developed haplotype-segregation analysis for clinical and diagnostic use in Marfan syndrome. The process involves characterizing three new intragenic sites in the normal DNA sequence and finding variations (polymorphism) that can be used as markers to follow inheritance patterns of the fibrillin gene (alleles) in patients with Marfan syndrome. The normal intragenic microsatellite polymorphisms (genetic markers) are widely interspersed in the FBN1 gene. Consequently, with typing of each family member for these genetic polymorphic markers, the inheritance pattern can be followed to determine haplotypes associated with disease-producing mutations. Although the genetic markers for the haplotype (haplotype segregation) must be determined for each family, this is considerably easier than identifying the exact mutation in the FBN1 gene.

Pereira and colleagues[37] used haplotype-segregation analysis in 14 families and found that in 11 families a definite presymptomatic diagnosis could be made in family members with equivocal clinical manifestations. Curiously, in two families, members who would have been considered to have Marfan syndrome by clinical criteria alone were found not to carry the haplotype and therefore did not have associated aortic disease. Thus patients who have mild features, such as myopia, of Marfan syndrome within affected families, may not have Marfan syndrome and thus may not be at equal risk of developing life-threatening cardiovascular manifestations. These latter patients may not require prophylactic beta-blockers and such intensive follow-up, although some watchfulness is clearly in order. Similarly, because of the great intrafamilial clinical variability of Marfan syndrome, even with the same FBN1 mutation,[36] patients who might be considered not to have Marfan syndrome by clinical criteria within an affected kindred may, in fact, be shown to be at great risk by haplotype-segregation typing criteria and thus require beta-blocker therapy as well as careful follow-up.

Histology

On histological examination of aortic wall specimens in patients with Marfan syndrome, medial degeneration of elastic tissue and medial necrosis of smooth muscle cells of the aortic wall is the usual finding.[38] In our own patients, histological study of the aorta has always revealed medial degeneration.[15] This further evidence supports the tenet that loss and disruption of elastic fibers are central to the clinical phenotype of Marfan syndrome.[33, 39] In addition, there appears to be a loss of the normal distensibility and increased stiffness of the aorta because of the loss of aortic tissue.[40] Of interest, in the usually fatal form of neonatal Marfan syndrome, the microfibrillar protein fibrillin is not only abnormal, as in adults, but is almost completely absent and is associated with a marked reduction of decorin in the extracellular matrix.[41] The genetic mutation in this form has not yet been reported.

Incidence

The prevalence of Marfan syndrome is 4 to 6 per 100,000 people,[2, 33] although in China the incidence appears to be much higher and is reported to be about 17 per 100,000.[31]

Clinical Manifestations

Until the recent advent of haplotype-segregation analysis, the initial diagnosis of Marfan syndrome has been based soley on the clinical findings at the time of presentation. The clinical manifestations of Marfan syndrome have been classified into major and minor criteria by Pyeritz, McKusick, and their colleagues.[2, 33]

The Berlin Nosology Meeting in 1986[42] established criteria for the diagnosis of Marfan syndrome based on the criteria of McKusick and Pyeritz.[2, 33] In patients with no affected primary relatives, the musculoskeletal system and at least two other systems must be involved (total of three systems) with at least one a major manifestation as identified by an asterisk (*) in the discussion that follows. If a primary relative is affected, two systems at least should be involved, with preferably one major manifestation (*), depending on the family phenotypes.[2-4, 15, 33]

Major Criteria

The four major systems are (1) ocular, (2) musculoskeletal deformities, (3) a family history of the syndrome, and (4) cardiovascular abnormalities.

1. The most common **ocular abnormality** is a displaced and subluxated lens, known as ectopia lentis,* and is present in 87% of patients (Fig. 5–1).[31] Myopia, flat cornea, elongated globe, cataracts, and retinal detachment due to an increased axial globe length may also be present.

2. The **musculoskeletal deformities** include pectus excavatum or carinatum (Fig. 5–2), long fingers and narrow fingernails (arachnodactyly in 77% of patients,[31] Fig. 5–3), joint hypermobility, including the Walker-Murdoch wrist sign,[43] recurrent dislocations (shoulder, hip, patellar), a positive Steinberg thumb sign (the maximally opposed thumb

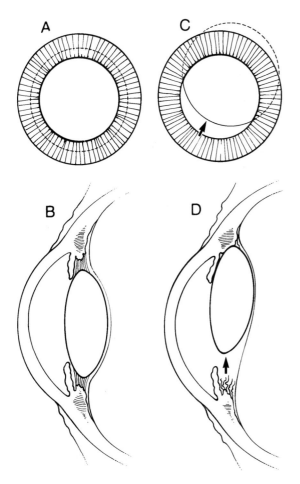

FIGURE 5–1 Illustration of centrally located eye lens (**A, B**) and (**C**) dislocated lens (ectopia lentis). **B, D** show the lateral view and how the loss of the normal suspensory ligaments of the lens results in dislocation of the lens. (From Svensson LG, Crawford ES. Curr Probl Surg 1993;30:1–172.)

protrudes beyond the other fingers wrapped around the thumb, Fig. 5-3),[44] joint flexion contractures (hammer toes), discrepancy in limb length versus torso length (dolichostenomelia), tall stature, scoliosis (72% of females, 50% of males),[45] kyphoscoliosis, thoracic lordosis, protrusio acetabulae, genu recurvatum, pes planus, spina bifida occulata or dural ectasia* (Fig. 5-4), dilated cisterna magna, lumbosacral meningocele, and narrow, high arched palate (Fig. 5-5). Typically, arm span exceeds height by 3 inches (7.62 cm). The distance between the crown of the head to the pubis is less than a ratio of 0.86 compared with the distance from the pubis to the floor in a standing patient.

3. A family history of Marfan syndrome or similar clinical characteristics in family members should be investigated by careful attention to medical family records, information from the family physician, and also by asking the patient about his or her grandparents, parents, siblings, and progeny. Approximately 25% of patients, however, report no family history of the disease and, therefore, their condition may be the result of a new spontaneous mutation in the fibrillin gene.

4. The **cardiovascular abnormalities** include mitral valve or aortic valve disease. Mitral valve prolapse (2 mm posterior mitral leaflet displacement during late systole on M-mode tracings confirmed by billowing on two-dimensional echocardiography) occurs in 90% of patients, and floppy valve, annular enlargement, or mitral valve regurgitation may be present in one third to one half, depending on age and reason for presentation. Dyspnea may be associated with mitral valve or aortic valve regurgitation (33%), although such symptoms as palpitations (50% of patients), light-headedness (25% of patients), and chest pain not due to pneumothorax or aortic dissection (75% of patients) are difficult to explain but may be partly related to mitral valve disease, including prolapse.[40] Aortic disease includes aortic valve regurgitation, a dilated aortic root* in about 80% of patients,[31] annuloaortic ectasia,* aortic dissection,* and aneurysmal disease. The severity of the damage to the aorta depends on how late patients are seen (Fig. 5-6). Roman and colleagues[45] demonstrated that generalized ascending aortic dilatation was present in 58% of males and grew more rapidly (0.11 mm/y) than in females; males usually had marked

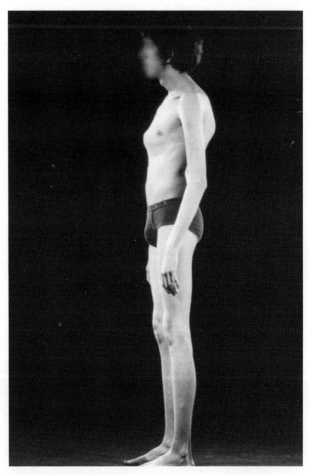

FIGURE 5–2 Patient with Marfan syndrome. Note the short chest in comparison to arm and leg length (dolichostenomelia), pectus carinatum, kyphosis, flat feet, arachnodactly, and height. (From Svensson LG, Crawford ES. Curr Probl Surg 1993;30:1–172.)

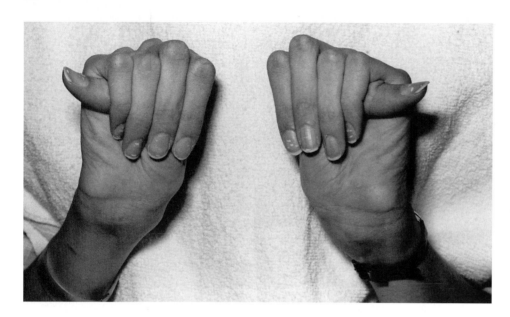

FIGURE 5–3 Positive thumb sign. (From Svensson LG, Crawford ES. Curr Probl Surg 1993;30:1–172.)

FIGURE 5–4 CT scan of patient with sacral and lumbar dural ectasia. Note also the calcified aneurysm wall (lower windows).

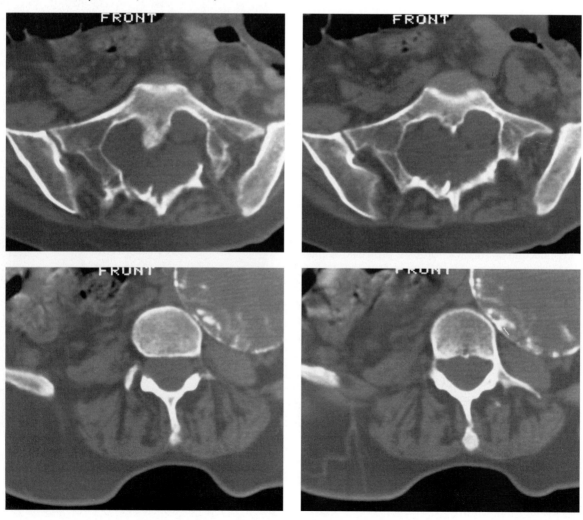

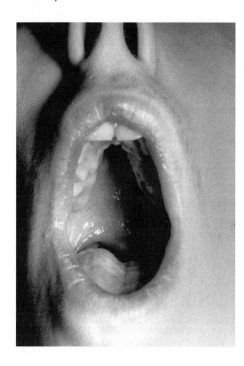

FIGURE 5–5 Narrow, high arched palate with dental crowding. (From Svensson LG, Crawford ES. Curr Probl Surg 1993;30:1–172.)

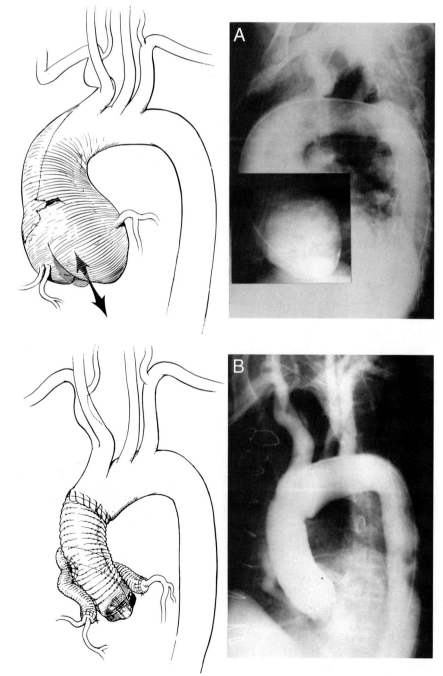

FIGURE 5–6 A, Diagram and angiogram showing limited aortic dissection (type II) associated with annuloaorticectasia and aortic valve regurgitation. B, Postoperative angiogram after insertion of composite valve graft by the Cabrol technique. (From Svensson LG, Crawford ES. Curr Probl Surg 1993; 30:1–172.)

aortic valve regurgitation (36%). Overall, in 19% of patients, or one third of those with generalized dilatation, aortic complications developed during an average of 49 months of follow-up. Of those patients in whom complications developed, 95% initially had generalized aortic dilatation. Typically, the course of progression is dilatation of the sinuses of Valsalva, followed by dilatation of the sinotubular ridge and then progressively of the ascending aorta and the aortic arch (Fig. 5-7). Rarely is the distal ascending aorta, the abdominal aorta, or the descending thoracic aorta involved first by aneurysm formation. Type III aortic dissection, however, is not uncommon (Fig. 5-8), but this is usually associated with a dilated proximal aorta (Fig. 5-9). Aortic dissection may occur at any time, particularly in patients with a family history of

aortic dissection, and it may even develop occasionally in patients with no significant aortic dilatation.[15] An important caveat is that aortic dissection in patients with the syndrome is often painless and it is not unusual to see a patient with no history of pain or hemodynamic compromise who has aortic dissection.[7]

Minor Criteria

The minor criteria include myopia, flat cornea (keratometer reading < 42), retinal detachment, cataracts, narrow chest with an acute subcostal angle, genu valgus, skin stretch marks (striae distensae), hernias (particularly inguinal), muscular hypotonia, peptic ulcer disease, cardiac arrhythmias, left ventricular diastolic dysfunction, cardiac

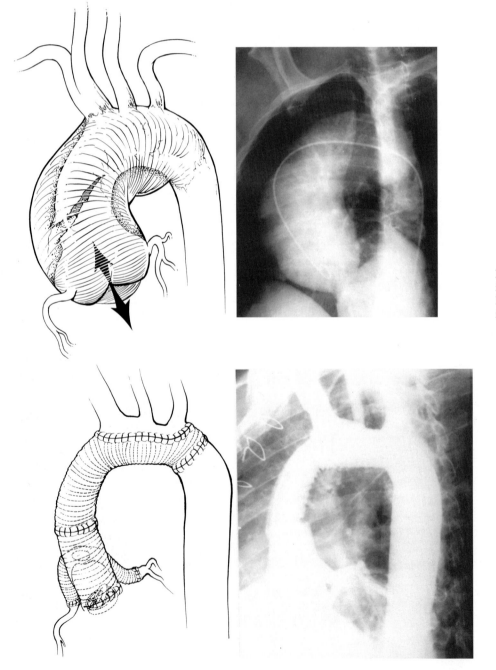

FIGURE 5–7 Dissection extending into the aortic arch repaired with hypothermic circulatory arrest and insertion of a composite valve graft.

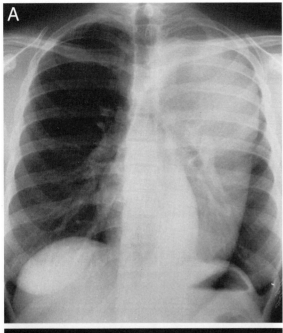

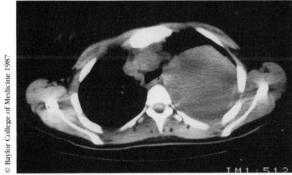

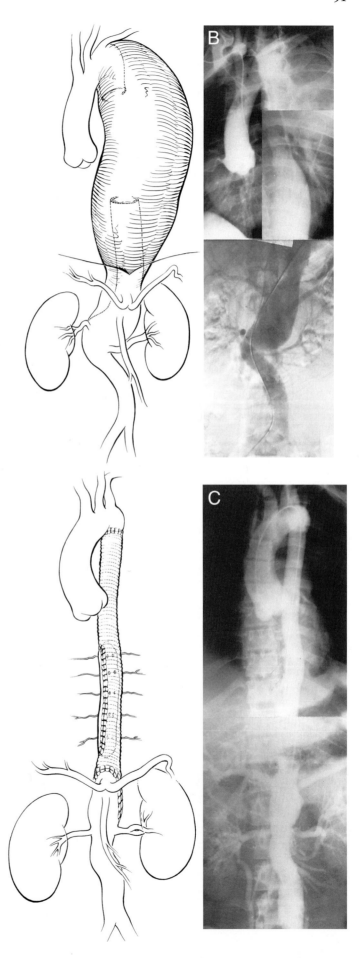

FIGURE 5–8 **A,** Chest radiograph of aneurysm occupying most of the left pleural cavity and CT scan through the chest. **B,** Angiogram showing type III aortic dissection. **C,** Postoperative angiogram after thoracoabdominal repair and reimplantation of the intercostal arteries. (From Svensson LG, Crawford ES. Curr Probl Surg 1993; 30:1–172.)

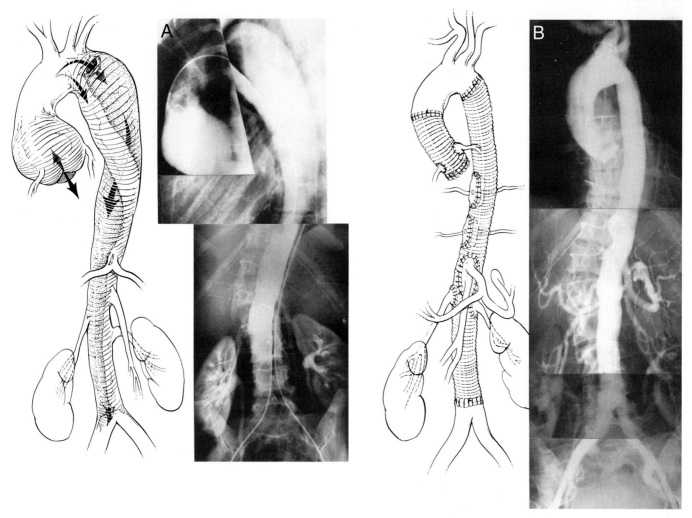

FIGURE 5–9 **A,** Angiogram of ascending aortic dilatation and aortic valve regurgitation associated with type III aortic dissection. **B,** Angiogram after repair by ascending aortic composite valve graft insertion with the button technique and thoracoabdominal repair with re-implantation of intercostal, celiac, and superior mesenteric arteries and separate attachment of renal arteries. In patients with Marfan syndrome, ostia of visceral arteries often require separate reimplantation both because the ostia are far apart and because visceral Carrel patches tend to dilate more with time in patients with Marfan syndrome. Later aneurysm formation at the Carrel patch can result in rupture or the need for reoperation. (From Svensson LG, Crawford ES. Curr Probl Surg 1993;30:1–172.)

myopathy, bleeding tendency, psychiatric problems such as obsessive-compulsive behavior, learning disability, hyperactivity, pulmonary dysfunction, spontaneous pneumothorax, apical blebs, and joint dislocations.[7, 15]

Diagnosis

For those patients who come to our Marfan Syndrome Clinic at the Lahey Clinic, we perform a full clinical examination, obtain an ophthalmologic examination if one has not been recently done, and request an echocardiogram and a CT scan with contrast of the chest and abdomen. Other findings, such as arrhythmias and orthopedic problems, may require additional screening studies. Family members, including siblings and children, are examined by our geneticist.

The cardiac and aortic surgeon should particularly look for the presence of mitral valve disease, aortic valve disease, aortic dissection, the extent of aneurysmal disease, cardiac arrhythmias, the adequacy of pulmonary function, and the patient's coagulation status.[7, 15] It should be noted, however, that patients with less severe phenotypic characteristics of Marfan syndrome may have the disease. With time, the course of the disease may progress and thus the patients require at least a yearly follow-up. If there are other affected family members within a kindred, then further genetic research, such as haplotype-segregation analysis, may confirm that these patients have Marfan syndrome.

Management

The importance of early surgical treatment of Marfan syndrome is evident from the fact that the average age at death used to be 32 years without treatment. Nevertheless, we

have seen previously untreated patients in their 70s with the syndrome, suggesting that other factors, such as the type of elastic tissue abnormality, play a role in long-term prognosis.[15] Newer and safer surgical interventions have considerably improved long-term survival, as will be discussed.[15]

A report from the Cleveland Clinic indicates that the presence of a diastolic murmur or cardiomegaly is associated with decreased survival.[46] Death usually occurs as a result of serious cardiovascular complications of the syndrome. Thus prolongation of life is dependent on both prevention and early control of complications.[15, 18] Currently, and for the foreseeable future, the only definitive method of treatment is surgical repair of cardiovascular abnormalities.[15, 18, 47]

Medical therapy with beta-blockers may retard the rate of dilatation of the aorta.[7, 33, 48] Shores and colleagues[49] randomly assigned 70 patients to beta-blocker therapy ($n = 32$) or to a control group ($n = 38$). The rate of dilatation was significantly lower ($p < 0.001$) in the treated group, and the Kaplan-Meier survival curve was better. The effect of beta-blockers may be due to the negative inotropic effect and reduced dP/dt and possibly also to increased crosslinking of collagen fibers.[50] Of interest, aortic dissection occurred in these Marfan syndrome patients with normal aortas (ratio 1:1 of Marfan patients' aorta diameter to normal) but most often at a ratio greater than 1:4 to normal. Thus the size ratio of twice the normal aorta as an indication for surgery may be too conservative.

A problem frequently encountered involves advising female patients with Marfan syndrome who wish to have children. The incidence of transfer of genes is one in two, and potential parents should be made aware of this by genetic counseling. Pyeritz[51] advises that although the risk of dissection is increased in patients with an aorta less than 4.0 cm in diameter, the risk is small. Aortic dissection, however, can occur in an aorta of any size during pregnancy, and thus frequent monthly aortic echocardiograms and blood pressure monitoring are essential. The patients should thus plan to have children early, while their aortic dimensions are smallest. An alternative is to insert an aortic homograft or, failing that, to perform either a composite valve graft with a pericardial valve or a separate biological valve with an ascending aortic tube graft. The patient should be clearly informed, however, that the repair will have to be redone at a later date. The option of a separate valve and graft makes a reoperation easier, although the risk of rupture or dissection in the sinotubular section cannot be ignored. The technique proposed by David and Feindel[52] of preserving the aortic valve but replacing the aortic wall with an inner tube graft may also be preferred in selected patients. In patients in whom the aortic root, including the sinotubular ridge, is not markely enlarged and the length of the free margin of the aortic valve cusps does not exceed that of the aortic root circumference, this technique appears to function well in early reports. Long-term results confirming continued good results would make this technique more applicable to a wider group of patients with Marfan syndrome.

From our experience, there are some principles concerning management that are worth considering. Patients with mitral valve disease or prolonged QT intervals are prone to malignant ventricular arrhythmias and sudden death, although most patients with mitral valve disease will have a progressive increase in dyspnea, warning them to seek medical advice. Therefore, we routinely screen patients with echocardiograms and perform preoperative 24-hour Holter monitoring. It should be noted that patients with mitral valve prolapse are more prone to sudden death, particularly if there is evidence of one or more of the following: the mitral valve circumference is increased, the leaflets are larger, the posterior leaflet is thickened, and extensive endocardial plaque is present.[53-57]

Of greater concern in patients with Marfan syndrome are the complications of the aorta, namely, aortic dissection, rupture, or both. Not infrequently in patients with advanced disease, aortic dissection may occur in the proximal aorta, with other segments being aneurysmal (Fig. 5-10). Aortic aneurysms most often affect the ascending aorta in young patients, and the second most frequent site of aneurysm development is the abdominal aorta. The latter usually occurs in older patients with Marfan syndrome who have undergone repair of the ascending aorta or who may have appeared to have escaped aortic complications involving the proximal aorta. We have observed an increased frequency of aortic dissection within certain identified kindreds with Marfan syndrome, and thus we recommend that these patients undergo operations earlier for ascending aortic dilatation. It is noteworthy, however, that careful examination of our patients revealed that only two of 151 developed aortic dissection without aortic dilatation being present. Although these two patients were treated with separate replacement of the aortic valve and graft replacement of the ascending aorta, the residual sinus segment dilated and required reoperation and repair with a composite graft. Consequently, although it is a rare occurrence in our experience, dissection may occur even when there is a gross appearance of a normal aorta, although at the histological level the aorta is structurally abnormal. Dilatation often occurs first in the sinuses of Valsalva, followed by dilatation of the aortic annulus above the sinuses (sinotubular ridge), and thereafter dilatation progresses distally into the ascending aorta and later the aortic arch. Patients with only sinus of Valsalva dilatation appear to be less prone to dissection and also tend to have a slower rate of dilatation (Fig. 5-11). If the entire root is dilated, however, then the rate of expansion is greater and the risk of dissection is also greater. In such patients, the dilated sinus can rupture into a cardiac chamber, usually the right ventricular outflow tract.

We firmly maintain that any operation short of composite valve graft insertion with a mechanical valve in patients with Marfan syndrome will be prone to a high rate of failure over a period of time. The reason for this is that the aorta is diseased, with medial degeneration, mucoid accumulation

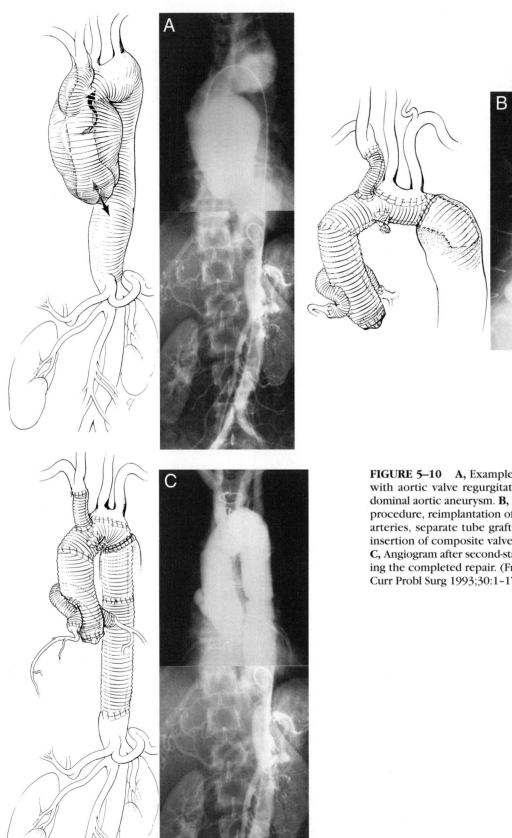

FIGURE 5–10 **A,** Example of ascending aortic dissection with aortic valve regurgitation and associated thoracoabdominal aortic aneurysm. **B,** Angiogram after elephant trunk procedure, reimplantation of the left carotid and subclavian arteries, separate tube graft to the innominate artery, and insertion of composite valve graft by the Cabrol technique. **C,** Angiogram after second-stage elephant trunk repair showing the completed repair. (From Svensson LG, Crawford ES. Curr Probl Surg 1993;30:1–172.)

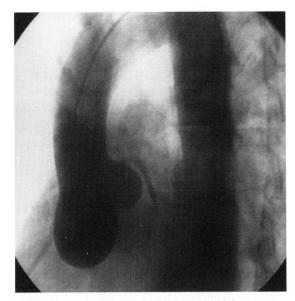

FIGURE 5–11 A 34-year-old nurse observed for several years for sinus of Valsalva aneurysm; she had a strong history of Marfan syndrome with aortic dissection. A composite valve graft was inserted with a tube graft to the left main artery and reimplantation of the right coronary artery as a button without the need for a homologous blood transfusion.

("cysts"), and smooth muscle necrosis, and the aortic valve invariably shows myxomatous degeneration. Figs. 5-12 to 5-14 show examples of operations that failed because of inadequate initial operative repairs done elsewhere.

Indications for Repair

Dissection involving the ascending aorta, particularly acute dissection, requires immediate repair. Distal acute dissections, however, are initially treated medically; however, if the patient does not respond to medical treatment or if complications arise, then the patient should undergo an operation. We tend to be more aggressive in operating earlier in these particular patients than in patients without Marfan syndrome who have type III dissection because of the younger age of patients with Marfan syndrome and their greater potential for subsequent aortic rupture and more rapid aneurysm growth rates.

Mitral or aortic valve regurgitation resulting in heart failure or left ventricular deterioration requires surgical intervention. The mitral valve may be repaired by standard techniques, or it may have to be replaced.

The rate of growth of the aortic diameter averages 2 mm per year,[58] and when this exceeds 5 to 7 mm or more per year we recommend repair. For those patients with asymptomatic aneurysms either twice the size of the normal aorta or exceeding 4.7 cm to 5 cm in diameter, we advise operative repair because of the particularly high risk of rupture or dissection in these patients.[15] These recommendations, however, should not be considered absolutes but should be influenced by the patient's gender, age, height, expected normal aortic size, rate of aortic growth, and family history of aortic dissection, as discussed later.

Clearly, knowledge of the average normal aortic size in patients with Marfan syndrome is of critical importance in establishing when surgery is necessary, especially in younger patients. Reed and colleagues[59] studied the dimensions of the aorta at the aortic root in men and women taller than the 95th percentile for height (189 cm in men, 175 cm in women). Simple linear regression showed that aortic diameter correlated significantly ($p < 0.0001$) with body surface area, height, weight, and systolic blood pressure but not with age or diastolic blood pressure. Multiple regression analysis showed that after adjustment for height ($p = 0.035$), the other variables were not significant. The equation for aortic root diameter for height was

$$\text{aortic diameter} = -45.9 + 0.493 \text{ height (cm)} - 0.001 \times 2.$$

The value of $r = 0.65$, $p < 0.0001$. For body surface area (m^2), the equation was

$$\text{aortic diameter} = -1.915 + 3.826 \text{ body area} - 0.704 \times 2$$

The value of $r = 0.52$, $p < 0.0001$. The 95th percentile or the 5th percentile were 0.75 cm greater or less, respectively, than the mean. Henry and colleagues[60] reported an equation for

$$\text{aortic root diameter} = 24 \text{ (BSA } m^2)^{1/3} + 0.1 \text{ (age)} - 4.3$$
$$\text{or} = 11.8 \text{ (weight kg)}^{0.213} + 0.1 \text{ (age)} - 4.3.$$

We find the latter equation is particularly useful in children and still growing teenagers.

FIGURE 5–12 Patient who had a circumferential aortoplasty for type I aortic dissection that required reoperation and complete repair.

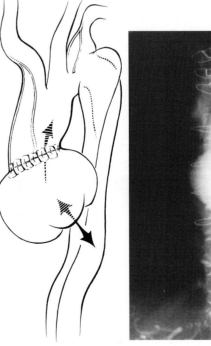

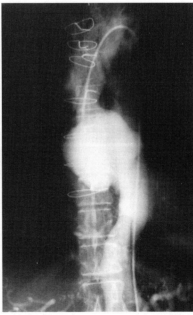

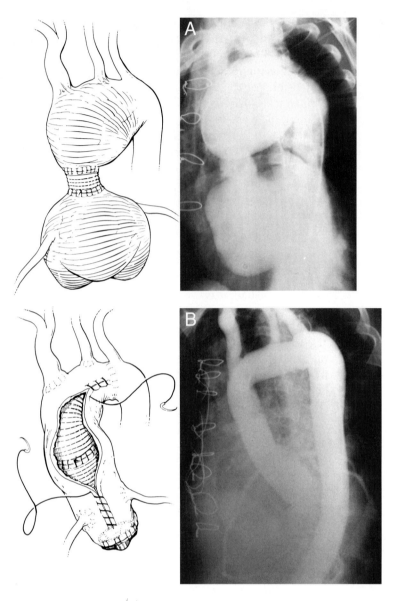

FIGURE 5–13 **A,** Patient with only ascending graft replacement complicated by later proximal root aneurysm and arch aneurysm formation. **B,** Angiogram after insertion of a composite valve graft by the button technique and replacement of the proximal aortic arch. Note the distal anastomosis between the left carotid and subclavian arteries and also the separate reimplantation of the innominate arteries because of the wide spacing between the arterial ostia.

FIGURE 5–14 **A,** Patient with separate graft and aortic valve replacement complicated by aortic root aneurysm formation and dissection beyond the previous repair. **B,** Result after insertion of composite valve graft, elephant trunk procedure, and descending aortic second-stage elephant trunk repair.

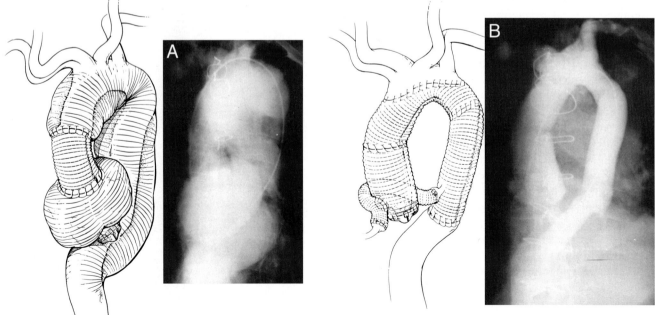

Jeremy and colleagues[61] studied the relationship between age and aortic dilatation. They found that aortic pulse pressure and velocity were greater in patients with Marfan syndrome. Also, aortic distensibility was less, and stiffness increased with age and aortic diameter. The significant independent predictors for aortic dilatation were systolic blood pressure and aortic stiffness. Thus the larger the aortic diameter, the greater the risk of rupture because of increasing pulse pressure, velocity, and loss of distensibility to accommodate cardiac systolic ejection. These changes are probably due to loss of elastic fibers. Roman and colleagues[45] have shown that initial aortic size and generalized ascending aortic dilatation are the best predictors of aortic dissection and progressive aortic regurgitation. Furthermore, higher systolic blood pressure, increased height and aortic growth rate, and older age were also associated with a greater risk. Patients with aortic complications had a supraaortic ridge size of 4 to 6 cm versus 2.9 cm in patients without complications. Treasure's group[62] observed 148 patients. Of the 11 patients who presented with aortic dissection, the average ridge size was 5.1 cm compared with 3.7 cm in those who remained well ($p < 0.05$). Pyeritz performed an analysis of 55 patients with aortic dissection (Abstract, International Marfan Symposium, 1992) and found that 36% of the patients who developed dissection had an aortic diameter less than 6 cm at the time of last follow-up. The predictors were aortic diameter and family history of dissection. These reports further support earlier surgical intervention, when the aorta is smaller, particularly now that surgery has become safer, with elective composite valve graft insertions having a 98% survival rate. Certainly, most recent reports support surgical intervention if the aorta exceeds 5 cm in diameter, but in the high-risk patient with an aorta in the 4.7 to 5 cm range, aortic surgery may also have to be considered.

Operations

The operative technique for repair of aortic aneurysms in patients with Marfan syndrome is similar to that used for other medial degenerative aneurysms and dissection aneurysms, with certain provisions (see chapters on operative techniques). Great care must be taken in suturing graft prostheses in position because the aorta is particularly prone to tearing.[15, 18] To minimize trauma to the aorta, 4–0 Prolene on a small needle (RB) is used for aortic anastomoses. Excessive postoperative bleeding, atrial and ventricular arrhythmias, and respiratory failure are potential postoperative complications.[15, 18, 47, 63] The diseased mitral valve can be either repaired or replaced, including through the aortic annulus.[15, 63, 64] The latter procedure is a relatively easy method of replacing the mitral valve. Patients with Marfan syndrome require careful long-term monitoring for the development of subsequent aortic or valvular disease since multiple operative procedures may be required to treat cardiovascular problems[15] (Fig. 5–15). Ultimately, some patients will require replacement of the entire aorta.

RESULTS

We examined the results of surgery in 151 patients who underwent a total of 280 operations.[15, 65, 66] The aortic valve was replaced in 135, the mitral valve in 13, the entire aorta was replaced in 10 (often after multiple operations, Fig. 5–15), most of the aorta in 26, and the entire thoracic aorta in seven. Despite the complexity and frequent reoperations in these patients to correct previous operations attempted elsewhere, the 30-day survival was 94% and the 5- and 10-year Kaplan-Meier analysis survival rates were 75% and 56%, respectively, with 95% in New York Heart Association class I or II. Aortic dissection was present in 102 (67%), of which 61 (60%) were type I. It is noteworthy that five patients had new acute dissections in the presence of chronic dissections. These new dissections were usually in different segments. Before surgery, 105 (70%) had aortic valve regurgitation, 76 (50%) had mitral valve prolapse, and 29 (20%) had mitral valve insufficiency. Thirty-five (23%) had preoperative ventricular or atrial arrhythmias. Ascending aortic lacerations (three acute) were found in 10 patients although frank aortic dissection was not present (Figs. 5–16 and 5–17). These lacerations may be precursors of more extensive aortic dissections. Thirty-four patients (23%) underwent reoperations because of inadequate repairs done elsewhere at the first operation, such as separate valve and aortic grafts instead of composite valve grafts, or because of complications of older operative techniques. In some patients aortic disease may also have progressed beyond the location of earlier repairs, particularly after aortic dissection type I, and required reoperation at a later date (Fig. 5–18).

Smith and colleagues[67] from Stanford University examined the results of surgical management in 40 patients with aortic dissection and Marfan syndrome. Sixteen had acute type A (DeBakey type I or II) dissection, two had acute type B (DeBakey type III), 18 had chronic type A, and four had chronic type B. Four patients died (10%)—three with acute and one with chronic dissection. Of the 15 late deaths, seven were due to aortic sequelae. Actuarial survival was 71%, 54%, and 22% at 5, 10, and 15 years, respectively. In analysis of their patients who required late reoperation, Smith and colleagues[67] also concur with us that composite valve graft insertion is the preferable procedure in patients with Marfan syndrome with ascending aortic disease, including mechanical aortic valve replacement in all patients. They suggest that a homograft aortic root replacement is an option in young female patients who are planning to have children or when Coumadin is contraindicated. In patients who have Marfan syndrome with acute type B (type III) dissection, unless otherwise contraindicated, Smith and colleagues also advocate aggressive early operation, particularly when the patients have large localized aneurysms and refractory hypertension.

We subscribe to a new, precise method for insertion of composite grafts[16, 17] that appears to avoid the problems of earlier methods by placing a graft to the left main coronary artery and using a button technique for the right coronary

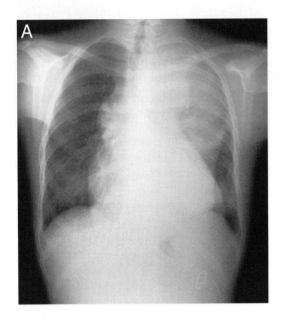

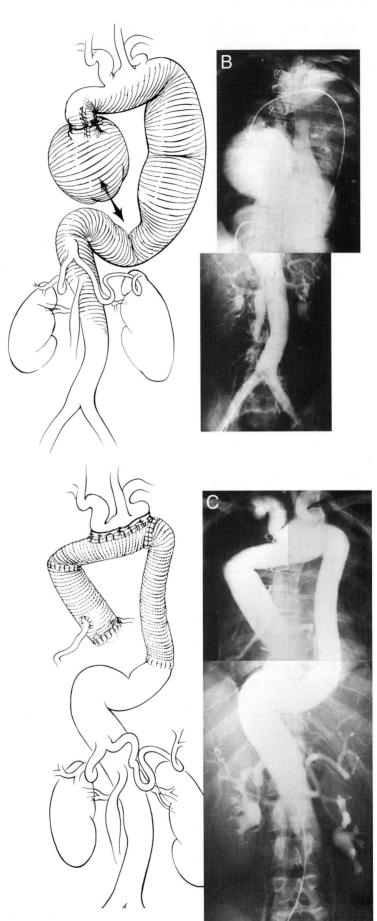

FIGURE 5–15 **A,** Chest radiograph of patient with Marfan syndrome and extensive aneurysm. **B,** Angiogram after repair was attempted elsewhere with intraluminal graft followed by root aneurysm formation and aortic regurgitation and distal aneurysm formation. **C,** Angiogram after insertion of composite valve graft (classic Bentall technique), replacement of the aortic arch, and descending aortic repair.

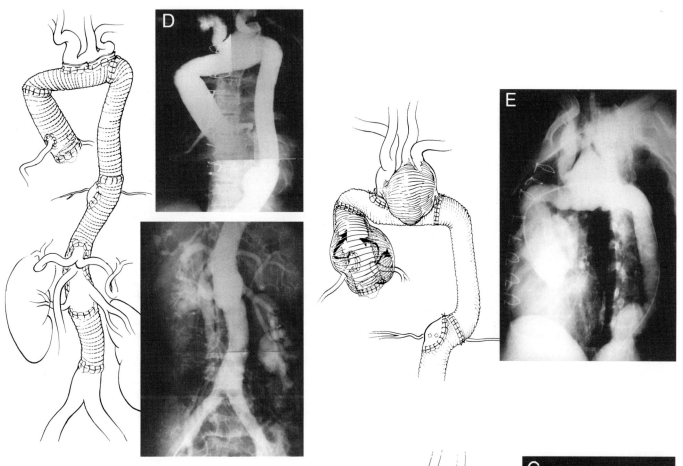

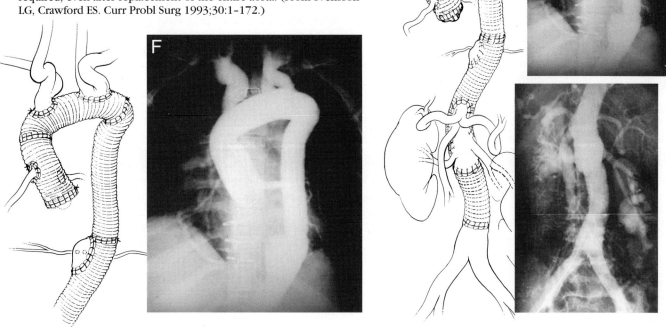

FIGURE 5–15 *Continued* **D,** Angiogram after thoracoabdominal repair with reimplantation of intercostal and visceral arteries. **E,** Later false aneurysm formation at the coronary ostia after classic Bentall wrap repair and aneurysm formation of the aortic arch Carrel patch. **F,** Angiogram after repair of the coronary ostia and separate implantation of the innominate artery and the combined left carotid and subclavian arteries. **G,** Angiogram after replacement of the entire aorta with reoperation on the aortic arch. Note that there is some dilatation of the visceral Carrel patch, emphasizing that continued follow-up is required, even after replacement of the entire aorta. (From Svensson LG, Crawford ES. Curr Probl Surg 1993;30:1–172.)

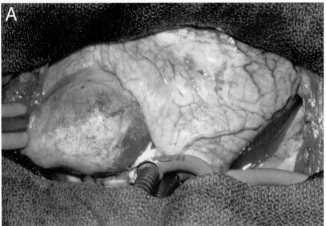

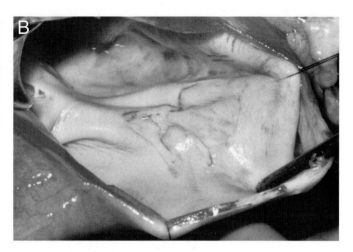

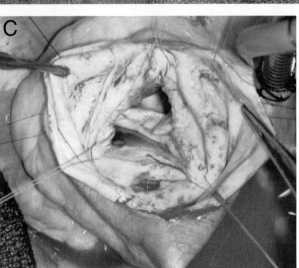

FIGURE 5–16   **A,** Intraoperative photograph of patient with Marfan syndrome and acute limited ascending aortic dissection. Note hemorrhages in the aortic adventitia. **B,** Photograph of the inside of the aorta. Note that the intima is torn; however, there is not the classic undermining of the intima that is usually seen with aortic dissection in patients without Marfan syndrome. These limited tears of the aorta are not infrequently seen with Marfan syndrome. **C,** Different view of the tears after excision of the aortic valve.

artery. This procedure has been used in 46 patients, 21 with aortic dissection and four with acute dissection. The 30-day survival rate was 100%, with only 27% of the patients requiring intraoperative blood transfusions despite the fact that half of the patients also required aortic arch repairs. There has been one late death due to hepatitis.

EHLERS-DANLOS SYNDROME

Ehlers-Danlos syndrome, sometimes referred to as the "India rubber man" disorder, is characterized by an increased range of motion of the joints, frequent joint dislocations, and an increased propensity for elasticity or fragility of the skin. Other features include kyphoscoliosis, diverticular disease of the colon, and a fragile ocular globe.

The syndrome has ten distinct phenotypes, of which two are of interest to the surgeon[42, 68]:

1. Type I (Gravis or the classical form) is inherited as an autosomal dominant trait with the clinical features of skin hyperextensibility, skin scarring, joint hypermobility, skeletal deformities, mitral valve prolapse, and uncommon involvement of the arteries. When the aorta is involved, it is usually the sinuses of Valsalva that are affected.

2. Type IV (Sack-Barabas syndrome or the arterial-ecchymotic form) is characterized by autosomal dominance (occasionally, recessive transmission in 4% of patients with Ehlers-Danlos syndrome), severe bruising with minor trauma, a thin transparent skin with prominent venous plexus without hyperextensibility, premature aging of hand and facial skin, hyperpigmentation, severe scarring, mild joint hypermobility except for finger joint hypermobility, colonic

FIGURE 5–17   Intraoperative photographs of a patient with Marfan syndrome who had acute inferior myocardial infarction associated with limited ascending aortic dissection with hematoma in the aortic wall. The intima is torn, but undermining of it is limited. A tube graft has been sutured to the left main coronary artery ostium for the composite valve graft repair. The patient received no homologous blood products, was extubated the next day, and went home 6 days after surgery.

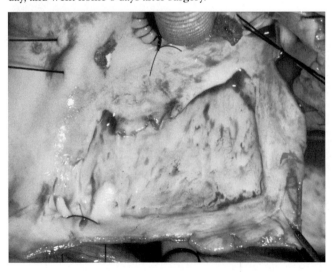

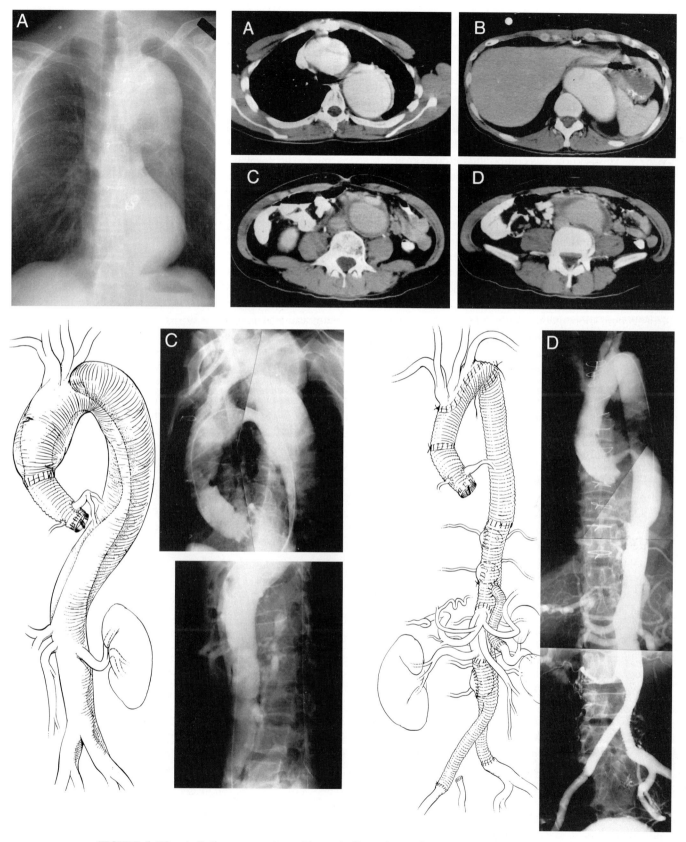

FIGURE 5–18 **A,** Patient presenting with aortic dissection and aneurysm formation beyond previous composite valve graft insertion as seen on the chest radiograph, **(B)** CT scans (A, chest; B, suprarenal aorta; C, infrarenal aorta; and D, at the aortic bifurcation), and **(C)** angiogram. **D,** Postoperative angiogram after replacement of the aortic arch, elephant trunk procedure, thoracoabdominal aneurysm repair with separate graft to the left renal artery, and aortic bifurcation graft to the right external iliac artery and to the left common iliac artery.

rupture, characteristic facial appearance, and frequent arterial involvement. This type has been further subdivided into IV-A acrogeric, IV-B acrogeric autosomal recessive, IV-C ecchymotic, and IV-D others (speculative). Type III collagen deficiency is found in this group of patients.

Rarely, aortic rupture has been reported in type VI (ocular scoliotic form).[7, 69] Type VI can result from a mutant allele inherited from each parent causing an additive effect of each mutant allele and resulting in clinical expression in a patient. This is known as compound heterozygosity.[70]

Pathology

Several gene and biochemical problems have been found in patients with Ehlers-Danlos syndrome, including enzymatic problems with the conversion of procollagen to collagen. The aortic wall disease is characterized by loss of collagen and loss of elastin in a narrow band of the aortic media. The internal elastic lamina is also disrupted and fragmented. The net result of the aortic involvement is the occurrence of aortic dissection, spontaneous rupture of the aorta, formation of arteriovenous fistulae, and multiple aneurysms.[69]

Female patients with Ehlers-Danlos syndrome, similar to those with Marfan syndrome, are particularly prone to aortic dissection or rupture during the third trimester of pregnancy, and during labor and delivery. Pregnant patients should have any cardiac valvular and/or aortic lesions repaired before the third trimester or should undergo Cesarean delivery.[7, 71]

Management

Aortic aneurysms in this group of patients are treated similarly to those in patients with Marfan syndrome; however, the operations can be technically very demanding with respect to maintenance of hemostasis. Cikrit and colleagues[72] reported that, in a series of 36 patients, postoperative bleeding occurred 38 times and was usually related to the aorta and its branches. In 15 of the 36 patients, a total of 29 aneurysms were detected, involving predominantly the aorta, the visceral arteries, and the carotid arteries. Of the 36 patients who underwent operations, 15 had ligation of bleeding vessels. Only one of four patients had a successful bypass procedure. Seven patients died after operation. Similarly, arteriography was complicated by bleeding, hematoma formation, femoral artery occlusion, and death. Thus, when operations are undertaken, ligation of bleeding vessels may be the best course of action because of the high risk of bleeding. Nevertheless, we have successfully repaired thoracoabdominal aneurysms in these patients, including a physician who continues to do well in active practice.

PSEUDOXANTHOMA ELASTICUM

A rare disease, pseudoxanthoma elasticum is classified by its transmission being inherited as either an autosomal recessive or a dominant trait. Like Marfan syndrome, it affects the elastic tissue of the body, although on skin biopsy the elastic tissue is fragmented and often calcified.[42] Clinically, the disease is characterized by the following: cardiovascular involvement, including the coronary arteries, and media of medium-sized arteries, with calcification, occlusions, or occasional rupture; ocular complications, usually retinal hemorrhages and angioid streaks; skin lesions, yellow in appearance, maximally in flexures; and gastrointestinal hemorrhage.

The cardiovascular manifestations, in contrast to Marfan syndrome, are usually those of occlusive disease. Thus coronary artery disease is frequently observed, as is occlusive disease of the intrarenal arteries, the distal upper extremity arteries, and the lower extremity arteries.[73-76] Involvement of the aorta and the proximal part of the arterial branches, however, is rare. Calcification of arteries is common and must be differentiated from Mönckeberg's sclerosis. In most patients, the deposition of fragmented elastic tissue in the skin, particularly in areas of stress such as the axillae, groin, neck, popliteal fossa, and cubital fossae, results in raised plaques.[73-76] Fractures in Bruch's membrane result in bleeding and scar formation in the retina and can progress to blindness. This results in angioid red or dark brown streaks, which radiate from the optic disc.[73-76] Thinning of vessels in the gastric mucosa results in a high incidence of upper gastrointestinal hemorrhage.[73-76] Similarly, uterine hemorrhage requiring hysterectomy is common in women.[76] Occlusive disease is treated by surgery as indicated.

MENKES' SYNDROME

Menkes' syndrome is a rare disorder characterized by lax skin, hypermobile joints, severe brain dysfunction, abnormal hair, decreased serum copper and ceruloplasmin levels, and vascular rupture.[42]

REFERENCES

1. McKusick VA. The cardiovascular aspects of Marfan syndrome: a heritable disorder of connective tissue. Circulation 1955;2:321-41.
2. Pyeritz RE, McKusick VA. The Marfan syndrome: diagnosis and management. N Engl J Med 1979;300:772-7.
3. Pyeritz RE, Murphy EA, McKusick VA. Clinical variability in the Marfan syndromes. Birth Defects 1979;15:155-78.
4. Pyeritz RE. Diagnosis and management of cardiovascular disorders in the Marfan syndrome. Cardiovasc Med 1980;5:759-69.
5. Etter LE, Glover LP. Arachnodactyly complicated by dislocated lens and death from rupture of dissecting aneurysm of aorta. JAMA 1943;123:88-9.
6. Baer RW, Taussig HB, Oppenheimer EH. Congenital aneurysmal dilatation of the aorta associated with arachnodactyly. John Hopkins Med J 1943;72:309-31.
7. Svensson LG, Crawford ES. Aortic dissection and aortic aneurysm surgery: clinical observations, experimental investigations, and statistical analyses. Part III. Curr Probl Surg 1993;30:1-172.
8. Muller WH, Damman JF Jr., Warren WG. Surgical correction of cardiovascular deformities in Marfan's syndrome. Ann Surg 1960;152:506-17.
9. Starr A, Edwards ML. Clinical experience with ball-valve prosthesis. Ann Surg 1961;154:726-40.
10. Starr A. Clinical experience with semirigid ball-valve prosthesis. Circulation 1963;27:779-83.
11. Groves LK, Effler DB, Hawk WA, Guliti R. Aortic insufficiency secondary to aneurysmal changes in the ascending aorta: surgical management. J Thorac Cardiovasc Surg 1964;48:362-79.

12. Wheat MN Jr, Wilson JR, Bartley TD. Successful replacement of the entire ascending aorta and aortic valve. JAMA 1964;188:717-9.

13. Bentall H, DeBono A. A technique for complete replacement of the ascending aorta. Thorax 1968;23:338-9.

14. Crosby IK, Ashcroft WC, Reed WA. Surgery of proximal aorta in Marfan's syndrome. J Thorac Cardiovasc Surg 1973;66:75-81.

15. Svensson LG, Crawford ES, Coselli JS, Safi HJ, Hess KR. Impact of cardiovascular operation on survival in the Marfan patient. Circulation 1989;80(3 Pt 1):i233-42.

16. Svensson LG. Approach to the insertion of composite valve graft. Ann Thorac Surg 1992;54:376-8.

17. Svensson LG, Crawford ES, Hess KR, et al. Composite valve graft replacement of the proximal aorta: comparison of techniques in 348 patients. Ann Thorac Surg 1992;54:427-39.

18. Gott VL, Pyeritz RE, Cameron DE, et al. Composite graft repair of Marfan aneurysm of the ascending aorta: results in 100 patients. Ann Thorac Surg 1991;52:38-44.

19. Kouchoukos NT. Composite graft replacement of the ascending aorta and aortic valve with the inclusion-wrap and open techniques. Semin Thorac Cardiovasc Surg 1991;3:171-6.

20. Kouchoukos NT, Wareing TH, Murphy SF, Perrillo JB. Sixteen-year experience with aortic root replacement: results of 172 operations. Ann Surg 1991;214:308-18.

21. Cabrol C, Pavie A, Mesnildrey P, et al. Long-term results with total replacement of the ascending aorta and reimplantation of the coronary arteries. J Thorac Cardiovasc Surg 1986;91:17-25.

22. Dietzmann RH, Peter ET, Wang Y, Lillehei RC. Mitral insufficiency in Marfan's syndrome. Dis Chest 1967;51:650-3.

23. Gillinov AM, Hulyakar A, Cameron DE, et al. Mitral valve operation in patients with the Marfan syndrome. J Thorac Cardiovasc Surg 1994;107:724-31.

24. DeBakey ME, Cooley DA, Crawford ES, Morris GC Jr. Aneurysms of the thoracic aorta: analysis of 179 cases treated by resection. J Thorac Surg 1958;36:393.

25. DeBakey ME, Crawford ES, Garret HE, et al. Surgical considerations in the treatment of aneurysms of the thoracoabdominal aorta. Ann Surg 1965;162:650-62.

26. Crawford ES. Thoracoabdominal and abdominal aortic aneurysm involving renal, superior mesenteric, and celiac arteries. Ann Surg 1974;179:763-72.

27. Crawford ES, Snyder DM, Cho GC, et al. Progress in treatment of thoraco-abdominal and abdominal aortic aneurysms involving celiac, superior mesenteric, and renal arteries. Ann Surg 1978;188:404-22.

28. Crawford ES, Walker HJ, Saleh SA, Normann NA. Graft replacement of aneurysm in descending thoracic aorta: results without bypass or shunting. Surgery 1981;89:73-85.

29. Crawford ES, Saleh SA. Transverse aortic arch aneurysm: improved results of treatment employing new modifications of aortic reconstruction and hypothermic cerebral circulatory arrest. Ann Surg 1981;194:180-8.

30. Crawford ES, Snyder DM. Treatment of aneurysms of the aortic arch: a progress report. J Thorac Cardiovasc Surg 1983;85:237-46.

31. Sun QB, Zhang KZ, Cheng TO, et al. Marfan syndrome in China: a collective review of 564 cases among 98 families. Am Heart J 1990;120:934-48.

32. Kainulainen K, Pulkkinen L, Savolainen A, et al. Location on chromosome 15 of the gene defect causing Marfan syndrome. N Engl J Med 1990;323:935-9.

33. Pyeritz RE. Editorial: Marfan syndrome. N Engl J Med 1990;323:987-9.

34. Aoyama T, Francke U, Dietz HC, Furthmayr H. Quantitative differences in biosynthesis and extracellular deposition of fibrillin in cultured fibroblasts distinguish five groups of Marfan syndrome patients and suggest distinct pathogenic mechanisms. J Clin Invest 1994;94:130-7.

35. Milewicz DM, Pyeritz RE, Crawford ES, Byers PH. Marfan syndrome: defective synthesis, secretion, and extracellular matrix formation of fibrillin by cultured dermal fibroblasts. J Clin Investig 1992;89:79-86.

36. Dietz HC, Saraiva JM, Pyeritz RE, et al. Clustering of fibrillin (FBN1) missense mutations in Marfan syndrome patients at cysteine residues in EGF-like domains. Human Mutation 1992;1:366-74.

37. Pereira L, Levran O, Ramirez F, et al. A molecular approach to the stratification of cardiovascular risk in families with Marfan's syndrome. N Engl J Med 1994;331:148-53.

38. Trotter SE, Olsen EG. Marfan's disease and Erdheim's cystic medionecrosis: a study of their pathology. Eur Heart J 1991;12:83-7.

39. Hollister DW, Godfrey M, Sakai LY, Pyeritz RE. Immunohistologic abnormalities of the microfibrillar-fiber system in the Marfan syndrome. N Engl J Med 1990;323:152-9.

40. Hirata K, Triposkiadis F, Sparks E, et al. The Marfan syndrome: abnormal aortic elastic properties. J Am Coll Cardiol 1992;18:57-63.

41. Raghunath M, Superti-Furga A, Godfrey M, Steinmann B. Decreased extracellular deposition of fibrillin and decorin in neonatal Marfan syndrome fibroblasts. Hum Genet 1993;5:511-5.

42. Beighton P, de Paepe A, Danks D, et al. International nosology of heritable disorders of connective tissue, Berlin, 1986. Am J Med Genet 1988;29:581-94.

43. Walker BA, Murdoch JL. The wrist sign: a useful physical finding in the Marfan syndrome. Arch Intern Med 1970;126:276-7.

44. Steinberg I. A simple screening test for the Marfan syndrome. Am J Roentgenol 1966;97:118-24.

45. Roman MJ, Rosen SE, Kramer-Fox R, Devereux RB. Prognostic significance of the pattern of aortic root dilation in the Marfan syndrome. J Am Coll Cardiol 1993;22:1470-6.

46. Marsalese DL, Moodie DS, Vacante M, et al. Marfan's syndrome: natural history and long-term follow-up of cardiovascular involvement. J Am Coll Cardiol 1989;14:422-8.

47. Crawford ES, Coselli JS. Marfan's syndrome: combined composite valve graft replacement of the aortic root and transaortic mitral valve replacement. Ann Thorac Surg 1988;45:296-302.

48. Taherina AC. Cardiovascular anomalies in Marfan's syndrome: the role of echocardiography and beta-blockers. South Med J 1993;86:305-10.

49. Shores J, Berger KR, Murphy EA, Pyeritz RE. Progression of aortic dilatation and the benefit of long-term b-adrenergic blockade in Marfan's syndrome. N Engl J Med 1994;330:1335-41.

50. Brophy CM, Tilson JE, Tilson MD. Propanolol stimulates the crosslinking of matrix components in skin from the aneurysm-prone blotchy mouse. J Surg Res 1989;46:330-2.

51. Pyeritz RE. Maternal and fetal complication of pregnancy in the Marfan syndrome. Am J Med 1981;71:784-90.

52. David TE, Feindel CM. An aortic valve-sparing operation for patients with aortic incompetence and aneurysm of the ascending aorta. J Thorac Cardiovasc Surg 1992;103:617-21.

53. Chesler E, King RA, Edwards JE. The myxomatous mitral valve and sudden death. Circulation 1983;67:632-9.

54. Pocock WA, Bosman CK, Chesler E, et al. Sudden death in primary mitral valve prolapse. Am Heart J 1984;107:378-82.

55. Nishimura RA, McGoon MD, Shub C, et al. Echocardiographically documented mitral valve prolapse: long term follow-up of 237 patients. N Engl J Med 1985;313:1305.

56. Farb A, Tang AL, Atkinson JB, et al. Comparison of cardiac findings in patients with mitral valve prolapse who die suddenly to those who have congestive heart failure from mitral regurgitation and to those with fatal noncardiac conditions. Am J Cardiol 1992;70:234-9.

57. Farb A, Tang AL, Atkinson JB, Virmani R. Morphological differences in mitral valve prolapse patients who die suddenly. Cardiol Board Rev 1993;10:53-8.

58. Hwa J, Richards JG, Huang H, et al. The natural history of aortic dilatation in Marfan syndrome. Med J Austral 1993;158:558-62.

59. Reed CM, Richey PA, Pulliam DA, et al. Aortic dimensions in tall men and women. Am J Cardiol 1993;71:608-10.

60. Henry WL, Gardin JM, Ware JH. Echocardiographic measurements in normal subjects from infancy to old age. Circulation 1980;62:1054-61.

61. Jeremy RW, Huang H, Hwa J, et al. Relation between age, arterial distensibility, and aortic dilatation in the Marfan syndrome. Am J Cardiol 1994;74:369-73.

62. Treasure T, Naftel DC, Conger KA, et al. The effect of hypothermic circulatory arrest time on cerebral function, morphology, and biochemistry. J Thorac Cardiovasc Surg 1983;86:761-70.

63. Crawford ES, Coselli JS, Svensson LG, et al. Diffuse aneurysmal disease (chronic aortic dissection, Marfan, and mega aorta syndromes) and multiple aneurysm: treatment by subtotal and total aortic replacement emphasizing the elephant trunk operation. Ann Surg 1990;211:521-37.

64. Gillinov AM, Hulyalkar A, Cameron DE, et al. Mitral valve operation in patients with the Marfan syndrome. J Thorac Cardiovasc Surg 1994;107:724-31.

65. Svensson LG. Rationale and technique for replacement of the ascending aorta, arch, and distal aorta using a modified elephant trunk procedure. J Cardiac Surg 1992;7:301-12.

66. Crawford ES, Coselli JS, Svensson LG, et al. Diffuse aneurysmal disease (chronic aortic dissection, Marfan, and mega aorta syndromes) and multiple aneurysm: treatment by subtotal and total aortic replacement emphasizing the elephant trunk technique. Ann Surg 1990;211:521-37.

67. Smith JA, Fann JI, Miller C, et al. Surgical management of aortic dissection in patients with the Marfan syndrome. Circulation 1994;90: II-235-II-242.

68. Serry C, Agomuoh OS, Goldin MD. Review of Ehlers-Danlos syndrome: successful repair of rupture and dissection of abdominal aorta. J Cardiovasc Surg (Torino) 1988;29:530-4.

69. Steinberg AG, Bearn AG, et al. Progress in Medical Genetics, New Series. Vol 5. Genetics of Cardiovascular Disease. Philadelphia: WB Saunders, 1983:5.

70. Ha VT, Marshall MK, Elsas LJ, et al. A patient with Ehlers-Danlos syndrome type VI is a compound heterozygote for mutations in the lysyl hydroxylase gene. J Clin Invest 1994;93:1716-21.

71. Williams GM, Gott VL, Brawley RK, et al. Aortic disease associated with pregnancy. J Vasc Surg 1988;8:470-5.

72. Cikrit DF, Miles JH, Silver D. Spontaneous arterial perforation: the Ehlers-Danlos specter. J Vasc Surg 1987;5:248-55.

73. Carlborg U, Ejrup B, Gronblad E, Lund F. Vascular studies in pseudoxanthoma elasticum and angoid streaks; with a series of color photographs of the eyeground lesions. Acta Med Scand 1959;166 (Supp 350):1-84.

74. Connor PJJ, Juergens JL, Perry HO, et al. Pseudoxanthoma elasticum and angoid streaks: a review of 106 cases. Am J Med 1961;30:537-43.

75. Altman LK, Fialkow PJ, Parker F, Sagebiel RW. Pseudoxanthoma elasticum: an underdiagnosed genetically heterogeneous disorder with protean manifestations. Arch Intern Med 1974;134:1048-54.

76. Mendelsohn G, Buckley BH, Hutchins GM. Cardiovascular manifestations of pseudoxanthoma elasticum. Arch Pathol Lab Med 1978;102:298-302.

Aortitis and Inflammatory Aneurysms

AORTITIS

The presence of inflammatory cells in the aortic media or adventitia is indicative of aortitis. Macroscopically, the aorta often has a thickened aortic wall, which changes from an edematous appearance during the acute phase of aortitis to a scarred, white, glistening appearance when observed later in the disease process. In both Takayasu's disease and giant cell arteritis, although the cause is not known, the immune system clearly is an important factor. There are two main categories of aortitis: (A) infective and (B) with no known infective agent. Infections of the aortic wall usually are not discussed together with other forms of aortitis, and thus this category is explained under mycotic aneurysms and infected prostheses. The noninfective aortitis group can be further divided into two subclassifications: (1) those in which the aorta is mainly involved; and (2) those that predominantly involve other organ systems but may also involve the aorta and the arterial tree.[1]

Noninfective Aortitis Group Involving Predominantly the Aorta

The most well-known disorder in this subgroup is Takayasu's disease, which is characterized by an acute episode of systemic manifestations, usually in a young female, associated with neurological symptoms and stenoses of aortic side branches, often those of the aortic arch. Other types of aortitis in this subgroup are the chronic inflammatory aneurysms of unknown cause, generally involving the infrarenal abdominal aorta but occasionally the thoracic aorta. We have occasionally seen ascending aortic inflammatory aneurysms that do not appear to be associated with Takayasu's disease or other systemic collagen vascular disease; however, the causes of these rare inflammatory aneurysms are unknown, although the ascending aorta has a rich lymphatic plexus, as does the abdominal aorta (see Etiology of Inflammatory Aneurysms of the Abdominal Aorta). The inflammatory aneurysms found in the chest are frequently associated with the autoimmune type of collagen vascular disease. A caveat is that some of these inflammatory aneurysms of the thoracic aorta can be very difficult to distinguish clinically or histologically from those associated with or caused by tuberculosis.[1] Chronic inflammatory aneurysms involving the infrarenal aorta are discussed at the end of this chapter.

Takayasu's Disease

HISTORY AND CLASSIFICATION

In 1908 Takayasu,[2] a Japanese ophthalmologist, described a 21-year-old woman with characteristic retinal artery arteriovenous anastomoses and microaneurysms. In a discussion of the presentation, Ohnishi and Kagoshima reported that they, too, had observed patients with similar clinical signs including notably the absence of radial artery pulses.[2] Further funduscopic abnormalities found were venous engorgement, neovascularization, hemorrhage, and a pale papilla. Subsequently, different presentations and manifestations of the disease have been reported (Fig. 6-1). As a result, the disease has acquired numerous synonyms, including pulseless disease, idiopathic medial aortopathy, aortitis syndrome, giant cell arteritis of the aorta (this term is better reserved for giant cell arteritis, per se, particularly temporal arteritis), aortic arch syndrome, primary arteritis of the aorta, brachiocephalic arteritis, panaortitis, reverse coarctation, occlusive thromboaortopathy, and nonspecific aortitis. The so-called middle aortic syndrome in adults, which is not of a congenital origin and is characterized by a long coarctation from the descending thoracic aorta into the abdomen, may also be a form of Takayasu's arteritis.[1, 3, 4]

Several reports have classified Takayasu's disease according to various aspects of the disorders, including anatomical sites affected, acuity of the disease, patterns of presentation, or criteria for diagnosis. We find it most useful to classify the disease according to the anatomical sites affected, since this determines the symptom complexes at time of presentation, and also according to the acuity (activity) of the disease.

First, the classification of Takayasu's obliterative disease has been described in terms of five anatomical sites affected (Fig. 6-1).

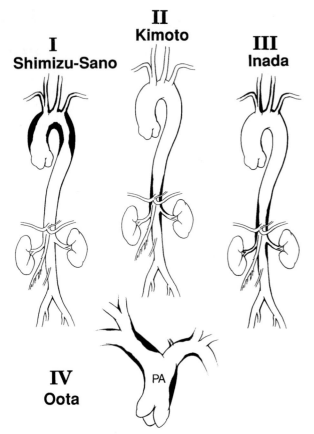

FIGURE 6–1 Classification of Takayasu's disease. (From Svensson LG, Crawford ES. Curr Probl Surg 1993;30:1–172.)

Anatomical Classification of Takayasu's Disease

Type I: Aortic arch involvement

Reported by Shimizu[5] in 1951: Classical "pulseless disease" presenting with brain ischemia, visual disturbances, and reduced blood flow to the upper extremity.[1]

Type II: Thoracoabdominal involvement

Reported by Kimoto[6] in 1979: Presentation with atypical coarctation of the thoracoabdominal aorta with associated arterial hypertension, often renovascular hypertension, and mesenteric ischemia.[1]

Type III: Diffuse involvement

Described in 1965 by Inada[7]: Diffuse inflammatory involvement of the aorta.[1]

Type IV: Pulmonary involvement

Noted by Oota[8] in 1940 and detailed by Lupi-Herrera[9] in 1977: Presentation with hemoptysis or pulmonary hypertension from stenoses and inflammation of the central pulmonary arteries.

Type V: Aneurysmal type

Described by Ueno[10] in 1967: In this type, the aorta is diffusely aneurysmal as are the side branches from the aorta.[1] A study of Japanese patients with Takayasu's disease reported that 32% had aneurysms, usually involving the

ascending aorta, and that aortic regurgitation was present in half the patients with ascending aortic aneurysms.[11]

Classification by Acuity, Aortic Morphology, Site, and Clinical Pattern. Pokrovskii of the USSR,[12] on the basis of his observations in 300 patients, classified patients according to

- Three *stages of the disease:*
    1. Acute
    2. Subacute recurrent
    3. Chronic
- Three *morphologic types:*
    1. Stenosing
    2. Deforming
    3. Aneurysmic
- Three *sites:*
    1. Aortic branches
    2. Thoracoabdominal aorta
    3. Aortic branches *and* thoracoabdominal aorta
- Ten *clinical patterns:*
    1. Generalized inflammatory reaction
    2. Lesions of the aortic arch with brain symptoms
    3. Descending thoracic aorta involvement
    4. Renovascular hypertension
    5. Visceral ischemia
    6. Aortoiliac occlusive disease
    7. Coronary artery disease
    8. Aortic valve insufficiency
    9. Pulmonary arterial involvement
    10. Aortic aneurysm formation

The symptoms and signs associated with these ten clinical patterns may vary according to the arteries involved and the resultant end-organ ischemia.[1]

Although the preceding classifications emphasise the wide spectrum of the disease, we have consistently found that the most useful grouping of patients with the disease is according to the five anatomical types (arch, thoracoabdominal, diffuse, pulmonary, and aneurysmal) and also the degree of acuity, namely, acute (active disease), subacute (remission from acute disease), and chronic (inactive disease that is quiescent and "burnt out" but has resulted in arterial damage).

HISTOLOGY

Histological examination of the aorta in patients with Takayasu's disease may demonstrate a thickened aortic wall, intimal thickening from fibrosis, medial degeneration with loss of smooth muscle cells and elastic tissue, hemorrhage, proliferation of the vasa vasorum, and enlargement of the adventitia. In the acute phase, there is infiltration by inflammatory cells such as lymphocytes, histiocytes, giant cells, plasma cells, and polymorphonuclear cells. The typical adventitial histologic pattern shows infiltration by perivascular mononuclear cells in the vasa vasorum with an onion-skin-like appearance. In the chronic stage, the vasa vasorum of the adventitia are obliterated by the dense fibrosis. Unlike the findings in syphilitic aortitis, plasma cells are absent and granulomas may occur but are rare.[13] The changes of all the layers may affect the aorta diffusely or involve the aorta in patches with areas of normal aorta in between. Near old areas of scarring there may be new areas of active lesions suggesting that the disease is progressive. When necrosis predominates there is a tendency toward aneurysm formation, whereas if the intimal proliferative component is prominent occlusive disease of aortic branches occurs.[1, 14-16] Arterial stenosis or occlusion, atheroma formation, and thrombus formation may also be found.[13]

DEMOGRAPHICS

The ratio of female patients to male patients with Takayasu aortitis is about 4 to 1 although 7 to 1 has been reported.[9, 13, 17, 18] Most commonly, the disease occurs in the Orient and India at an incidence of 1% to 2%, whereas the disease in the United States has been noted by Restrepo and associates,[19] based on autopsy studies, to have a considerably lower incidence of 0.11%. The reasons for the higher incidence of the disease in certain racial groups may partly be that there may be a genetic hereditary component to the disease related to HLA haplotypes.[20] Kerr and colleagues have calculated that in the United States Takayasu's disease occurs in 2.6 patients per million people per annum.[21] Aortitis in our own patients, as indicated by the presence of inflammatory cells found in histological specimens of the aorta, accounts for approximatley 12% of patients, although not all of these patients have Takayasu's aortitis. A similar incidence has also been reported in Minnesota.[22]

Compared with patients elsewhere, patients in the United States tend to have more extensive diffuse disease of the aorta and its branches similar to that observed to a lesser extent in patients from India, Thailand, and Mexico, whereas in Japan aortic arch disease is more prevalent. In South Africa, Korea, and Singapore, midaortic disease and renal artery disease appear to be more frequent.[21] The reasons for these reported differences have not been explained; the differences are possibly spurious, or there may be complex environmental factors involved.

CLINICAL PRESENTATION

Acute clinical manifestations of Takayasu's syndrome tend to occur according to certain patterns, namely, systemic, neurological, and either predominantly cardiac or pulmonary symptoms.

The systemic symptoms include malaise, low-grade fever, weight loss, fatigability, sweating, weakness, elevated erythrocyte sedimentation rate, leukocytosis, and elevated C-reactive protein. In addition, Ueda[23] found that 74% of

patients had detectable levels of antiaortic antibodies in the serum. Neurological symptoms include dizziness, headache, syncope, and visual disturbances. Cardiac manifestations include dyspnea, palpitations, precordial oppression, angina, heart failure, and arrhythmias. Pulmonary symptoms are usually coughing, hemoptysis, pleuritic chest pain, and symptoms suggestive of pulmonary embolism. It should be noted that pulmonary symptoms may be related to acute interstitial disease that is independent of large vessel involvement and may have the appearance of adult respiratory distress syndrome.[24]

Precipitation of an acute episode is often related to a minor infection, such as tonsillitis, or stress, such as pregnancy.[1] Of interest, Ueda and colleagues[13] noted that of 197 patients, 22% had a history of tuberculosis, 9% had a history of nephritis, and, more rarely, 3% had various infective diseases such as pneumonia, rheumatic disease, diphtheria, cholecystitis, and pancreatitis, although the majority of patients (> 66%) had no antecedent history of infections or inflammatory disease. Ulcerative colitis is also associated with Takayasu's disease.[25] The relationship between infections and the causation of aortitis is discussed later in this chapter.

The systemic manifestations of the acute phase may go unnoticed, however, and only several years later, during the chronic phase, when clinical evidence of occlusive disease, aneurysms, or both becomes apparent, is the diagnosis made.

The location of the arterial disease process determines the clinical signs. Thus coronary involvement results in myocardial ischemia; aortic valve involvement or cardiomyopathy causes heart failure; carotid disease leads to tender carotid arteries; brachiocephalic arterial occlusion results in neurologic deficits, signs, and funduscopic abnormalities; renal artery stenosis causes either renal failure or renovascular hypertension; limb artery occlusions result in limb arterial deficits and evidence of ischemia; abdominal visceral occlusions cause bowel ischemia; and pulmonary artery stenosis leads to pulmonary hypertension.

Aneurysms are usually associated with manifestations related to where they are found, such as abdominal aortic tenderness, backache, and signs of compression of adjacent structures. Ultimately, if aneurysms continue to grow, rupture of aneurysms will occur and, it should be noted, that aortic dissection may also develop. As a rule, intraparenchymal organ arteries and distal arteries of the upper or lower limb are not involved.[1]

DIAGNOSIS

The diagnosis of Takayasu's disease should be suspected when a young female patient presents with symptoms and signs of occlusive disease, particularly the absence of carotid, subclavian, brachial, or radial pulses (left radial absent in 76%[13]) and a history of fever of unknown origin. In 72% of patients (94 of 130), Ueda and associates[13] found a discrepancy greater than 10 mm Hg in blood pressure between the right and left arms. In a study of 60 patients in the United States, Kerr and colleagues[21] noted that 97% were female, mostly of Asian extraction, with a median age of 25 years. Only 33% had systemic symptoms, and a bruit was the most common clinical finding. Apparently, 57% of patients did not have constitutional symptoms. Stenotic lesions were present in 98% and aneurysms in 27%. Even during clinically inactive disease, 44% of arterial biopsies revealed active disease.

While some adults with the middle aortic syndrome do have Takayasu's, there is clearly a small group of patients who have true congenital coarctation of the aorta that has to be differentiated.[1, 3, 4,] Eibenberger and colleagues,[26] who evaluated nine of their own patients with middle aortic syndrome and reviewed 108 patients from the literature, pointed out that there is a slight male predominance, patients are

less than 20 years of age, and the stenosis is short and usually suprarenal with renal ostial involvement.

In children, the diagnosis can be difficult to make because there are several childhood diseases that are similar in presentation but are more common, although they rarely involve the aorta. The differential diagnosis includes Henoch-Schonlein purpura, microscopic polyarteritis, Wegener's granulomatosis, Churg-Strauss syndrome, Kawasaki disease, and polyarteritis nodosa.[27]

The blood tests to confirm the diagnosis should include the erythrocyte sedimentation rate, levels of C-reactive protein and complement, serum protein electrophoresis, antinuclear and DNA antibodies, rheumatoid factor, lupus erythematosus antibodies, and elevated white blood cell count. A tuberculin skin test is also required.

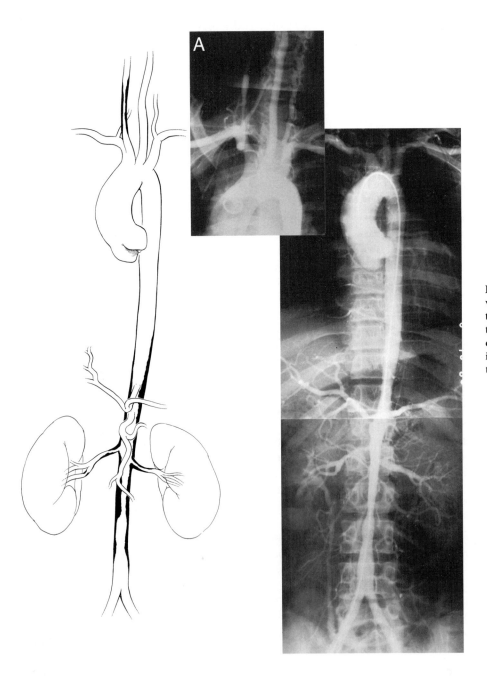

FIGURE 6–2 A, Extensive aortitis with diffuse narrowing of the aorta treated by **(B)** placing a tube graft from the ascending aorta to the aortic bifurcation with side grafts to the renal arteries and also by placing a tube graft to the right common carotid artery.

Illustration continued on following page

To define the extent of the aortic involvement, angiography of the entire aorta and the major aortic branches, particularly those to the brain, is necessary. In those patients who have evidence of right-sided heart failure, pulmonary hypertension, or a history of hemoptysis, pulmonary angiography and pulmonary hemodynamic studies should also be performed. We observed a young pregnant woman who presented with hemoptysis and a positive ventilation perfusion scan suggestive of pulmonary embolic disease. During pulmonary angiography, however, a large ascending aortic aneurysm was noted on delayed films. Subsequent to a cesarean delivery of a normal baby, the patient underwent successful replacement of the ascending aorta with prosthetic bypass grafts to beyond tight stenoses of her common carotid arteries.[1]

Ishikawa[28] has proposed that, for acute Takayasu's disease to be diagnosed, certain criteria should be met:

1. The patient is usually under 40 years of age.

2. Presence of either left or right subclavian artery lesions.

3. Four or more minor criteria should be present. These include an elevated erythrocyte sedimentation rate (ESR), common carotid artery tenderness, hypertension, aortic regurgitation, annuloaortic ectasia, pulmonary artery lesions, left common carotid artery lesion, brachiocephalic trunk lesion, or involvement of the thoracic or abdominal aorta. Usually the left common carotid or left subclavian arteries are involved; however, if both subclavian arteries are involved, then only two minor criteria are required for a diagnosis.[1] Clearly, in those patients

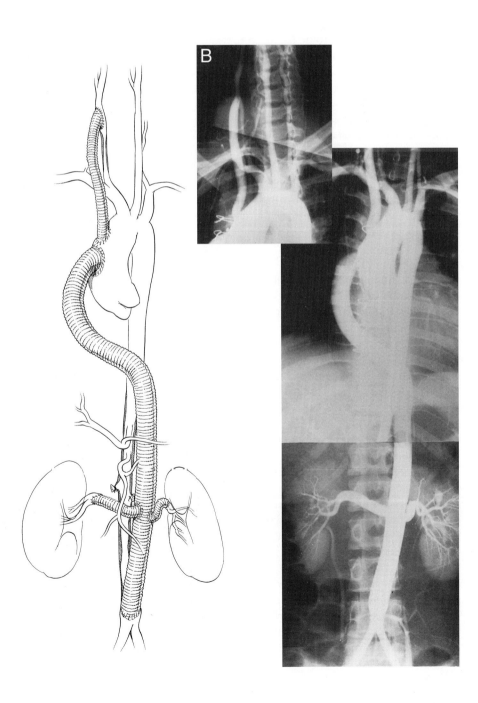

FIGURE 6–2 *Continued*

presenting with chronic Takayasu's aortitis, these criteria are less likely to be met.

MEDICAL TREATMENT

Treatment with steroids is controversial because steroids may delay wound healing after operations and increase the risk of sepsis. Nevertheless, steroids may be necessary to control acute manifestations preoperatively. Indeed, steroids will control the systemic symptoms of the disease in up to 75% of patients.[18] In the study by Kerr and colleagues[21] of 60 patients in the United States, medical therapy with steroids or other cytotoxic agents (cyclophosphamide or methotrexate) was necessary in 80% of patients to control the acute phase, while the remaining 20% had monophasic self-limiting disease. It should be noted that, overall, 23% of patients failed to respond to medical therapy, and restenosis after surgical bypass or angioplasty was common. Methotrexate and dapsone appear to be useful steroid-sparing agents and newer biological, immunomodulatory agents may also become useful in clinical management.[29, 30]

Occlusive disease or aneurysmal disease may progress despite medical therapy and apparent remission of the acute phase into a subacute phase, and for aneurysmal segments, the rate of dilatation may be accelerated because of steroid use. Administration of steroids should control the acute phase of the disease and thus allow for operations to be performed at a later stage when the aorta is less inflamed and scar tissue has formed. An important caveat is that there is evidence that steroids may increase the risk of rupture of aneurysms.[1, 31]

SURGICAL AND INTERVENTIONAL TREATMENT

Surgical and interventional indications for operation are hypertension from stenotic coarctation of the aorta or renovascular disease (Fig. 6-2), end-organ ischemia or peripheral limb ischemia, and aneurysm formation. Tyagi and associates[32] reported on 36 patients with aortic stenosis treated with balloon angioplasty. Dilatation was successful in 34, with a marked decrease in gradient pressure from 75.3 mm Hg to 24.8 mm Hg ($p < 0.0001$). In 20 patients, at an average of 7.7 months later (range, 3 to 24 months), the gradients further decreased in seven and stayed the same in 12, and restenosis occurred in one patient. Patients with stenoses that were less than 4 cm long had the best results. Sharma and colleagues[33] performed angioplasty in 10 patients and found that in patients with discrete concentric lesions angioplasty was successful; however, in the five patients with eccentric lesions, two operations failed, four patients had large intimal flaps, and an aneurysm developed in one. Sometimes we will refer patients who have short stenoses of the aorta, renovascular hypertension, and stenoses of the aortic branches for angioplasty (particularly if there are factors that preclude surgical intervention). Tyagi and colleagues[34] evaluated transluminal angioplasty in 54 patients with hypertension and renovascular disease. Angioplasty was successful in 89.3% attempted arterial

lesions, hypertension was reduced within 48 hours to normal or lower than before in 93%, and an average of 14.2 months later 13.5% had restenosis. The stenotic lesions were successfully redilated.

The definitive treatment of occlusive disease of arteries and aneurysms is operative, because even small saccular aneurysms may rupture. In both our experience (Fig. 6-3) and that of Haga and colleagues[35] aortic dissection may also occur, albeit rarely, and thus require surgical intervention. The surgical techniques are similar to those undertaken for other aneurysms, although stenotic branch arteries will often require bypass, endarterectomy, or both (Figs. 6-4 to 6-6).[1, 31, 36] We prefer a mediastinal approach with prosthetic bypasses from the aorta to the branch arteries of the aortic arch,[37] including bypasses to the subclavian arteries. Occlusion or a stenosis of a brachiocephalic artery or left carotid artery is best treated with a prosthetic bypass graft because saphenous veins tend to fail. The graft should be connected to the artery by an end-to-end distal anastomosis. The reason for this is that if there is an end-to-side distal anastomosis, then platelet emboli and thrombus can build up in an occluded segment of an artery and cause embolization to the brain. We recommend that abdominal visceral stenoses be treated either by endarterectomy if the lesion is ostial, or by a prosthetic bypass if the lesion is more distal.[1] In selected patients with hypertension, renal autografting may be an option.[29] Aortic valve replacement alone may occasionally be needed, although in our experience[1] and that of Ohteki and colleagues,[38] in most patients aortic repairs or bypasses are usually required either at the same time as the aortic valve replacement or later (Fig. 6-6). Often the disease progresses and new aneurysms or branch artery stenoses have to be treated at a later date.

LONG-TERM PROGNOSIS

After onset of symptoms, long-term survival in all patients is reported to be 91% and 84% at 5 years and 10 years, respectively.[39] Predictors of death or adverse events include severe hypertension, functional disability, and cardiac involvement.[39] The causes of death may be stroke, sudden death, heart failure, myocardial infarction, aortic valve insufficiency, cardiomyopathy, heart failure, renal failure, and rupture of aneurysms.[1] Ishikawa and Maetaric[40] observed 120 patients, for as long as 20 years in some cases, and found by multivariate Cox analysis that the predictors for a poor long-term survival rate were major complications (retinopathy, hypertension, aortic regurgitation, or aneurysm), a progressive course of active disease, and an abnormal ESR. The poorest prognosis of 43% 15-year survival applied to those patients with complications and a progressive course of the disease, as opposed to a 96.4% survival rate in patients with no major complications. Thus, because active disease and complications are important predictors of long-term survival, patients should be regularly observed for progression of disease. Robbs and colleagues[41] found that, of 134 patients they operated on, four patients (5%) had progression of disease

Text continued on page 116

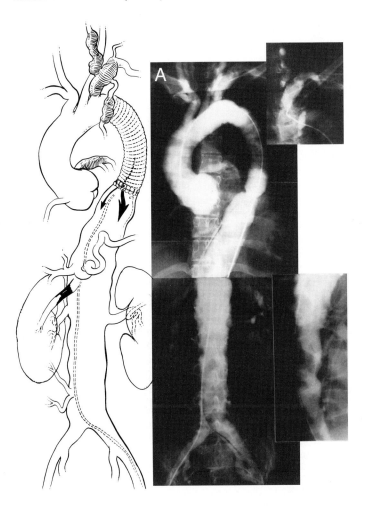

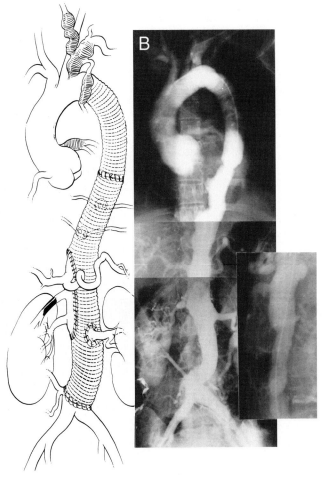

FIGURE 6–3 **A,** Patient with aortitis and previous descending aortic repair with distal aneurysm formation associated with aortic dissection. Note also the aneurysm formation of the aortic arch branches. **B,** Aortogram after thoracoabdominal aortic repair with separate reimplantation of the left renal artery.

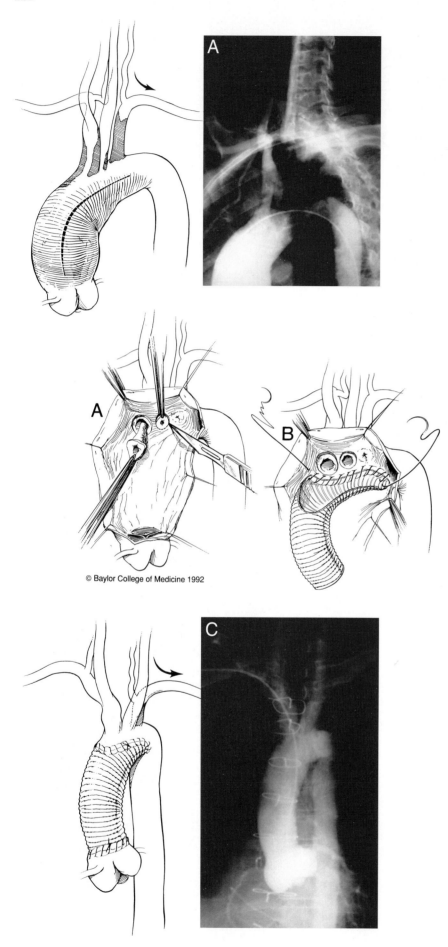

© Baylor College of Medicine 1992

FIGURE 6–4 **A,** Patient who had neurological symptoms associated with innominate artery and left common carotid artery stenoses, left subclavian artery steal, and aneurysm formation of the aorta due to aortitis. **B,** Intraoperative diagrams of repair including endarterectomies of the innominate and left common carotid arteries. **C,** Aortogram of postoperative repair.

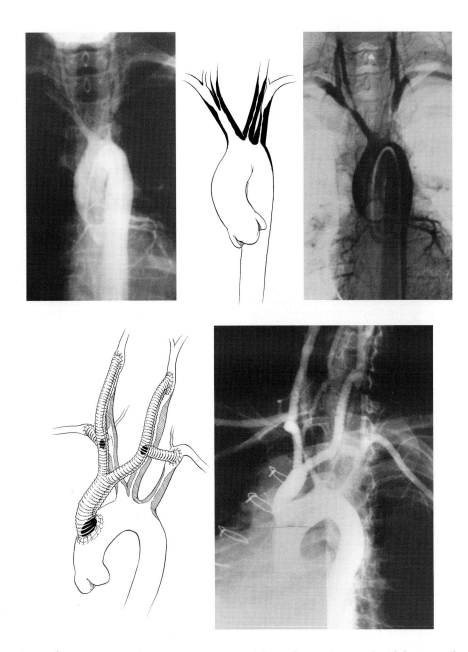

FIGURE 6–5   Patient with extensive stenoses of the arch vessels treated with bypasses from the ascending aorta to the right and left carotid arteries and to the left and right subclavian arteries. (From Svensson LG, Crawford ES. Curr Probl Surg 1993;30:1–172.)

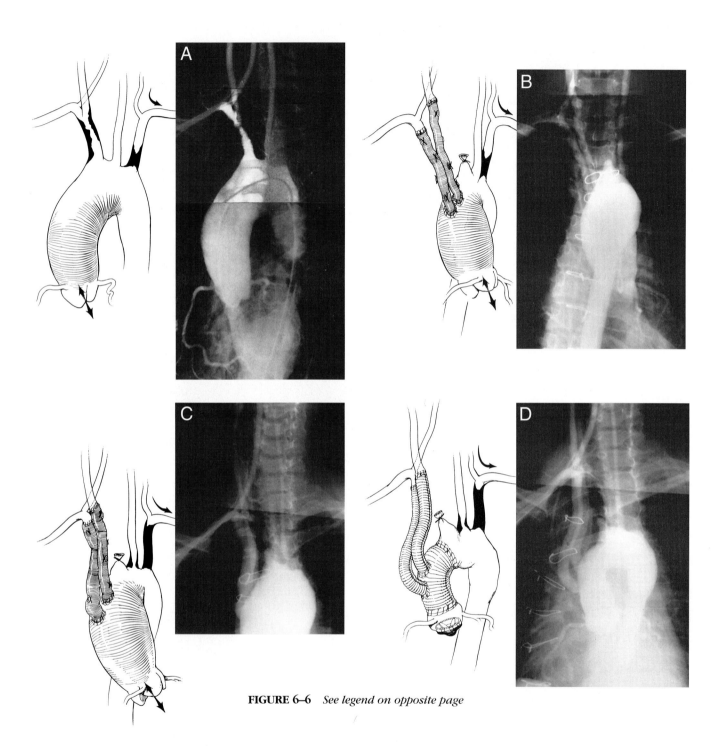

FIGURE 6–6 *See legend on opposite page*

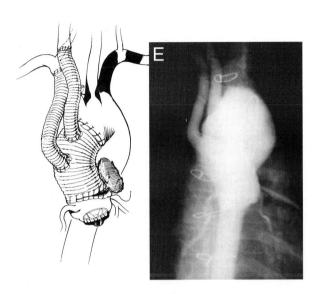

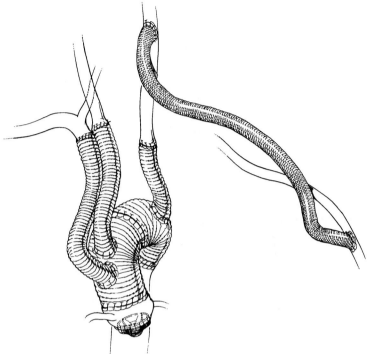

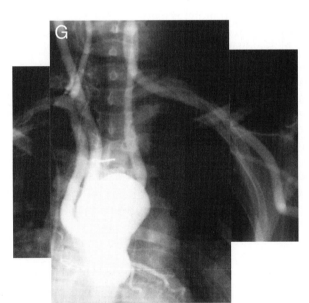

FIGURE 6–6 **A,** Patient with innominate artery stenosis and left subclavian artery steal. **B,** Arteriogram after vein interposition grafts. **C,** Later arteriogram with progression of disease and new left common carotid artery stenosis. The saphenous vein grafts have dilated and kinked. **D,** Arteriogram after ascending aortic repair, insertion of aortic valve, and prosthetic graft bypasses to the right common carotid and subclavian arteries. **E,** Later progression of the disease with increased left common carotid stenosis, occlusion of the left subclavian artery beyond the vertebral artery, and false aneurysm formation at the proximal suture line. **F,** Diagram after repair of the false aneurysm, replacement of the rest of the aortic arch, tube graft to the left common carotid artery, and polytetrafluoroethylene bypass from the left common carotid artery to the left subclavian artery. **G,** Postoperative arteriogram. (From Svensson LG, Crawford ES. Curr Probl Surg 1993; 30:1–172.)

that resulted in death and seven (8.9%) had progression without death; however, three patients in this group required further surgery. Angiography is still the gold standard, although magnetic resonance imaging (MRI) with magnetic resonance angiography and spiral computed tomography (CT) are useful noninvasive adjuncts for follow-up of patients. None of these studies, however, can determine which of the vascular lesions are active.

Noninfective Aortitis with Incidental Involvement of the Aorta

A diverse group of patients often have autoimmune diseases, including the involvement by arteritis (usually by arterial stenoses) of medium-sized arteries, but occasionally they will also have involvement with aortitis of the aorta. The list includes giant cell arteritis (granulomatous aortitis, Horton's disease), rheumatoid arthritis, relapsing polychondritis, Sjögren's disease, Reiter's disease, ankylosing spondylitis, systemic lupus erythematosus, Cogan's syndrome (associated with ocular and auditory involvement), polymyalgia rheumatica, rarely Kawasaki's disease, Crohn's disease, ulcerative colitis, sarcoid, and Behçet's disease. Others not typically associated with autoimmune disease are ergotism and radiation fibrosis. The most commonly seen of this group of patients with involvement of the aorta is giant cell arteritis.[1]

Giant Cell Arteritis

Giant cell arteritis, like the other types of arteritis, is an autoimmune disease that involves medium-sized arteries and sometimes the aorta. The name is derived from the histological finding that giant cells are present within inflammatory granulomas of the aortic wall. The condition is more widely known for its involvement of the temporal arteries ("temporal arteritis"), which results in severe headaches and blindness in half of affected patients. Two other synonyms for this disorder are *temporal arteritis* and *Horton's disease*. There is a close relationship between polymyalgia rheumatica and giant cell arteritis in some patients, with polymyalgia rheumatica sometimes preceding the development of giant cell arteritis.

HISTOLOGY

Histological findings are similar to those of other autoimmune diseases involving the aorta, although involvement of smaller arteries, including the cranial arteries and temporal arteries of the upper torso, should not be overlooked. Histological findings include intimal thickening by inflammatory cells and infiltration of the aortic media by granulomas, multinucleated giant cells, epithelial cells, T-lymphocytes, mononuclear cells and various types of other white cells. Granulocytes do not seem to be involved, as they are in other vasculitides.[42] The internal elastic lamina often appears necrotic and fragmented, and there may be focal hemorrhage in the aortic wall. Frequently segments of involvement alternate with histologically normal areas, and sometimes either perivasculitis of the vasa vasorum or vena comitantes phlebitis is present.

INCIDENCE

The incidence of giant cell arteritis (temporal arteritis) is reported to be 17.4 patients per 100,000 of the population per annum.[43-45] The prevalence, however, increases with age, and females predominate at a ratio of 2:1. The incidence in patients older than 50 years of age is believed to be up to 30 cases per 100,000 per annum.[42] The disease is more common in northern European countries and in Minnesota, possibly because of a common heritage. The disease may also be increasing in frequency.[46] In Iceland the incidence between 1984 and 1990 was 27 per 100,000 per year in patients over 50 years of age; 36 per 100,000 and 18 per 100,000 per year, respectively, for women and men.[47]

CLINICAL PRESENTATION

Patients usually have headaches or visual disturbances associated with a fever of unknown origin. In approximately 60% of patients the temporal pulses are not palpable. Besides temporal artery tenderness, jaw claudication, myalgia, arthritis, or partial or total loss of vision (either unilateral or bilateral) may occur. Loss of vision is usually due to ischemic optic neuritis. Amaurosis fugax, transient ischemic attacks, strokes, acute confusional states, ischemic cervical myelopathy, and ocular muscle abnormalities may also occur. Such symptoms as nausea, general malaise, loss of appetite, and tenderness over arteries, particularly the temporal, occipital, and carotid arteries, may be present. Patients are usually over the age of 60 years.

The erythrocyte sedimentation rate is markedly elevated in most patients, particularly during the early phase of the disease. Other serum abnormalities include an elevated prothrombin time and alpha-2 globulin, transaminase, and alkaline phosphatase levels. Anticardiolipin antibody levels may also be raised in 50% of patients. The alpha 1-antichymotripsin level appears to remain elevated while the disease is active, and when the levels return to below 0.7 g/L, the disease is less active and prednisone levels can be tapered.[48]

DIAGNOSIS

The diagnosis is confirmed by temporal artery biopsy. It is interesting that corticosteroid treatment does not appear to have any effect on the incidence of positive findings for temporal arteritis on temporal artery biopsy.[49] With high-dose treatment and longer courses, however, findings are more atypical. The presentation may be quite similar to that associated with Takayasu's aortitis, although the following signs support the diagnosis of giant cell arteritis: older age of the patients, slightly higher male incidence, positive temporal artery biopsy, normal aortic valve, and formation of an ascending aortic aneurysm without a densely inflamed, thickened ascending aorta.

On color Doppler imaging of orbital blood flow, central retinal and short posterior ciliary arterial flow velocities are reduced, there is increased turbulence, and vascular resistance is significantly increased.[50] Arteriography should reveal evidence of occlusive disease, particularly of the carotid arteries, the subclavian arteries, and their branches. In the more chronic phase of giant cell arteritis, the aortic manifestations occur in approximately 10% of patients, often several years after the initial acute illness, which may have been forgotten by the patient. Secondary to the pattern of aortic arch vessel involvement is the presentation of lower limb ischemia as a result of superficial femoral artery or profunda femoris involvement. More rarely, the abdominal visceral arteries, the vertebral arteries, the coronary arteries, and the intracranial branches of the carotid arteries are involved.[43-45] Aortic rupture may occur infrequently.[45] Despite the inflammatory involvement of the aorta with scar tissue formation, patients may also have acute dissection associated with aortic valve prolapse.[43-45, 51] On angiography, the aortic branch arteries tend to be more distally involved than in Takayasu's disease.

TREATMENT

During the acute phase, treatment with steroids should relieve visual disturbances and headaches and may even prevent blindness. Symptoms caused by branch artery stenoses, such as claudication, also usually resolve with administration of steroids.[45] Therapy, however, should be maintained indefinitely; as with Takayasu's disease, there is the theoretical possibility that this will lead to an increased risk of aneurysm formation or aortic rupture. Aortic lesions in the chronic phase are treated surgically, much like other atherosclerotic or degenerative conditions; the often thickly scarred aorta is easy to suture to an aortic prosthesis. During the acute phase, the aorta is often more friable and likely to tear and more caution must be exercised during suturing.[45, 52-59] In our experience, once aneurysms occur (primarily in the ascending aorta, although also in the descending aorta), progressive dilatation of the rest of the aorta occurs, resulting in what is commonly referred to as a mega-aorta. In fact, in a patient with giant-cell arteritis, one of us (L.G.S.) had to replace the entire aorta from the aortic valve to the bifurcation during one operation (Fig. 6-7).[60] The patient also had renal artery stenosis, celiac artery stenosis, and iliofemoral artery setnoses.

Rheumatoid Aortitis

Typically, involvement of the aorta in patients with rheumatoid arthiritis is rare, although when it is present the ascending aorta or aortic valve is involved. More rarely, the aortic arch or the descending thoracic aorta is involved. Calcification of the ascending aorta is not infrequent in later

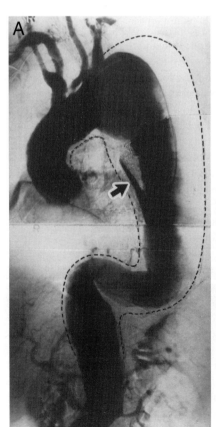 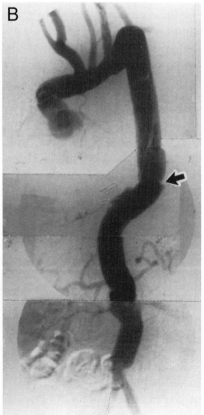

FIGURE 6–7 **A,** Aortogram of patient with giant cell aortitis with an extensive aneurysm from the aortic valve to the aortic bifurcation resulting in dysphagia, hoarseness, and severe pain not relieved by narcotics. *Arrow* indicates contrast material tracking under clot within the aorta. **B,** Postoperative aortogram after replacement of the entire aorta from the aortic valve to the aortic bifurcation during one operation. The *arrow* indicates where two 60 cm tube grafts were joined for a sufficiently long graft for the repair (see chapter on entire aorta replacements for details). (Reprinted with permission from the Society of Thoracic Surgeons. From Svensson LG, Shahian DM, Davis FG, et al. Ann Thorac Surg 1994;58:1164-6.)

stages of the disease. The histological findings are similar to those of other forms of inflammatory aortitis. Occasionally, rheumatoid lesions of the aorta may be found.[54, 55] Associated lesions, such as digital pad ulcers, gangrene of digits, Raynaud's phenomenon, and mesenteric gangrene, may occur.

Relapsing Polychondritis

Late in relapsing polychondritis vascular complications can occur and often result in the patient's death. As suggested by the name, the lesions predominantly affect cartilage. Thus manifestations are characterized by joint polyarthritis, nasal chondritis, auricular chondritis, involvement of the major airways, and evidence of inflammatory disease. Fevers of unknown origin, malaise, and an elevated ESR are frequent findings, particularly in the early phases of the disease. Aneurysms may occur in any segment of the aorta and dissection of the ascending aorta is not uncommon.[61]

Ankylosing Spondylitis

Rarely, aortitis may develop in patients with ankylosing spondylitis. Aortic valve involvement is reported to occur in 5% of patients.[62] The risk appears to be time-dependent, with aortic involvement developing in 12% of patients who have had the disease for more than 30 years compared with only 2% of those who have had the disease less than 10 years. Replacement of the aortic valve and the ascending aorta has infrequently been reported.[52, 53, 63] In 1958 Graham reported a series of 519 patients, 24 of whom developed aortic insufficiency at an average age of 39 years. In this seminal series, an association with conduction defects, cardiac enlargement, pericarditis, and an anginal type of pain of obscure origin was also noted. Other findings included annuloaortic ectasia, dilatation of the sinuses, focal degenerative changes of the elastic lamina and muscle cells of the aortic media, and patchy inflammatory lesions in all layers of the aorta. Cardiac and aortic involvement was more common with peripheral arteritis, iritis, and pericarditis.

Behçet's Disease

The most common manifestations of Behçet's disease are the presence of aphthous ulcers of moist membranes, such as the mouth and genitalia, uveitis, and frequent occurrence in men between the ages of 20 and 40 years. Other manifestations include skin lesions comparable to those observed in erythema nodosum, skin pustules, gastrointestinal disease similar to Crohn's disease, pancreatitis, pneumonitis, joint synovitis, arthritis, hypopyon, epididymo-orchitis, glomerulonephritis, polyneuropathy, and meningoencephalitis. In the later stages of the disease, blindness occurs and patients are seen with cardiac or vascular complications. Cardiac complications include endo-, myo-, or pericarditis, conduction defects, valve destruction, and coronary aneurysms or stenoses.[64] Vascular lesions include thoracic and abdominal aneurysms, thrombophlebitis (migrans and saltans), thromboses of large veins such as the superior and inferior venae cavae, pulmonary artery stenoses, and occlu-sive disease of medium-sized arteries. Isolated aneurysms in medium-sized arteries, including those in the pulmonary vasculature, may occur and, in the latter instance, may be accompanied by hemoptysis.

Behçet's disease appears to be of autoimmune etiology, and thus the disease does respond to immunosuppressive therapy with such agents as steroids and chlorambucil.[65] In the few patients with this disease on whom we have operated we have observed that the aorta has the appearance of inflammatory aneurysms, and a standard operative repair has been used successfully with suturing of grafts to normal-appearing aortic tissue. These patients are often prone to postoperative thrombosis, and some may require anticoagulation to prevent venous or graft thrombosis.

Polymyalgia Rheumatica and Uncommon Causes

Rarely, in 10% to 15% of patients, polymyalgia rheumatica involves the aorta by either aortic dissection, aneurysm formation, or occlusive disease of the aortic branches.[42] The disease is characterized by aching in the shoulder, neck, and hip muscles, morning stiffness, and associated systemic features. As indicated previously, the disease appears to progress to a form of giant cell arteritis. The vascular lesions are then treated as indicated by the angiographic findings and the patient's clinical symptoms and signs.

Of interest is the rare involvement of the aorta in patients with systemic lupus erythematosus (SLE). Although occasionally these patients have aortic aneurysms, a patient who has total occlusion of the aorta should be suspected of having SLE, particularly if the thrombosis extends into or involves the renal arteries. The reason for this is the presence of a lupus inhibitor called "lupus anticoagulant" that inhibits either synthesis or release of PGI_2, the latter preventing platelet aggregation. Lupus inihibitor may also affect protein C and hence the coagulation system. The net result is a tendency for coagulation to occur in larger arteries or veins. Patients with SLE, particularly if they are taking steroids, are at increased risk of mycotic aneurysms.

Bacharach and colleagues[66] have suggested that cocaine abuse may result in a distinct form of lymphoplasmocytic aortitis that histologically is different from Takayasu's disease or syphilis. Other rare causes of aortis are Buerger's, Cogan's, and Kawasaki's disease.

Possible Etiological Factors in Aortitis

The diverse group of diseases that may cause aortitis raises the question of etiology. Clearly, aortic wall injury, as evidenced by the inflammatory response, is a common denominator. The cause of the aortic wall injury, however, is only beginning to be elucidated. Probably the inciting event is unique for each disease; perhaps the cause is multifactorial.

Weyand and colleagues[42] studied tissue cytokines in 34 patients with polymyalgia rheumatica (no arteritis) or giant-cell arteritis. In giant-cell arteritis specimens, interleukin-1β,

interleukin-6, and transforming growth factor-β1 mRNA transcripts were produced from macrophage activation, whereas interferon-γ and interleukin-2 mRNAs were produced from T cell activation. Macrophage and T cell–derived cytokines were similar from patients with polymyalgia rheumatica, although lymphokine profiles were distinctive. Interferon-γ was thus found in 67% of patients with giant cell arteritis in addition to interleukin-2, although patients with polymyalgia rheumatica had only interleukin-2. The authors, therefore, concluded that because patients who have polymyalgia without arteritis had no interferon-γ production and interferon-γ was associated with giant cell arteritis, interferon-γ may be involved in the progression to overt arteritis. These lymphokines are derived from T helper cells (TH1), and therefore giant cell arteritis appears to be related to TH1 cells. Of interest, tuberculoid leprosy has also been associated with a TH1-like disease. In those patients who develop arteritis (10% to 15%) in association with polymyalgia rheumatica, it appears that an exogenous triggering antigen (the source of which is unknown) causes TH1 cells to produce pro-inflammatory interferon-γ. TH1 cells are known to suppress TH2 cells; the significance of this is that TH2 cells are of primary importance in regulating the pathogenic effects of TH1 cells, and TH2 cells are also anti-inflammatory.[67] Arterial specimens with giant cell arteritis show evidence of classic complement, alternative complement, and lytic complex activation.[67]

Although the cause of these diseases is unclear, we can theorize that infective agents may be precipitating the autoimmune reaction that results in aortic disease. Of interest is the finding that heat-shock protein 65 (hsp 65) is produced from injured arteries and that hsp 65 results in binding of dendritic γ T cells and an immune reaction. Furthermore, hsp 65 is part of the antigen of both *Mycobacterium leprae* and *Mycobacterium tuberculosis*. Human T cells can recognize bacteria, particularly mycobacterial hsp 65.[68] Thus it is intriguing to speculate that T cells activated by tuberculous hsp 65 may then be attracted to areas of minimal arterial injury, resulting in chromic cellular immune damage of arteries. Hence the frequent association of aortitis, particularly in Takayasu's disease, with a past history of tuberculosis infection. This is further supported by the fact that Kawasaki arteritis, resulting in coronary or aortic aneurysms, is associated with toxic shock syndrome *Staphyloccccus aureus* infection[69] (see Chapter 3). Moreover, inflammatory infrarenal aneurysms may be associated with cytomegalovirus infection (see below).

INFLAMMATORY ANEURYSMS OF THE INFRARENAL AORTA

The cause of inflammatory aneurysms of the infrarenal aorta has not been established. Gaylis[70] has proposed that inflammatory aneurysms of the infrarenal aorta arise because of obstruction of the rich lymphatic plexus that courses over the infrarenal aorta. Sterpetti and colleagues[71] support this theory by stating that reactive lymphatic hyperplasia is a notable factor that may result in inflammatory aneurysms. A more recent intriguing possibility is that cytomegalovirus may play a role; Tanaka and colleagues[72] have reported a correlation between inflammatory disease and the presence of cytomegalovirus DNA. Furthermore, this may be an ongoing active infection.[73] Van der Wal and colleagues[74] examined specimens of descending thoracic aorta and found that atherosclerosis was associated with inflammatory infiltrates of macrophages and T lymphocytes surrounding the vasa vasorum and that the infiltrate was more extensive with greater amounts of atherosclerotic penetration of the aorta. There was also loss of smooth muscle cells, collagen, and extensive remodeling. This type of inflammation, however, is more characteristic of atherosclerotic or aneurysms of the medial degenerative type than of inflammatory aneurysms per se; the latter sometimes has very little evidence of atherosclerosis, suggesting that atherosclerosis probably is not an etiological factor in the grossly characteristic inflammatory type of aneurysms.

In contrast to inflammatory aneurysms of the autoimmune type, the systemic constitutional symptoms and signs are minimal. When they occur, fever of unknown origin, malaise, and weight loss are the most frequent. An elevated ESR is often detected. Most patients have associated abdominal tenderness or pain in the vicinity of or over the aneurysm. On CT or MRI scan, the anterior surface of the aneurysm characteristically appears to be thickened and homogeneous[75] (Figs. 6–8 to 6–10). If calcification is present, it tends to be located on the inner surface of the aortic wall. By contrast, if thrombus is found in the aortic wall in patients with noninflammatory infrarenal aortic aneurysms, the calcification tends to be found on the outer circumference of the wall.[75] It is noteworthy that the posterior wall of the aneurysm is often thin. The importance of this finding is that this is the area in which rupture usually occurs. After either CT scanning or aortography of the aneurysm, delayed films should be obtained to observe the position of the ureters. The surrounding fibrosis may draw the ureters toward or incorporate them into the aortic wall. This can easily lead to injury of the ureters during operations.[1]

Tennant and colleagues[76] reviewed their MRI findings in 15 patients. They observed that inflammatory aneurysms appeared to have distinctively laminated walls that were present in all 15 patients but were not seen in 45 other patients who did not have inflammatory aneurysms. Even MRI scans of the aortic wall specimens revealed the laminated bands, although in the illustrative MRI these are not clearly seen (Fig. 6–8).

The aorta looks shiny and pink and has a plaquelike appearance in the anterior wall. The aorta is also firm from the fibrosis. The dense inflammatory involvement of the retroperitoneum can extend laterally as far as the flanks and encase retroperitoneal structures. Microscopic examination of the aortic wall reveals a dense infiltration of fibrous tissue,

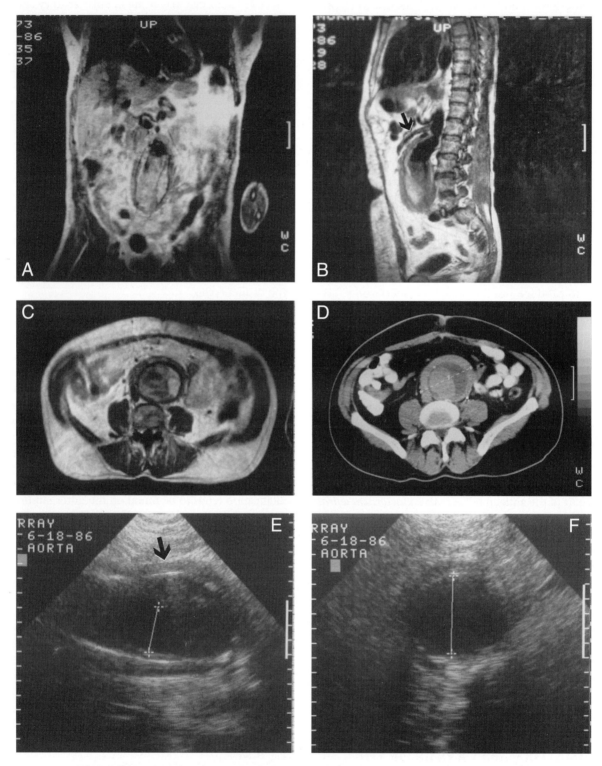

FIGURE 6–8   Findings in a patient with inflammatory aneurysm. **A, B,** and **C,** MRI images. Note that *arrow* indicating superior mesenteric artery is stretched over the anterior wall of the aneurysm. **D,** CT image. Note the thick anterior and lateral walls of the aneurysm but thinner posterior wall. **E** and **F,** Ultrasound findings also showing the thickened aortic wall and superior mesenteric artery *(arrow).* (From Svensson LG, Crawford ES. Curr Probl Surg 1993;30:1–172.)

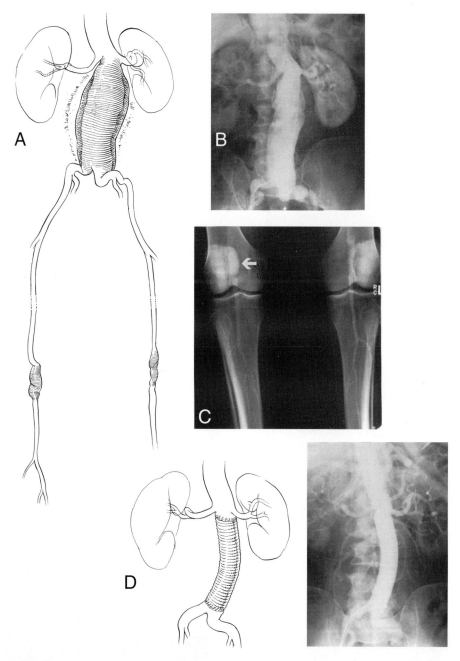

FIGURE 6–9   A, Diagram of arteriogram of the same patients as in Figure 6-8 showing the infrarenal aneurysm **(B)** and the popliteal aneurysm **(C). D,** Diagram and arteriogram of post-operative repair. (From Svensson LG, Crawford ES. Curr Probl Surg 1993;30:1–172.)

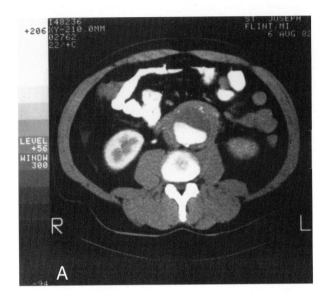

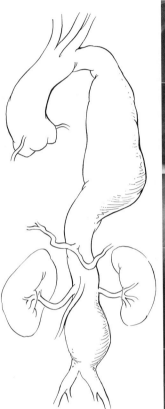

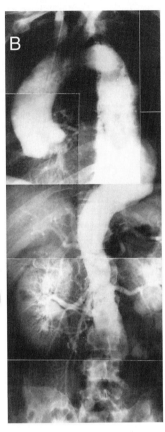

FIGURE 6–10 Patient with inflammatory aneurysm of the abdominal and descending aorta. **A,** CT scan. Note the thick anterior and lateral walls and internal luminal thrombus. **B,** Diagram of aneurysm and arteriogram. **C,** Delayed films showing evidence of obstructive hydronephrosis with calyceal loss and medial displacement of the ureters.

Illustration continued on following page

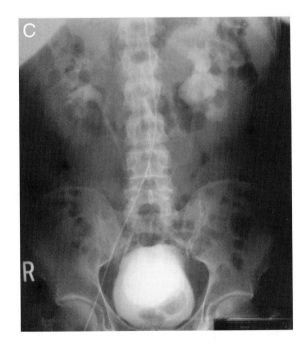

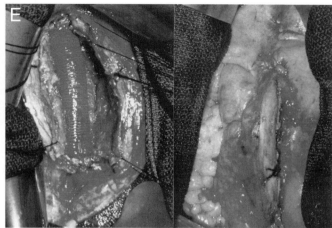

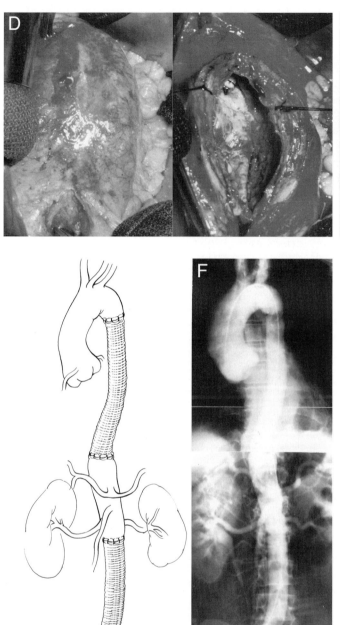

FIGURE 6–10 *Continued* **D,** Intraoperative photographs of glistening surface *(left window)* and thick aortic wall after incision of the aneurysm *(right window).* **E,** Photograph of tube graft after repair *(left window)* and after closure of the retroperitoneum *(right window).* Note that the duodenum was not dissected free from the aneurysm. **F,** Postoperative diagram and arteriogram. (From Svensson LG, Crawford ES. Curr Probl Surg 1993;30:1–172.

inflammatory cells, and plasma cells. The tunica media shows medial degeneration of elastic tissue and necrosis of smooth muscle cells. The adventitia is usually the thickest layer with lymphocytic aggregates, perhaps because of the rich plexus of lymphatics in this layer.

SURGICAL TREATMENT

Shumacker and Garrett[77] reported the first repair of an inflammatory type of infrarenal aortic aneurysm on May 7, 1955. The inflamed abdominal aortic aneurysm was replaced with a tube graft, and both ureters were drained and mobilized to relieve ureteric obstruction. The operative technique for repairing infrarenal inflammatory aneurysms consists of minimal dissection of surrounding tissue, including leaving the duodenum attached to the anteriolateral surface of the aneurysm.[75, 78]

A cautionary note is that the duodenal wall is often incorporated in the inflammatory process and thus may be inadvertently entered during any mobilization attempts. In fact, the only death in the series of 10 patients reported by Goldstone and colleagues[78] in 1978 was from duodenal breakdown. Moreover, because the surrounding tissues are usually involved in the inflammatory process, attempts at freeing the aorta can result in extensive retroperitoneal bleeding.

Because of the fibrosis surrounding the infrarenal aorta, the aorta is cross-clamped at the diaphragm in approximately half our patients.[75] The graft is then sutured into position within the aneurysm by the inclusion technique. The ureters are not mobilized since the inflammatory process surrounding the aorta resolves in time in most patients.[75] Pennell and colleagues[79] have reported that the operative mortality rate for infrarenal inflammatory aortic aneurysm repairs is increased in comparison to noninflammatory procedures (7.9% versus 2.4%, $p < 0.002$).

REFERENCES

1. Svensson LG, Crawford ES. Aortic dissection and aortic aneurysm surgery: clinical observations, experimental investigations, and statistical analyses. Part III. Curr Probl Surg 1993;30:1–172.
2. Takayasu M. A case with unusual changes of the central vessels in the retina. Acta Soc Ophthal Jap 1908;12:554–5.
3. Trench FN, Lengyel I, Maffei EW. Coartacoes e estonoses segmentares da aorta toracica e abdominal de localizacao atipica. Arg Hosp Santa Casa Sao Paulo 1957;3:33–128.
4. Lande A. Takayasu's arteritis and congenital coarctation of the descending thoracic and abdominal aorta: a critical review. Am J Roentgenol 1978;127:227–33.
5. Shimizu K, Sano K. Pulseless disease. J Neuropathol Clin Neurol 1951;1:37–47.
6. Kimoto S. The history and present status of aortic surgery in Japan particularly for aortitis syndrome. J Cardiovasc Surg 1979;20:107–26.
7. Inada K. A typical coarctation of the aorta with a special reference to its genesis. Angiology 1965;16:608.
8. Oota K. Ein seltner Fall von beiderseitigen Carotis-Subclaviaverschluss. Trans Soc Pathol Jap 1940;30:680.
9. Lupi-Herrera E, Sanchez-Torres G, Marcushamer J, et al. Takayasu's arteritis: clinical study of 107 cases. Am Heart J 1977;93:94.
10. Ueno A, Awane Y, Wakabayashi A, Shimizu K. Case reports: successfully operated obliterative brachiocephalic arteritis (Takayasu) associated with the elongated coarctation. Jpn Heart J 1967;8:538–44.
11. Matsumura K, Hirano T, Takeda K, et al. Incidence of aneurysms in Takayasu's arteritis. Angiology 1991;42:308–15.
12. Pokrovskii AV. Nonspecific aortoarteritis (classification and surgical treatment). Kardiologiia 1986;26:5–12.
13. Ueda H, Ishikowa K, Kirisowa N, et al. Clinical and pathological studies of aortitis syndrome: a committee report. Jpn Heart J 1968;9:76–87.
14. Nasu T. Pathology of pulseless disease: systemic study and critical review of 21 autopsy cases reported in Japan. Angiography 1962;14:225.
15. Rose AG, Sinclair-Smith CC. Takayasu's arteritis: a study of 16 autopsy cases. Arch Pathol Lab Med 1980;104:231–7.
16. Saito Y, Hirota K, Ito I, et al. Clinical and pathological studies of five autopsied cases of aortitis syndrome. Part I. Findings of the aorta and its branches, peripheral arteries and pulmonary arteries. Jpn Heart J 1992;13:20–33.
17. Ueda H, Morooka S, Ito I, et al. Clinical observation of 52 cases of aortitis syndrome. Jpn Heart J 1969;10:277–88.
18. Morooka S, Ito I, Yamaguchi H, et al. Follow-up observations of aortitis syndrome. Jpn Heart J 1972;13:201–13.
19. Restrepo C, Jejeda C, Correa P. Non-syphilitic aortitis. Arch Pathol 1969;87:1.
20. Numano F. Hereditary factors of Takayasu arteritis. Heart Vessels Suppl 1992;7:68–72.
21. Kerr GS, Hallahan CW, Giordano J, et al. Takayasu arteritis. Ann Intern Med 1994;120:919–29.
22. Bickerstaff LK, Pairolero PC, Hollier LH, et al. Thoracic aortic aneurysms: a population-based study. Surgery 1982;92:1103–8.
23. Ueda H. Renovascular hypertension as a manifestation of arteritis syndrome. Jpn Heart J 1967;8:209.
24. Kreidstein SH, Lytwyn A, Keystone EC. Takayasu arteritis with acute interstitial pneumonia and coronary vasculitis: expanding the spectrum. Arthritis Rheum 1993;36:1175–8.
25. Ishikawa H, Kondo Y, Ejiri Y, et al. An autopsy case of ulcerative colitis associated with Takayasu's disease with review of 13 Japanese cases. Gastroenterol Jpn 1993;28:110–7.
26. Eibenberger K, Dock W, Metz V, et al. Stenosen und Verschlusse der Aorta abdominalis bei Patienten unter 40 Jahren. Rofo Fortschr Geb Rontgenstr Neuen Bildgeb Verfahr 1993;159:388–92.
27. Roberti I, Reisman L, Churg J. Vasculitis in childhood. Pediatr Nephrol 1993;7:479–89.
28. Ishikawa K. Diagnostic approach and proposed criteria for the clinical diagnosis of Takayasu's arteriopathy. J Am Coll Cardiol 1988;12:964–72.
29. Kerr G. Takayasu's arteritis. Curr Opin Rheumatol 1994;6:32–8.
30. Hoffman GS. Treatment of chronic idiopathic systemic vasculitides. Adv Exp Med Biol 1993;336:227–34.
31. Takagi A, Kajiura N, Tada Y, Ueno A. Surgical treatment of nonspecific inflammatory arterial aneurysms. J Cardiovasc Surg (Torino) 1986;27:117–24.
32. Tyagi S, Kaul UA, Nair M, et al. Balloon angioplasty of the aorta in Takayasu's arteries: initial and long-term results. Am Heart J 1992;124:876–82.
33. Sharma S, Shrivastava S, Kothari SS, et al. Influence of angiographic morphology on the acute and longer-term outcome of percutaneous transluminal angioplasty in patients with aortic stenosis due to nonspecific aortitis. Cardiovasc Intervent Radiol 1994;17:147–51.
34. Tyagi S, Singh B, Kaul UA, et al. Balloon angioplasty for renovascular hypertension in Takayasu's arteritis. Am Heart J 1993;125:1386–93.
35. Haga Y, Yoshizu H, Okuda E, et al. Surgical resection of an ascending aortic dissection in Takayasu's arteritis. Ann Thorac Surg 1992;54:359–60.
36. Robbs JV, Human RR, Rajaruthnam P. Operative treatment of nonspecific aortoarteritis (Takayasu's arteritis). J Vasc Surg 1986;3:605–16.
37. Crawford ES, DeBakey ME, Cooley DA, et al. Surgical treatment of occlusions of the innominate, common carotid and subclavian arteries: a ten year experience. Surgery 1969;65:17.
38. Ohteki H, Itoh T, Natsuaki M, et al. Aortic valve replacement for Takayasu's arteritis. J Thorac Cardiovasc Surg 1992;104:482–6.
39. Subramanyan R, Joy J, Balakrishnan KG. Natural history of aortoarteritis (Takayasu's disease). Circulation 1989;80:429–37.
40. Ishikawa K, Maetani S. Long-term outcome for 120 Japanese patients with Takayasu's disease—clinical and statistical analyses of related prognostic factors. Circulation 1994;90:1855–60.
41. Robbs JV, Abdool-Carrim AT, Kadwa AM. Arterial reconstruction for non-specific arteritis (Takayasu's disease): medium to long term results. Euro J Vasc Surg 1994;8:401–7.
42. Weyand CM, Hicok KC, Hunder GG, Goronzy JJ. Tissue cytokine patterns in patients with polymyalgia rheumatica and giant cell arteritis. Ann Intern Med 1994;121:484–91.
43. Hunder GG, Sheps SG, Allen GL, Joyce JW. Daily and alternate-day corticosteroid regimens in treatment of giant cell arteritis: comparisons in a prospective study. Ann Intern Med 1975;82:613–8.
44. Huston KA, Hunder GG, Lie JT, et al. Temporal arteritis: a 25-year epidemiologic, clinical and pathologic study. Ann Intern Med 1978;88:162–7.
45. Klein RG, Hunder GG, Stanson AW, Sheps SG. Large artery involvement in giant cell (temporal) arteritis. Ann Intern Med 1975;83:806–12.
46. Nordborg E, Andersson R, Bengtsson BA. Giant cell arteritis. Drugs Aging 1994;4:135–44.
47. Baldursson O, Steinsson K, Bjornsson J, Lie JT. Giant cell arteritis in Iceland: an epidemiologic and histopathologic analysis. Arthiritis Rheum 1994;37:1007–12.
48. Pountain GD, Calvin J, Hazleman BL. Alpha 1-antichymotripsin, C-reactive protein, and erythrocyte sedimentation rate in polymyalgia rheumatica and giant cell arteritis. Br J Rheumatol 1994;33:550–4.
49. Achkar AA, Lie JT, Hunder GG, et al. How does previous corticosteroid treatment affect the biopsy findings in giant cell (temporal) arteritis? Ann Intern Med 1994;120:987–92.
50. Ho AC, Sergott RC, Regillo CD, et al. Color Doppler hemodynamics of giant cell arteritis. Arch Ophthalmol 1994;112:938–45.
51. Save-Soderbergh J, Malmvall B-E, Andersson R, Bengtsson BA. Giant cell arteritis as a cause of death: report of nine cases. JAMA 1986;255:493–6.
52. Austen WG, Blennerhassett JB. Giant-cell aortitis causing an aneu-

rysm of the ascending aorta and aortic regurgitation. N Engl J Med 1965;272:80-3.

53. Gula G, Pomerance A, Bennett M, et al. Homograft replacement of aortic valve and ascending aorta in a patient with non-specific giant cell aortitis. Br Heart J 1977;39:581-5.

54. Hollenhorst RW, Brown JR, Wagenor HP, et al. Neurologic aspects of temporal arteritis. Neurology 1960;10:490-8.

55. Honig HS, Weintraub AU, Goures MN, et al. Severe aortic regurgitation secondary to idiopathic aortitis. Am J Med 1977;63:623-33.

56. McMillan GC. Diffuse granulomatous aortitis with giant cells associated with partial rupture and dissection of the aorta. Arch Pathol 1950;49:63-9.

57. Rivers SP, Baur GM, Inahara T, et al. Arm ischemia secondary to giant cell arteritis. Am J Surg 1982;143:554-8.

58. Salisbury RS, Hazleman BL. Successful treatment of dissecting aortic aneurysm due to giant cell arteritis. Ann Rheum Dis 1981;40:507-8.

59. Soorae AS, McKeown F, Cleland J. Aortic valve replacement for severe aortic regurgitation caused by idiopathic giant cell aortitis. Thorax 1980;35:60-3.

60. Svensson LG, Shahian DM, Davis FG, et al. Replacement of entire aorta from aortic valve to bifurcation during one operation. Ann Thorac Surg 1994;58:1164-6.

61. Michet CJ, McKenna CH, Luthra HS, O'Fallon WM. Relapsing polychondritis: survival and predictive roles of early disease manifestations. Ann Intern Med 1986;104:74-8.

62. Schilder DP, Harvey WP, Hufnagel CA. Rheumatoid spondylitis and aortic insufficiency. N Engl J Med 1956;255:11-7.

63. Spangler RD, McCallister BD, McGoon DC. Aortic valve replacement in patients with severe aortic valve incompetence associated with rheumatoid spondylitis. Am J Cardiol 1970;26:130-4.

64. Mickley V, Kogel H, Gaschler F, et al. Infrarenales aortenaneurysma bei morbus Behcet. VASA 1992;21:233-40.

65. O'Duffy JE, Robertson DM, Goldstein NP. Chlorambucil in the treatment of uveitis and meningoencephalitis of Behçet's disease. Am J Med 1984;76:75-84.

66. Bacharach JM, Colville DS, Lie JT. Accelerated atherosclerosis, aneurysmal disease, and aortitis: possible pathogenetic association with cocaine abuse. Int Angiol 1992;11:83-6.

67. Getsy JA, Phillips SM. Cytokines in polymyalgia and giant cell arteritis. Ann Intern Med 1994;121:536-37.

68. Heng MK, Heng MCY. Heat-shock protein 65 and activated γ/δ T cells in injured arteries. Lancet 1994;344:921-23.

69. Leung DYM, Meissner HC, Fulton DR, et al. Toxic shock syndrome toxin-secreting Staphyloccus aureus in Kawasaki syndrome. Lancet 1993;342:1385-8.

70. Gaylis H. Etiology of abdominal aortic "inflammatory" aneurysms: hypothesis (letter). J Vasc Surg 1985;23:643.

71. Sterpetti AV, Hunter WJ, Feldhaus RJ, et al. Inflammatory aneurysms of the abdominal aorta: incidence, pathologic, and etiologic considerations. J Vasc Surg 1989;9:643-9.

72. Tanaka S, Tohy Y, Mori R, et al. Possible role of cytomegalovirus in the pathogenesis of inflammatory aortic disease: a preliminary report. J Vasc Surg 1992;16:274-9.

73. Tanaka S, Komori K, Okadome K, et al. Detection of active cytomegalovirus infection in inflammatory aortic aneurysms with RNA polymerase chain reaction. J Vasc Surg 1994;20:235-43.

74. Van der Wal AC, Becker AE, Das PK. Medial thinning and atherosclerosis-evidence for involvement of a local inflammatory effect. Atherosclerosis 1993;103:55-64.

75. Crawford JL, Stowe CL, Safi HJ, et al. Inflammatory aneurysms of the aorta. J Vasc Surg 1985;2:113-24.

76. Tennant WG, Hartnell GG, Baird RN, Horrocks M. Radiologic investigation of abdominal aortic aneurysm disease: comparison of three modalities in staging and the detection of inflammatory change. J Vasc Surg 1993;17:703-9.

77. Shumacker HB Jr, Garrett R. Obstructive uropathy from abdominal aortic aneurysm. Surg Gynecol Obstet 1955;100:758-61.

78. Goldstone J, Malone JM, Moore WS. Inflammatory aneurysms of the abdominal aorta. Surgery 1978;83:425-30.

79. Pennell RC, Hollier LH, Lie JT, et al. Inflammatory abdominal aortic aneurysms: a thirty-year review. J Vasc Surg 1985;2:859-69.

7

Aortic Infections

Aortic infections can be divided into three groups and include those associated with (1) chronic infections by bacteria, not necessarily of the aorta per se, but often associated with chronic inflammatory changes of the aorta; and (2) acute primary infections of the aorta (mycotic aneurysms); and (3) aortic infections associated with previous operations, usually involving aortic grafts.

CHRONIC BACTERIAL INFECTIONS

The two most commonly associated bacterial infections are syphilitic aortitis and tuberculous aortitis. Tuberculous aortitis is discussed in Chapter 6.

Syphilitic Aortitis

Historical Note

Ambrose Paré[1] first noticed the association between syphilis and aortic aneurysms in the sixteenth century after performing an autopsy on a patient who died of a ruptured descending aortic aneurysm. In the past, before the antibiotic era, up to 75% of abdominal aortic aneurysms were the result of syphilis.[2] In the extreme form, often seen prior to this century, painless aneurysms eroded through the sternum and patients would present with massive exsanguinating hemorrhages through aortocutaneous fistulae.

Pathology

Aneurysms associated with tertiary syphilis most commonly affect the ascending aorta, and sometimes the aortic sinuses may also be involved. Occasionally, aneurysms of the aortic arch and abdominal aorta occur, as observed by Astley Cooper in 1817 in the first report of an attempted ligation of the aorta.[3] If involvement of the aorta is focal, with irregularly shaped scars, then these aneurysms appear saccular, whereas if the affected area is more circumferential the aneurysms may be more fusiform in shape. As the aneurysms enlarge, involvement of the aortic valve is more likely, with the concomitant problem of aortic valve regurgitation. Furthermore, the coronary ostia are prone to ostial stenotic lesions resulting in myocardial ischemia. Of interest, aortic dissection has not been documented, probably because of scar tissue formation in the aortic wall.

Histologically, the aortic media is destroyed, and there is evidence of loss of elastic fibers and smooth muscle necrosis. Both the intima and the adventitia are thickened. Classically, the adventitial changes are characterized by perivascular inflammation of the vasa vasorum with plasma cells and endarteritis obliterans of the arteries. This is probably an important factor in the loss of the aortic media and the development of aneurysms. Spirochetes are not found in the aortic lesions.

Clinical Presentation and Management

Patients with syphilitic aortic aneurysms are usually otherwise healthy. On careful questioning, a history of having been treated for syphilis or other venereal disease will probably be obtained. Chancres may also have been noted in the past, and serologic testing for syphilis antibodies is usually positive. Management of the patients is similar to that of patients with other types of aneurysm, aside from the treatment of any possible active syphilitic disease.

MYCOTIC ANEURYSMS

Historical Note and Definition

Mycotic aneurysm, the name first used by Sir William Osler,[4] describes the fungus-like appearance of the aneurysmal wall. A mycotic aneurysm can be defined as a dilated segment of the aorta infected by a microorganism from a distant site without the presence of contiguous infections (for example, endocarditis), aortic trauma, or foreign graft prostheses in the aneurysm.[5] Despite the name, infections are usually caused by bacteria and only very rarely by a fungus. Except for bacterial endocarditis involving the aortic valve, the aortic valve annulus, and the surrounding tissue, bacterial infections of the aorta are unusual. During an 8½ year period, mycotic aneurysms in our practice, excluding endocarditis, accounted for only 0.85% (22 of 2585) of aneurysm repairs.[5]

Although endocarditis associated with an aortic annulus abscess is, by definition, not considered to be a mycotic aneurysm, Sir William Osler[4] documented the association between bacterial endocarditis and the development of peripheral infected aneurysms resulting from peripheral embolization. These infected mycotic aneurysms were often noted to rupture. Subsequently, in 1923, Stengel and Wolferth[6] reported that mycotic aneurysms could occur in 14% of patients without evidence of bacterial endocarditis. Later Crane,[7] further supported by Revell,[8] demonstrated that abnormalities of the aorta such as coarctation, hypoplastic aorta, and diseased segements of the aorta were predisposed to the development of mycotic aneurysms if bacteremia occurred. Two groups of researchers, Zak and colleagues[9] and Sommerville and associates[10] noted the association of infection with the *Salmonella* organism and atherosclerotic lesions. In addition, mycotic aneurysms can arise from infection of preexisting aneurysms or of posttraumatic false aneurysms.[11] Both Ernst and coworkers[12] and Williams and Fisher[13] found that a high proportion of the thrombus found in nonmycotic abdominal aortic aneurysms was coincidentally colonized by bacteria at the time of aneurysm repairs. Furthermore, the incidence of positive cultures was higher with ruptured aneurysms (38%) than with either symptomatic aneurysms (13%) or asymptomatic aneurysms (9%). The significance of these positive bacterial cultures and of the origin of the bacteria is not known, but it does not appear to influence the risk of postoperative sepsis. Steed and colleagues[14] routinely cultured thrombus from 116 patients undergoing abdominal aortic aneurysm repair

and found a lower than usual incidence of only 5.2% positive cultures, and none of those affected developed late graft infections. Similarly, Farkas and colleagues[15] found in the evaluation of 500 operative cultures that 37% were positive for bacteria, mostly related to skin flora; only one patient developed a late graft infection 6 years after surgery, and that was from an unrelated organism. Both of these studies concluded that routine cultures are not necessary and that positive cultures have no pathogenic significance.

Pathology

There are two sites at which mycotic sacciform aortic aneurysms most frequently occur. These are (1) the aortic arch and (2) the abdominal visceral arteries (Figs. 7–1 and 7–2). Although these are the two most usual sites, multiple sites may also be involved.[5] Most often there is penetration by the infection through the aortic wall, resulting in a false aneurysm or frank rupture.

Commonly, the organisms include *Staphylococcus aureus, Staphylococcus epidermidis, Salmonella* sp., *Streptococcus*

FIGURE 7–1   A, Diagram and aortogram of a patient with a rapidly expanding mycotic aneurysm. **B,** Postoperative diagram and aortogram after replacement of the lower descending thoracic aorta distally to the iliac arteries with reimplantation of the visceral arteries. (Reprinted with permission of the Society of Thoracic Surgeons. From Chan FY, Crawford ES, Coselli JS, et al. Ann Thorac Surg 1989;47:193–203).

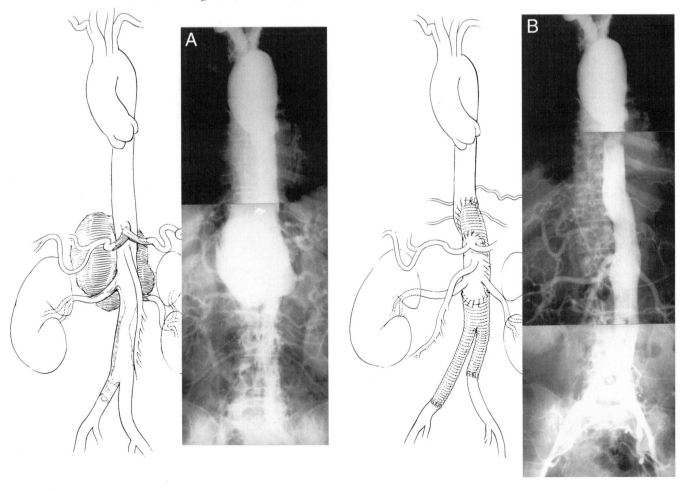

sp., *Haemophilus influenzae*, *Pseudomonas* sp., *Enterobacter* sp., *Proteus* sp., *Yersinia* sp., *Campylobacter fetus*, *Bacteroides fragilis*, *Candida* sp., and *Escherichia coli*.[5, 16, 17] Most of the *Salmonella* infections are due to *Salmonella Choleraesuis* and *Salmonella Typhimurium*.[11] Rarer infections, such as *Mycobacterium bovis* from bacilli Calmette-Guérin (BCG) vaccine, have been reported.[18] It is noteworthy that, in contrast to valvular endocarditis, mycotic aneurysms are associated with a broader range of bacteria, with *Salmonella* sp. accounting for up to 50%.[17] Furthermore, in our patients, positive blood cultures are less frequent and were present in only 6 of 22 patients (27%), although 17 (77%) had bacteria cultured from intraoperative specimens.[5]

Etiology

The bacteria appear to seed either by embolization of infected material or during episodes of bacteremia to the aortic wall at sites of congenital lesions, such as at the coarctation site of the aorta, patent ductus arteriosus, atherosclerotic plaques, or intraluminal clots.[5] Bacteremia may arise from infections of the urinary tract; heart valves; ear, nose, throat, or skin infections; dental manipulations; intravenous line sepsis; and distant wound infections.[5] For example, we have treated a 15-month-old child in whom a thoracoabdominal aneurysm developed after an umbilical catheter placed for hyperalimentation became infected and caused a mycotic aneurysm (Fig. 7–3).[19] Aortic aneurysms

FIGURE 7–2   **A,** Patient with a hemolytic *Streptococcus* mycotic aneurysm at the origin of the superior mesenteric artery from the abdominal aorta that involves the renal arteries. **B,** Treatment entailed extensive debridement, in situ graft replacement of the aorta, reimplantation of the left renal artery, bypass to the superior mesenteric artery, and antibiotics. (Reprinted with permission of the Society of Thoracic Surgeons. From Chan FY, Crawford ES, Coselli JS, et al. Ann Thorac Surg 1989;47:193–203).

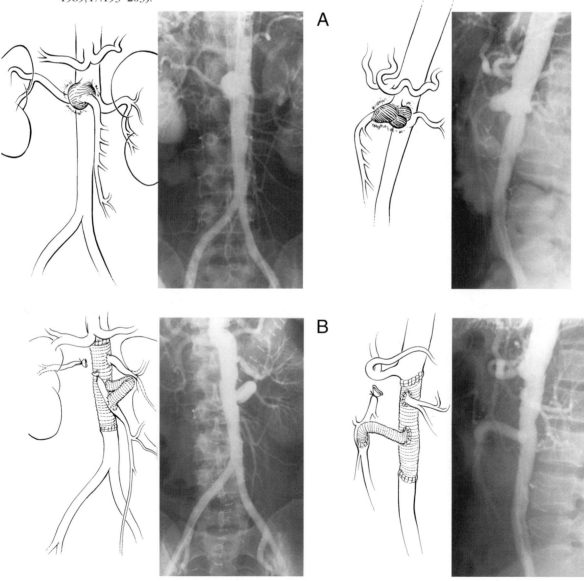

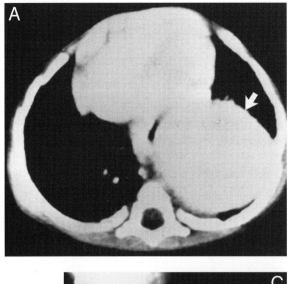

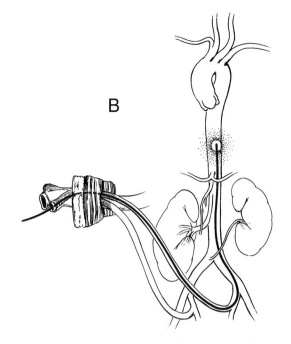

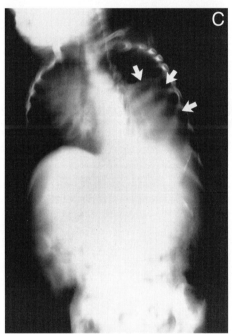

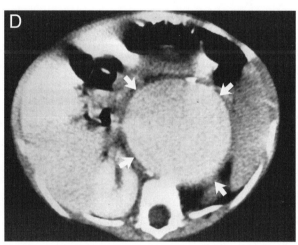

FIGURE 7–3 **A,** CT scan of 15-month-old child with a large thoracoabdominal aortic aneurysm as a result of an umbilical artery catheter infection **(B). C,** Radiograph showing the extent of the aneurysm in the chest. **D,** Scan showing the abdominal component. **E,** Diagram of aneurysm and aortogram.

Illustration continued on following page

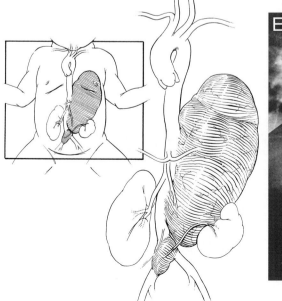

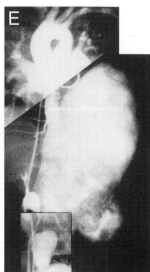

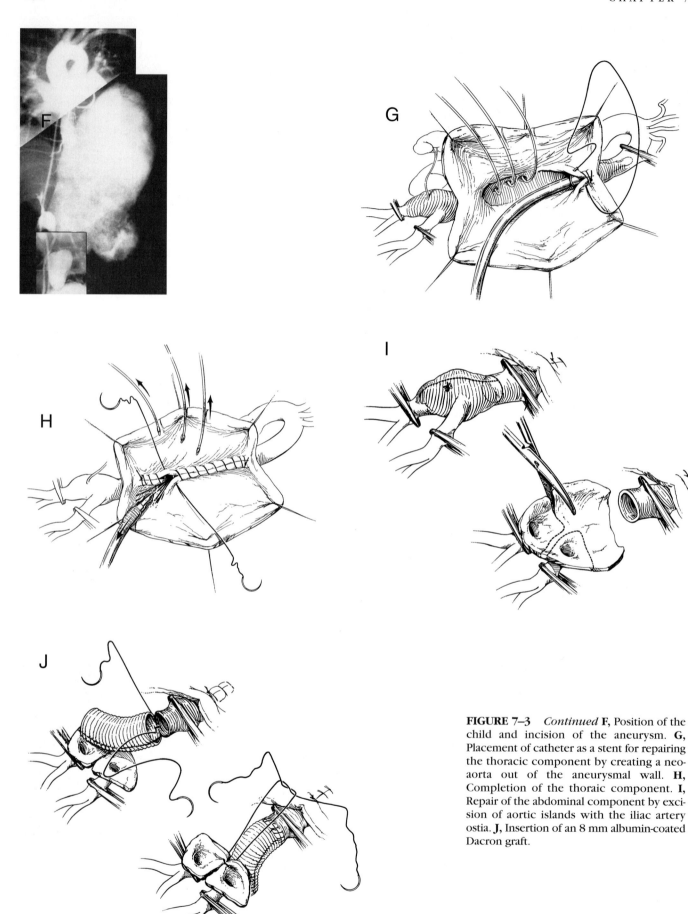

FIGURE 7–3 *Continued* **F,** Position of the child and incision of the aneurysm. **G,** Placement of catheter as a stent for repairing the thoracic component by creating a neo-aorta out of the aneurysmal wall. **H,** Completion of the thoraic component. **I,** Repair of the abdominal component by excision of aortic islands with the iliac artery ostia. **J,** Insertion of an 8 mm albumin-coated Dacron graft.

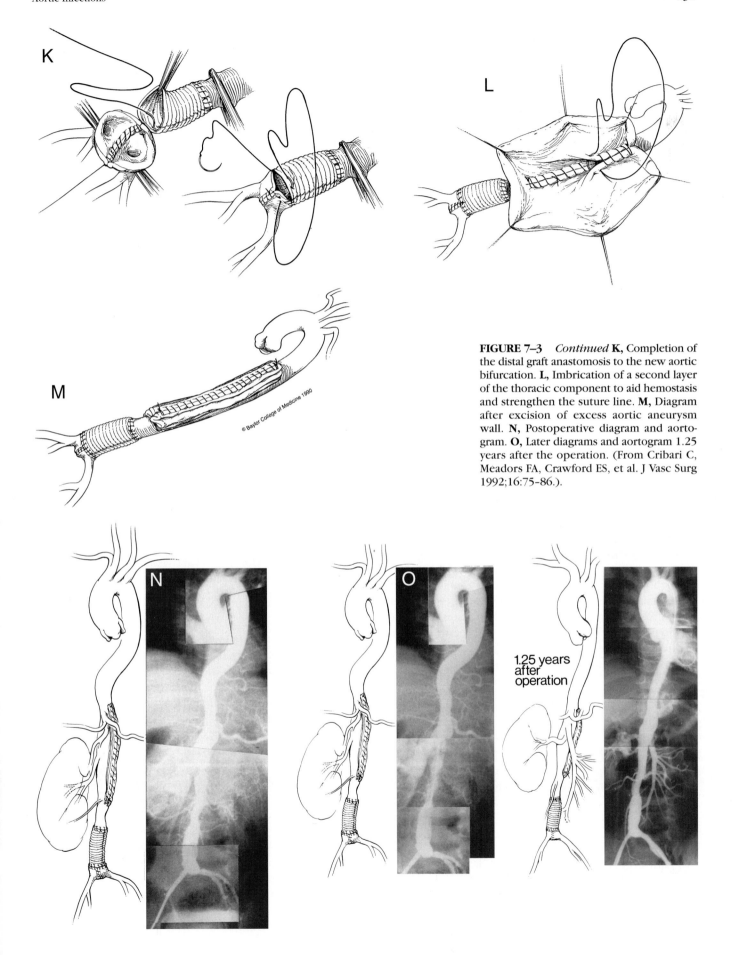

© Baylor College of Medicine 1990

FIGURE 7–3 *Continued* **K,** Completion of the distal graft anastomosis to the new aortic bifurcation. **L,** Imbrication of a second layer of the thoracic component to aid hemostasis and strengthen the suture line. **M,** Diagram after excision of excess aortic aneurysm wall. **N,** Postoperative diagram and aortogram. **O,** Later diagrams and aortogram 1.25 years after the operation. (From Cribari C, Meadors FA, Crawford ES, et al. J Vasc Surg 1992;16:75–86.).

1.25 years
after
operation

in children are extremely rare, and most are due to infections, usually related to umbilical catheters, but occasionally are the result of trauma (Fig. 7–4). Lobe and colleagues[20] evaluated five of their patients with mycotic complications of umbilical artery catheters. They noted that methicillin-resistant *Staphylococcus aureus* was always the bacterium involved and was associated with thrombocytopenia, anemia, renal failure, hypertension, and embolization to the toes. The initial thrombosis of the aorta with progression to aneurysm formation was documented in three patients by ultrasonography. Only one patient had a surgical repair of the aorta, with polytetrafluoroethylene (PTFE), and this patient was the only survivor of the mycotic infection.

Predisposing factors for the development of mycotic aneurysms associated with depressed host immunity include steroid use, chemotherapeutic drugs, alcoholism, chronic renal failure, diabetes, cancer, tuberculosis, chronic pancreatitis, collagen vascular disease, and irradiation.[21] In our series of 22 patients, 19 (87%) had predisposing depressed immunity.[5] Patients with the acquired immune deficiency syndrome (AIDS) are a new risk group, and any patient with a mycotic aneurysm should have an HIV test.[22, 23] Clearly, aortic infections can also be caused by direct aortic trauma, such as penetrating injuries, intraaortic balloon pumps, arterial catheters, and adjacent abdominal or thoracic operations. We do not, however, classify these latter aortic infections as mycotic aneurysms.

Clinical Presentation

The triad of fever, abdominal pain, and a pulsatile mass should alert the surgeon to the possibility of an abdominal mycotic aneurysm. Lethargy, rigors, and anorexia are common. Fever, recent onset of chest or back pain, and an enlarged aortic knuckle or widened mediastinum also suggest the possibility of a mycotic aneurysm of the aortic arch, although aortic dissection can have a similar presentation. Hoarseness, dysphagia, and respiratory stridor may occur. Also, there may be distal embolization of infected material, causing pain or tenderness over peripheral arteries. The white blood cell count may be elevated, but with *Salmonella* infections the reverse can occur and very low leukocyte counts are sometimes observed.

FIGURE 7–4 Summary of results with management of umbilical artery catheter-induced infections of the aorta.

Results: Cases in the Literature (35 Patients)

	Number of Patients	Survival*
Medical	16	4** (25%)
Surgical	19	16 (84%)

*Hospital survival
**Includes one patient who underwent left nephrectomy but not direct aortic procedure

Diagnosis

On computed tomography (CT) or magnetic resonance imaging (MRI) scans, the usual finding is a saccular aneurysm with a pouchlike appearance that is lined with thrombus. Vertebral osteomyelitis may be present, and on occasion the aneurysm might be multiloculated. Typically, calcification of the aneurysm, per se, is absent, whereas penetration through the aortic wall, particularly if the wall is calcified, is often seen. Thus it is not unusual to observe rapid growth of abdominal mycotic aneurysms and for aortic studies performed a few days apart to show rapid progression in size. Most mycotic aneurysms should be considered false aneurysms and could be classified as contained ruptures.[23] Sometimes the aneurysms are more fusiform in shape. Although not usually considered to be mycotic aneurysms, extensive aortic root destruction by contiguous endocarditis can lead to large aneurysms and rupture, including rupture into the cardiac chambers. In those patients with a fever, chest or back pain, and suspected endocarditis or mycotic aneurysms, transesophageal echocardiography (TEE) can be of great value. In one of our patients with such a presentation, a mycotic aneurysm of the thoracoabdominal aorta was suspected and was clearly confirmed on TEE. A large chest and upper abdominal abscess false aneurysm cavity ruptured when the patient's chest was opened; nevertheless she survived and was discharged 10 days later without any complications. One year after surgery she is still taking antibiotics for a *Streptococcus pneumonia* infection and will continue to do so for the rest of her life. A further advantage of TEE is that the heart can be more fully assessed, as for ruling out the possibility of an aortic root abscess and evaluating the compression of surrounding structures by the abscess cavity. A caveat, though, is that visualization of the more distal abdominal aorta is not possible and that the proximal aortic arch is not clearly seen.

Management

Patients with suspected mycotic aneurysm should be given antibiotics immediately after blood samples for cultures have been drawn. The reason for this is that bacterial cultures are not always positive and waiting for the results of them may unnecessarily delay surgery in patients who are often systemically very ill.

How mycotic aneurysms should be surgically managed intraoperatively is controversial. The central issue is whether an in situ graft should be placed or whether the aorta should be bypassed by extraanatomical grafts. We prefer to operate in situ without delay because of the high risk of death with medical therapy alone and because of the frequent presence of rupture.[5] Furthermore, all the potentially infected tissues can be debrided, including any infected clot, and this measure enables quicker recovery of the patient. Omentum or surrounding tissue should be used to surround the graft, fill dead space, and protect adjacent organs or structures. Tissue specimens for Gram staining need to be obtained because antibiotic therapy may require modification according to the pathogen found. In addition, one of us (L.G.S.) recommends placement of at least two thoracic chest tubes alongside the graft for both thoracic and abdominal infections. With separate antibiotic irrigation catheters placed into the debrided area, we alternate antibiotic irrigation with chest tube drainage of the fluid effluent. Our reported results with immediate in situ repair have been satisfactory, with 19 of 22 patients (86%) surviving surgery,[5] and similar success has been reported by others.[21, 24] This is also supported by Fichelle and colleagues,[25] who performed in situ reconstructions in 21 patients, including omental flaps in 19, with three early deaths and no late recurrences of infections.

Postponement of surgery while awaiting isolation of bacteria and response to antibiotics entails the risk rupture of the false aneurysm, spread of the infection, and development of septic multiple organ dysfunction. After surgery, we advise our patients to continue taking suppressive antibiotics for the rest of their lives because we believe that this may reduce the risk of a recurrent graft infection.[5]

INFECTED AORTIC PROSTHESES

Prevention

Once an aortic graft has become infected, it becomes insidiously difficult to manage. Thus central to management is the prevention of graft infections whenever possible. As in the case of mycotic aneurysms, graft infection is due to seeding of microorganisms to the graft from a distant site, to direct graft contamination at the time of surgery, or to surrounding contiguous tissues causing contamination such as enteric fistula. Meticulous surgical techniques and judicious administration of prophylactic antibiotics are the most important factors for guarding against infection. Also, whenever possible, potential sources of bacteria must be eliminated before surgery; these include urinary tract infections, respiratory tract infections, infected gangrene of toes, and infected skin ulcers.[26]

The choice of antibiotics for prophylaxis has been evolving over time. Cefazolin and cefamandole are currently the two most frequently administered antibiotics for major vascular surgery. Another option is to use vancomycin and ceftazidime for vascular and cardiovascular surgery. In our patients, both vancomycin, 1 g, and ceftazidime, 1 g, are given intravenously before the operation. At the end of the operation, a further dose of 1 g of vancomycin and 1 g of ceftazidime is given, and thereafter ceftazidime is given at a dosage of 1 g every 8 hours for 48 hours and vancomycin at 500 mg every 6 hours for 48 hours. The wounds should also be irrigated with a gentamicin solution because we have previously shown in a prospective randomized study that the topical antibiotic, if different from the systemic antibiotics, has a further beneficial effect.[27] In our experience with the latter regimen since 1991, there has not been an increased incidence of renal dysfunction or resistance to the antibiotics. Of particular note is that neither superficial nor deep wound infection of any clinical significance has developed in any patients, including those with infected grafts, prosthetic aortic valve infections, and mycotic aneurysms. Although this antibiotic combination would be excessive for many situations, the regimen should be considered for those patients undergoing high-risk major aortic surgery, particularly if past experience has revealed a problem with staphylococcal or gram-negative bacterial infections.[26]

One of the reasons vancomycin is a better prophylactic antibiotic is that staphylococcal species (particularly *Staphylococcus epidermidis*) that are highly sensitive to vancomycin have become increasingly common causes of postoperative graft infection. A prospective randomized double-blind study reported in 1992 by Maki and colleagues[28] demonstrated that vancomycin is better than cefazolin or cefamandole in the prevention of wound infections after cardiac or major vascular surgery. Nonetheless, because vancomycin does not inhibit the gram-negative organisms, gram-negative antibiotics such as ceftazidime or an aminogylcoside will have to be administered for operations that involve the potential risk of gram-negative infections. This should particularly include operations involving the groin, where gram-negative infections are more common.

Whether prophylactic antibiotic therapy should be continued in the intensive care unit after the first 48 hours, particularly in patients with chest tubes or on ventilators, remains an unanswered question. One risk of continuing with antibiotics is the possibility that organisms resistant to the antibiotics might develop in the sputum, the gastrointestinal tract, and eventually the urinary tract. Furthermore, there is the potential problem of increasing renal dysfunction because of prolonged vancomycin use. At present we advise against prolonged use of prophylactic antibiotics unless there is a strong indication for continuing them postoperatively, as in treatment of infections such as bacterial endocarditis or mycotic aneurysms. However, patients who are undergoing invasive procedures, such as transesophageal echocardiograms, should be given prophylactic antibiotics before the procedure. Edwards[29] has documented that patients who have infections of either the urinary tract or the lower respiratory tract have a respective incidence of wound infections of 30% and 25%.[26]

In the final analysis, prevention of graft infection depends on careful surgical technique, drainage of all dead spaces, and prudent use of prophylactic antibiotics. In addition to intravenous prophylactic antibiotics, a different topical antibiotic in the wound is also of value.[27]

LATE GRAFT INFECTIONS

The late development of graft infections is probably due either to direct contamination with indolent organisms at the time of surgery or to postoperative episodes of bacteremia or septicemia, particularly in the intensive care unit. These later developing infections can often be treated successfully with antibiotics without resorting to operative procedures. Nevertheless, the unwelcome legacy of these episodes of septicemia are pseudoaneurysms, a potentially shortened life span, and progressive organ dysfunction, such as renal failure.[26]

Delayed prevention of graft infections in patients who have prosthetic material is similar to that in patients with mechanical valve prostheses. Thus the prevention of these graft infections is based on the intuitive premise that prophylactic antibiotics prevent the seeding of bacteria to the graft. However, there are no controlled clinical studies documenting a definite beneficial effect of antimicrobial prophylaxis for graft infections or mechanical heart valve infections as opposed to wound infections.[26]

The prophylactic antibiotics should be selected on the basis of those organisms that are most likely to seed at the time of the invasive procedure. The patient's allergies to antibiotics should also be considered. It is a matter of concern that minor oral manipulations involve a high incidence of bacteremia and include brushing of teeth, as high as 40%; periodontal surgery, 88%; tooth extraction, 82%; and tonsillectomy, 38%.[26] Furthermore, with urinary catheter manipulation and gastroesophageal procedures, the respective incidences of bacteremia are 50% and 54%.[26] The American Heart Association recommends an antibiotic regimen to protect against the most likely bacteria involved in procedures.[30] Thus, for most patients who are able to take oral antibiotics, a course of 3 g of amoxicillin before the procedure followed by 1 g 6 hours later should be adequate. Intravenous antibiotics are required for patients who are unable to take oral antibiotics.[26]

Definition and Incidence

A graft infection can be defined as proven graft colonization by bacteria, the presence of pus surrounding the graft, or both.[26] The diagnosis is confirmed by positive bacterial cultures and, usually, a false aneurysm.

The incidence of aortic postoperative graft infection is 0.86% to 3%.[5, 26, 31, 32] Although it is uncommon, when it does occur the consequences are serious. Of 13 patients with early or late graft infections after 1509 thoracoabdominal repairs by us,[33] 12 died.[26]

Clinical Presentation

Clinical signs that should alert the surgeon to the possibility of a graft infection include postoperative sepsis, as evidenced by fever and leukocytosis; septicemia or bacteremia; secondary bleeding at anastomoses; clinical or occult bleeding from the gastrointestinal tract; aortointestinal fistula; draining pus from operative wounds; delayed wound healing; suture line abscesses; rupture of anastomoses; detection of false aneurysms on late follow-up; distal septic emboli; thrombosis of the aortic graft or its branches; and systemic symptoms such as fever, loss of weight, lassitude, loss of appetite, and malaise. Once bacteria have been cultured from the blood, urine, sputum, wound drainage, and surgical specimens of tissue and explanted prosthetic material, the sensitivity of the organisms to antimicrobials is determined and the antibiotic treatment is optimized for the patient.[16, 26, 32]

Diagnostic Studies

False aneurysms and perigraft fluid collections are detected by CT, aortography, or echocardiography. TEE is particularly useful for the detection of aortic root destruction or annular abscesses. MRI has the greatest reported accuracy and can distinguish between perigraft fluid and blood and can detect perigraft inflammation.[34, 35] Indium III–labeled leukocyte scans in the late postoperative period have a reported sensitivity of up to 100%.[26] Fiorani and colleagues[36] have reported that in those patients who have no CT evidence of graft infection but who have clinical findings suggestive of infection, the sensitivity of technetium 99m-hexametazime (99mTc) is 100% and the specificity 94.4%. When readily accessible, fluid collections around the graft that are not false aneurysms can be aspirated with CT-aided guidance for definitive diagnosis of a graft infection and the extent can be demarcated by injection of contrast material.

The bacterial cultures usually reveal that *Staphylococcus* species are the cause of infection (gram-negative organisms are sometimes found) and probably portend a poor outcome.[37] Organisms may include *Staphylococcus aureus, Staphylococcus epidermidis, Acinetobacter, Enterobacter, Klebsiella, Corynebacterium, Citrobacter, Pseudomonas, Escherichia coli, Bacteroides fragilis, Streptococcus* species, enterococci, *Salmonella, Klebsiella, Proteus,* and rarely fungi and *Candida.*[26]

Management

The management of the aortic prosthesis that is infected is usually achieved by three methods, the use of which depends on various factors such as the condition of the patient, the result of bacterial cultures, and available options. Thus a plan of action should be implemented early, particularly since the treatment strategy may require prolonged care and multiple procedures.[26]

CONSERVATIVE MANAGEMENT

The first approach is conservative management with the use of antibiotics directed at the organism and, in some cases, also the use of CT scan–guided drainage of infected fluid collections with a percutaneous catheter. This technique, including drainage, can often be used for low-grade infections involving the abdominal aortic grafts. It is not always successful, however, as illustrated by the case shown in Fig. 7-5. Matley and colleagues[38] have reported successful treatment of a *Klebsiella* infection of a thoracoabdominal graft by insertion of a percutaneous drainage catheter with ultrasound guidance and also the administration of systemic antibiotics. After 2 years of follow-up of their patient, there has been no evidence of sepsis on either clinical examination, hematologic studies, CT or Indium III scans. Morris and colleagues[39] were more aggressive and debrided surrounding tissue but left the aortic graft intact and then irrigated the cavity with antibiotic solution. Of their 10

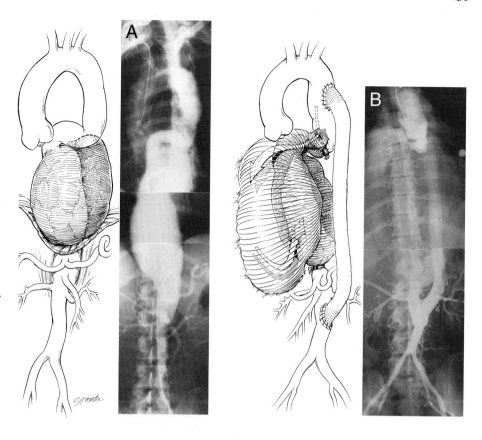

FIGURE 7–5 **A,** Original aortogram of a patient with Marfan syndrome and large thoracoabdominal aneurysm treated elsewhere **(B)** with attempted aneurysm inflow and outflow occlusion and bypass. **C,** The thoracoabdominal aneurysm was repaired by us, but 6 weeks later the patient developed a *Staphylococcus epidermidis* infection that was treated with intravenous antibiotics and placement of a percutaneous catheter alongside the graft for gentamicin irrigation of the cavity. **D,** Subsequently the patient underwent an ascending aorta-to-abdominal aorta bypass and, 2 weeks later, removal of the old infected graft. (From Svensson LG. In: Calligaro KD, Veith FJ, eds. Management of Infected Arterial Grafts. St. Louis, MO: Quality Medical Publishing Inc; 1994:65–81).

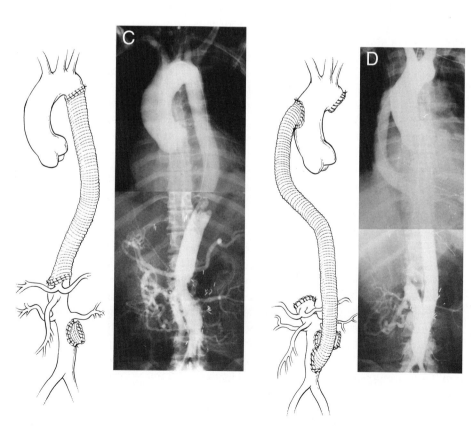

patients, two died of graft infection. For more peripheral graft infections, debridement with or without closure of the wound with muscle flaps can also be successful.[26, 40, 41] We have found that, for patients with infrarenal grafts (particularly aortobifemoral grafts with only one limb infected), debridement and irrigation with antibiotics may be successful with less aggressive infections such as those caused by *Staphylococcus epidermidis*. If needed, local extraanatomical grafts can be placed to prevent limb ischemia when only a limb of an aortobifemoral graft is removed.[26] In an extensive review of the subject, Calligaro and Veith[42] came to the same conclusion.

In Situ Repair with
Prosthetic or Biological Material

The second approach is operation at the site of the previous graft insertion with removal of the old graft and in situ replacement with a new prosthesis or homologous aortic graft.

In situ replacement of infected aortic prosthesis has been reported in some large series, including cardiac valve procedures.[5, 21, 24, 26, 32, 37, 43–47] It is worthwhile to examine the results of aortic valve procedures, since there are some similarities to aortic graft prosthesis infections. Haydock and colleagues[44] reported a series of 30 patients all of whom had bioprosthetic or mechanical prostheses inserted (homografts were inserted in 8 of the 30 patients). Although such patients can be very difficult to manage, Haydock's group was able to achieve a 5-year survival rate of 64%. In this group of patients, the actuarial freedom from reinfection was 80% at 10 years. The 30-day mortality rate in the same series was 18%.

When an in situ repair is performed, there has been controversy as to whether a biological or a prosthetic substitute should be used. David and associates[48] reported aortic root repair with autologous pericardium after debridement of the aortic root for endocarditis followed by prosthetic valve replacement in 21 patients, with one postoperative death (4.8%). Fiore and associates[49] had similar results with a Dacron patch, which is a technique we have also used (Fig. 7-6). Danielson and colleagues[50] reported successful placement of an aortic valve in the ascending aorta with bypass grafts to the coronary arteries, for severe aortic root endocarditis. As reported by Chan and associates[5] and Coselli and coworkers[32] from our group, the results of using in situ prosthetic material and valves for both aortic repairs and replacement of ascending aortic graft infections were also satisfactory without the use of allografts. Similarly, in the illustrative cases shown (Fig. 7-7),[26] good results have been achieved, even in the face of *Staphylococcus aureus* infection, with composite valve grafts inserted in areas of frank and pustular infections.

Ralph-Edwards and colleagues[47] from the Toronto group reported on 12 patients who had infective endocarditis that arose from previous composite valve grafts (including four homografts) inserted to replace the aortic root. The patients were treated with debridement, bovine pericardial left ven-

tricular flow tract repair, and insertion of new valved prosthetic conduits. Despite the severity of the disease, there was only one postoperative death. These authors suggest that radical debridement is of more value than the insertion of conduits. It would appear from their report that the surrounding root destruction was worse when a biological homograft had been used for the original operation. Ergin and colleagues[46] describe extensive aortic root repairs with prosthetic material (Teflon felt) and composite valve grafts in 15 patients in whom an aortic root had been destroyed by endocarditis, with only one death (1 of 15, 6.7%). Clearly, according to these findings, prosthetic material can be safely used, provided that any infected material is thoroughly debrided; thus we continue to favor this in situ composite graft replacement approach (Fig. 7-8).[26]

The alternative to the use of prosthetic grafts is the use of biological grafts such as homografts. Although Haydock and colleagues[44] report a preference for homografts in the replacement of the ascending aorta, it is noteworthy that in a subsequent paper from that same group the mortality rate exceeded 50% in patients who required homografts for the replacement of the aortic valve and ascending aorta because of infections.[51] It is worth noting that even the author with the greatest experience with this type of procedure, Ross of England, had an early mortality rate of 33%.[52] The Mayo Clinic group has reported a 20% (2/10) early mortality rate for homograft insertions for infections.[53] In the study by McGiffin and colleagues[54] from O'Brien's group, which showed that the use of a subcoronary homograft (allograft) was associated with a reduced risk of early death in 195 patients undergoing native or prosthetic valve endocarditis operations ($n = 209$). These findings are unusually favorable when compared with all other reports and may reflect patient-selection biases as indicated by them. Moreover, McGiffin's group was unable to show a significantly lower risk of recurrent endocarditis with homografts than with mechanical valves or porcine valves, although trends favored the homografts.

Patients who have undergone coronary artery bypass operations may have infections of the aorta associated with rupture or false aneurysm formation at the saphenous vein graft anastomotic sites or at the cannulation sites (Fig. 7-9). These ruptures or false aneurysms are mostly associated with postoperative mediastinal infection, and frequently the localization of the infection is at the site of previously placed Teflon felt pledgets. These patients require prompt surgery because of the risk of rupture. The operative technique usually entails femero-femoral bypass with deep hypothermic arrest, thorough debridement of the aorta, repair of the aorta with a patch, reanastomosis of bypasses, rotation of muscle and omental flaps, and antibiotic irrigation of the area. Follis and colleagues[55] have reported that these types of infections are more common after heart and lung transplantation, presumably because of immunosuppression.

Kieffer and colleagues[45] have recently advocated the use of homografts for infected abdominal prostheses. DeBakey, Crawford, and Szylagi, however, have been critical of the

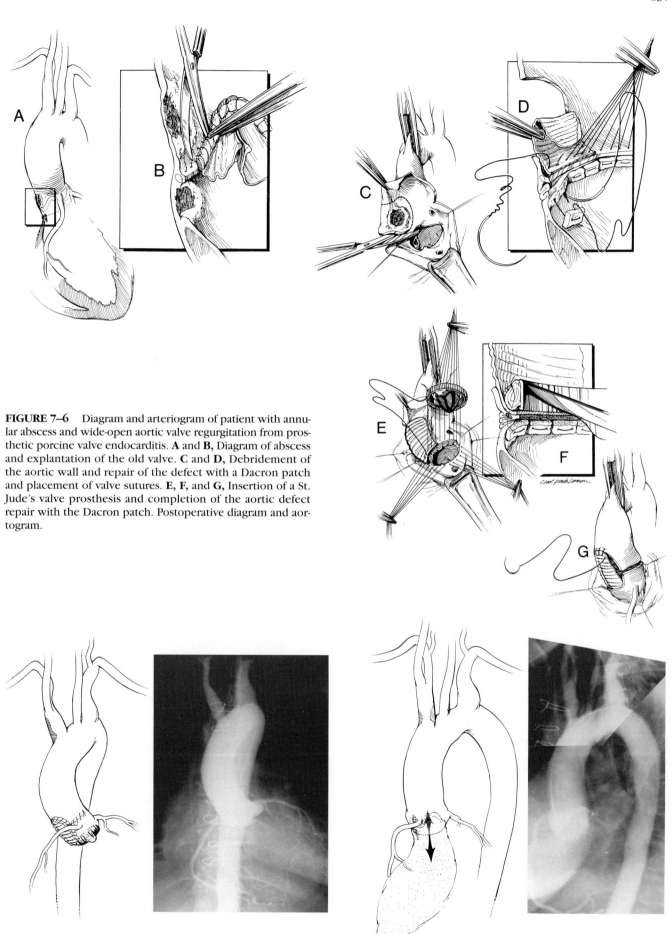

FIGURE 7–6 Diagram and arteriogram of patient with annular abscess and wide-open aortic valve regurgitation from prosthetic porcine valve endocarditis. **A** and **B,** Diagram of abscess and explantation of the old valve. **C** and **D,** Debridement of the aortic wall and repair of the defect with a Dacron patch and placement of valve sutures. **E, F,** and **G,** Insertion of a St. Jude's valve prosthesis and completion of the aortic defect repair with the Dacron patch. Postoperative diagram and aortogram.

use of homografts in the abdominal and thoracoabdominal position because of the deterioration of the grafts.[26] Similarly, Ernst has reported poor results with homografts. Nevertheless, it is of interest that Kieffer and colleagues, in their experience with 43 patients, achieved an 88% operative sur-

vival rate in these difficult-to-manage patients. Three patients required reoperation for homograft-related complication.[26]

Integral to the management of infected aortic grafts by in situ repairs is the use of appropriate antibiotics. The infected and inflamed tissues have to be thoroughly debrided and

FIGURE 7–7   A, Patient with porcine aortic valve replacement who subsequently experienced aortic dissection that was treated elsewhere with ascending aortic graft repair that was followed by *Staphylococcus aureus* infection. **B,** At the time of the third operation, pus surrounded the graft, and a large abscess involving most of the annulus required debridement and obliteration of the cavity with pledget sutures. **C,** Diagram and aortogram after insertion of composite valve graft and beveled repair into the aortic arch using deep hypothermia with circulatory arrest.

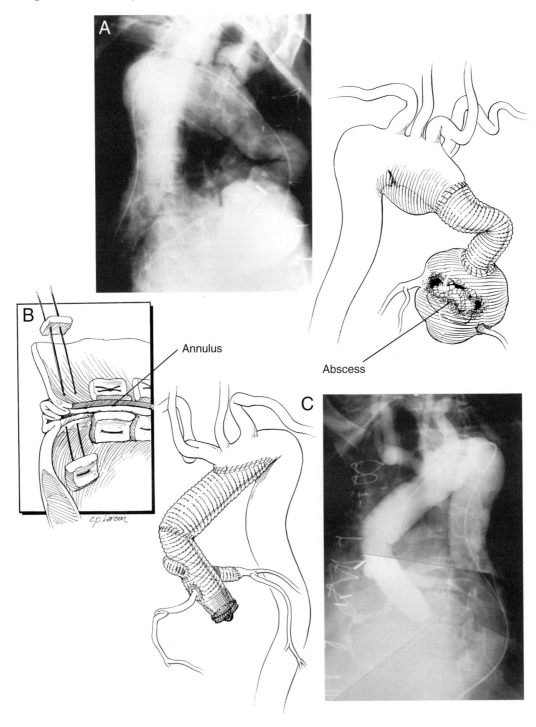

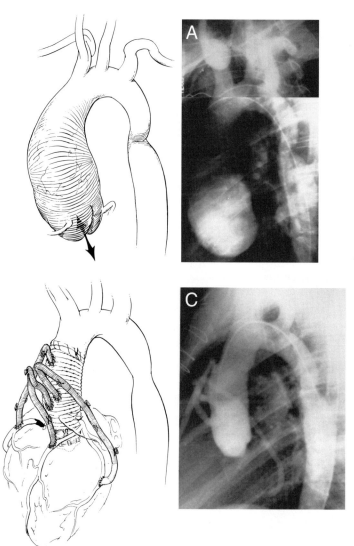

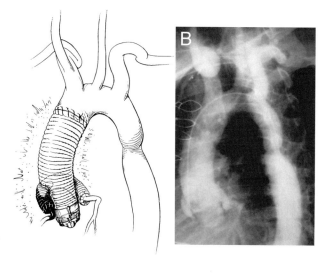

FIGURE 7–8 A, Patient with aortic valve regurgitation, aortic root and ascending aortic aneurysm, and mild coarctation. B, Postoperative arteriogram after development of a composite valve graft infection with occlusion of the right coronary artery bypass, caused by *Pseudomonas aeruginosa* septicemia. C, Diagram and aortogram after insertion of a new composite valve graft, oversewing of the coronary ostia, and distal coronary artery saphenous bypasses. (Reprinted by permission from the Society of Thoracic Surgeons. From Svensson LG, Crawford ES, Hess KR, et al. Ann Thorac Surg 1992; 54:427–39.)

sent for bacterial cultures to establish sensitivities for antibiotic administration. The appropriate antibiotics then are selected on the basis of antimicrobial sensitivities.[26]

An important component of preventing reinfection of the graft is the placement of tissue to fill the dead space created by both removal of false aneurysms and debridement surrounding infected tissue. If the dead space is not obliterated, then fluid and blood accumulate around the graft and serve as a culture medium for bacteria to again propagate with reinfection of the new graft. For mediastinal infections, the omentum and muscle flaps, such as flaps of the pectoral, rectus, serratus, latisimus, and intercostal muscles (see illustrations), can be used (Fig. 7-10). For infections involving the left side of the chest after descending thoracic or thoracoabdominal aortic graft infections, similar flaps can be used and, in addition, a thoracoplasty can be performed. When tissue is required to obliterate dead space in the abdomen, the omentum or perinephric fat can conveniently be used (Figs. 7-11 and 7-12).[26, 43]

Thus, in our opinion, like mycotic aneurysms, infected prostheses are best primarily treated by graft removal, in situ repair, coverage of the new graft with viable tissue, and

suppressive antibiotics (Fig. 7-13).[5, 26, 32] Good results have also been reported by others.[26, 31, 56-58]

EXTRAANATOMICAL BYPASSES

The third alternative is the insertion of extraanatomical bypasses, such as axillobifemoral, ascending-descending, ascending-abdominal, ascending bifemoral, or descending thoracic aorta–to-bifemoral bypasses, followed by removal of the infected graft at a later stage and oversewing of the aortic stumps.[26]

Two of the reasons we prefer in situ repairs to extraanatomical bypasses, particularly axillobifemoral bypasses, are that there is an increased incidence of aortic stump blowout when the aortic stump is oversewn and the extraanatomical bypasses are prone to failure over the course of time. The reported incidence of stump blowout is as high as 50% for the abdominal aorta. If extraanatomical bypasses are used, removal first of the infected grafts followed by extraanatomical bypass is reported to involve a lower risk of recurrence of infection and a lower amputation rate.[58-60] In agreement with Bove and associates[61] and Hargrove and colleagues,[31] we find that an ascending aorta–to-retroperitoneal

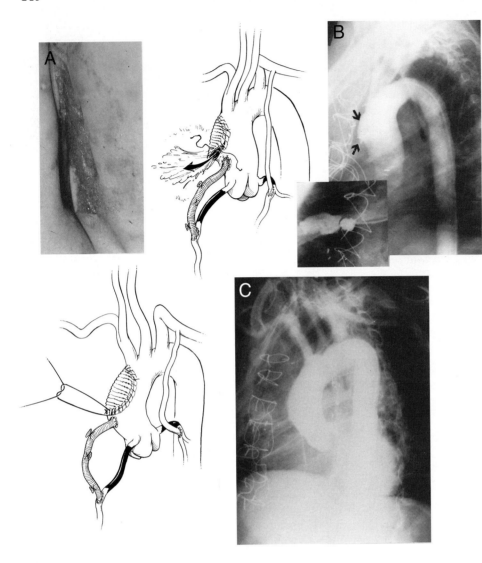

FIGURE 7–9 **A** and **B,** Patient with infection at cannulation site after coronary artery operation, treated elsewhere with debridement and Dacron patch repair of the ascending aorta. **C,** Arteriogram showing postoperative false aneurysm.
*Illustration continued on
following page*

abdominal aorta bypass graft technique can be used for infected descending or thoracoabdominal aortic grafts once infection of the left side of the chest has been eliminated or controlled.[26] If need be, the left side of the chest can be entered after the initial procedure to remove the old infected graft, as illustrated in Fig. 7–5.[23, 26] An advantage of an initial end-to-side proximal anastomosis for aortoiliac disease is that often the old graft can be removed without the need for immediate replacement. This allows the infection to be cleared before a repeat bypass is performed. Muscle flaps, the omentum, or both are used to bring viable tissue and blood supply to the debrided tissue and eliminate dead space.[5, 23, 26, 32, 62]

CONCLUSION. Whichever of the three procedures is used, when the infected prosthesis is removed it is important to extensively debride the area and then fill all dead spaces with viable tissue (either omentum or muscle flaps). The omentum can be mobilized to reach the upper extent of a mediastinal incision or up to the aortic arch when approached through a left thoracotomy. Similarly, the omentum can be used for infected abdominal prostheses, and muscle flaps

are particularly beneficial for filling in the pleural cavity to minimize the risk of leaving dead space that accumulates fluid and becomes infected. Similarly, muscle flaps are very useful for management of mediastinal infected tissue. A technique that is rarely used today, but one that in our opinion is worth remembering, involves an aortorrhaphy of the old aortic wall to repair chronic infected aneurysms. We described this in a 15-month-old child with a thoracoabdominal aneurysm (Fig. 7–3).[19, 26]

LONG-TERM MANAGEMENT. Postoperatively, patients are treated with intravenous antibiotics for 6 weeks on the basis of bacterial sensitivities and, thereafter, with oral suppressive antibiotics for the rest of their lives.[5, 23, 26, 32]

OPERATIVE STRATEGY. Entry into pleural or mediastinal space can be hazardous with extensive false aneurysm or extensive graft infections. Under these circumstances, particularly if lateral chest radiographs or CT scans reveal posterior sternal or manubrial involvement, femorofemoral bypass with deep hypothermic circulatory arrest may be required. For femorofemoral bypass, we cannulate the groin
Text continued on page 151

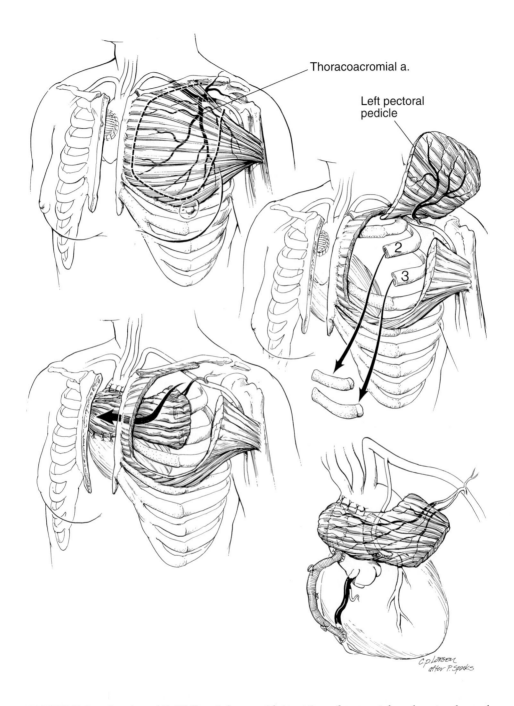

Thoracoacromial a.

Left pectoral pedicle

C.P.Larsen
after P.Sparks

FIGURE 7–9 *Continued* **D–H,** Repair by us with insertion of new patch and pectoral muscle flaps. Recurrent infection was later treated with ascending aortic and proximal aortic arch tubular graft repair and rectus abdominus muscle flaps.

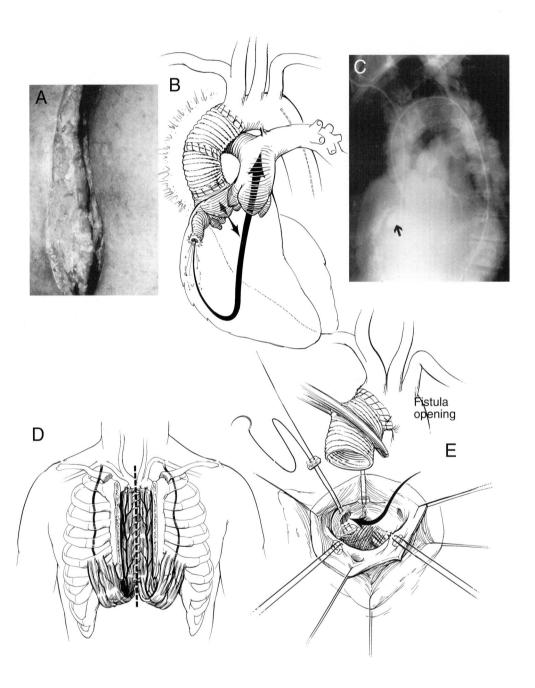

FIGURE 7–10 **A–D,** Diagrams, photographs, and aortogram of a patient who underwent repair of acute aortic dissection followed by ascending aortic graft infection, aortic valve regurgitation, and a fistula into the right ventricle. The *arrow* indicates the site of the fistula. The infection and associated mediastinitis were treated with rectus flaps elsewhere. **D** and **E,** Operative repair undertaken by division of the rectus muscles, insertion of a new proximal aortic arch graft (**F**) with hypothermic circulatory arrest, and closure of the fistula with pledgets.

Illustration continued on following page

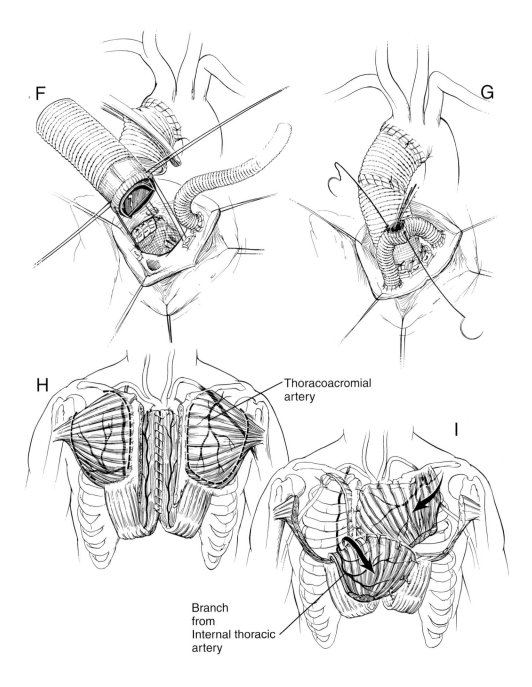

Thoracoacromial
artery

Branch
from
Internal thoracic
artery

FIGURE 7–10 *Continued* **F** and **G,** The aortic root was then repaired with insertion of a composite valve graft by the Cabrol technique. **H–M,** Diagrams of the muscle flaps used to cover the composite graft in the same patient, including the latissimus dorsi, the pectoral, and in addition the previously placed rectus abdominus muscles.

Illustration continued on following page

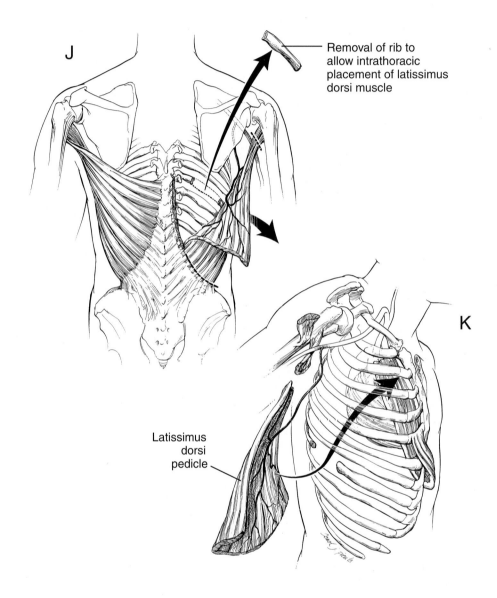

J

Removal of rib to
allow intrathoracic
placement of latissimus
dorsi muscle

K

Latissimus
dorsi
pedicle

FIGURE 7–10   *Continued* **H–M,** Diagrams of the muscle flaps used to cover the composite
graft in the same patient, including the latissimus dorsi, the pectoral, and in addition the previously placed rectus abdominus muscles.

Illustration continued on following page

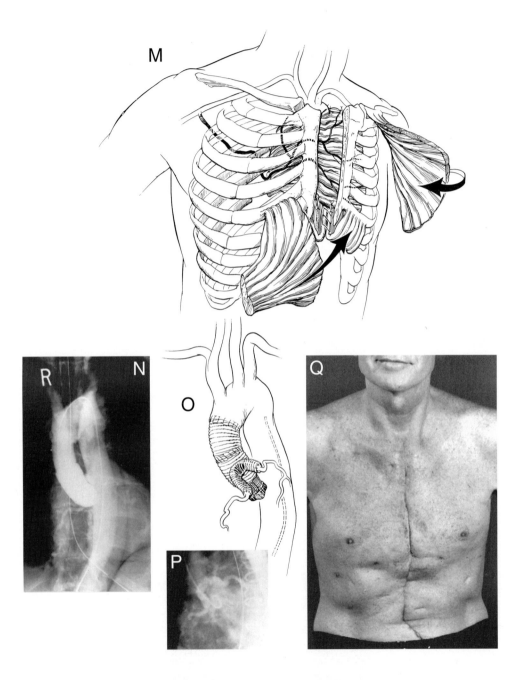

FIGURE 7–10 *Continued* **H–M,** Diagrams of the muscle flaps used to cover the composite graft in the same patient, including the latissimus dorsi, the pectoral, and in addition the previously placed rectus abdominus muscles. **N–Q,** Postoperative diagram and aortogram after successful repair and postoperative photograph 6 months after the operation. (Reprinted with permission from the Society of Thoracic Surgeons. From Coselli JS, Crawford ES, Williams TW Jr, et al. Ann Thorac Surg 1990;50:868–86.).

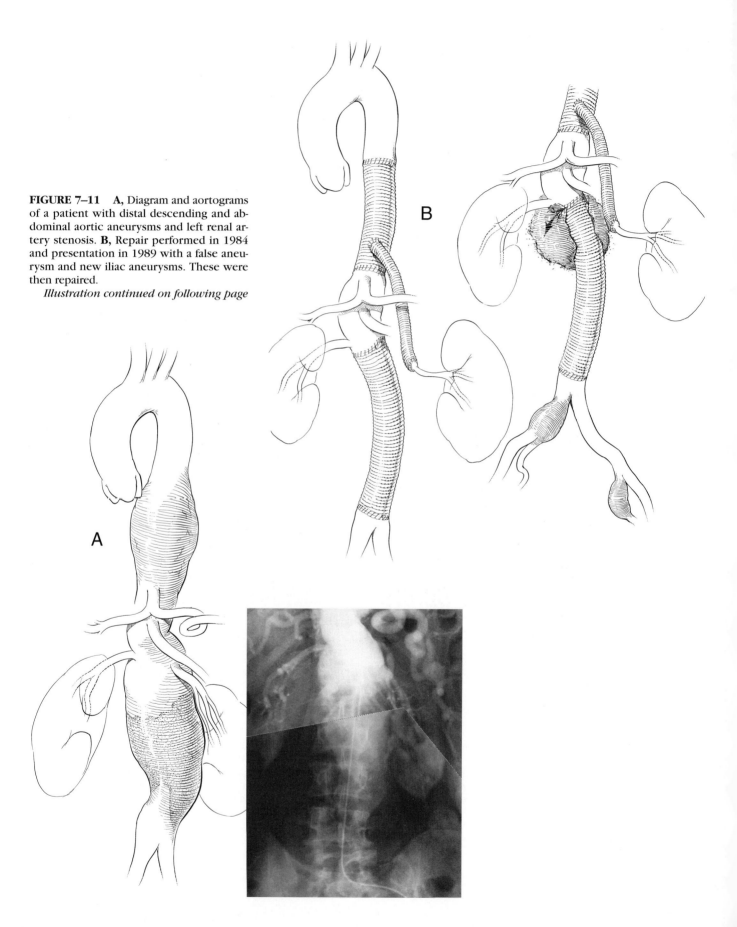

FIGURE 7–11 **A,** Diagram and aortograms of a patient with distal descending and abdominal aortic aneurysms and left renal artery stenosis. **B,** Repair performed in 1984 and presentation in 1989 with a false aneurysm and new iliac aneurysms. These were then repaired.

Illustration continued on following page

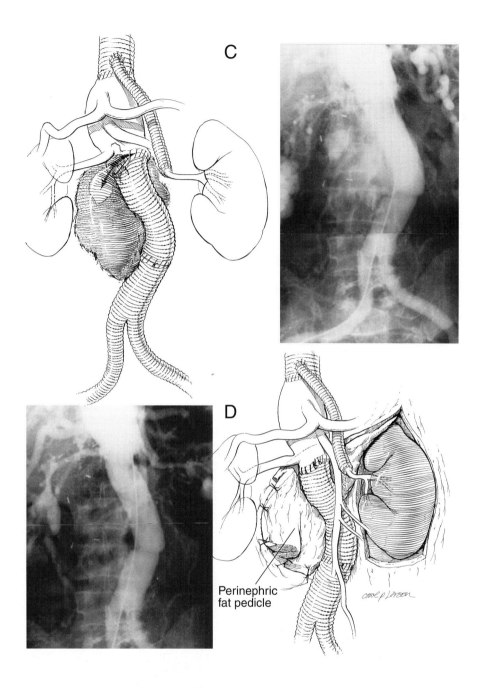

C

D

Perinephric
fat pedicle

FIGURE 7–11 *Continued* **C,** Presentation in 1990 with graft infection and repair with omental flap over the graft. **D,** Repair of false aneurysm and closure with perinephric fat flap **(E, F, and G).** (From Svensson LG. In: Calligaro KD, Veith FJ, eds. Management of Infected Arterial Grafts. St. Louis, MO: Quality Medical Publishing Inc; 1994:65–86.)

Illustration continued on following page

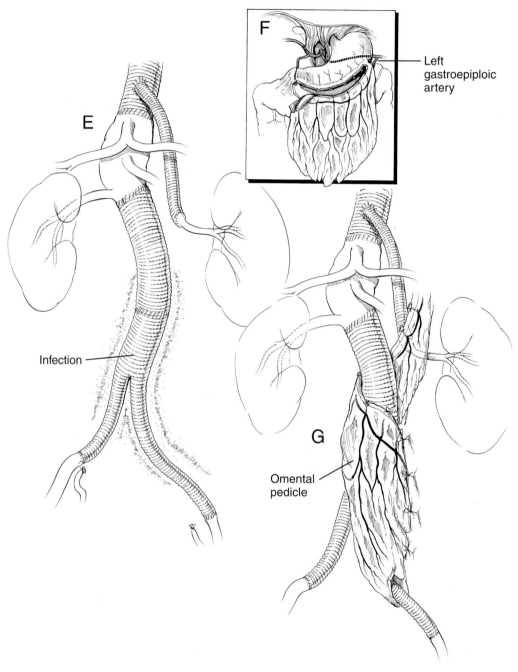

E

F

Left
gastroepiploic
artery

Infection

G

Omental
pedicle

FIGURE 7–11   *Continued*

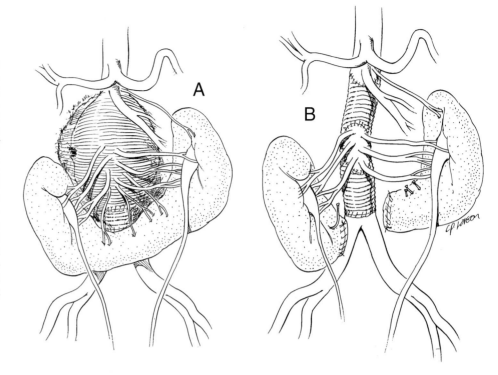

FIGURE 7–12 A, Patient with attempted partial repair of abdominal aortic aneurysm below renal arteries supplying a horseshoe kidney complicated by infection and rupture of the unresected part of the abdominal aneurysm. **B,** Diagram of repair after extensive debridement, division of the horseshoe kidney, placement of a beveled graft behind the celiac and superior mesenteric artery, and reimplantation of an aortic wall patch containing the origin of the renal arteries. The cavity and graft were packed with omentum and irrigated with antibiotic solution. (From Svensson LG, Persson LA, Cohen PM, Gaylis H. S Afr J Surg 1987;25:161–3.)

FIGURE 7–13 **A–F,** Diagram, arteriogram, and chest radiographs of a patient with two previous descending aorta-to-abdominal aorta bypasses for diffuse coarctation caused by Takayasu's aortitis of the thoracoabdominal aorta followed by lung erosion and aortopulmonary fistula.

Illustration continued on following page

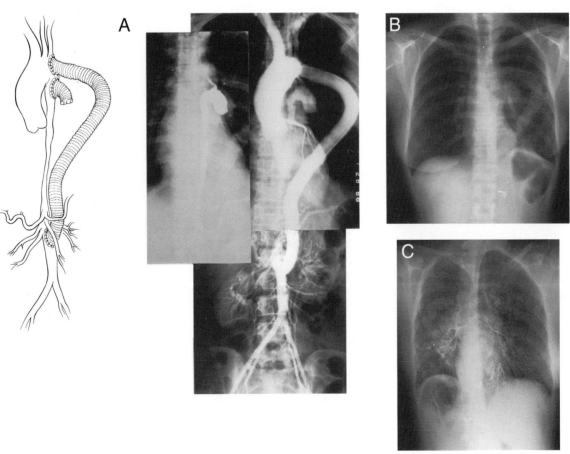

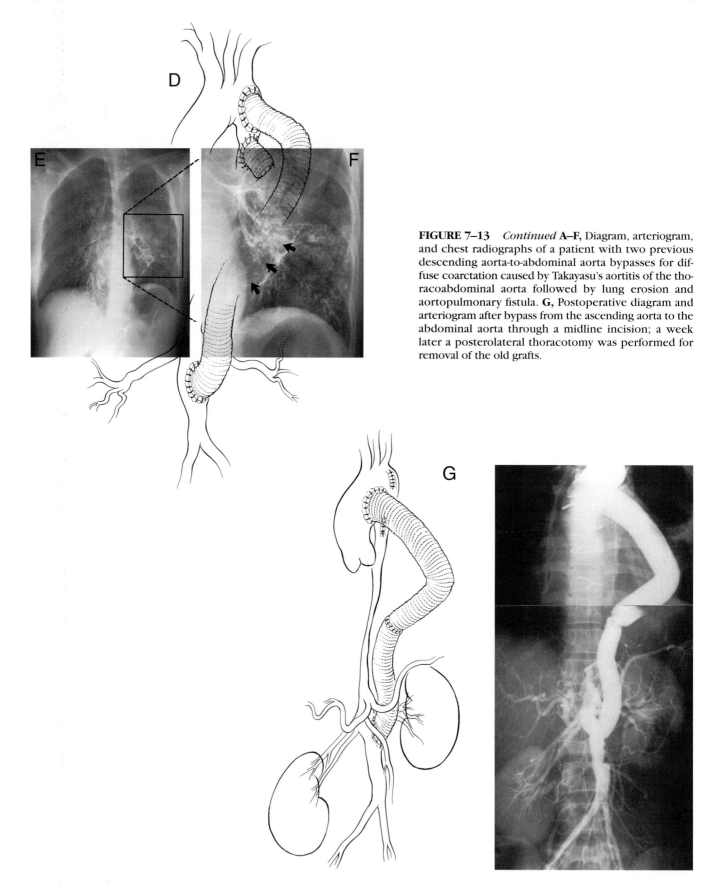

FIGURE 7–13 *Continued* **A–F,** Diagram, arteriogram, and chest radiographs of a patient with two previous descending aorta-to-abdominal aorta bypasses for diffuse coarctation caused by Takayasu's aortitis of the thoracoabdominal aorta followed by lung erosion and aortopulmonary fistula. **G,** Postoperative diagram and arteriogram after bypass from the ascending aorta to the abdominal aorta through a midline incision; a week later a posterolateral thoracotomy was performed for removal of the old grafts.

artery and vein, cool the patient until the electroencephalogram shows no electrical activity, and then open the mediastinum. The operative repair is then performed as described above, including extensive debridement, graft insertion, filling of all areas of dead space, and insertion of antibiotic perfusion catheters. We describe the operative techniques in greater detail in subsequent chapters.

REFERENCES

1. Paré A. In the apologie and treatise containing the voyages made into divers places with many of his writings upon surgery. Birmingham, Ala: The Classics of Surgery Library; 1984.
2. Estes JE Jr. Abdominal aortic aneurysm: a study of one hundred and two cases. Circulation 1950;2:258-64.
3. Brock RC. The life and work of Sir Astley Cooper. Ann R Coll Surg Engl 1969;44:1-18.
4. Osler W. The Gulstonian lectures on malignant endocarditis. Br Med J 1885;1:467-70.
5. Chan FY, Crawford ES, Coselli JS, et al. In situ prosthetic graft replacement for mycotic aneurysm of the aorta. Ann Thorac Surg 1989;47:193-203.
6. Stengel A, Wolferth CC. Mycotic (bacterial) aneurysms of intravascular origin. Arch Intern Med 1923;31:527.
7. Crane AR. Primary multilocular mycotic aneurysm of the aorta. Arch Pathol 1937;24:634-41.
8. Revell STR. Primary mycotic aneurysms. Ann Intern Med 1945;22:431-40.
9. Zak FG, Strauss L, Saphra I. Rupture of diseased large arteries in the course of enterobacterial (salmonella) infection. N Engl J Med 1958;258:824.
10. Sommerville RI, Allen EV, Edwards JE. Bland and infected arteriosclerotic abdominal aortic aneurysms: a clinicopathologic study. Medicine 1959;38:207.
11. Wilson SE, Van Wagenen P, Passaro E. Arterial infection. Curr Probl Surg 1978;15:1-89.
12. Ernst CB, Campbell HC J., Daugherty ME, et al. Incidence and significance of intra-operative bacterial cultures during abdominal aortic aneurysmectomy. Ann Surg 1977;185:626-33.
13. Williams RD, Fisher FW. Aneurysm contents as a source of graft infection. Arch Surg 1977;112:415-6.
14. Steed DL, Higgins RS, Pasculle A, Webster MW. Culture of intraluminal thrombus during abdominal aortic aneurysm resection: significant contamination is rare. Cardiovasc Surg 1991;1:494-8.
15. Farkas JC, Fichelle JM, Laurian C, et al. Long-term follow-up of positive cultures in 500 abdominal aortic aneurysms. Arch Surg 1993;128:284-8.
16. Reddy DJ, Shepard AD, Evans JR, et al. Management of infected aorto-iliac aneurysms. Arch Surg 1991;126:873-8.
17. Kearney RA, Eisen HJ, Wolf JE. Nonvalvular infections of the cardiovascular system. Ann Intern Med 1994;121:219-30.
18. Woods JM 4th, Schellack J, Stewart MT, et al. Mycotic abdominal aortic aneurysm induced by immunotherapy with bacille Calmette-Guerin vaccine for malignancy. J Vasc Surg 1988;7:808-10.
19. Cribari C, Meadors FA, Crawford ES, et al. Thoracoabdominal aneurysm associated with umbilical artery catheterization: case report and review of the literature. J Vasc Surg 1992;16:75-86.
20. Lobe TE, Richardson CJ, Boulden TF, et al. Mycotic thrombo-aneurysmal disease of the abdominal aorta in preterm infants: its natural history and its management. J Pediatr Surg 1992;27:1054-9.
21. Johansen K, Devin J. Mycotic aortic aneurysms: a reappraisal. Arch Surg 1983;118:583-8.
22. Dupont JR, Bonavita JA, DiGiovanni RJ, et al. Acquired immunodeficiency syndrome and mycotic abdominal aortic aneurysms: a new challenge? Report of a case. J Vasc Surg 1989;10:254-7.
23. Svensson LG, Crawford ES. Aortic dissection and aortic aneurysm surgery: clinical observations, experimental investigations, and statistical analyses. Part III. Curr Probl Surg 1993;30:1-172.
24. Hollier LH, Money SR, Creely B, et al. Direct replacement of mycotic thoracoabdominal aneurysms. J Vasc Surg 1993;18:477-85.
25. Fichelle JM, Tabet G, Cormier P, et al. Infected infrarenal aortic aneurysms: when is in situ reconstruction safe? J Vasc Surg 1993;17:635-45.
26. Svensson LG. Thoracoabdominal graft infections. In: Calligaro KD, Veith FJ, eds. Management of Infected Arterial Grafts. St. Louis, MO: Quality Medical Publishing Inc 1994:65-81.
27. Svensson LG, Wellsted M, Hinder RA, Myburgh JA. Improved prevention of abdominal wound sepsis by parenteral and topical antibiotics. J R Coll Surg Edinb 1986;31:7-12.
28. Maki DG, Bohn MJ, Stolz SM, et al. Comparison study of cefazolin, cefamandole, and vancomycin for surgical prophylaxis in cardiac and vascular operations: a double-blind randomized study. J Thorac Cardiovasc Surg 1992;104:1423-34.
29. Edwards LD. The epidemiology of 2056 remote site infections and 166 surgical wound infections occurring in 1864 patients. Ann Surg 1976;184:758-66.
30. Dajani AS, Bisno AL, Chung KJ, et al. Prevention of bacterial endocarditis: recommendations by the American Heart Association. JAMA 1990;22:2919-33.
31. Hargrove WC 3d., Edmunds L Jr. Management of infected thoracic aortic prosthetic grafts. Ann Thorac Surg 1984;37:72-7.
32. Coselli JS, Crawford ES, Williams TWJ, et al. Treatment of postoperative infection of ascending aorta and transverse aortic arch, including use of viable omentum and muscle flaps. Ann Thorac Surg 1990;50:868-81.
33. Svensson LG, Crawford ES, Hess KR, et al. Experience with 1509 patients undergoing thoracoabdominal aortic operations. J Vasc Surg 1993;17:357-70.
34. Olofsson PA, Auffermann W, Higgins CB, et al. Diagnosis of prosthetic aortic graft infection by magnetic resonance imaging. J Vasc Surg 1988;8:99-105.
35. Spartera C, Morettini G, Petrassi C, et al. Role of magnetic resonance imaging in the evaluation of aortic graft healing, perigraft fluid collection, and graft infection. Eur J Vasc Surg 1990;4:69-73.
36. Fiorani P, Speziale F, Rizzo L, et al. Detection of aortic graft infection with leukocytes labeled with technetium 99m-hexametazime. J Vasc Surg 1993;17:87-96.
37. D'Agostino RS, Miller DC, Stinson EB, et al. Valve replacement in patients with native valve endocarditis: what really determines operative outcome? Ann Thorac Surg 1985;40:429-38.
38. Matley PJ, Beningfield SJ, Lourens S, Immelman EJ. Successful treatment of infected thoracoabdominal aortic graft by percutaneous catheter drainage. J Vasc Surg 1991;13:513-15.
39. Morris GE, Friend PJ, Vassallo DJ, et al. Antibiotic irrigation and conservative surgery for major aortic graft infection. J Vasc Surg 1994;20:88-95.
40. Perler BA, Vander Kolk CA, Manson PM, Williams GM. Rotational muscle flaps to treat localized prosthetic graft infection: long-term follow-up. J Vasc Surg 1993;18:358-65.
41. Calligaro KD, Veith FJ, Schwartz ML, et al. Selective preservation of infected prosthetic arterial grafts: analysis of a 20-year experience with 120 extracavitary-infected grafts. Ann Surg 1994;220:461-71.
42. Calligaro KD, Veith FJ. Diagnosis and management of infected prosthetic aortic grafts. Surgery 1991;110:805-13.
43. Svensson LG, Persson LA, Cohen PM, Gaylis H. Successful management of ruptured septic aortic aneurysm and horseshoe kidney with multiple renal arteries: a case report. S Afr J Surg 1987;25:161-3.
44. Haydock D, Barrat-Boyes B, Macedo T, et al. Aortic valve replacement for active infectious endocarditis in 108 patients: a comparison of freehand allograft valves with mechanical prostheses and bioprostheses. J Thorac Cardiovasc Surg 1992;103:130-9.
45. Kieffer E, Bahnini A, Koskas F, et al. In situ allograft replacement of infected infrarenal aortic prosthetic grafts: results in forty-three patients. J Vasc Surg 1993;17:349-56.
46. Ergin MA, Raissi S, Follis F, et al. Annular destruction in acute bacterial endocarditis: surgical techniques to meet the challenge. J Thorac Cardiovasc Surg 1989;97:755-63.
47. Ralph-Edwards A, David TE, Bos J. Infective endocarditis in patients who had replacement of the aortic root. Ann Thorac Surg 1994;58:429-33.
48. David TE, Komeda M, Brofman PR. Surgical treatment of aortic root abscess. Circulation 1989;80((suppl I)):I-269-74.
49. Fiore AC, Ivey TD, McKeown PP, et al. Patch closure of aortic annulus mycotic aneurysms. Ann Thorac Surg 1986;42:372-9.
50. Danielson GK, Titus JL, DuShane JW. Successful treatment of aortic

valve endocarditis and aortic root abscesses by insertion of prosthetic valve in ascending aorta and placement of bypass grafts to
coronary arteries. J Thorac Cardiovasc Surg 1974;67:443-9.

51. Kirklin JK, Smith D, Novick W, et al. Long-term function of cryopreserved aortic homografts: a ten year study. J Thorac Cardiovasc
Surg 1993;106:154-66.

52. Belcher P, Ross D. Aortic root replacement—20 years experience of
the use of homografts. Thorac Cardiovasc Surg 1991;39:117-22.

53. Tuna IC, Orszulak TA, Schaff HV, Danielson GK. Results of homograft aortic valve replacement for active endocarditis. Ann Thorac
Surg 1990;49:619-24.

54. McGiffin DC, Galbraith AJ, McLachlan GJ, et al. Aortic valve infection: risk factors for death and recurrent endocarditis after aortic
valve replacement. J Thorac Cardiovasc Surg 1992;104:511-20.

55. Follis FM, Paone RF, Wernly JA. Mycotic aneurysms of the ascending
aorta after coronary revascularization. Ann Thorac Surg 1994;58:
236-8.

56. Jacobs MJ, Reul GJ, Gregoric I, Cooley DA. In situ replacement and
extra-anatomic bypass for the treatment of infected abdominal aortic grafts. Eur J Vasc Surg 1991;5:83-6.

57. Robinson JA, Johansen K. Aortic sepsis: is there a role for in situ
graft reconstruction? J Vasc Surg 1991;13:677-82.

58. Bahnini A, Ruotolo C, Koskas F, Kieffer E. In situ fresh allograft
replacement of an infected aortic prosthetic graft: eighteen months'
follow-up. J Vasc Surg 1991;14:98-102.

59. O'Hara PJ, Hertzer NR, Beven EG, Krajewski LP. Surgical management of infected abdominal aortic grafts: review of a 25-year experience. J Vasc Surg 1986;3:725-31.

60. Reilly LM, Stoney RJ, Goldstone J, Ehrenfeld WK. Improved management of aortic graft infection: the influence of operation
sequence and staging. J Vasc Surg 1987;5:421-31.

61. Bove EL, Parker MDJ, Marvasti MA, Randall PA. Complete extra-
anatomic bypass of the aortic root: treatment of recurrent mediastinal infection. J Thorac Cardiovasc Surg 1983;86:932-4.

62. Pairolero PC, Arnold PG, Piehler JM, McGoon DC. Intrathoracic
transposition of extrathoracic skeletal muscle. J Thorac Cardiovasc
Surg 1983;86:809-17.

63. Svensson LG, Crawford ES, Hess KR, et al. Composite valve graft
replacement of the proximal aorta: comparison of techniques in
348 patients. Ann Thorac Surg 1992;54:427-39.

64. Coselli JS, Crawford ES, Williams TW Jr, et al. Treatment of postoperative infection of ascending aorta and transverse aortic arch,
including use of viable omentum and muscle flaps. Ann Thorac
Surg 1990;50:868-81.

Congenital Abnormalities of the Aorta in Adults

COARCTATION OF THE AORTA

Coarctation of the aorta is characterized by congenital stenosis of a site in the descending thoracic, distal aortic arch or abdominal aorta associated with a pressure gradient across the stenosis. The incidence is approximately 40 to 50/100,000 live births, with a male:female ratio of 2:1. Three major subgroups of coarctation of the descending thoracic aorta are recognized: preductal, juxtaductal (paraductal), and postductal. The type usually found in infants is the preductal type, with the patent ductus arteriosus supplying blood to the distal aorta. The juxtaductal form tends to progress with time and with growth to a postductal form (adult type). In most patients who have preductal coarctation of the aorta at the aortic isthmus, the condition is diagnosed in infancy either because of other congenital lesions, hypertension, or cardiac failure or because of routine medical examinations. As the ductus closes in these patients, if the coarctation is not treated, the mortality rate is reported to be over 80%.[1-4] The pioneering work by surgeons such as Crafoord, Kirklin, and Waldhausen resulted in successful relief of the coarctation and improved survival.[3-6] More recently balloon angioplasty has come in vogue.

Detection of untreated coarctation of the aorta in adults is now uncommon. In most patients the presence of the coarctation will be detected during routine physical examinations if they have not previously had symptoms or signs related to the coarctation. Thus adults are seen more commonly with late complications associated with previous repairs such as aneurysm formation, restenosis, inadequate graft size, or graft infection (Fig. 8-1). Occasionally they present with undetected postductal coarctation, including poststenotic dilatation, pseudocoarctation formation, and bacterial infection at the site of the stenosis. Patients may also have rupture or aortic dissection, and the risk appears to be increased during pregnancy.[7] With the increasing use of angioplasty to dilate coarctation and the recurrence of coarctation after some types of operative procedures, patients may be seen with residual or recurrent coarctation.

The classic symptoms and signs may be found. These include proximal hypertension, decreased femoral pulses, radiofemoral delay, parascapular pulsation or thrill, systolic murmurs over the back (classically intrascapular), discrepancy of lower extremity growth, left ventricular hypertrophy, heart failure, nosebleed, leg claudication, leg weakness, and rib notching visible on chest radiographs. Rib notching is noted more frequently in older patients and correlates inversely with the coarctation diameter (Fig. 8-2).[8] Asymptomatic aneurysms that form in association with the coarctation may be detected on chest radiographs or, more rarely, on echocardiography, either transthoracic or transesophageal.

Untreated, 80% of adult patients with undiagnosed coarctation will die of complications associated with hypertension. Abbott[9] found that the cause of death was hypertensive in most, cardiac in 50%, and included valvular and atherosclerotic heart disease. Death was caused by cerebral hemorrhage in 13%. Aortic causes of death were rupture in 22% (from either proximal dissection or rupture of poststenotic aneurysms) and rupture of a mycotic aneurysm at the coarctation site in 7%.[10] Rarely, patients may have paraplegia or paraparesis from enlargement and compression of the spinal cord or rupture of the spinal arteries, particularly the anterior spinal artery.[11]

Operative Techniques

In infants, four basic operative techniques are used:

1. The classic method performed first by Crafoord in October 1944[12] consisted of mobilizing the aorta above and below the coarctation, dividing the intercostal arteries to get sufficient mobility, and then performing an end-to-end repair after resecting the coarctation (Fig. 8-3). In infants who undergo end-to-end repair with absorbable polydioxanone sutures (PDS), the results are excellent.[13] This procedure has been advocated by some authors as the preferred technique for infants under 1 year of age, although this is controversial.[14-16] The initial operative methods to reduce the risk of recoarctation appear to be an aggressive and extensive arch anastomosis with absorbable PDS or with polypropylene suture.[15, 16]

2. The procedure introduced by Waldhausen[3, 4] entailed the mobilization of the left subclavian artery and division of the left subclavian artery immediately before the internal mammary artery and vertebral arteries, followed by reflection of the left subclavian artery down as a flap to bridge

artery flap, is not used because of the likely development of ischemia in the left arm. Nor do we recommend the technique of Crafoord[12] because of the increased risk of paraplegia in adults. In a review of 12,532 coarctation repairs, Brewer and colleagues[11] reported that 0.41% developed postoperative neurological deficits. In adults, however, the segmental intercostal or lumbar arteries that formerly supplied the spinal cord with blood via radicular arteries atrophy, and thus potential alternate pathways of blood supply to the spinal cord are not as readily available. The dependency of the spinal cord blood supply on fewer radicular arteries increases the risk of paraplegia developing during the postoperative period. Repair of the coarctation with a synthetic patch is not advised in adults because of the increased incidence of aneurysm formation.[23] Post-stenotic dilatation and even aneurysm formation are not unusual (Fig. 8–4). The aneurysm formation is due, in part, to the loss of elastic tissue and smooth muscle cells beyond the coarctation.[24]

Pseudocoarctation may also be present without a pressure gradient because of elongation of the aorta with kinking of it (Fig. 8–5). The cause of aneurysms in these patients is unclear, but it is noteworthy that the elastic tissue, on his-

tological examination, shows evidence of degeneration and loss of elastic tissue.

One of the postoperative problems after coarctation repairs, and occasionally after repair of aortic dissection or degenerative aneurysm, is severe hypertension, possibly related to interference with aortic baroreceptors and abnormally set mechanisms to maintain renal blood flow. Sealy[25] reviewed this complication and found that it develops in half of the patients during the first 24 hours after coarctation repairs. Hypertension is sometimes associated with abdominal pain and occasionally with small-bowel necrosis, and it may be due to arteritis. During the postoperative period, norepinephrine excretion increases and angiotensin levels increase. Beta-blockers, nitroprusside, and angiotensin-converting enzyme blockers are effective in controlling the postoperative hypertension. An alternative method of repair in adults is the technique of Blalock, which consists of inserting an interposition end-to-side graft from the left subclavian artery to the descending aorta. This method has the potential advantage of a lower risk of paraplegia or renal failure. Similarly, a tube graft can be placed from the distal aortic arch to the descending aorta, as shown in Figure 8–6.

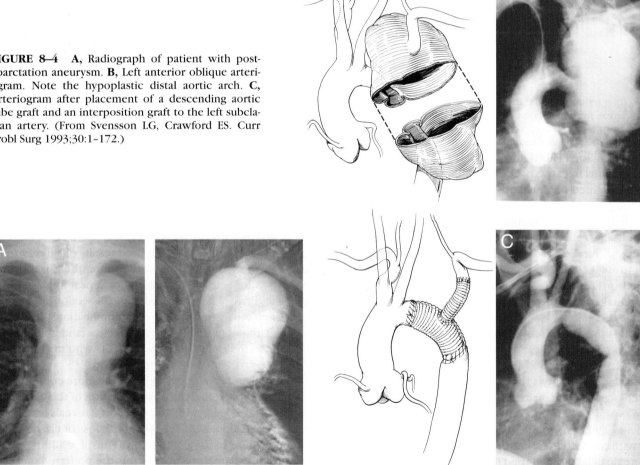

FIGURE 8–4 **A,** Radiograph of patient with post-coarctation aneurysm. **B,** Left anterior oblique arteriogram. Note the hypoplastic distal aortic arch. **C,** Arteriogram after placement of a descending aortic tube graft and an interposition graft to the left subclavian artery. (From Svensson LG, Crawford ES. Curr Probl Surg 1993;30:1–172.)

Congenital Abnormalities of the Aorta in Adults

COARCTATION OF THE AORTA

Coarctation of the aorta is characterized by congenital stenosis of a site in the descending thoracic, distal aortic arch or abdominal aorta associated with a pressure gradient across the stenosis. The incidence is approximately 40 to 50/100,000 live births, with a male:female ratio of 2:1. Three major subgroups of coarctation of the descending thoracic aorta are recognized: preductal, juxtaductal (paraductal), and postductal. The type usually found in infants is the preductal type, with the patent ductus arteriosus supplying blood to the distal aorta. The juxtaductal form tends to progress with time and with growth to a postductal form (adult type). In most patients who have preductal coarctation of the aorta at the aortic isthmus, the condition is diagnosed in infancy either because of other congenital lesions, hypertension, or cardiac failure or because of routine medical examinations. As the ductus closes in these patients, if the coarctation is not treated, the mortality rate is reported to be over 80%.[1-4] The pioneering work by surgeons such as Crafoord, Kirklin, and Waldhausen resulted in successful relief of the coarctation and improved survival.[3-6] More recently balloon angioplasty has come in vogue.

Detection of untreated coarctation of the aorta in adults is now uncommon. In most patients the presence of the coarctation will be detected during routine physical examinations if they have not previously had symptoms or signs related to the coarctation. Thus adults are seen more commonly with late complications associated with previous repairs such as aneurysm formation, restenosis, inadequate graft size, or graft infection (Fig. 8-1). Occasionally they present with undetected postductal coarctation, including poststenotic dilatation, pseudocoarctation formation, and bacterial infection at the site of the stenosis. Patients may also have rupture or aortic dissection, and the risk appears to be increased during pregnancy.[7] With the increasing use of angioplasty to dilate coarctation and the recurrence of coarctation after some types of operative procedures, patients may be seen with residual or recurrent coarctation.

The classic symptoms and signs may be found. These include proximal hypertension, decreased femoral pulses, radiofemoral delay, parascapular pulsation or thrill, systolic murmurs over the back (classically intrascapular), discrepancy of lower extremity growth, left ventricular hypertrophy, heart failure, nosebleed, leg claudication, leg weakness, and rib notching visible on chest radiographs. Rib notching is noted more frequently in older patients and correlates inversely with the coarctation diameter (Fig. 8-2).[8] Asymptomatic aneurysms that form in association with the coarctation may be detected on chest radiographs or, more rarely, on echocardiography, either transthoracic or transesophageal.

Untreated, 80% of adult patients with undiagnosed coarctation will die of complications associated with hypertension. Abbott[9] found that the cause of death was hypertensive in most, cardiac in 50%, and included valvular and atherosclerotic heart disease. Death was caused by cerebral hemorrhage in 13%. Aortic causes of death were rupture in 22% (from either proximal dissection or rupture of poststenotic aneurysms) and rupture of a mycotic aneurysm at the coarctation site in 7%.[10] Rarely, patients may have paraplegia or paraparesis from enlargement and compression of the spinal cord or rupture of the spinal arteries, particularly the anterior spinal artery.[11]

Operative Techniques

In infants, four basic operative techniques are used:

1. The classic method performed first by Crafoord in October 1944[12] consisted of mobilizing the aorta above and below the coarctation, dividing the intercostal arteries to get sufficient mobility, and then performing an end-to-end repair after resecting the coarctation (Fig. 8-3). In infants who undergo end-to-end repair with absorbable polydioxanone sutures (PDS), the results are excellent.[13] This procedure has been advocated by some authors as the preferred technique for infants under 1 year of age, although this is controversial.[14-16] The initial operative methods to reduce the risk of recoarctation appear to be an aggressive and extensive arch anastomosis with absorbable PDS or with polypropylene suture.[15, 16]

2. The procedure introduced by Waldhausen[3, 4] entailed the mobilization of the left subclavian artery and division of the left subclavian artery immediately before the internal mammary artery and vertebral arteries, followed by reflection of the left subclavian artery down as a flap to bridge

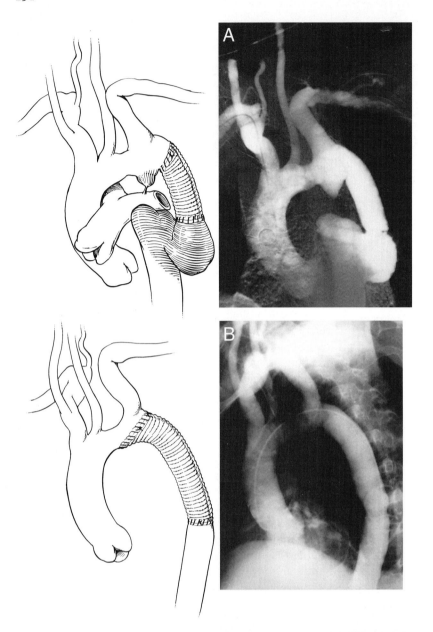

FIGURE 8–1   A, Patient with previous tube graft repair of coarctation of the aorta with later postcoarctation aneurysm formation. B, Postoperative arteriogram after placement of a new tube graft.

FIGURE 8–2   Young man who presented with coarctation of the aorta and ascending aortic dissection. *Left,* MRI view of aneurysm in ascending aorta and coarctation in proximal descending aorta. *Right,* Chest radiograph with rib notching; *arrow* indicates the 3 sign seen at the site of coarctation.

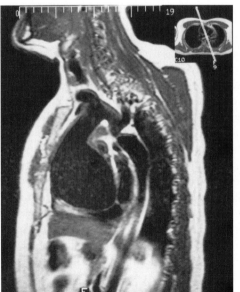

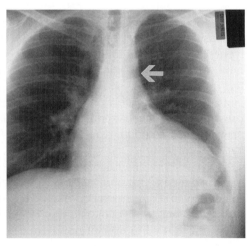

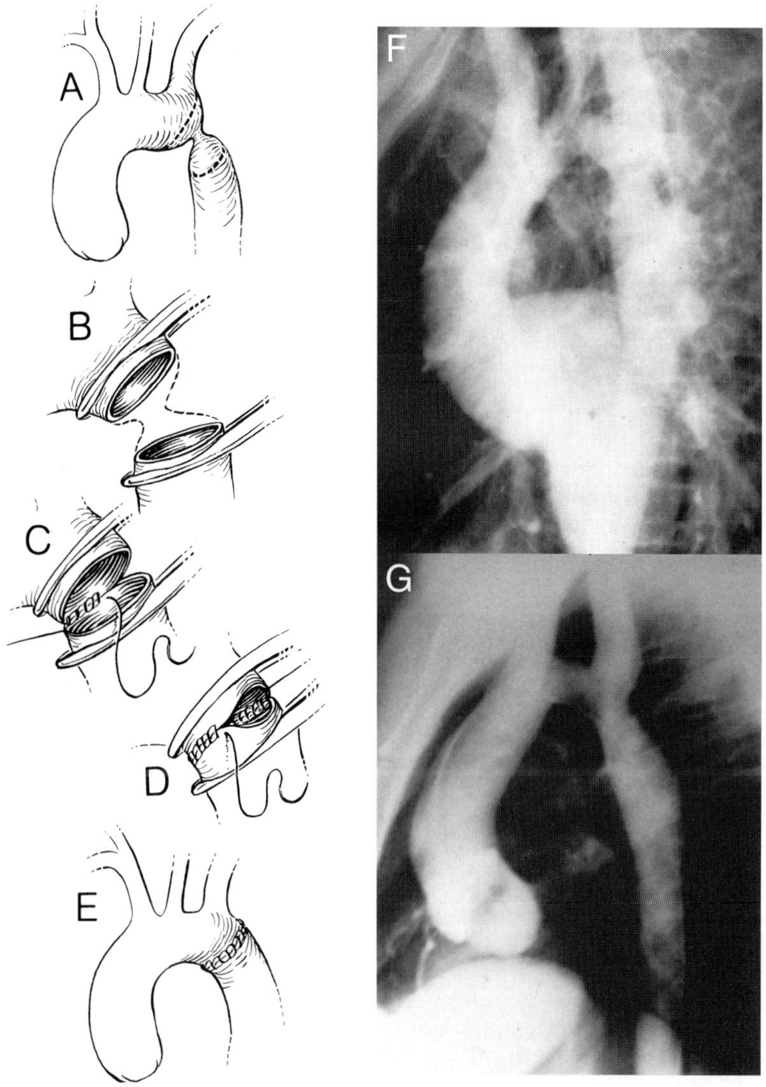

FIGURE 8–3   A–E. Steps in the Crafoord type of coarctation repair and postoperative arteriograms in an adult (F and G).

the coarctation. This is advocated as the preferred method for neonates because of the low recurrence rate.[17] Jonas[18] has highlighted potential problems with the technique that the surgeon should be aware of at the time of surgery. These include the possibility that the juxtaductal shelf of smooth muscle may subsequently fibrose and predispose to aneurysm formation, a hypoplastic distal aortic arch is difficult to augment, and a second coarctation membrane in the distal aortic arch may be missed.

3. Blalock advocated turning the left subclavian artery down and anastomosing it to the aorta or performing an interposition graft between the left subclavian artery and the descending thoracic aorta.

4. A simple method that was used extensively was to open the aorta across the coarctation and then to place a patch of prosthetic material across the coarctation. The septum of the coarctation could also be excised at the same time. In children, good long-term results have been reported without recoarctation or aneurysm formation when a Gortex patch has been used in conjunction with excision of the posterior fibrous ridge.[19]

Increasingly, balloon angioplasty for coarctation of the aorta is being used in infants. However, its exact role in management is still being debated,[20] although some large series have been reported.[21] Rao and Chopra[22] reviewed the results and, despite a recoarctation rate of 31% in children, advocated angioplasty instead of surgery. The study, however, was biased against surgery since it used results of surgery from the 1970s for comparison. Furthermore, there is a risk of aneurysm formation, particularly for repeat angioplasty, a continued risk of infection and aortic dissection, and a high incidence of catheterization site complications, including limb length discrepancies.[20] A prospective randomized study is required to better define the patients who might benefit and the risks from this procedure.

For adults, the coarctation is usually more complicated, particularly since there is often dilatation of the aorta, and histological examination of the aorta reveals extensive medial degeneration of the aorta with loss of elastic tissue in the vicinity of the coarctation. Thus, for adults, aortic repair with an interposition graft is the preferred method. The technique of Waldhausen,[3, 4] involving a subclavian artery flap, is not used because of the likely development of ischemia in the left arm. Nor do we recommend the technique of Crafoord[12] because of the increased risk of paraplegia in adults. In a review of 12,532 coarctation repairs, Brewer and colleagues[11] reported that 0.41% developed postoperative neurological deficits. In adults, however, the segmental intercostal or lumbar arteries that formerly supplied the spinal cord with blood via radicular arteries atrophy, and thus potential alternate pathways of blood supply to the spinal cord are not as readily available. The dependency of the spinal cord blood supply on fewer radicular arteries increases the risk of paraplegia developing during the postoperative period. Repair of the coarctation with a synthetic patch is not advised in adults because of the increased incidence of aneurysm formation.[23] Post-stenotic dilatation and even aneurysm formation are not unusual (Fig. 8–4). The aneurysm formation is due, in part, to the loss of elastic tissue and smooth muscle cells beyond the coarctation.[24]

Pseudocoarctation may also be present without a pressure gradient because of elongation of the aorta with kinking of it (Fig. 8–5). The cause of aneurysms in these patients is unclear, but it is noteworthy that the elastic tissue, on histological examination, shows evidence of degeneration and loss of elastic tissue.

One of the postoperative problems after coarctation repairs, and occasionally after repair of aortic dissection or degenerative aneurysm, is severe hypertension, possibly related to interference with aortic baroreceptors and abnormally set mechanisms to maintain renal blood flow. Sealy[25] reviewed this complication and found that it develops in half of the patients during the first 24 hours after coarctation repairs. Hypertension is sometimes associated with abdominal pain and occasionally with small-bowel necrosis, and it may be due to arteritis. During the postoperative period, norepinephrine excretion increases and angiotensin levels increase. Beta-blockers, nitroprusside, and angiotensin-converting enzyme blockers are effective in controlling the postoperative hypertension. An alternative method of repair in adults is the technique of Blalock, which consists of inserting an interposition end-to-side graft from the left subclavian artery to the descending aorta. This method has the potential advantage of a lower risk of paraplegia or renal failure. Similarly, a tube graft can be placed from the distal aortic arch to the descending aorta, as shown in Figure 8–6.

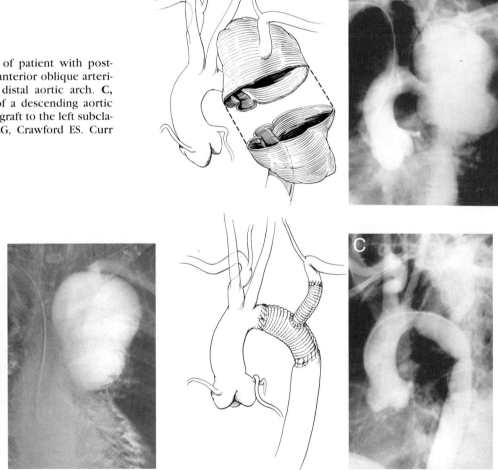

FIGURE 8–4 A, Radiograph of patient with post-coarctation aneurysm. **B,** Left anterior oblique arteriogram. Note the hypoplastic distal aortic arch. **C,** Arteriogram after placement of a descending aortic tube graft and an interposition graft to the left subclavian artery. (From Svensson LG, Crawford ES. Curr Probl Surg 1993;30:1–172.)

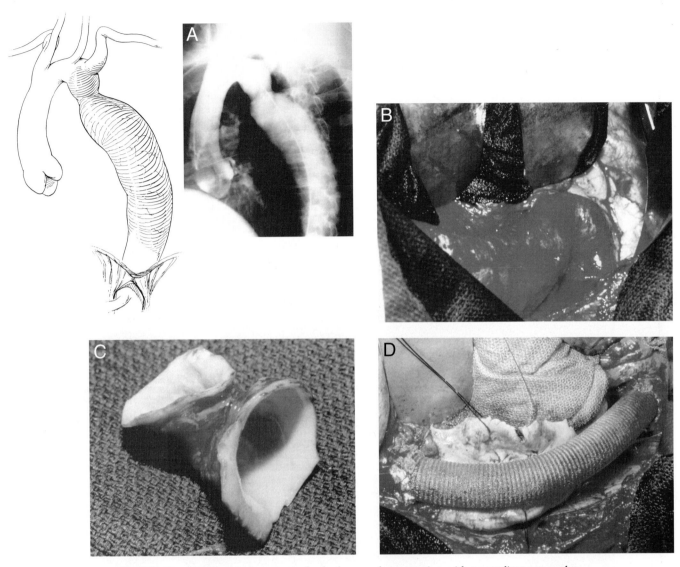

FIGURE 8–5   **A,** Young male patient who had a pseudocoarctation with no gradient across the narrowing and an aneurysm more distally in the descending aorta. **B,** Intraoperative photograph showing the waist in the descending aorta. **C,** Photograph of the resected specimen. **D,** Photograph of the repair with a tube graft.

When patients have had multiple previous repairs of the descending aorta and scar tissue formation presents a formidable barrier to conventional methods of repair, an alternative technique is to perform a bypass from the ascending aorta to the abdominal aorta (Figs. 8-7 to 8-9). We have used this method also for patients who have ascending aortic dissection in combination with coarctation of the aorta.[26] In these patients it is best to try to repair both lesions at the same time; by repairing the ascending aorta with cardiopulmonary bypass and doing an ascending aorta-to-abdominal aorta bypass, both problems are solved. Figure 8-10 and Figures 2-1 and 2-2 illustrate a patient in whom this was done with the use of a composite valve graft.[26] The patient required no homologous blood transfusion. Thus, for selected patients, we advise this latter technique, which is safe and appears to entail a minimal risk of renal failure or para-

plegia. Similarly, this procedure can be used for the rare patient who has coarctation of the upper abdominal aorta (middle aortic syndrome) (Fig. 8-11).

Abdominal Coarctation Associated with Von Recklinghausen's Neurofibromatosis

The association between Von Recklinghausen's neurofibromatosis and aortic coarctation is rare. The more frequent association is between this condition and renal artery stenosis.[27] The aorta is involved in 30% of patients with either renal artery stenosis or aneurysms.[27] Usually the associated condition is coarctation of the abdominal aorta. However, other lesions can include coarctation of the aorta at the isthmus and the descending thoracic aorta and the

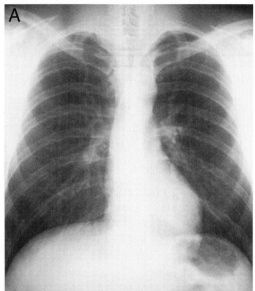

FIGURE 8–6 **A,** Chest radiograph of a young ice hockey player with increasing leg heaviness. Note the rib erosion and 3 sign. **B,** MRI scan showing abrupt cutoff of the distal aortic arch and large left subclavian artery. **C** and **D,** Posteroanterior aortogram showing the distal aortic arch terminating in the left subclavian artery with no visible flow through the coarctation. **E,** Concurrent injection into the blind distal aortic pouch and the distal descending aorta, showing complete coarctation of the aorta. Note the large artery coming off the proximal pouch, which is the anterior spinal artery. This large anterior spinal artery was also seen on transverse MRI views of the spinal cord and vertebral column.

Illustration continued on following page

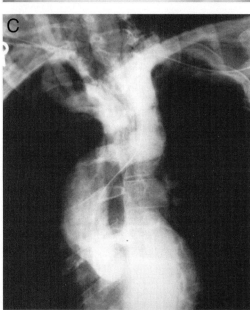

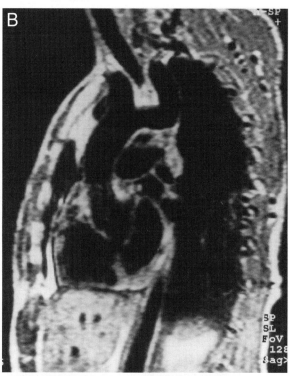

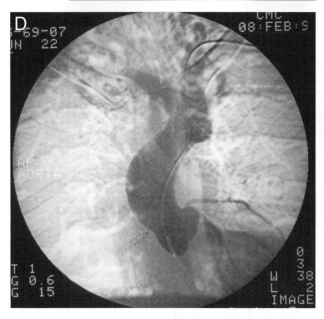

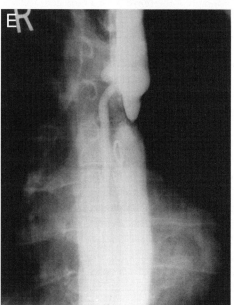

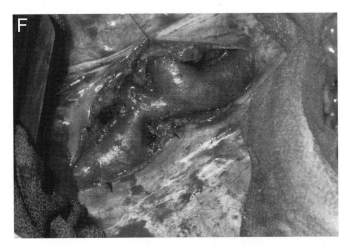
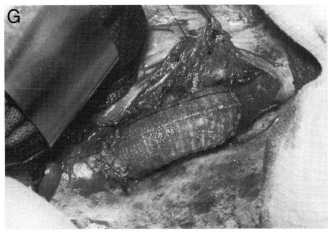

FIGURE 8–6 *Continued* **F,** Intraoperative photograph of the coarctation. Note that the distal aortic arch, under the traction suture and the left vagus nerve, turns superiorly to the right into the left subclavian artery. The distal descending aorta is to the left. **G,** Intraoperative photograph showing the operative repair with the tube graft originating from the distal aortic arch and the left subclavian artery extending down onto the descending aorta. Intraoperative and postoperative pressure measurements revealed no residual gradient across the repair.

development of aortic aneurysms or dissection of the thoracic aorta.[28–30] Stenosis of the pulmonary valve or artery has also been reported.[31, 32] Most of the patients have been young, mostly in the first three decades of life.

The classic features of Von Recklinghausen's neurofibromatosis are usually present. These include the classic café au lait spots on the skin, neurofibromas, a positive family history in 50% of patients, freckles in the groin or axilla, and pigmented hamartomas (Lisch nodules) of the iris. Other features may include macrocephaly, short stature, learning disability, and speech defects. Diagnosis is made on the basis of café au lait spots larger than 1.5 cm in diameter and the finding of Lisch nodules on the iris. The hereditary hamartomas are believed to be of neural crest origin with involvement of the neuroectoderm, mesoderm, and endoderm, and the potential involvement of many organs. The ascending aorta and aortic arch are also believed to be of neural crest origin and thus may partly account for the association with coarctation of the aorta.[33] The histologic findings are not characteristic. Features include intimal proliferation, increased ground substance, and loss of elastic fibers. Neurogenic tissue of various types may be found in vessel walls. Death has been reported to occur by the age of 34 years in one third of patients who have abdominal coarctation.[27–29, 34–37]

Abdominal Coarctation

Coarctation of the abdominal aorta is best treated surgically when hypertension becomes uncontrollable with medications.[38, 39] Other surgical options are either aorto-aorto bypass of the distal aorta[40] or patch repair. Figure 8-11 illustrates the use of an ascending aorta–to–abdominal aorta bypass for this type of problem.

Occasionally young patients are seen with abdominal coarctation that is not due to Takayasu's aortitis. Eibenberger and colleagues[41] reviewed 108 cases reported in the literature and concluded that in patients with congenital coarctation there was a male predominance, patients were younger than 20 years of age, and the stenosis was short, suprarenal, and involved the renal arteries.

Results of Operations in Adults

A 30-year experience with 190 consecutive patients (mean age, 25 years) was reported by Lawrie and colleagues.[42] The patients underwent a variety of procedures for aortic coarctation. Dacron prostheses were used in 65% of the patients. Postoperative moderate or severe hypertension continued in 20% of the patients, although this was less frequent in patients less than 13 years of age. Patients over 21 years of age more frequently had persistent hypertension and experienced cardiovascular complications. Most serious of these was the development of aneurysms either in association with the coarctation or at distant sites. Heikkinen and colleagues[23, 43] noted, on late follow-up of 130 patients who had undergone surgical repairs between the ages of 6 and 23 years, that five developed later ascending aortic complications including rupture, dissection, and aneurysms, emphasizing the need for long-term follow-up.

Balloon angioplasty in adolescents and adults has been reported.[44–47] Shaddy and colleagues[47] randomly assigned 36 patients to either surgery (*n* = 16) or angioplasty (*n* = 20). The success rate for relieving the aortic gradient was similar, with no deaths with either procedure. On follow-up, 20% of the patients who underwent angioplasty developed aneurysms and 25% had restenosis. Fawzy and colleagues[46] used balloon angioplasty in 23 adolescents or adults. Restenosis occurred in two, and aneurysms developed in two patients. One patient, however, developed aortic dissection contained only by a layer of adventitia and required an emergency operation. Erbel and colleagues[44, 45] also reported the development of aortic dissection detected during transesophageal echocardiography (TEE) monitoring of the

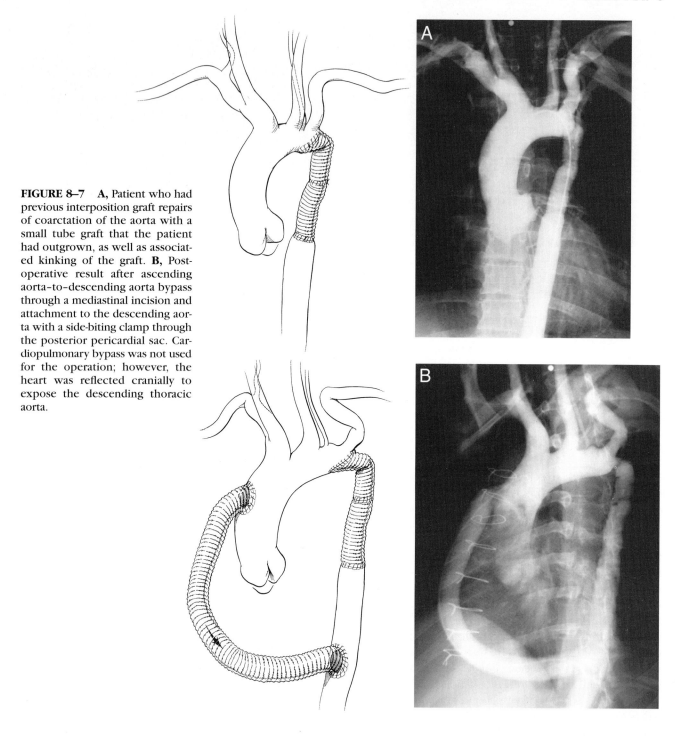

FIGURE 8–7 **A,** Patient who had previous interposition graft repairs of coarctation of the aorta with a small tube graft that the patient had outgrown, as well as associated kinking of the graft. **B,** Postoperative result after ascending aorta–to–descending aorta bypass through a mediastinal incision and attachment to the descending aorta with a side-biting clamp through the posterior pericardial sac. Cardiopulmonary bypass was not used for the operation; however, the heart was reflected cranially to expose the descending thoracic aorta.

dilatation. The indications for angioplasty in adults have to be established and, although feasible, the risks may be higher.[48]

ABNORMAL DEVELOPMENT OF THE AORTIC ARCH

Embryology

During the fourth to fifth weeks of gestation the aortic sac gives rise to six paired aortic arches that supply the branchial arches. The pair of dorsal aortas fuse to form a single dorsal aorta that has some 30 intersegmental arteries, and the latter in turn give rise to the intercostal and lumbar arteries and, in the neck, form part of the vertebral arteries. The aortic sac produces the proximal aortic arch, and the distal aortic arch is formed from the dorsal aorta. It is believed that the heart outflow tract and the aortic arch may originally be derived from the neural crest to account for the association of the bicuspid aortic valve with aortic anomalies, particularly coarctation of the aorta.[33] The seventh intersegmental arteries contribute to the subclavian arteries. During normal development the right fourth

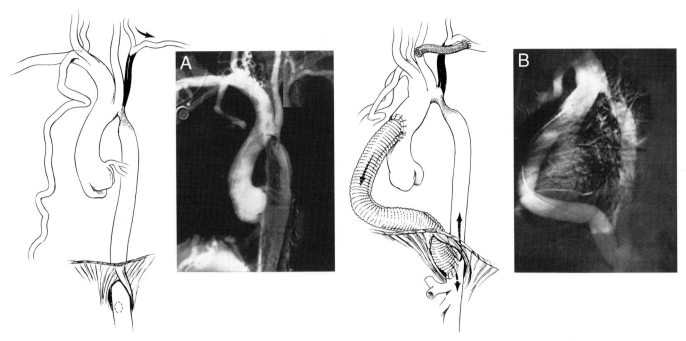

FIGURE 8–8 **A,** Patient with coarctation of the aorta associated with occlusion of the left subclavian artery and left vertebral artery steal to the left arm. **B,** Postoperative arteriogram after ascending aorta to upper abdominal aorta bypass and placement of an interposition graft from the left common carotid artery to the left subclavian artery. (From Svensson LG, Crawford ES. Curr Probl Surg 1993;30:1–172.)

arch in the embryo forms the innominate artery and the proximal part of the right subclavian artery, and the seventh intersegmental artery forms the distal part of the right subclavian artery. On the left side, the fourth arch forms the segment of the aorta between the left common carotid artery and the left subclavian artery. The proximal left subclavian artery is formed from the left seventh intersegmental artery that arises directly from the aorta. The recurrent laryngeal nerves pass around the sixth aortic arches. Thus, because the sixth aortic arch involutes or contributes to the pulmonary arteries, the right recurrent nerve passes around the right subclavian artery and the left recurrent nerve passes around the ductus arteriosus, since this segment persists. In the case of a right aberrant subclavian artery, the origin is from the distal left fourth aortic arch, namely beyond the left carotid artery and the left subclavian artery.[10]

Double Aortic Arch

If the right and left fourth arches persist, then a double aortic arch occurs and forms a vascular ring around the trachea and esophagus. Usually the anterior left arch is smaller and gives rise to the left common carotid and subclavian arteries, whereas the right arch gives rise to the right subclavian and carotid arteries. To correct this problem and the resulting compression of the trachea and esophagus, the smaller anterior aortic arch is divided and tacked to the back of the sternum.

Interrupted Aortic Arch

An interrupted aortic arch is usually associated with varying degrees of cardiac pathologies, such as ventricular septal defect. The problem becomes apparent early in life and the infant requires intubation, correction of acidosis, and infusion of prostaglandin E1 to maintain perfusion through the ductus arteriosus. The prognosis is poor without surgical correction of the aortic deformity and associated cardiac lesions.

Aberrant Right Subclavian Artery

An aberrant right subclavian artery occurs in less than 1% of the population[49] and may result in so-called dysphagia lusoria. Bayford,[50] in 1794, called this "lusoria" because of the Latin term *lusus naturae* meaning a "freak of nature." In 1946 Gross[51] performed the first division of a right anomalous subclavian artery to relieve compression of the esophagus.

Pathology

The aberrant right subclavian artery is usually (78%) posterior to the esophagus where compression of the esophagus can cause dysphagia, known as dysphagia lusoria. In 18% of patients it is between the trachea and the esophagus, and in 4% it is anterior to the trachea. Barium swallow shows that the esophagus is indented at the level of T3 or T4. The site of origin from the aorta is usually dilated and is

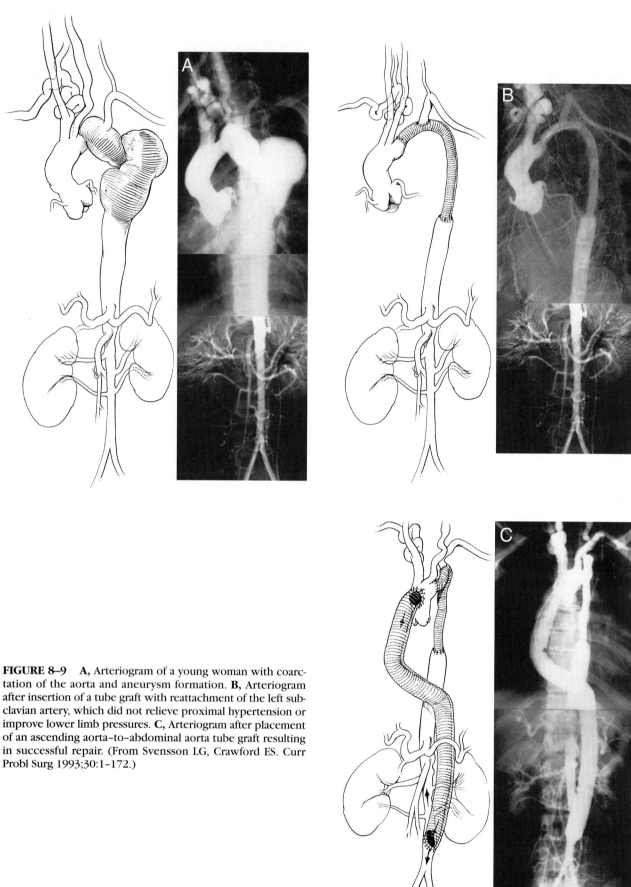

FIGURE 8–9 **A,** Arteriogram of a young woman with coarctation of the aorta and aneurysm formation. **B,** Arteriogram after insertion of a tube graft with reattachment of the left subclavian artery, which did not relieve proximal hypertension or improve lower limb pressures. **C,** Arteriogram after placement of an ascending aorta–to–abdominal aorta tube graft resulting in successful repair. (From Svensson LG, Crawford ES. Curr Probl Surg 1993;30:1–172.)

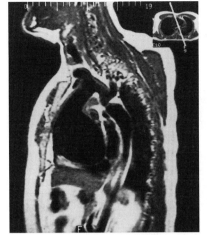

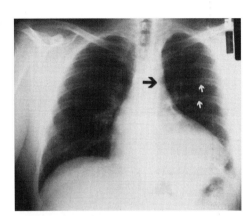

FIGURE 8–10 Upper left window shows MRI scan of a patient with an ascending aortic aneurysm and coarctation of the aorta. Right upper window shows the chest radiograph with rib notching, a 3 sign *(black arrow),* and a large heart silhouette. Lower windows show the arteriogram, which revealed an aortic dissection of the ascending aorta. Repair consisted of placement of an ascending aortic composite valve tube graft and a tube graft from the ascending aorta to the abdominal aorta. (Reprinted with permission from the Society of Thoracic Surgeons. From Svensson LG. Ann Thorac Surg 1994;58:241–3.)

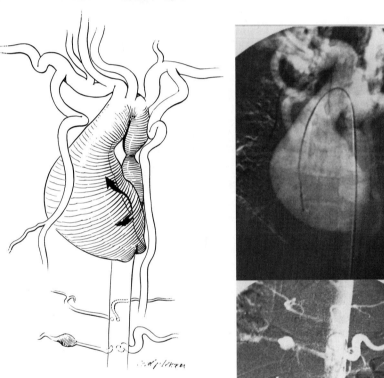

known as Kommerell's diverticulum. A varying extent of the proximal aberrant right subclavian artery is also often dilated, and if it is neglected the other arteries arising in the vicinity may also become involved in the aneurysm.[10] It should be noted that the right inferior laryngeal nerve is not recurrent.

Clinical Management

Although the aberrant right subclavian artery is a rare congenital malformation, it should be suspected when dysphagia occurs in infancy or early childhood. Patients who do not have early dysphagia or dyspnea may later present with aneurysmal enlargement of the distal aortic arch at the site of Kommerel's diverticulum. Occasionally, patients have limb ischemia.[52] In infants an aberrant right subclavian

artery may be detected earlier because of an interrupted aortic arch.[53] Magnetic resonance imaging (MRI) for pediatric thoracic aorta imaging is particularly useful,[54] although three-dimensional echocardiography also has advantages for cardiac evaluation. In adults, our usual approach to correction of this congenital abnormality is to repair both the distal aortic arch and the proximal descending aorta with an interposition graft and then oversew the stump of the right subclavian artery (Figs. 8–12 to 8–14). If the origin of the left subclavian artery, which most often arises proximal to the origin of the right subclavian artery, also needs to be divided, then it is reimplanted by means of an interposition tube graft. The patient is then turned on his or her back and either the right subclavian artery is anastomosed directly to the right common carotid artery through a right

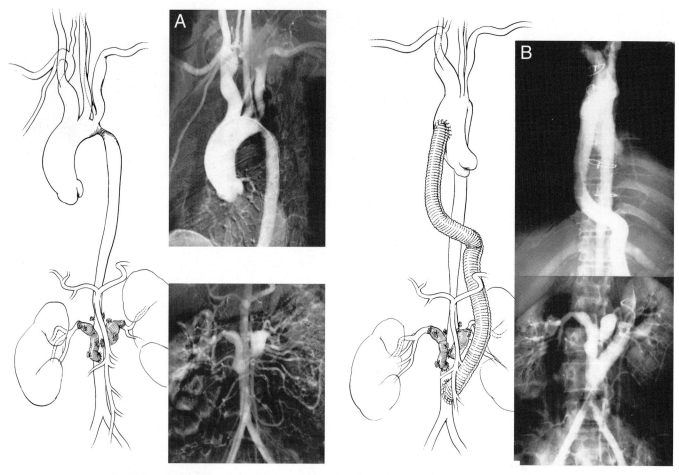

FIGURE 8–11 **A,** Patient with a long coarctation from the left subclavian artery to the abdominal aorta where previously vein bypasses to the two renal arteries had been performed. **B,** Postoperative arteriogram after placement of a tube graft from the ascending aorta, through the diaphragm, behind the pancreas, and down to the abdominal aorta below the renal artery bypasses. (From Svensson LG, Crawford ES. Curr Probl Surg 1993;30:1–172.)

supraclavicular incision or an interposition graft is inserted between the two vessels. Flow to the left subclavian artery can also be reestablished with a left carotid artery–to–left subclavian artery bypass if it has been divided in the chest (Figs. 8–12 to 8–14). An approach that has been proposed by Spencer's group[55] is to first place an interposition graft between the distal right subclavian artery and the left common carotid artery with a supraclavicular incision and then resect and oversew Kommerell's diverticulum with a side-biting clamp. Attempts at repair through the right side of the chest have not met with much success.[10, 55] Verkroost and colleagues[56] have advocated a mediastinal incision, deep hypothermia with circulatory arrest, and repair. We believe, however, that for most patients this method has greater risks than repair through the left side of the chest as described above. Nevertheless, cardiopulmonary bypass should be available if required.

Right-sided Aortic Arch

A right-sided arch is uncommon (0.05% of the population), and lesions that require surgical repair are even more

rare. The lesions that may require repair include an enlarged Kommerell's diverticulum from the aberrant left subclavian artery that arises from the distal right-sided arch or constriction of the esophagus resulting in dysphagia. These patients may also be more prone to aortic dissection in the right-sided aortic arch. In patients with a right-sided arch, the entire right dorsal aorta has persisted and the left dorsal aorta has involuted. The ductus arteriosus, however, is left-sided, which results in a complete vascular ring around the esophagus and trachea that may cause symptoms because of compression of these structures. An MRI scan may detect this.[57] More rarely, bilateral ductus arteriosus may be present.[58] The methods of treatment are similar to those used for lesions of the left-sided arch, although deep hypothermia with circulatory arrest is required more often to repair the sometimes complex lesions of the distal arch.[59, 60] Midulla and colleagues[61] reported on a patient with a double aortic arch and a right descending aorta with dissection for which deep hypothermia with circulatory arrest was required to divide the left arch and insert a descending aortic graft.

A tubular graft is used to repair the distal aortic arch, and then the aberrant left subclavian artery is reattached to the

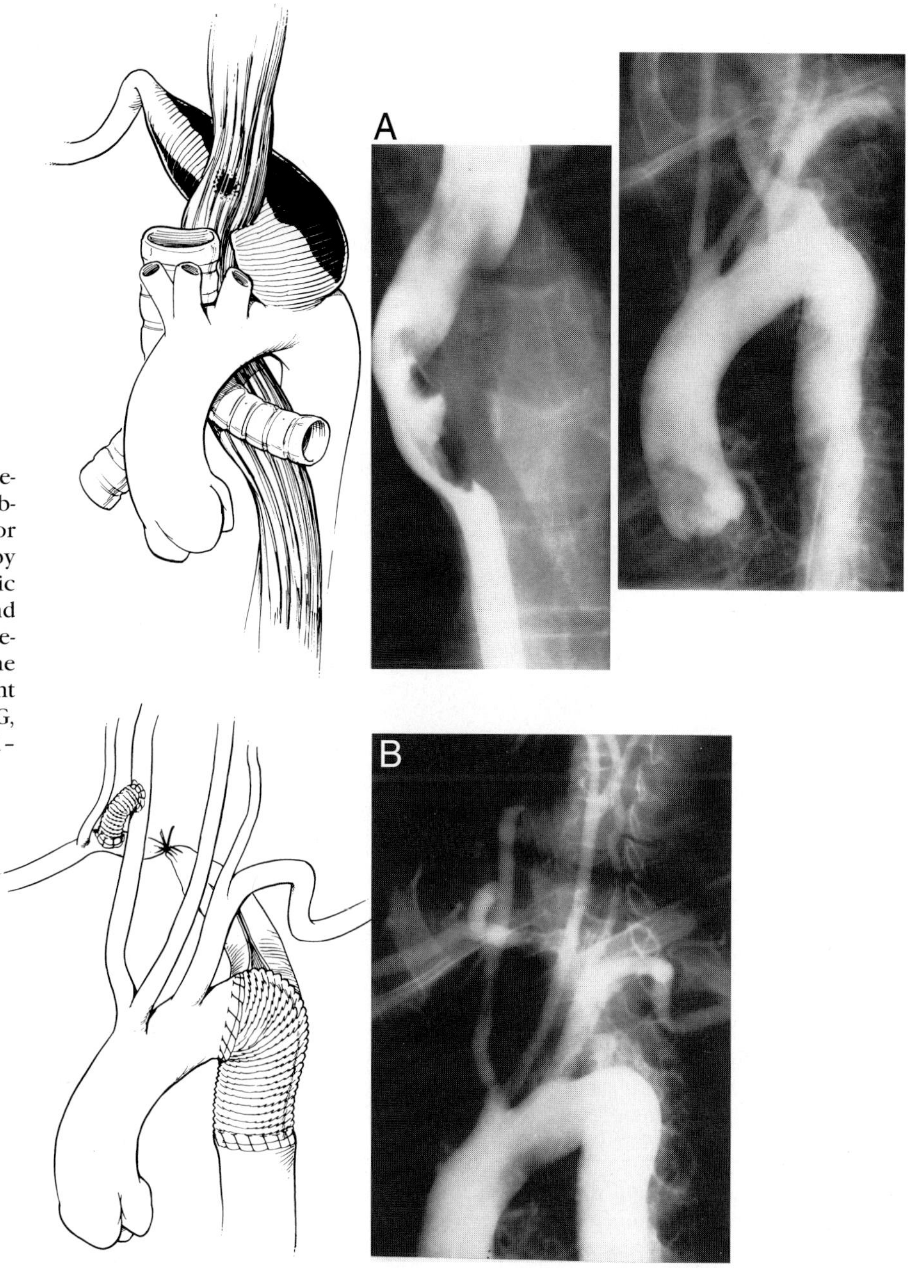

FIGURE 8–12 **A,** Barium swallow and arteriogram of patient with aberrant right subclavian artery and erosion of the posterior esophagus. **B,** Arteriogram after repair by placement of a descending thoracic aortic tube graft through a left thoracotomy and placement of an interpostion tube graft between the right subclavian artery and the right common carotid artery through a right supraclavicular incision. (From Svensson LG, Crawford ES. Curr Probl Surg 1993;30:1–172.)

tubular graft with an interposition graft (Figs. 8-15 and 8-16). Alternatively, the origin of the left subclavian artery can be oversewn and an interposition graft can be placed between the left common carotid artery and the distal left subclavian artery through a left supraclavicular incision.[10]

Cervical Aortic Arch

Very rarely the fourth aortic arch migrates caudally or it involutes, leaving the third aortic arch to form the aortic arch high in the chest or lower neck. There may be other aortic anomalies, particularly a right-sided aortic arch, but the compression of surrounding stuctures is usually not severe enough to require surgical intervention.

SUPRAVALVULAR AORTIC STENOSIS

Supravalvular aortic stenosis (SAS) and the association with elfin facies in affected patients were described by Williams, Barratt-Boyes, and Lowe[62] in 1961. Although the syndrome is associated with mental retardation in the nonfamilial form,[63] patients often have language and musical abilities far greater than expected for their level of intelligence. Presentation is similar to that of aortic valve stenosis with either increasing dyspnea or angina. Sudden death may also occur. Only 40% to 50% of patients with SAS have Williams syndrome; in the remaining patients either there is an autosmal dominant familial transmission or the syndrome is sporadic.[64-67] Successful treatment of SAS

Text continued on page 170

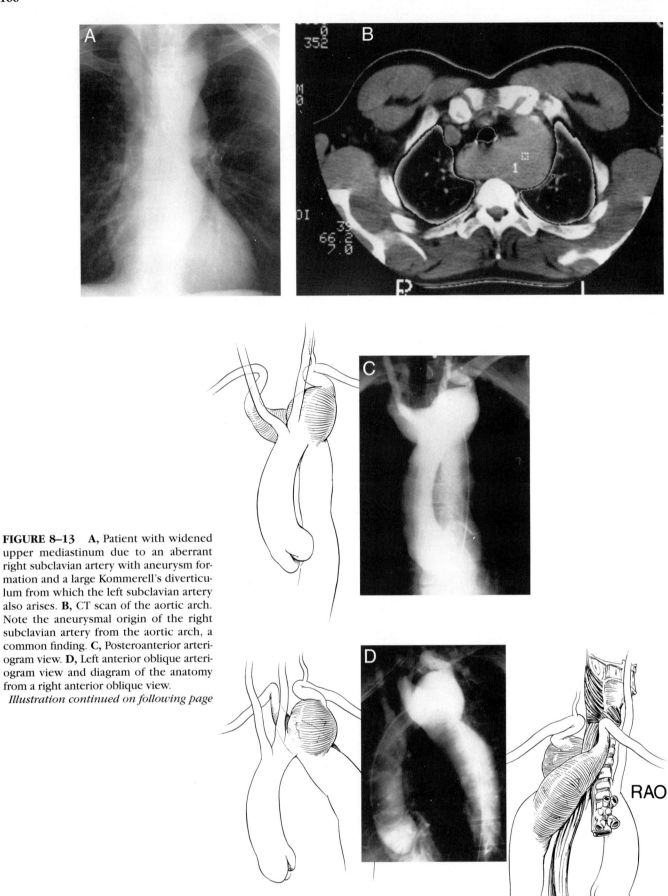

FIGURE 8–13 **A,** Patient with widened upper mediastinum due to an aberrant right subclavian artery with aneurysm formation and a large Kommerell's diverticulum from which the left subclavian artery also arises. **B,** CT scan of the aortic arch. Note the aneurysmal origin of the right subclavian artery from the aortic arch, a common finding. **C,** Posteroanterior arteriogram view. **D,** Left anterior oblique arteriogram view and diagram of the anatomy from a right anterior oblique view.

Illustration continued on following page

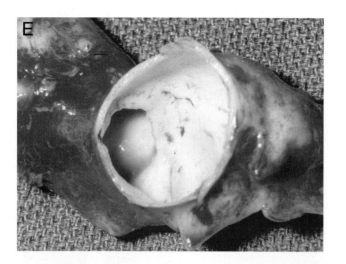

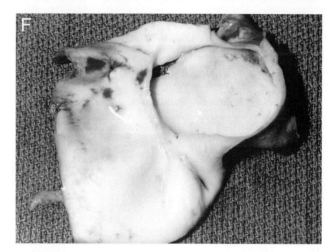

FIGURE 8–13 *Continued* **E** and **F,** Operative specimens showing origin of the large Kommerell's diverticulum and right subclavian artery. **G,** Arteriogram after repair by placement of a descending thoracic aortic tube graft, an interposition tube graft to the left subclavian artery, and an interposition tube graft between the right subclavian artery and the right common carotid artery. (From Svensson LG, Crawford ES. Curr Probl Surg 1993;30:1–172.)

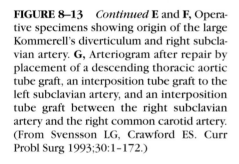

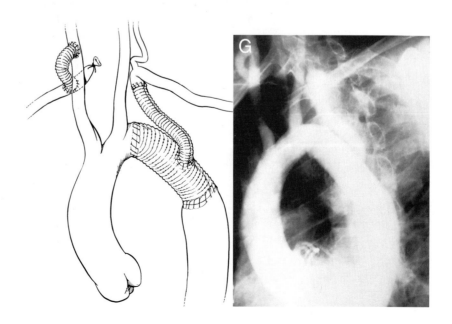

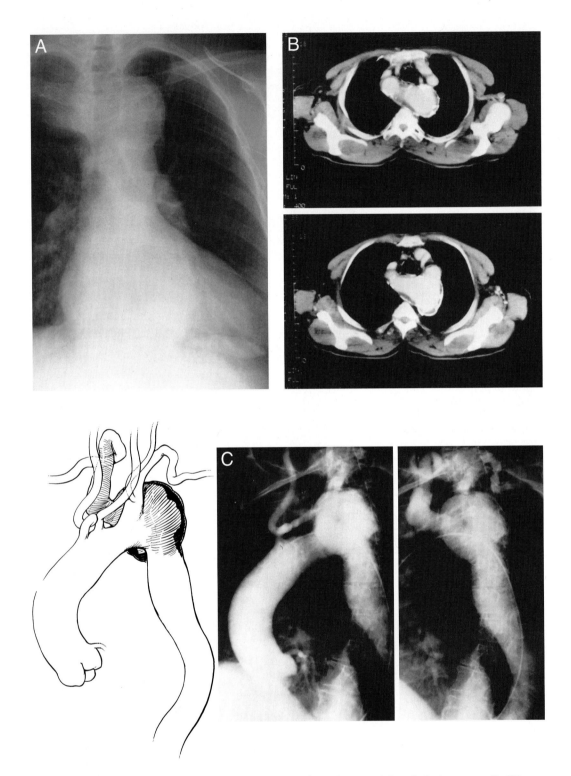

FIGURE 8–14 **A,** Chest radiograph of a patient with an aberrant right subclavian artery. **B,** CT scan of the aortic arch. **C,** Left anterior oblique arteriogram with aneurysm formation.

Illustration continued on following page

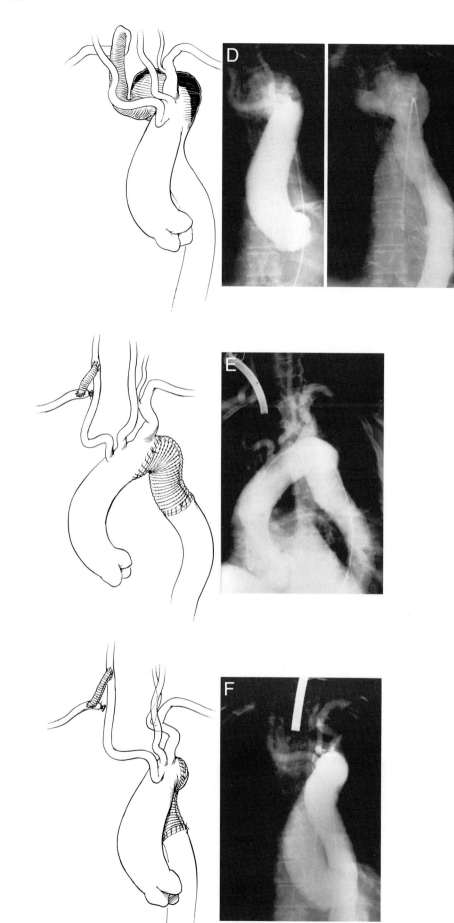

FIGURE 8–14 *Continued* **D,** Posteroanterior view. **E** and **F,** Postoperative arteriogram after placement of a descending aortic tube graft and an interposition tube graft between the right subclavian and the right common carotid artery.

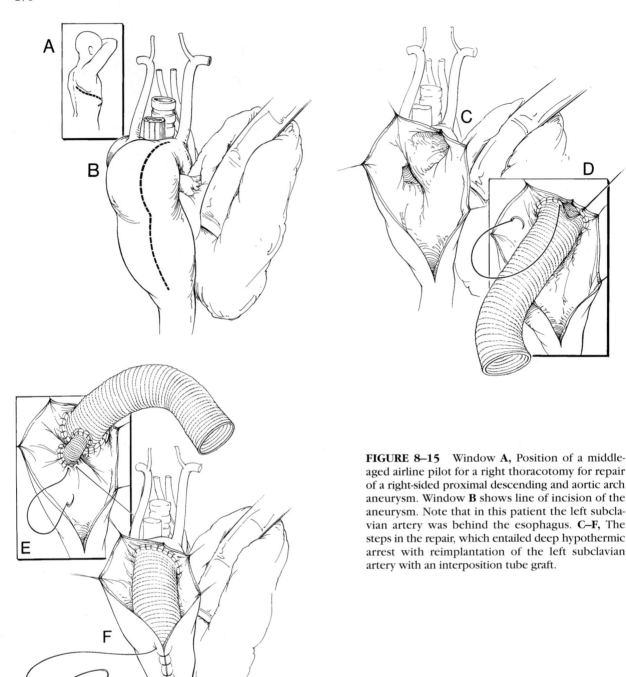

© Baylor College of Medicine 1987

FIGURE 8–15 Window **A,** Position of a middle-aged airline pilot for a right thoracotomy for repair of a right-sided proximal descending and aortic arch aneurysm. Window **B** shows line of incision of the aneurysm. Note that in this patient the left subclavian artery was behind the esophagus. **C–F,** The steps in the repair, which entailed deep hypothermic arrest with reimplantation of the left subclavian artery with an interposition tube graft.

by enlargement of the aorta with a patch was reported in 1961 by Williams and colleagues[62] and by McGoon and colleagues.[65]

The SAS is usually localized, although a more diffuse narrowing or waist in the ascending aorta may be present.[62, 65] In addition, there is an internal circumferential shelf, which further increases the gradient across the stenosis. Often the aortic valve commissures are attached to the undersurface of this shelf, sometimes obstructing flow to the left main

coronary artery, and this can complicate the repair, particularly in the one third of patients who have associated aortic valve stenosis. Fig. 8–17 shows a patient who had this type of SAS and required shelf excision, commissure resuspension, commissurotomy, and then patch closure of the ascending aorta. Coronary artery disease may be accelerated in these patients because of the coronary hypertension,[63] and therefore coronary catheterization should be performed in older patients. Rarer associated anomalies

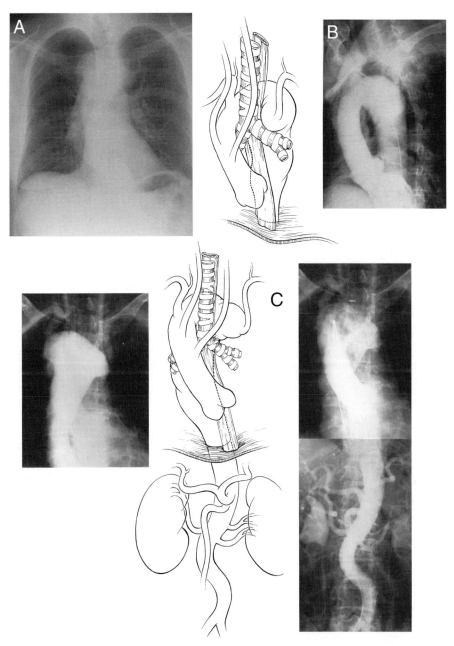

FIGURE 8–16   Patient with dysphagia and a right-sided aortic arch as seen on chest radiograph **(A). B,** The anatomy and the arteriograms in left anterior oblique view. **C,** The posterior anterior view.

Illustration continued on following page

include pulmonary artery stenosis, greater vessel stenosis, coarctation, abdominal aorta anomalies, and ventricular septal defect. An association with Marfan syndrome has been reported in 5% of patients[64]; however, because the genetic molecular defects are different between the syndromes, this has yet to be confirmed by either RFLP or PCR analysis. In patients without Williams syndrome, an elastic gene deletion in the 7q region has been associated with SAS.[66] Ewart and colleagues[67] have found that disruption of the elastin

genes causes familial SAS; however, deletion of the entire elastin locus is associated with Williams syndrome.

Operative Repair

The classical method of repair is to incise the ascending aorta and extend the incision into the noncoronary or right coronary cusp sinus. After the aortic shelf is excised, the incision is repaired with a teardrop or diamond-shaped patch. Alternatively, if the incision has been extended into

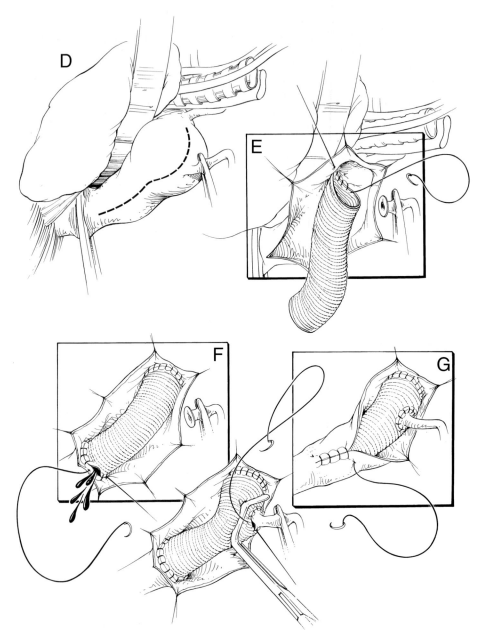

FIGURE 8–16 *Continued* **D,** The findings at the time of operation through a right thoracotomy with deep hypothermic circulatory arrest. **E,** Anastomosis of the tube graft to the distal aortic arch followed by anastomosis to the descending aorta **(F)** and finally reimplantation of the left subclavian artery into the graft **(G).**

Illustration continued on following page

both sinuses, the repair is performed with an inverted Y or pantaloon patch, as described by Doty and colleagues.[68] In another technique described by Brom the aorta is transected circumferentially and then the sinuses of Valsalva are incised.[69] The sinuses and sinotubular ridge are then enlarged with triangular patches. A further modification that Myers, Waldhausen, and colleagues have described involves making corresponding incisions into the ascending aorta and then interdigitating the incisions, thus repairing the aorta entirely with autologous aortic tissue.[69]

Figure 8–17 shows a patient with more extensive SAS that required also an aortic valve repair.

Long-term Results

Of 80 patients operated on at the Mayo Clinic[63]—67 with the localized and 13 with the diffuse form and 31 with Williams syndrome—two died (2.5%). The 10-year and 20-year survival rates were, respectively, 94% and 91%. On Cox multivariate analysis, the only predictor of late death was aortic valve involvement. There was no difference accord-

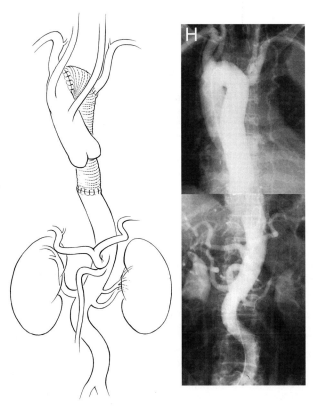

FIGURE 8–16 *Continued* **H,** The completed PA arteriogram view of the repair.

FIGURE 8–17 **A,** Preoperative arteriogram of a patient with Williams syndrome and supravalvular stenosis with a 50 mm Hg gradient across the aortic valve and a 55 mm Hg gradient across the supravalvular shelf. **B,** Window A shows the intraoperative findings of a shelf, stenosis of the aortic valve, and fusion of the commissures. Window B shows the commissurotomy being performed. **C,** Closure of the incision with a teardrop patch after resuspension of the commissures and excision of the supravalvular shelf. Postoperative TEE showed a trace of aortic valve regurgitation and an insignificant gradient.

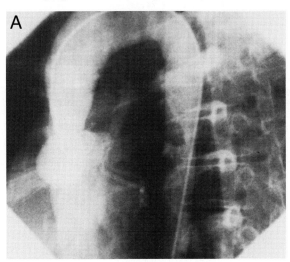

ing to patch shape, but diffuse disease required an extensive patch.

REFERENCES

1. Blalock A, Park EA. The surgical treatment of experimental coarctation (atresia) of the aorta. Ann Surg 1944;119:445-56.
2. Trummer MJ, Mannix EPJ. Abdominal pain and necrotizing mesenteric arteritis following resection of coarctation of the aorta. J Thorac Cardiovasc Surg 1963;45:198.
3. Waldhausen JA, King H, Nahrwold DL, et al. Management of coarctation in infancy. JAMA 1964;187:220.
4. Waldhausen JA, Nahrwold DL. Repair of coarctation of the aorta with a subclavian flap. J Thorac Cardiovasc Surg 1966;51:532-3.
5. Crafoord C, Nylin F. Congenital coarctation of aorta and its surgical treatment. J Thorac Surg 1945;14:347-61.
6. Kirklin JW, Burchell HB, Pugh DC, et al. Surgical treatment of coarctation of the aorta in a ten-week old infant: report of a case. Circulation 1952;6:411-14.
7. Deal K, Wooley CF. Coarctation of the aorta and pregnancy. Ann Intern Med 1973;78:706.
8. Glancy DL, Morrow AG, Simon AL, Roberts WC. Juxtaductal aortic coarctation: analysis of 84 patients studied hemodynamically, angiographically, and morphologically after age 1 year. Am J Cardiol 1983;51:537-51.
9. Abbott ME. Coarctation of the aorta of the adult type, II. Am Heart J 1928;3:574-618.
10. Svensson LG, Crawford ES. Aortic dissection and aortic aneurysm surgery: clinical observations, experimental investigations, and statistical analyses. Part III. Curr Probl Surg 1993;30:1-172.
11. Brewer LA, Fosburg RA, Mulder GA, Verska JS. Spinal cord complications following surgery for coarctation of the aorta. J Thorac Cardiovasc Surg 1972;64:368.
12. Crafoord Ci, Ekstom G. The surgical treatment of patent ductus arteriosus: a clinical study of 290 cases. Acta Chir Scand 1952;169 (Supp):1-197.
13. Arenas JD, Myers JL, Gleason MM, et al. End-to-end repair of aortic coarctation using absorbable polydioxanone suture. Ann Thorac Surg 1991;51:413-7.
14. Rubay JE, Sluysmans T, Alexandrescu V, et al. Surgical repair of coarctation of the aorta in infants under one year of age: long-term results in 146 patients comparing subclavian flap angioplasty and modified end-to-end anastomosis. J Cardiovasc Surg (Torino) 1992;33:216-22.
15. Kappetein AP, Zwinderman AH, Bogers AJJC, et al. More than thirty-five years of coarctation repair: an unexpected high relapse rate. J Thorac Cardiovasc Surg 1994;107:87-95.

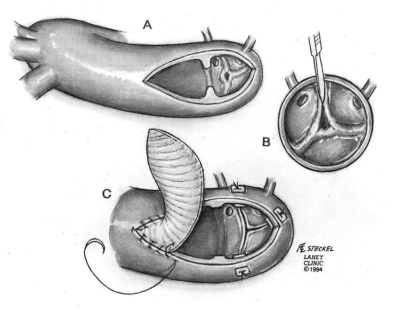

16. vanHeurn LWE, Wong CM, Spiegelhalter DJ, et al. Surgical treatment of aortic coarctation in infants younger than three months: 1985-1990. J Thorac Cardiovasc Surg 1994;107:74-86.

17. Merrill WH, Hoff SJ, Stewart JR, et al. Operative risk factors and durability of repair of coarctation of the aorta in the neonate. Ann Thorac Surg 1994;58:399-403.

18. Jonas RA. Coarctation: do we need to resect ductal tissue? Ann Thorac Surg 1991;52:604-7.

19. Bertolini A, Dalmonte P, Toma P, et al. Goretex patch aortoplasty for coarctation in children: nuclear magnetic resonance assessment at 7 years. J Cardiovasc Surg (Torino) 1992;33:223-8.

20. Svensson LG. Aortic surgery, coarctation of the aorta, and aortic dissection. Curr Opin Cardiol 1993;8:254-61.

21. Tynan M, Finley JP, Fontes V, et al. Balloon angioplasty for the treatment of native coarctation: results of Valvuloplasty and Angioplasty of Congenital Anomalies Registry. Am J Cardiol 1990;65:790-2.

22. Rao PS, Chopra PS. Role of balloon angioplasty in the treatment of aortic coarctation. Ann Thorac Surg 1991;52:621-31.

23. Heikkinen L, Sariola H, Salo J, Ala KK. Morphological and histopathological aspects of aneurysms after patch aortoplasty for coarctation. Ann Thorac Surg 1990;50:946-8.

24. Kukongviriyapan U, Gow BS. Morphometric analyses of rabbit thoracic aorta after poststenotic dilatation. Circ Res 1989;65:1774-86.

25. Sealy WC. Paradoxical hypertension after repair of coarctation of the aorta: a review of its cause. Ann Thorac Surg 1990;50:323-9.

26. Svensson LG. Management of acute dissection with coarctation of the aorta in single operation. Ann Thorac Surg 1994;58:241-3.

27. Flynn MP, Buchanan JB. Neurofibromatosis, hypertension, and renal artery aneurysms. South Med J 1980;73:618-20.

28. Glenn F, Keefer EBC, Speer DS, et al. Coarctation of lower thoracic and abdominal aorta immediately proximal to celiac axis. Surg Gynecol Obstet 1952;94:561-9.

29. Pentecost M, Stanley P, Takahoshi M, Isaacs H Jr. Aneurysms of the aorta and subclavian and vertebral arteries in neurofibromatosis. Am J Dis Child 1981;135:475-7.

30. Rowen M, Dorsey TJ, Kegel SM, Ostermiller WE. Thoracic coarctation associated with neurofibromatosis. Am J Dis Child 1975;129:113-5.

31. Itzchak Y, Ratznelson D, Boichis H, et al. Angiographic features of arterial lesions in neurofibromatosis. Am J Roentgenol Radium Ther Nucl Med 1974;122:643-7.

32. Watson GH. Pulmonary stenosis, café au lait spots, and dull intelligence. Arch Dis Child 1967;42:303-7.

33. Kappetein AP, Groot ACG, Zwinderman AH, et al. The neural crest as a possible pathogenetic factor in coarctation of the aorta and bicuspid aortic valve. J Thorac Cardiovasc Surg 1991;102:830-6.

34. DeBakey ME, Garrett HE, Howell JF, et al. Coarctation of the abdominal aorta with renal arterial stenosis: surgical considerations. Ann Surg 1965;165:830-43.

35. Greene SF, Fitzwater JE, Burgess J. Arterial lesions associated with neurofibromatosis. Am J Clin Pathol 1974;62:481-7.

36. Riccardi VM. Medical progress: Von Recklinghausen neurofibromatosis. New Engl J Med 1981;305:1617-27.

37. Senning A, Johannson L. Coarctation of abdominal aorta. J Thorac Cardiovasc Surg 1960;40:517.

38. Hodgkin JE, Dines DE, Didier EP. Preoperative evaluation of the patient with pulmonary disease. Mayo Clin Proc 1973;48:114-8.

39. Latimer RG, Dickman M, Day WC, et al. Ventilatory patterns and pulmonary complications after upper abdominal surgery determined by preoperative and postoperative computerized spirometry and blood gas analysis. Am J Surg 1971;122:622-32.

40. Roques X, Bourdeaud'hui A, Choussat A, et al. Coarctation of the abdominal aorta. Ann Vasc Surg 1988;2:138-44.

41. Eibenberger K, Dock W, Metz V, et al. Stenosen und Verschlusse der Aorta abdominalis bei Patienten unter 40 Jahren. Rofo Fortschr Geb Rontgenstr Neuen Bildgeb Verfahr 1993;159:388-92.

42. Lawrie GM, DeBakey ME, Morris GC Jr, et al. Late repair of coarctation of the descending thoracic aorta in 190 patients. Arch Surg 1981;116:1557-60.

43. Heikkinen LO, Ala-Kuliju KV, Salo JA. Dilatation of ascending aorta in patients with repaired coarctation. 1991;25:25-8.

44. Erbel R, Bednarczyk I, Pop T, et al. Detection of dissection of the aortic intima and media after angioplasty of coarctation of the aorta. Circulation 1990;81:805-14.

45. Erbel R, Sievert H, Bussman WD, et al. Aortenisthmusstenosendilatation im Erwachsenenalter eine deutsche kooperative Studie. Z Kardiol 1988;77:797-804.

46. Fawzy ME, Dunn B, Galal O, et al. Balloon coarctation angioplasty in adolescents and adults: early and intermediate results. Am Heart J 1992;124:167-71.

47. Shaddy RE, Boucek MM, Sturtevant JE, et al. Comparison of angioplasty and surgery for unoperated coarctation of the aorta. Circulation 1993;87:793-9.

48. Waldman JD, Karp RB. How should we treat coarctation of the aorta? Circulation 1993;87:1043-5.

49. Goldbloom AA. The anomalous right subclavian artery and its possible clinical significance. Surg Gynecol Obstet 1922;34:378-84.

50. Bayford D. An account of a singular case of obstructed deglutition. Memoirs Med Soc London 1794:275-86.

51. Gross RE. Surgical treatment of dysphagia lusoria. Ann Surg 1946;124:532-4.

52. Kieffer E, Bahnini A, Koskas F. Aberrant subclavian artery: surgical treatment in thirty-three adult patients. J Vasc Surg 1994;19:100-11.

53. Kutsche LM, Van Mierop L. Cervical origin of the right subclavian artery in aortic arch interruption: pathogenesis and significance. Am J Cardiol 1984;53:892-5.

54. Burrows PE, MacDonald CE. Magnetic resonance imaging of the pediatric thoracic aorta. Semin Ultrasound CT MR 1993;14:129-44.

55. Esposito RA, Khalil I, Galloway AC, Spencer FC. Surgical treatment for aneurysm of aberrant subclavian artery based on a case report and a review of the literature. J Thorac Cardiovasc Surg 1988;95:888-91.

56. Verkroost MW, Hamerlijnck RP, Vermeulen FE. Surgical management of aneurysms at the origin of an aberrant right subclavian artery. J Thorac Cardiovasc Surg 1994;107:1469-71.

57. Friese KK, Dulce MC, Higgins CB. Airway obstruction by right aortic arch with right-sided patent ductus arteriosus: demonstration by MRI. J Comput Assist Tomogr 1992;16:888-92.

58. Nair SK, Subramanyam R, Venkitachalam CG, Valiathan MS. Right aortic arch with isolation of the left subclavian artery and bilateral patent ductus arterioses: a case report. J Cardiovasc Surg (Torino) 1992;33:242-4.

59. Svensson LG, Labib S. Aortic dissection and aneurysm surgery. Curr Opin Cardiol 1994;9:191-9.

60. Svensson LG, Crawford ES, Hess KR, et al. Deep hypothermia with circulatory arrest: determinants of stroke and early mortality in 656 patients. J Thorac Cardiovasc Surg 1992;106:19-31.

61. Midulla PS, Dapunt OE, Sadeghi AM, et al. Aortic dissection involving a double aortic arch with a right descending aorta. Ann Thorac Surg 1994;58:874-5.

62. Williams JCP, Barratt-Boyes BG, Lowe JB. Supravalvular aortic stenosis. Circulation 1961;24:1311.

63. vanSon JAM, Danielson GK, Puga FJ, et al. Supravalvular aortic stenosis. J Thorac Cardiovasc Surg 1994;107:103-15.

64. Peterson TA, Todd DB, Edwards JE. Supravalvular aortic stenosis. J Thorac Cardiovasc Surg 1965;50:734-41.

65. McGoon DC, Mankin HT, Vlad P, et al. The surgical treatment of supravalvular aortic stenosis. J Thorac Cardiovasc Surg 1961;41:125-33.

66. Olson TM, Michels VV, Driscoll DJ, et al. Identification of elastin gene deletions in supravalvular aortic stenosis. J Am Coll Cardiol 1994;Abstract:43A.

67. Ewart AK, Jin W, Atkinson D, et al. Supravalvular aortic stenosis associated with a deletion disrupting the elastin gene. J Clin Invest 1994;93:1071-7.

68. Doty DB, Polansky DB, Jenson CB. Supravalvular aortic stenosis. J Thorac Cardiovasc Surg 1977;74:362-71.

69. Myers JL, Waldhausen JA, Cyran SE, et al. Results of surgical repair of congenital supravalvular aortic stenosis. J Thorac Cardiovasc Surg 1993;105:281-8.

Occlusive Disease of the Aorta

Aortic occlusive disease is clearly much less common than occlusive disease of the aortic branches. Most commonly, the aortic bifurcation and the proximal iliac arteries are involved by the development of atherosclerosis. Occasionally the innominate artery, the left common carotid artery, and the left subclavian artery are involved at their origin from the aortic arch. Although the cause of atherosclerosis of the aorta is not clearly established, it is associated with tobacco abuse, diabetes, hypertension, and hyperlipidemias. In women a "hypoplastic aorta syndrome" may occur, often associated with smoking. More rarely, the occlusive disease is of an inflammatory nature associated with such conditions as Takayasu's disease. The inflammatory diseases of the aorta are discussed elsewhere. Occlusive disease of the branches of the aorta, particularly of the lower extremities, is extensively covered in other texts. This chapter will concentrate on occlusive disease that directly affects the aorta and that requires aortic operations.

ATHEROSCLEROSIS AND CALCIFICATION OF THE ASCENDING AORTA

Rarely do patients have occlusive disease of the ascending aorta alone. When present, it takes the form of atherosclerotic lesions with associated fronds of tissue floating in the bloodstream. These fronds of atherosclerotic and thrombotic material may embolize and cause strokes or distal ischemic damage. Surgical removal of these lesions, when they are not associated with other cardiovascular disease, is debatable, and most patients are best treated with full anticoagulation with warfarin. On follow-up transesophageal echocardiography (TEE) examination, the lesions will usually have disappeared, either as a result of embolization or lysis.

Occasionally when aortic valve replacement is required, particularly for aortic valve stenosis in elderly patients, a calcified porcelain ascending aorta is found. The development of the calcification is often preceded by a history of radiation or inflammatory disease (for example, rheumatoid arthritis or severe arthritis). The options for managing this type of problem include placement of a left ventricular apex-to-descending aorta valved conduit; insertion of a composite graft and a distal ascending or arch anastomosis

with separate distal vein bypass grafts to the coronary arteries; or endarterectomy of the ascending aorta. In six patients we have performed endarterctomy of the ascending aorta, and in two patients we have performed endarterectomy of the entire aortic root (including the left main artery) to insert an aortic valve.[1] All six patients survived without any major complications. Figures 9-1 and 9-2 illustrate the preoperative and postoperative films of two patients.

OCCLUSIVE LESIONS OF THE AORTIC ARCH BRANCHES

Most of the lesions that affect the branches of the aortic arch at the origin of these arteries are due to the various types of aortitis. Atherosclerosis is uncommon and usually is not associated with ulceration but only with stenosis, most commonly of left subclavian artery origin. Aneurysms of the innominate or left subclavian arteries in association with aortic aneurysms occur with Marfan syndrome, congenital lesions, previous congenital heart operations, or trauma and are discussed elsewhere.

Patients with atherosclerotic stenoses or occlusion of the origin of the arch arteries often have no symptoms because of the extensive network of potential collateral arteries. Typically, when multiple arteries are involved, symptoms may include dizziness, loss of consciousness, visual disturbances due to posterior cerebral circulation disturbances, weakness, a heavy feeling in the limbs, limb tiredness, and, very occasionally, claudication of the upper extremities with exertion. Rarely, patients have symptoms of stroke, transient ischemic attacks, amaurosis fugax, cerebellar dysfunction, and gangrene of the extremities related to embolization, presumably of platelet aggregates. Signs may include absent pulses, limb weakness, secondary Raynaud's phenomena, and, rarely, digital gangrene. There may be a discrepancy between brachial artery pressures from the upper limbs. Auscultation over the arteries may reveal a bruit that must be differentiated from a murmur arising from a stenotic aortic valve. Classically, left subclavian artery stenosis is accompanied by a subclavian artery steal syndrome (Fig. 9-3). This is due to left arm exercise resulting in reversal of flow down the left vertebral artery to the left subclavian artery, stealing blood from the posterior circle of Willis

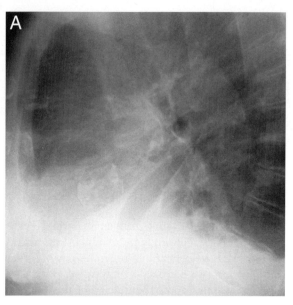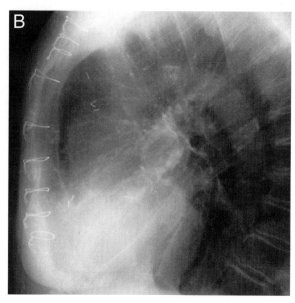

FIGURE 9–1   **A** and **B,** Preoperative and postoperative lateral chest radiographs illustrate the porcelain aorta before and after endarterectomy of the ascending aorta, aortic root, and left main coronary artery ostium. Note the leaflet of the St. Jude's mechanical valve prostheis.

and cerebellar arteries. These patient therefore have cerebellar signs, dizziness, and loss of consciousness. In the rare patient who has had an internal mammary artery bypass to a coronary artery and subsequently presents with subclavian artery stenosis, heart-to-limb steal syndrome may result in angina due to reversal of flow in the mammary artery.

Noninvasive studies, such as duplex carotid and subclavian artery scans, may identify turbulent flow, reversal of flow, and occasionally a stenosis, although the origin of the arteries from the aortic arch is usually not visualized. Not infrequently, associated tandem lesions of the internal carot-

id arteries are found. Possible lesions are best identified by angiography together with aortic studies as indicated. Delayed films are required to identify a subclavian steal syndrome and to determine whether the internal carotid artery is patent in patients with carotid artery occlusions.

Most patients with occlusive disease of only the arch branches and no aortic disease can be treated conservatively. If symptoms are disabling or embolization is occurring, if multiple arteries are involved, or if there are tandem lesions of the internal carotid arteries, operative repair, usually by extraanatomic bypasses with or without an internal carotid

FIGURE 9–2   **A** and **B,** Chest radiographs in a second patient in whom a pericardial valve was inserted after the same procedure.

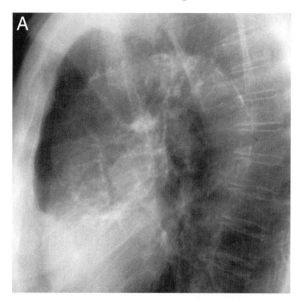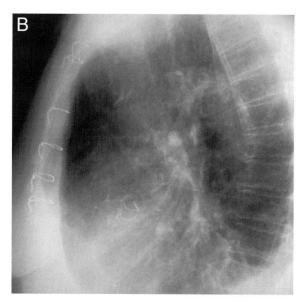

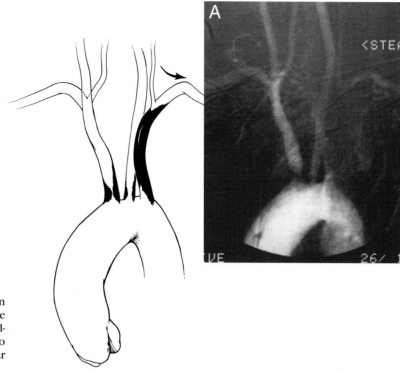

FIGURE 9–3 **A,** Female patient with left subclavian steal syndrome associated with stenosis of innominate artery origin. **B,** Postoperative angiogram after ascending aorta–to–innominate artery bypass and bypass to the left subclavian artery through a left supraclavicular incision.

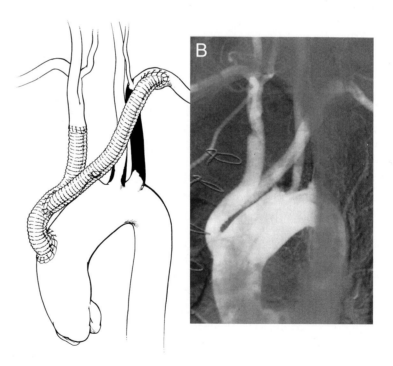

artery bypass, is performed because of the lower mortality and morbidity rates. The principles of repair include use of a disease-free donor artery, not leaving a blind pouch of occluded artery with stagnant blood flow because of the risk of thrombosis or generation of platelet thrombi, use of artery-to-artery anastomosis when feasible, and, when not feasible, the use of prosthetic material such as Dacron rather than vein grafts. Our preference has been to use Dacron.

Occasionally, because of associated aortic disease or the involvement of multiple arteries, a transthoracic procedure (usually a median sternotomy) is required. In younger patients transthoracic procedures should also be considered. Attachment of an end-to-side bifurcation graft to the ascending aorta with a side-biting clamp is a convenient way to perform end-to-end bypasses to two branch arteries, such as the right subclavian and right carotid arteries or the innominate and left carotid arteries. Although more difficult, even the origin of the left subclavian artery can be reached by a transthoracic approach. We prefer not to perform endarterectomy of the origin of the arch branches but have done so occasionally in association with aortic arch repairs.

In the reports by Crawford et al.,[2] Reul and colleagues,[3] Vogt and colleagues,[4] Cherry and colleagues,[5] and Brewster and colleagues,[6] transthoracic repairs with bypass grafts have had a low mortality and morbidity rate. Balloon dilatation of the origin of the brachiocephalic arteries is generally not indicated because of the associated risk of stroke and of recurrence of stenoses, particularly when compared with surgical series. Nevertheless, this approach is being explored in selected patients, including the use of stents, by our invasive cardiology colleagues.

In the 142 patients operated on by Crawford and colleagues[2] because of brachiocephalic artery disease, the survival rate was 98% with a 10-year survival rate of 58%; 8% of the patients died of strokes. In the series by Brewster and associates[6] the operative mortality rate in a series of 37 patients undergoing innominate artery repairs was 3.4%. Furthermore, the results with bypass procedures on late follow-up have been very good.[6, 7] In a study of 148 patients with innominate atherosclerosis who were operated on, Kieffer and colleagues[8] reported a 5.4% mortality rate and a 3.4% incidence of stroke. The 10-year survival rate was 51.9%, with a 98.6% freedom from ipsilateral stroke. A mediastinal approach was used in 91% of the patients, and 78% underwent bypasses rather than endarterectomies.

OCCLUSIVE DISEASE OF THE THORACOABDOMINAL AORTA

Patients who have blue toe syndrome as a result of microthromboembolic phenomena require careful examination to determine the site of origin (Fig. 9–4). If both feet are involved, then the likely site of origin is the aorta above the level of the aortic bifurcation. If the patient also has evidence of renal dysfunction with normal renal arteries, a more proximal site, such as the descending thoracic aorta, should be suspected. Atheroembolism to the other abdominal viscera may result in such symptoms as abdominal pain, diarrhea, loss of weight, and blood in the stools and may be confused with ischemic colitis, pancreatitis, peptic ulcer disease, and diverticulitis. Rarely, the ascending aorta or the aortic arch is the source of atheroembolic material, and then it is usually associated with amaurosis fugax, transient ischemic events, and strokes. Ophthalmic examination of the retina may reveal the presence of Hollenhorst plaques in the retinal arteries. The segment of aorta causing the atheroembolism should be replaced with a tube graft (Fig. 9–5) or, if only the abdominal aorta is involved, endarterectomy can be performed as an alternative method in selected patients. Figure 9–4 demonstrates the findings in a young male patient who had evidence of distal embolization asso-

ciated with descending aortic occlusive disease. The patient underwent successful descending aortic and thoracoabdominal aortic endarterectomy by one of us (L.G.S.).

Aortography will usually identify the site of origin of atheroembolic material, as shown by an irregular aortic lumen or penetrating ulcers.

PENETRATING ATHEROSCLEROTIC ULCERS OF THE DESCENDING AND THORACOABDOMINAL AORTA

Elderly hypertensive patients, particularly women, will sometimes have acute chest or back pain, left-sided effusion, and, on computed tomography (CT), magnetic resonance imaging (MRI), or TEE, a clot-filled limited "dissection" of the descending thoracic or thoracoabdominal aorta arising from an atherosclerotic penetrating ulcer (Fig. 9–6). In his classic review of aortic dissection in 1934, Shennan[9] first described the entity in six patients. Since the appearance is that of aortic dissection, these patients may be treated medically as described for De Bakey type III aortic dissections (see Chapter 4). These patients, however, have a more ominous prognosis than patients with classic aortic dissection. Whereas classic aortic dissection occurs typically in the medial plane of the aorta, in patients with penetrating ulcers who survive long enough to reach the hospital the adventitial layer is dissected from the media. The adventitia may also rupture, and then the hematoma is contained only by surrounding mediastinal tissues. The "dissection" in these patients typically arises from the penetrating ulcer and then tracks up and down the aorta, often limited by areas of severe calcification associated with the usually severe atherosclerotic disease. Whereas the tear causing classic type III dissection is at the base of the left subclavian artery, the site of entry into the "dissection" with penetrating ulcers is at the ulcer itself and may involve an extensive segment of the aorta. On postmortem examination, we have noted that there may be multiple atherosclerotic ulcers, often extending into the adventitia. The "false lumen," however, is small and may not be circumferential; there is no typical septum, and the lesion never exceeds the size of the true lumen, the latter being a common feature of classic aortic dissection. In a recent patient we operated on successfully, the penetrating ulcer was between the superior mesenteric artery and the right renal artery, with associated contained rupture, and the "dissection" extended from 3 cm distal to the left subclavian artery to the infrarenal aorta.

These patients are usually in shock and have associated advanced comorbid disease, and the mortality rate from surgery is high. Nevertheless, it should be borne in mind that the prognosis is worse than for classic aortic dissection. Examination of these patients before surgery is similar to that described for classic aortic dissection, and CT, MRI, or TEE can be used.[10-13]

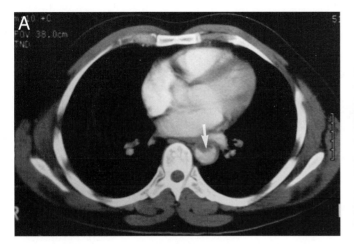

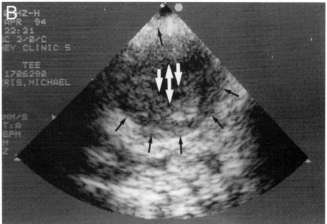

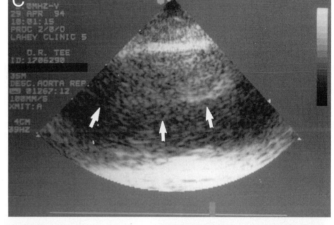

FIGURE 9–4 **A,** CT scan in a young male patient with "blue toe syndrome," repeated episodes of pancreatitis, abdominal ischemia, progessive renal failure with renal infarcts, and an intraluminal stenosis as indicated by the *white arrow.* **B,** Transverse view on TEE. The *black arrows* indicate the outer aortic wall, and the *white arrows* indicate the aortic lumen. **C,** TEE long-axis view, with the *white arrows* indicating the surface of the stenosis in the aortic lumen. **D,** Preoperative aortographic findings with *arrow* indicating site of stenosis. **E,** Postoperative angiogram after endarterectomy of the descending and thoracoabdominal aorta. Histologic study revealed that the stenosis was due to atherosclerotic material, and extensive test for hypercoagulability failed to reveal any evidence of a prothrombotic disease. On anticoagulation with warfarin, the patient has had no further problems.

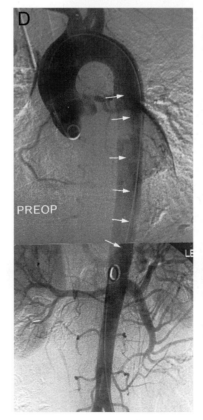

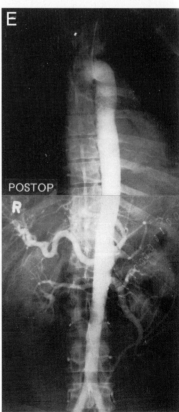

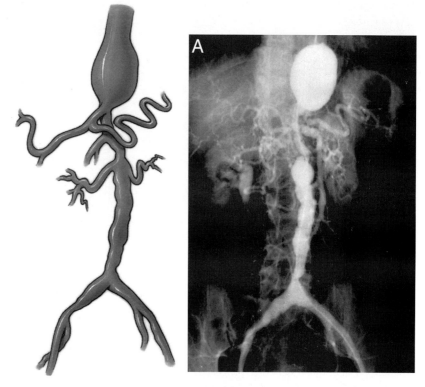

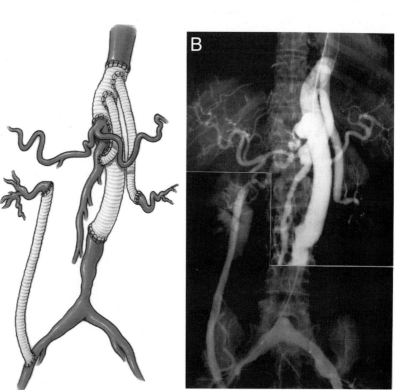

FIGURE 9–5   Aortogram of a patient with extensive occlusive disease of the abdominal aorta and a low aneurysm of the descending aorta. **B,** Postoperative arteriogram after thoracoabominal aorta repair with a tube graft and insertion of tube grafts to the left kidney, right kidney, and superior mesenteric artery.

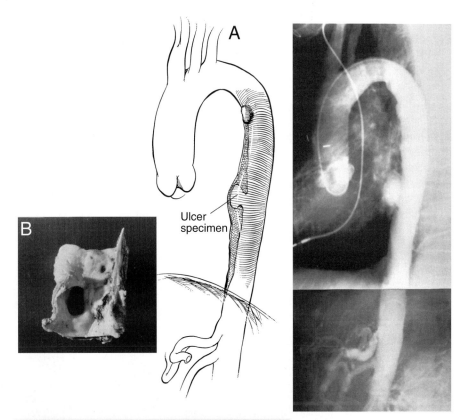

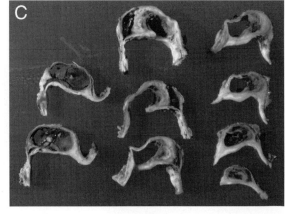

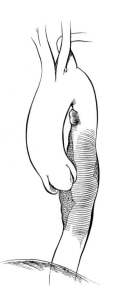

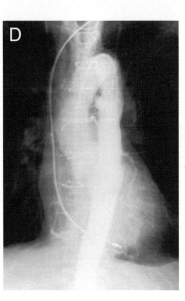

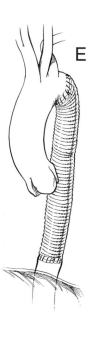

FIGURE 9–6   Patient with penetrating ulcer and the type of aortic dissection, typically with only a wall hematoma and without a septum, seen in older patients with this type of dissection. **A,** Diagram of the aorta and arteriogram. Note that the dissection is not seen on an arteriogram unless the wall is noted to be widened. The aortic wall, however, because of the extensive atherosclerosis, is typically irregular. **B,** Photograph of the excised specimen of the aorta containing the penetrating ulcer. **C,** Photographs of the transversely sliced ulcer and segments of the opened aorta with dissection extending up and down from the ulcer with extensive atherosclerosis. **D,** Preoperative anteroposterior arteriogram. **E,** Diagram of postoperative repair.

OCCLUSIVE DISEASE OF THE ABDOMINAL AORTA

In patients with occlusive disease of the infrarenal abdominal aorta the most common symptom is claudication, typically of the buttocks and upper thigh. When associated with impotence in men and decreased femoral pulses, the findings are referred to as the Leriche syndrome. Elevation pallor, dependent rubor, poor capillary circulation, skin pitting of digits, ulceration, gangrene, blue toe syndrome, loss of hair, and atrophic shiny skin may be other findings. The

claudication should not be confused with neurogenic claudication. Neurogenic claudication may be initiated by standing still, is relieved by sitting or lying down, and is associated with such findings as a positive straight leg-raising test. In contrast, vasuclar claudication is associated with the findings discussed above and is usually relieved by standing still.

Atherosclerosis of the distal aorta, either total occlusion of the aorta or significant stenosis resulting in distal ischemia, barring any contraindications, is treated with conventional aorto-bi-iliac or bifemoral bypass (Fig. 9–7). When tandem lesions of the aorta or iliac arteries are associated with occlusive disease in the femoropopliteal arterial segments, then

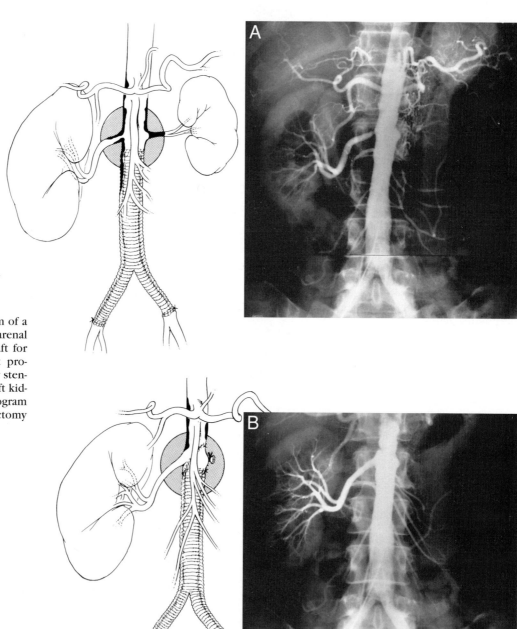

FIGURE 9–7 **A,** Aortogram of a patient who had an infrarenal repair with a bifurcated graft for atherosclerotic disease that progressed, causing renal artery stenoses and infarction of the left kidney. **B,** Postoperative aortogram after right renal endarterectomy and left renal nephrectomy.

the proximal disease of the aorta is treated first to ensure adequate outflow for later distal repairs. In many patients, a subsequent femoropopliteal or distal bypass is not necessary after the initial aortic operation, particularly if the patients stop smoking and start a regular exercise program.

An uncommon occurrence is acute occlusion of the abdominal aorta. This may be associated with atherosclerotic disease, but often it is also associated with a hypercoagulable state (for example, with systemic lupus erythematosis or polycythemia vera). Rarely the cause is aortic dissection, trauma, umbilical catheters (discussed elsewhere), or iatrogenic factors (for example, intraaortic balloon pumps). Suprarenal propagation of thrombus after axillofemoral bypass for infrarenal occlusive disease is also a rare cause. The natural history of infrarenal abdominal aortic occlusive disease, it should be recalled, is to progress proximally with time (Fig. 9–6). Babu and colleagues[14] reported on a series of 48 patients with limb ischemia, acute abdomen, paralysis, or hypertension. In 36 underlying atherosclerotic disease and cardiac disease or dehydration caused the thrombosis; however, in six patients the aorta was normal and thrombosis was caused by a hypercoagulable state. The hypercoagulable states were due to heparin-platelet antibodies in three patients, protein C deficiency in one, and anticardiolipin antibody in one, and in one patient the cause was not identified. The operative mortality rate in 45 patients operated on was 52%, and 29 patients required multiple procedures. Occlusive disease and stenoses of the aorta or its branches are also best identified with aortography; from the information gained, the operative procedure can be planned (see chapter on Aortography). In addition, Brewster and colleagues[15] have documented that, with appropriate biplane angiographic examination of the abdomen, renal artery occlusive disease is present in 19% of patients. More recently MRI has been advocated as a routine procedure in these types of patients because of its value in imaging the aorta and because of the ability to detect stenoses in aortic branches.

Aortography, particularly in patients with symptoms of abdominal occlusive disease such as abdominal angina (postprandial dull epigastric ache lasting about an hour and proportional to the size of the meal), weight loss, chronic diarrhea, and abdominal bruits, may reveal occlusive lesions or complete obstruction of the visceral arteries to the gastrointestinal tract. If these lesions should progress, disastrous complications such as gangrene of the intestines or renal failure may occur. Stenoses of the visceral arteries are seldom detected before they become symptomatic, except as an incidental finding during aortography. Clearly, for those patients who have symptoms and who can undergo an operation, operative repair of the occlusive segment is usually warranted.[16] In patients with distal aortic stenoses, typically above the aortic bifurcation,[17] insertion of an aortobifemoral graft is the operation of choice. As has been emphasized by Rutherford,[18] aortobifermoral bypass is the gold standard by which other treatments, such as endarterectomy, balloon angioplasty, stents, and axillobifemoral bypass, must be compared. An operative mortality rate of 2% to 4% and a 10-year patentcy rate of 75% should be expected. The methods of operative repair are described in later chapters.

REFERENCES

1. Svensson LG, Sun J, Cruz H, Shahian DM. Endarectomy for aortic valve stenosis and calcified porcelain aorta. Ann Thorac Surg 1996; 61:149–52.
2. Crawford ES, Stowe CL, Powers RWJ. Occlusion of the innominate, common carotid, and subclavian arteries: long-term results of surgical treatment. Surgery 1983;94:781–91.
3. Reul GJ, Jacobs MJHM, Gregoric ID, et al. Innominate artery occlusive disease: surgical approach and long-term results. J Vasc Surg 1991;14:405–12.
4. Vogt DP, Hertzer NR, O'Hara PJ, Beven EG. Brachiocephalic arterial reconstruction. Ann Surg 1982;196:541–52.
5. Cherry KJ, McCullough JL, Hallett JWJ, et al. Technical principles of direct innominate artery revascularization: a comparison of endarterectomy and bypass grafts. J Vasc Surg 1989;9:718–24.
6. Brewster DC, Moncure AC, Darling RC, et al. Innominate artery lesions: problems encountered and lessons learned. J Vasc Surg 1985;2:99–112.
7. Crawford ES, DeBakey ME, Cooley DA, ct al. Surgical treatment of occlusions of the innominate, common carotid and subclavian arteries: a ten year experience. Surgery 1969;65:17.
8. Kieffer E, Sabatier J, Koskas F, Bahnini A. Atherosclerotic innominate artery occlusive disease: early and long-term results of surgical reconstruction. J Vasc Surg 1995;21:326–37.
9. Shennan T. Dissecting Aneurysms. Medical Research Clinical Special Report Series No. 193. London: His Majesty's Stationery Office, 1934.
10. Stanson AW, Kazmier FJ, Hollier LH, et al. Penetrating atherosclerotic ulcers of the thoracic aorta: natural history and clinicopathologic correlations. Ann Vasc Surg 1986;1:15–23.
11. Kazeroomi EA, Bree R, Williams DM. Penetrating atherosclerotic ulcers of the descending thoracic aorta: evaluation with CT and distinction from aortic dissection. Radiology 1992;183:759–65.
12. Mohr-Kahaly S, Erbel R, Kearney P, et al. Aortic intramural hemorrhage visualized by transesophageal echocardiography: findings and prognostic implications. J Am Coll Cardiol 1994;23:658–64.
13. Movsowitz HD, Lampert C, Jacobs LE, Kotler MN. Penetrating atherosclerotic aortic ulcers. Am Heart J 1994;126:1210–17.
14. Babu SC, Shah PM, Nitahara J. Acute aortic occlusion—factors that influence outcome. J Vasc Surg 1995;21:567–75.
15. Brewster DC, Retana A, Waltman AC, Darling RC. Angiography in the management of aneurysms of the abdominal aorta: its value and safety. N Engl J Med 1975;292:822.
16. Svensson LG, Crawford ES, Hess KR, et al. Thoracoabdominal aortic aneurysms associated with celiac, superior mesenteric and renal artery occlusive disease: methods and analysis of results in 271 patients. J Vasc Surg 1992;16:378–90.
17. DeBakey ME, Creech OJ, Cooley DA. Occlusive disease of the aorta and its treatment by resection and homograft replacement. Ann Surg 1954;140:290–310.
18. Rutherford RB. Aortobifemoral bypass, the gold standard: technical considerations. Semin Vasc Surg 1994;7:11–6.

10

Traumatic Injuries of the Aorta

Most traumatic injuries of the aorta are due to penetrating trauma associated with either missiles or stabbing injuries or caused by blunt trauma. The resulting lesions in the aorta may include simple contusions, intramural hematomas, intimal tears, false aneurysms, rupture, or holes from which exsanguination can occur. Any potential injuries of the aorta should be investigated and treated; failure to do so can result in a fatal injury that might have been successfully treated with surgery.

PENETRATING INJURIES

Successful repair of a penetrating injury of the ascending thoracic aorta was reported by Dshanelidze of Russia in 1923.[1] Most penetrating injuries are due to either gunshot wounds or stab wounds with a knife. These require immediate operative repair, and the insertion of a graft is rarely necessary. Occasionally, as we have experienced with the abdominal aorta, the aorta has to be mobilized, circumferentially debrided, and then repaired with an end-to-end anastomosis or by insertion of a tube graft. For the repair of suprarenal abdominal aortic injuries, a retroperitoneal approach similar to that used for thoracoabdominal aneurysms can be used.[2] Patients who have been shot with high-velocity projectiles seldom survive long enough to undergo emergency operations, but even when they do, injuries are extensive because of the shock waves caused by the projectile. Of particular importance with penetrating injuries is the identification of injury to other structures, such as the airways, esophagus, veins, and adjacent organs. Operative results for penetrating injuries are dependent on the mechanism of injury, the time elapsed before treatment, blood loss, period of shock, and associated organ injuries.[2-3] In a review of 129 abdominal aortic penetrating injuries, Lopez-Viego's group[5] found that 50% involved the infrarenal aorta, that mortality was greater with free hemorrhage as opposed to contained retroperitoneal injuries, and that the overall mortality rate was 62%. Injuries involving the aortic arch and the greater vessels can be successfully treated with judicious use of hypotension and bypass shunts without the use of cardiopulmonary bypass, if needed.[6]

TRAUMATIC RUPTURE OF THE AORTA

In 1557 Vesalius noted the first patient with traumatic rupture of the aorta (TRA) after a fall from a horse.[7] In 1959, Passaro and Pace[8] reported the repair of a traumatic rupture of the aorta. With the advent of high-speed travel, the incidence of traumatic rupture of the aorta has increased. In some autopsy series, about one fifth of deaths resulting from motor vehicle accidents are associated with a TRA.[9] Parmley and associates[10] performed a classical study of 275 autopsies on patients with acute TRA and noted the high mortality rate if TRA is not diagnosed and treated immediately. Only 14% of the patients had reached a hospital alive; of those, only 20% lived longer than 1 hour and 30% died within 6 hours. Twenty-eight percent of the patients who lived longer than one hour went on to live longer than 8 days, and only 2% of patients with TRA survived longer than 4 months. The site of rupture, determined during autopsy, was the aortic isthmus in 45%; the ascending aorta in 23%; the descending thoracic aorta in 13%; the transverse aortic arch in 8%; the abdominal aorta in 5%, and multiple sites in 6%. The study by Parmley and coworkers has been criticized by several authors, most recently by Pate,[11] as probably representing an extreme situation, since the study included a wide variety of causes of injury; furthermore, although the mortality rate was high, many patients might have died of causes other than exsanguination from traumatic injuries of the aorta. Thus, the risk of rupture may not be quite as high, although clearly such patients require immediate treatment.

When the abdominal aorta is involved, this injury is often associated with lap seat belts.[12] In up to 10% of patients the tears have been reported to be at multiple sites.[13, 14] Cardiac valve tears, particularly of the aortic valve, may also occur.[15] Lundevall[13] has suggested that the reason for rupture occurring in the aorta, particularly at the aortic isthmus during rapid deceleration injuries, is that the aortic arch and diaphragm are fixed points in the thorax and during rapid deceleration these are the two sites that anchor the heart and descending thorax aorta during impact. Other possible mechanisms include upward displacement of the heart during deceleration, unfolding of the aortic arch and descending aorta, pinching of the aorta between the rib cage and the vertebral column, and tearing at the weakest part of the aorta where the ductus arteriosus arose.

In any patient who has sustained a deceleration or acceleration injury or has had blunt chest trauma, a traumatic rupture of the thoracic aorta should be suspected. Clinical signs suggestive of severe chest trauma should be carefully examined for. The triad of signs associated with acute coarctation, which includes upper limb hypertension, radio-femoral pulse delay with amplitude discrepancy, and a harsh systolic precordial or interscapular murmur is sometimes observed.[16] Occasionally, peripheral pulses may be lost, particularly if aortic dissection occurs. DeBakey and associates[17] and Katz and colleagues[18] have noted that this type of aortic dissection may progress retrograde into the ascending aorta.

Methods of Detection

Patients with suspected TRA need rapid triage. If the blood pressure is elevated, which may be the case if no other associated injuries are present, then control with intravenous beta-blockers and nitroprusside is required. A suspicious chest radiograph is usually the first indication that TRA may be present. The patient should then be immediately taken to the radiology suite for aortography with multiple views of the aortic arch[19] (Fig. 10-1). The gold standard for both the detection and exclusion of TRA is aortography of the aorta, particularly with multiple views of the area of the isthmus. This is best imaged with a left anterior oblique view, which shows the lesser curve of the distal aortic arch in profile. Thus, patients with a widened mediastinum on radiography require immediate aortography. Although computed tomography (CT) scans have been used as a screening procedure (Fig. 10-1), the consensus is that the technique is neither sensitive nor specific enough to detect TRA. However, the newer technique of spiral enhanced CT, which produces a three-dimensional image, may be more useful. The role of transesophageal echocardiography (TEE) for the diagnosis of TRA is being evaluated at some centers, and early reports are encouraging. Le Bret and colleagues[20] found that when TRA was performed in 22 patients with thoracic trauma, the sensitivity was 100% for detection of mediastinal hematoma but specificity was only 75% for assuring the presence of hematoma. They found a distance of more than 3 mm between the probe and the aortic wall, a double contour of the aortic wall, and visualization of the ultrasound signal between the aortic wall and the visceral pleura to be signs of mediastinal hematoma. In a study by Smith and colleagues,[21] 101 patients were scheduled to have TEE for the detection of TRA, and 88 underwent the procedure. TRA was found in 11 patients (12%), with a 100% sensitivity and a specificity of 98%. With TEE, however, there is a risk of free aortic rupture occurring, as has been reported in patients with aortic dissection, because of the TEE probe causing gagging and a rapid increase in intrathoracic pressure.[22] We have also seen rupture occur during the induction of anesthesia. It is possible that the risk of rupture with TEE will be greater with TRA than with

aortic dissection. In the case of TRA, the lesion is a false aneurysm, often with only mediastinal soft tissue and parietal pleura preventing free rupture into the chest cavities, and the adventitia is frequently disrupted. With aortic dissection, on the other hand, the adventitia is intact unless rupture has occurred (for example, into the pericardium or abdominal retroperitoneal tissue). The use of intravascular ultrasonography for the detection of TRA has also been reported.[23] In the final analysis, however, it is advisable that aortography be performed in all patients in whom TRA is suspected after blunt chest trauma.[19]

Besides the history of blunt chest trauma or rapid acceleration or deceleration injury, the chest radiograph obtained in the emergency room is critical to the initial management of the patient (Fig. 10-1). Preferably, the radiograph should be taken with a nasogastric tube in position, as this usually provides a fairly accurate diagnostic technique. This method has a better than 80% sensitivity for identifying TRA at the aortic isthmus. Even higher sensitivity rates have been reported.[24] The findings are similar to those observed for acute aortic dissection. A widened or abnormal mediastinum is detected in approximately 93% of radiographs obtained in the emergency room.[25] The signs associated with TRA include an enlarged or abnormal aortic contour, particularly if the thickness of the aortic wall is more than 0.7 mm; downward displacement of the left bronchus; displacement of the trachea to the right; an increase in the tracheo–left bronchus angle; narrowing of the left bronchus; a fluid cap above the lung, especially if it appears to track down to the aortic knuckle with blurring of the aortic outline and obliteration of the medial aspect of the left upper lung field; opacification of the aortopulmonary window; left pleural effusion; hemopneumothorax; fractured sternum, clavicle, and ribs, particularly the first or second ribs; unstable sternum or flail chest wall segment; widened mediastinum (> 8 cm); loss or displacement of the left paraspinal pleural border; and displacement of the nasogastric tube to the right.[19, 26]

In conclusion, as stated earlier, the most useful method for the detection of TRA is aortography of the aorta, particularly with multiple views of the area of the isthmus. Although this approach may result in a high number of negative aortograms, up to 80% in one series,[27] the consequences of missing a TRA are usually disastrous and will often result in the death of the patient. The medicolegal consequences are also serious. Apart from identifying the tear in the aortic wall on aortography, we recommend thorough inspection for any surrounding adventitial hematoma.[26] If patients are hemodynamically unstable, with evidence of shock, a negative peritoneal lavage, and evidence of TRA and left bloody pleural effusion (which can be confirmed by pleurocentesis), then an emergency left thoracotomy may be necessary before an aortogram can be performed.

Management

As soon as the diagnosis of TRA has been made, the patient is immediately taken to surgery because of the risk

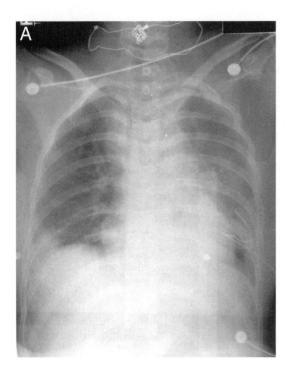

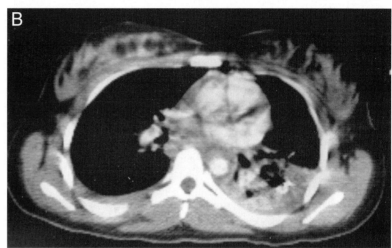

FIGURE 10–1 **A,** Chest radiograph after motor vehicle accident showing widened mediastinum, chest tube insertion for hemothorax, displaced trachea, and right effusion. **B,** CT scan showing subcutaneous air, mediastinal hematoma, hematoma around the descending aorta, and left pleural effusion and lung trauma.

Illustration continued on following page

of free rupture and exsanguination. A left thoracotomy is performed through the fourth intercostal space to obtain exposure. If additional exposure is needed, the posterior part of the rib either above or below the incision can be divided. The aorta proximal to the hematoma is carefully mobilized between the left carotid and left subclavian arteries. This is done by dividing the pleura and soft tissues both above and below the aorta and then gently using one's fingers to encircle the aorta. At the superior aspect of the gap between the aorta and the trachea there is often a band of tough tissue that has to be divided. The distal aorta is then encircled beyond the hematoma. Some surgeons also recommend opening the pericardium and mobilizing the ascending aorta so that, if required, it can be cannulated. We do not usually cannulate the ascending aorta in these patients but prefer to use the left atrial auricle for cannulation when atriofemoral bypass is used as discussed below. After the aorta is clamped both proximal and distal to the hematoma, the hematoma is entered and the aortic tear is identified either on the lesser curve of the aortic arch or as a circumferential tear at this level. Sometimes the tear may spiral, or multiple tears may be noted. If no tear is detected, then the anterolateral aorta on the lesser curve of the aorta beyond the subclavian artery is opened, and the tear is identified from inside the aorta. Once the tear has been identified, a decision is made as to whether it can be repaired either by primarily suturing the aorta with a running Prolene suture or by placing a patch or an interposition tubular graft.[19] If the tear is fresh and clean-cut and not circumferential, then a primary repair should be attempted because the aortic clamp time will usually be shorter and hemostasis is easier to obtain. Schmidt and colleagues[28] have advocated

primary repair as the preferred approach. In a recent patient of ours, a complex tear involved one third of the circumference of the aorta and was shaped like an H along the circumference of the aorta; yet it was successfully repaired by the primary technique, with a clamp time of 29 minutes (Fig. 10–2).[26] When a primary repair is performed, it is important to place the sutures deep so that the outer adventitial layers of the aorta are included in the primary repair. When prosthetic material is used to repair the aortic tear, most surgeons prefer to insert a tube graft rather than using a patch. A useful technique for rapid insertion of a tube graft involves cutting the tube graft along its length so that it becomes an open patch (Fig. 10–3).[29] The proximal and distal anastomoses are then performed, after which the cut along the tube graft is easily repaired by sewing a continuous suture along the cut edge, reestablishing a tube graft.[26]

The role of distal aortic perfusion for the prevention of paraplegia and renal failure during repair of TRA is controversial[19, 29-36] and is discussed further in subsequent sections. Of relevance to TRA repairs is our previous report[19] reviewing the world English-language literature on 596 TRA repairs. This meta-analysis showed that the mortality rate was highest with cardiopulmonary bypass (16.7%), slightly lower with shunts (11.4%), but still lower with simple aortic cross-clamping alone (5.8%, $p < 0.01$). There was no statistical difference in the rate of paraplegia or paraparesis according to the method used (2.2%, 2.3%, and 5.8%, respectively). This was also confirmed in a similar meta-analysis performed by Mattox and colleagues.[37] More recently von Oppel[38] reviewed the English-language literature published between 1972 and 1992 and found that in 1742 patients the mortality rate for cardiopulmonary pump

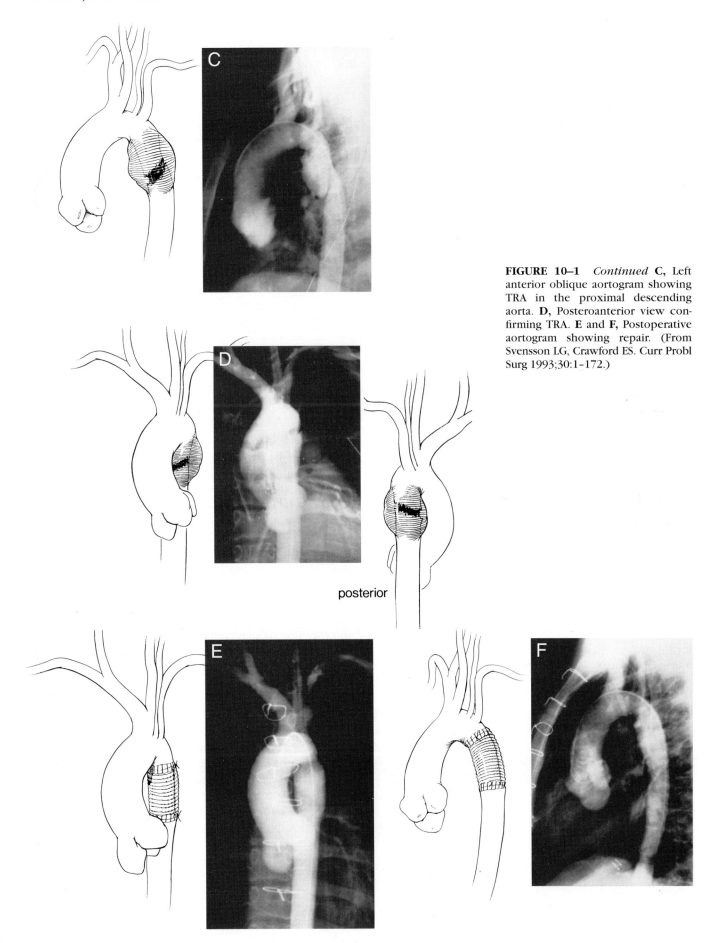

posterior

FIGURE 10–1 *Continued* **C,** Left anterior oblique aortogram showing TRA in the proximal descending aorta. **D,** Posteroanterior view confirming TRA. **E** and **F,** Postoperative aortogram showing repair. (From Svensson LG, Crawford ES. Curr Probl Surg 1993;30:1–172.)

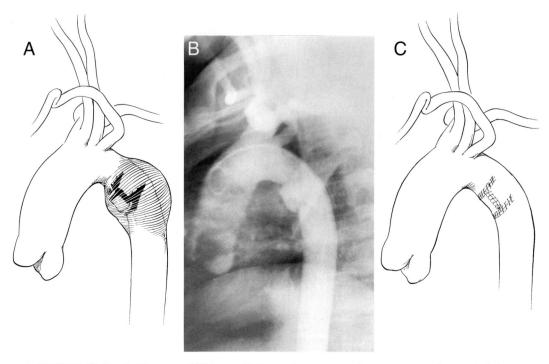

FIGURE 10–2 **A,** Diagram of TRA tear. **B,** Second aortogram showing tear at the aortic isthmus. The initial aortogram was nondiagnostic and therefore was repeated 3 days later. **C,** Diagram of primary repair.

perfusion of the distal aorta was 18.2%; the mortality rate was 11.9% for perfusion, without heparin, 12.3% for shunts, and 16% for aortic cross-clamping alone. The paraplegia rates were 2.4%, 1.7%, 11.1%, and 19.2%, respectively.

As first shown by Crafoord and Ekstom[39] in patients with aortic coarctation, the risk of a neurologic deficit increases with the aortic cross-clamp time in patients with TRA.[18] Hilgenberg and colleagues[40] have shown that the risk of neurological deficit occurring from increased aortic cross-clamp time may be even higher than previously documented. The curve showing the relationship between the aortic

FIGURE 10–3 Intraoperative photograph of a TRA repair after opening of the tube graft longitudinally for the anastomoses and then repair of the graft again as a means to reduce cross-clamp time.

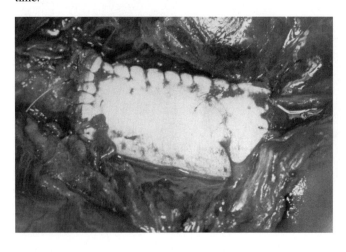

cross-clamp time and the risk of neurological injuries follows a sigmoid curve. Thus, for patients with TRA, there is a "window of safety" up to approximately 30 minutes.[41] Thereafter, the risk increases exponentially in the "window of vulnerability" and then plateaus to form a "window of virtual certainty" approximately 90 minutes after aortic clamping. Although superficial examination of this correlation may suggest that the faster the surgeon, the lower the risk of paraplegia, this is not entirely true. There are, for example, factors associated with the tear that may complicate the repair and thus prolong the clamp time. These factors may include more complicated tears, the need for interposition tubular grafts to be inserted, and the need for more intercostal arteries to be sacrificed. Our current practice is to use a centrifugal pump without heparin for TRA. This is based on our experience with 832 descending aortic repairs, including posttraumatic injuries, which showed that atriofemoral bypass with a centrifugal pump reduced the risk of renal failure and neurological injury if the clamp time exceeded approximately 40 minutes.[42] This has also been reported to be the method of choice by Walls and colleagues.[43] Pate and colleagues[44] recommend partial cardiopulmonary bypass with heparinization, and in 88 patients the survival rate was 90.9% without paraplegia.

Postoperative hypertension is a frequent occurrence after repairs for TRA and should be vigorously controlled; sometimes it is associated with diminished or absent distal pulses. The cause is not altogether clear but may be related to interference with aortic baroreceptors in the aortic arch in young patients with a vascular tree that is sensitive to neurohumoral vasoconstriction.[26]

If a complex tear is found at the time of angiography, an option is to first treat the patient conservatively with antihypertensives and then later to repair the aorta with deep hypothermia and circulatory arrest (Fig. 10–4).[19, 40] In our previous analysis, 44 patients were found to have been treated this way as reported in the English-language literature.[19] Thirty-six patients were subsequently operated on, and all the patients survived. In addition, low morbidity and mortality rates with medical therapy have also been reported in a large series of patients who were unsuitable candidates for surgery.[45]

Like descending aortic aneurysms, chronic traumatic aneurysms are managed by operative repair. Often on late follow-up the aneurysms are observed to have calcified (Fig. 10–5). Untreated, one third of all patients with chronic thoracic aneurysms die of the aortic lesion and 41% will have symptoms or an event related to the aneurysm within 5 years.[46] This high complication rate, the good survival rate (98% in our most recent experience[42]), and the low complication rate for descending thoracic aortic aneurysm operations (including operations for traumatic lesions), are

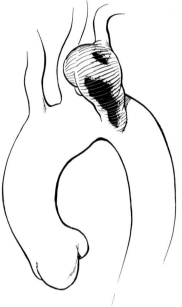

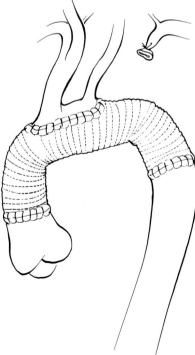

FIGURE 10–4 **A,** Complex TRA tear involving the origin of the left subclavian artery. **B,** Postoperative aortogram after repair involving deep hypothermia with circulatory arrest through a mediastinal incision (From Svensson LG, Crawford ES. Curr Probl Surg 1993;30:1–172.)

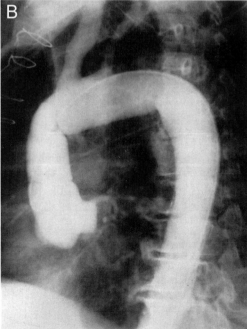

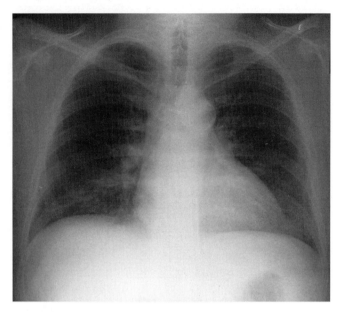

FIGURE 10–5 Chest radiograph of a patient who underwent urgent coronary artery bypass surgery; the patient had a past history of severe chest trauma and a calcified TRA, seen at the aortic knuckle on the radiograph

further reason to repair chronic aneurysms in most patients when detected.[42]

Ascending aortic tears, including aortic valve involvement, are repaired with cardiopulmonary bypass. When the aortic arch is involved, other associated injuries and the risk of deep hypothermia with circulatory arrest in the acute situation must be assessed. An option, as previously described in patients with head injuries, is to first treat them medically and later to repair the aortic arch.[47]

REFERENCES

1. Clarke CP, Brandt PWT, Cole DS, Barrat-Boyes BG. Traumatic rupture of the thoracic aorta: diagnosis and treatment. Br J Surg 1967; 54:353-8.
2. Mattox KL, McCollum WB, Beall AC, et al. Management of penetrating injuries of the suprarenal aorta. J Trauma 1975;15:808-12.
3. Billy LJ, Amato JJ, Rich NM. Aortic injuries in Vietnam. Surgery 1971;70:385-91.
4. Mattox KL, Shisennand HH, Espada R, et al. Management of acute combined injuries of the aorta and inferior vena cava. Am J Surg 1975;130:720-824.
5. Lopez-Viego MA, Snyder WH, Valentine RJ, Clagett GP. Penetrating abdominal aortic trauma: a report of 129 cases. J Vasc Surg 1992;16: 332-6.
6. Pate JW, Cole FH, Walker WA, Fabian TC. Penetrating injuries of the aortic arch and its branches. Ann Thorac Surg 1993;55:586-92.
7. Keen G. Closed injuries of the thoracic aorta. Ann R Coll Surg Engl 1972;51:137-56.
8. Passaro E, Pace WG. Traumatic rupture of the aorta. Surgery 1959;46:787-91.
9. Kirsh MM, Behrendt DM, Orringer MB, Gago O. The treatment of acute traumatic rupture of the aorta. Ann Surg 1976;184:308-16.
10. Parmley LF, Mattingly TW, Manion WC, Jahnke EJ Jr. Nonpenetrating traumatic injury of the aorta. Circulation 1958;17:1086-101.
11. Pate JW. Is traumatic rupture of the aorta misunderstood? Ann Thorac Surg 1994;57:530-1.
12. Randhawa MP Jr, Menzoian JO. Seat belt aorta. Ann Vasc Surg 1990;4:370-7.
13. Lundevall J. Mechanism of traumatic rupture of the aorta. Acta Pathol Microbiol Scand 1964;62:34-6.
14. Greendykle RM. Traumatic rupture of the aorta: special reference to automobile accidents. JAMA 1966;1966:527-30.
15. Nawa S, Kurozumi K, Teramoto S. Traumatic combined valve lesions with aneurysm of the sinus of Valsalva causing late onset of heart failure. Br Heart J 1987;57:377-9.
16. Symbas PN, Tyras DH, Ware RE, Dioro DA. Traumatic rupture of the aorta. Ann Surg 1973;178:6-12.
17. DeBakey ME, Kirsh MM, Behrendt DM, et al. The treatment of acute traumatic rupture of the aorta. Ann Surg 1976;184:308-16.
18. Katz NM, Blackstone EH, Kirklin JW, Karp RB. Incremental risk factors for spinal cord injury following operation for acute traumatic aortic transection. J Thorac Cardiovasc Surg 1981;81:669-74.
19. Svensson LG, Antunes MDJ, Kinsley RH. Traumatic rupture of the thoracic aorta: a report of 14 cases and a review of the literature. S Afr J Med 1985;67:853-7.
20. Le Bret FL, Ruel P, Rosier H, et al. Diagnosis of traumatic mediastinal hematoma with transesophageal echocardiography. Chest 1994; 105:373-76.
21. Smith MD, Cassidy JM, Souther S, et al. Transesophageal echocardiography in the diagnosis of traumatic rupture of the aorta. N Engl J Med 1995;332:356-62.
22. Silvey SV, Stoughton TL, Pearl W, et al. Rupture of the outer partition of aortic dissection during transesophageal echocardiography. Am J Cardiol 1991;68:286-7.
23. Read RA, Moore EE, Moore FA, et al. Intravascular ultrasonography for the diagnosis of traumatic aortic disruption: a case report. Surgery 1993;114:624-8.
24. Gundry SR, Burney RE, Mackenzie JR, et al. Clinical contact with the trauma patient enhances accuracy of chest roentgenogram interpretation in predicting traumatic rupture of the aorta. J Cardiovasc Surg (Torino) 1985;26:332-6.
25. Woodring JH. The normal mediastinum in blunt traumatic rupture of the thoracic aorta and brachiocephalic arteries. J Emerg Med 1990;8:467-76.
26. Svensson LG, Crawford ES. Aortic dissection and aortic aneurysm surgery: clinical observations, experimental investigations, and statistical analyses. Part III. Curr Probl Surg 1993;30:1-172.
27. Sturm JT, Hankins DG, Young G. Thoracic aortography following blunt chest trauma. Am J Emerg Med 1990;8:92-6.
28. Schmidt CA, Wood MN, Razzouk AJ, et al. Primary repair of traumatic aortic rupture: a preferred approach. J Trauma 1992;32: 588-92.
29. Antunes MJ. Acute traumatic rupture of the aorta: repair by simple aortic cross-clamping. Ann Thorac Surg 1987;44:257-9.
30. Pate JW. Traumatic rupture of the aorta: emergency operation. Ann Thorac Surg 1985;39:531-7.
31. Becker HM, Ramirez J, Echave V, Heberer G. Traumatic aneurysms of the descending thoracic aorta. Ann Vasc Surg 1986;1:196-200.
32. Marvasti MA, Meyer JA, Ford BE, Parker FB Jr. Spinal cord ischemia following operation for traumatic aortic transection. Ann Thorac Surg 1986;42:425-8.
33. Verdant A, Page A, Cossette R, et al. Surgery of the descending thoracic aorta: spinal cord protection with the Gott shunt. Ann Thorac Surg 1988;46:147-54.
34. Cowley RA, Turney SZ, Hankins JR, et al. Rupture of thoracic aorta caused by blunt trauma: a fifteen-year experience. J Thorac Cardiovasc Surg 1990;100:652-60.
35. DelRossi AJ, Cernaianu AC, Cilley J Jr, et al. Multiple traumatic disruptions of the thoracic aorta. Chest 1990;97:1307-9.
36. Zeiger MA, Clark DE, Morton JR. Reappraisal of surgical treatment of traumatic transection of the thoracic aorta. J Cardiovasc Surg (Torino) 1990;31:607-10.
37. Mattox KL, Holzman M, Pickard LR, et al. Clamp/repair: a safe technique for treatment of blunt injury to the descending thoracic aorta. Ann Thorac Surg 1985;40:456-*.
38. von Oppel UO. Traumatic aortic rupture: twenty-year metaanalysis of mortality and risk of paraplegia. Ann Thorac Surg 1994;58: 585-93.
39. Crafoord CI, Ekstom G. The surgical treatment of patent ductus arteriosus: a clinical study of 290 cases. Acta Chir Scand 1952;169 (supp):1-197.
40. Hilgenberg AD, Logan DL, Akins CW, et al. Blunt injuries of the thoracic aorta. Ann Thorac Surg 1992;53:233-8.

41. Svensson LG, Loop FD. Prevention of spinal cord ischemia in aortic surgery. In Bergan JJ, Yao JST, eds. Arterial Surgery: New Diagnostic and Operative Techniques. New York: Grune & Stratton. 1988:273-85.

42. Svensson LG, Crawford ES, Hess KR, et al. Variables predictive of outcome in 832 patients undergoing repairs of the descending thoracic aorta. Chest 1993;104:1248-53.

43. Walls JT, Boley TM, Curtis JJ, Schmaltz RA. Experience with four surgical techniques to repair traumatic aortic pseudoaneurysm. J Thorac Cardiovasc Surg 1993;106:283-7.

44. Pate JW, Fabian TC, Walker WA. Acute traumatic rupture of the aortic isthmus: repair with cardiopulmonary bypass. Ann Thorac Surg 1995;59:90-9.

45. Walker WA, Pate JW. Medical management of acute traumatic rupture of the aorta. Ann Thorac Surg 1990;50:965-7.

46. Finkelmeier BA, Mentzer R Jr, Kaiser DL, et al. Chronic traumatic thoracic aneurysm. Influence of operative treatment on natural history: an analysis of reported cases, 1950-1980. J Thorac Cardiovasc Surg 1982;84:257-66.

47. Svensson LG, Antunes JDJ, Kinsley RH. Traumatic rupture of the thoracic aorta: a report of 14 cases and a review of the literature. S Afr Med J 1985;67:853-7.

11

Primary Aortic Tumors

Involvement of the aorta by tumor can occur in one of four ways: (1) primary aortic tumor, (2) secondary metastatic involvement, (3) direct extension to the aorta by adjacent tumors, and (4) embolic obstruction by necrotic material from a distant tumor.

Primary aortic tumors are rare. By January 1984, Crawford and Crawford[1] had been able to collect only 23 cases from the world literature. The types included fibrosarcoma in six patients, fibromyxosarcoma in three, fibromyxoma in two, fibroxanthosarcoma in one, myxosarcoma in two, leiomyosarcoma in two, spindle cell sarcoma in one, angiosarcoma in one, malignant histiocytoma in one, sarcoma in three, and myxoma in one. Subsequently, in an updated series, Fonseca and colleagues[2] were able to find reports on a total of 31 patients. Most of the tumors were of connective tissue origin, and only one of them was not malignant. Tumors either diffusely involved the aorta or were polypoidal in nature; they are also described as intimal (spreading as plaques), intraluminal (polypoidal), or adventitial (resulting in local invasion). The tumors were associated with aortic occlusion or with distal aortic embolization. There does not appear to be any particular segment of the aorta that is prone to tumor formation, and the incidence is evenly distributed along the length of the aorta.

In the series collected by Crawford and Crawford,[1] 61% of the patients were male and ages ranged between 16 weeks and 70 years, although 69% were older than 50 years of age. The most common symptom, present in 70%, was pain. The pain was caused by local tumor invasion, metastatic disease, ischemia resulting from occlusion of arterial branches, or pain from distal ischemia due to embolic occlusion of arteries. Other signs included evidence of end-organ ischemia, such as stroke and hypertension, systolic murmurs, changing peripheral pulse status, and claudication. Anorexia, fevers, general malaise, and weight loss are also features. Mesenteric infarction from tumor embolization is also not infrequent.[3]

Of interest, malignant fibrous histiocytomas have been reported in association with Dacron grafts. Griepp's group[4] reported the development of such a tumor involving the adventitia at the proximal anastomosis 4 years after repair of an aortic dissection. These authors were able to find six additional reports in the English-language literature of this association with Dacron grafts. In a collected series of 32 patients reported by Weiss and colleagues,[5] four patients had Dacron-associated tumors. Oppenheimer and colleagues[6] found in animal studies that the incidence of sarcomas developing was 7% to 50% in animals that had plastic polymer exposure and that 85% of the sarcomas were fibrosarcomas. Furthermore, plastics without pores were more carcinogenic. Clearly, the association with Dacron grafts is extremely rare in humans and is probably fortuitous.

In most patients an aortic tumor is not diagnosed until an autopsy is performed. Occasionally, a tumor is found on histologic examination of an embolus, although a cardiac origin has to be excluded. Other than primary tumors, the aorta can be involved by direct extension of adjacent tumors, metastatic tumors, and embolism from distant neoplastic tumors.

Treatment modalities for primary tumors of the aorta have included surgery,[1,7] radiation therapy, and chemotherapy.[1,8] Unfortunately, most patients succumb to the aortic tumor or die of metastatic disease, even if the primary tumor in the aorta is controlled by radiation or is successfully excised. Nevertheless, Busby and colleagues[9] reported resection of a malignant fibrous histiocytoma in the descending aorta with repair, treatment 8 months later with triple chemotherapy, and long-term follow-up for 6 years without recurrence. Chemotherapy agents that have been tried include doxorubicin, vincristine, methotrexate, DTIC, ifosfamide, and cyclophosphamide.[10]

REFERENCES

1. Crawford ES, Crawford JL. Diseases of the Aorta Including an Atlas of Angiographic Pathology and Surgical Technique. Baltimore: Williams & Wilkins. 1984.
2. Fonseca JL, Fernandez-Valderrama I, Gesto R, et al. Malignant fibrous histiocytoma of the aorta complicated by anuria. Ann Vasc Surg 1992;6:164-7.
3. Higgins R, Posner MC, Staley C, et al. Mesenteric infarction secondary to tumor emboli from primary aortic sarcoma: guidelines for diagnosis and management. Cancer 1991;68:1622-7.
4. Fyfe BS, Quintana CS, Kaneko M, Griepp RB. Aortic sarcoma four years after Dacron graft insertion. Ann Thorac Surg 1994;58: 1752-4.
5. Weiss WM, Riles TS, Gouge TH, Mizrachi HH. Angiosarcoma at the site of a Dacron vascular prosthesis: a case report and literature review. J Vasc Surg 1991;14:87-91.
6. Oppenheimer BS, Oppenheimer ET, Stout AP, et al. The latent period in carcinogensis by plastics in rats and its relation to the presarcomatous stage. Cancer 1958;11:204-12.

7. Kattus AA, Longmire WP, Cannon JA, et al. Primary intraluminal tumor of the aorta producing malignant hypertension: successful surgical removal. N Engl J Med 1960;262:694-700.

8. Hernandez FJ, Staley TM, Ranganoth RA, et al. Primary leiomyosarcoma of the aorta. Am J Pathol 1979;3:251-6.

9. Busby JR, Ochsner JL, Emory WB, et al. Malignant fibrous histiocytoma arising from descending thoracic aorta. Ann Vasc Surg 1990; 4:185-8.

10. Burke AP, Virmani R. Sarcomas of the great vessels: a clinicopathologic study. Cancer 1993;71:1761-73.

12

Ischemia, Reperfusion, and No-Reflow Phenomenon

With Jianping Sun, M.D., Ph.D.

Three potential sources of injury to cells during surgery are (1) ischemia, (2) reperfusion, and (3) microcirculation flow dysfunction with no-reflow phenomenon. Such damage is a frequent, complex consequence of surgery. Of particular interest to physicians dealing with aortic diseases is the deleterious effect of such processes on the brain and spinal cord, although other organs at risk for hypoxia following aortic clamping include the kidneys, intestines, and liver. It should be recalled that for any type of aortic surgery, transient ischemia occurs as a result of aortic cross-clamping or circulatory arrest. If the cross-clamp or circulatory arrest time is prolonged, the resulting ischemia leads to considerable morbidity and often to death.[1-3] Neuronal tissue is particularly sensitive to periods of ischemia, and irreversible injury may occur within only a few minutes of hypoxia, compared, for example, with skeletal muscle that can recover following several hours of ischemia. It appears that many neurons may survive a brief time of ischemia but will remain dysfunctional for many hours or even days. Thus the principal means of of reducing the duration and degree of ischemia include

- At the mechanical level such devices as bypass pumps, shunts, retrograde brain perfusion, and cerebrospinal fluid drainage
- Improved and more efficient surgical techniques, including the reattachment of the spinal cord blood supply
- Slowing of metabolic activity with hypothermia
- Use of pharmacological adjuncts at the time of surgery such as steroids, pentothal, newer agents, and lidocaine to prevent ischemia-reperfusion injury.

This chapter will review the cause of, and events associated with, ischemia with particular reference to those factors believed to play a role in the development of neurologic injury.

DEFINITIONS

Ischemia, the lack of adequate blood flow, is the pathological process whereby the blood supply fails to keep up with tissue oxygen and metabolic substrate demands. Ischemia may be acute, as in stroke and cardiac infarction, or chronic, as in claudication. The injury sustained depends on both the depth and duration of the hypoxia. It can affect any organ, tissue, or cell as a result of embolization, thrombosis, occlusion of the blood vessel, or simply lack of adequate blood flow for a variety of reasons. The principal issues that underly the pathogenesis of cell injury in ischemia are hypoxia from lack of oxygen and the loss of energy stores.

Reperfusion is the reestablishment of blood flow and, hence, of oxygenation to ischemic tissue. The obvious advantages of reperfusion are the restoration of the energy supply and the return to cellular homeostasis. There is, however, an apparently contradictory effect in that reperfusion adds to the damage already inflicted by the ischemia.[4, 5] The term *ischemia-reperfusion injury* is used to describe this phenomenon. This deleterious effect is attributed predominantly to oxygen-derived free radicals that arise transiently during the process of reperfusion.[1, 4, 5] The highly toxic oxygen free radicals possibly are produced because of incomplete oxygenation during the initial stage of blood flow restoration. Lipid peroxidation is the chief mechanism by which oxygen free radicals injure cells. Cell membranes, which are composed of polyunsaturated fatty acid and phospholipid, are decomposed by lipid peroxidation.

Siesjö et al.,[6-8] Demopoulos et al.,[9] and Kontos et al.[10] have done much research on the production of these radicals, their association with brain damage, and the edema resulting from ischemia. Kontos et al.[10] have shown that superoxide dismutase (SOD) and mannitol, both of which are superoxide radical scavengers, may protect the brain after ischemia and reduce reperfusion edema. Edema is caused by increased cell permeability after ischemic injury.[5] Since oxygen free radicals are implicated in reperfusion injuries to the brain, the biochemistry of radical production is summarized.

Essentially the **no-reflow phenomenon** occurs when there is a failure in the reperfusion attempt because of blockage at the microcirculatory level, and the degree of this blockage seems proportional to the length of ischemia. What causes this effect is not clear, although evidence suggests that changes in the brain microcirculation may be of major consequence in posthypoxic, postischemic damage. Nitric oxide also appears to play an important role in the regulation of the microcirculation and neural injury.

NEURAL INJURY

The severity and duration of ischemia determine the extent of nervous tissue injury. The ischemia can be complete with no blood flow or incomplete with some blood flow, usually from collaterals, to the neural tissue. Normal cerebral blood flow in humans is about 50 ml/100 g/min, and the threshold at or below which ischemia occurs is 18 ml/100 g/min. The CA1 pyramidal cells of the hippocampus and neocortex, neurons of the caudoputamen, thalamus, and subcortical nuclei involving cortical function and memory, somatostatin neurons, and mossy cells of the dentate hilus are the most sensitive to ischemia.[11-13] In the spinal cord the anterior horn cells are the most sensitive; injury to them produces motor deficits.[11-13]

Most research on brain injury from ischemia has been based on stroke and cardiac arrest models. Research on deep hypothermia with circulatory arrest is less extensive. Spinal cord injury at the biochemical and metabolic level is probably similar to that which occurs in the brain. In fact, a rabbit spinal cord ischemia model is used for brain ischemia studies. Increasingly, research is being conducted on spinal cord ischemia after aortic operations. Although paralysis is uncommon after infrarenal aortic operations (0.2% for elective and 2.5% for ruptured aneurysms[14]), the incidence after some types of thoracoabdominal aortic operations can exceed 40%. Following are the causes of neural injury during aortic surgery:

1. Ischemia due to inadequate oxygen and substrate delivery by blood or blood flow: This may occur because of embolization to the brain by atherothrombotic material, inadequate brain perfusion during cardiopulmonary bypass, and lack of adequate cerebral protection during deep hypothermia with prolonged circulatory arrest. Causes of spinal cord ischemia include no or minimal blood flow during aortic cross-clamping and embolization, thrombosis, occlusion, or oversewing of segmental intercostal or lumbar arteries.

2. Reperfusion injury of ischemic tissue with reestablishment of blood flow.

3. Failure to reestablish microcirculatory blood flow to the brain or spinal cord.

ISCHEMIA

Oxygen is a basic fuel crucial to intracellular aerobic oxidative respiration, which replenishes the high-energy adenosine 5'-triphosphate (ATP) required for normal cellular function and homeostasis, including protein synthesis, membrane integrity, ion transportation, lipogenesis, and deacylation-reacylation reactions necessary for phospholipid turnover. Hypoxia caused by ischemia forces the cell to maintain energy sources by generating ATP anaerobically from glycogen through glycolysis and, to a lesser extent, from creatine phosphate through the action of the enzyme creatine kinase. Thus aerobic glycolysis stops and anaerobic glycolysis continues, only producing 7% of the ATP that is produced per molecule of glucose by aerobic metabolism.[15] The accumulation of lactic acid and other inorganic phosphates from glycolysis reduces intracellular pH. Intracellular acidosis alters normal enzyme kinetics and damages lysosomal membranes. Lysosomes contain RNAases, DNAases, proteases, phosphatases, glucosidases, and cathepsins. Leakage of these enzymes from lysosomes leads to enzymatic digestion of cell components.

At normothermia, 3 to 4 minutes of complete ischemia results in depletion of ATP and phosphocreatine high-energy phosphate stores and failure of energy-dependent membrane ion pumps with loss of normal ion gradients.[16] In particular, ouabain-sensitive Na^+-K^+-ATPase is responsible for the exchange and gradient of K^+ and Na^+ across the membrane. Failure of this active transport, owing to diminished ATP concentration, causes accumulation of sodium intracellularly with diffusion of potassium out of the cell. Cell edema and cell death ensue because of increased concentrations of water, sodium, and chloride and a decreased concentration of potassium. Thus the crucial events are ATP depletion resulting in dissipation of ion gradients, loss of intracellular communication, and halting of the synthesis of molecules.[8]

Extracellular ions show two major phases: (1) the gradual rise of potassium to 10 to 15 mmol/L in the first 2 minutes of ischemia, and (2) an abrupt increase in the potassium concentration accompanied by a precipitous fall in calcium, sodium, and chloride.[8] The second phase corresponds to the intracellular depletion of ATP to a level where ATP-dependent pumps cannot maintain adequate transmembrane transport of ions.

It is believed that calcium ions are the mediators of cell injury during ischemia of the brain.[17-19] The influx of calcium ions into the cell and the failure of mitochondria to deal with the excess calcium trigger the activation of phospholipase A_2 and nucleases, conversion of xanthine dehydrogenase to oxidase, and the release of excitatory neurotransmitters.[16] This results in catabolism of ATP to hypoxanthine. Membrane phospholipids are degraded to fatty acids with the release of arachidonic acid, resulting in prostaglandin production. Double-stranded DNA is fractured or denatured, yielding single-stranded segments.

Lactic acid causes acidosis, resulting in cellular damage and permanent neurological damage.[20] The levels of lactic acid produced in anaerobic tissues after a period of ischemia depend on glucose and glycogen levels prior to ischemia.[21] Recovery from a period of ischemia depends on the level of lactic acid present in the ischemic tissue.[20-22] Why acidosis accentuates neural injury is unclear, but it may be because lipid peroxidation is enhanced, magnifying the reperfusion injury.[7]

Chemical Mediation of Cellular Injury during Ischemia

Several factors associated with cellular damage that may result in cell death are calcium, neuronal transmitters, free fatty-acids, prostaglandins, and DNA breakage.

Calcium

Brierly and Brown described the stages of brain cell damage. Mitochondria and synaptic vesicles are destroyed, resulting in destruction of cellular membranes followed by development of cell edema. Meldrum[19] later proposed that high intracellular concentrations of calcium ion may account for the cellular damage. During ischemia there is abnormal influx of calcium across the cellular membrane. The normal cell has an entry channel for calcium and an exit channel. During ischemia, the exit channel is disrupted and phosphate concentrations in the cytosol rise and draw calcium out of the mitochondria into the cytosol.[23]

Because calcium appears to be a factor in cell membrane destruction, theories have arisen as to how this occurs and include that

1. Calcium stimulates calcium ion–dependent, energy-consuming events such as uncontrolled transmitter release.[18]

2. Mitochondria have to scavenge excess calcium at the expense of ATP production with resultant inadequate energy for other processes.

3. Calcium-dependent phospholipases and proteinases are activated, resulting in degradation of membranes and intracellular proteins.[24]

Of interest, Happel et al.[25] found that there is massive calcium influx in the spinal cord after contusion and that levels may rise to four times normal. It should be noted, however, that more recently the theory that calcium is the mediator of injury has been questioned[8] because neuronal death can occur without increased intracellular calcium levels.[26] The failure of calcium channel blockers to prevent neuronal damage after cardiac arrest in a large clinical study[27] and in our[28] own experience in nonhuman primates where paralysis was not prevented would corroborate evidence that calcium is not the sole mediator of neuronal cell death.

Intracellular calcium is an important second messenger mediating cellular communication and regulation. It is critical in excitation-contraction coupling in muscle, secretion, neurotransmitter release, metabolism, membrane permeability, cell integrity, adhesion, excitability, growth and differentiation, gene expression, and the control of calcium-dependent enzymes.[29-32]

The concentration of intracellular calcium must be closely controlled by living cells if they are to achieve their physiological roles. There are several mechanisms to maintain intracellular calcium homeostasis, most of which require ATP for function, such as calcium-activated ATPase and sodium-calcium exchange and uptake into the endoplasmic reticulum.[33] Under physiological conditions the cell maintains a low intracellular concentration of free ionized calcium, approximately 10^{-8} mol/L, and this rises to between 10^{-7} to 10^{-6} mol/L during cell excitation. An important route for calcium entry into neurons under physiological and even more so under pathological conditions is assumed to be voltage-gated calcium channels.[34]

Of particular interest are the role of Ca^{2+} molecules in the control of neurotransmitter release.[35, 36] and the possible involvement of Ca^{2+} in the death of neurons associated with cerebral ischemia.[37] Ischemia triggers a number of cytotoxic reactions, some of which are believed to be due to gross disturbances of calcium homeostasis. It has in fact been suggested that uncontrolled, excessive intracellular calcium accumulation represents the final common pathway for ischemia-induced cell death.[38]

There are at least four major voltage-gated calcium channels, namely, L-, T-, N-, and P-, which have been identified according to their electrophysiological and pharmacological properties[39-44] (Table 12–1). L-type Ca^{2+} channels, the best known class, have large, long-lasting conductances and are widely distributed in all excitable and nonexcitable cells, including cardiac cells, vascular and nonvascular smooth muscle, skeletal muscle, and neuronal tissues. They are the major pathway for voltage-gated Ca^{2+} entry into the heart and smooth muscle, and they help control transmitter release from endocrine cells and some neuronal preparations.[45] The L-type channels play a key role in excitation-contraction coupling processes both in cardiac muscle and vascular smooth muscle. The functions of L-type channels in the nervous system are less well defined, but include roles in the release of neurotransmitter at some synapses,[46] gene expression in cortical neurons,[47] and certain aspects of long-term potentiation.[48] Another important characteristic of L-type channels is that they are sensitive to the clinically available Ca^{2+} channel antagonists (e.g., nifedipine, verapamil, and diltiazem) and can thus be distinguished from T-, N-, and P-type Ca^{2+} channels, which are generally dihydropyridine resistant. Also found in all types of excitable tissues (usually along with L-type channels), the T-type Ca^{2+} channel is a transient channel and likely responsible for pacemaker activities in cardiac and neuronal tissues. Octanol and amiloride selectively block the low-threshold T-type calcium channels.[49-50] N-type and P-type Ca^{2+} channels are common in that they are selectively localized in neuronal tissues and involved in neurotransmitter release.[51, 52] There are currently no synthetic drugs for these two channels with the potency and specificity of those available for the L-type channel.[53] However, the w-conotoxin from the fish-eating Conus genus of molluscs and the agatoxins from funnel-web spider toxin (FTX) are potent and specific peptide toxins that block N-type and P-type Ca^{2+} channels, respectively.[54-56] These toxins are of great significance to the understanding of the molecular heterogeneity of calcium channels, and they are potentially useful in drug design

TABLE 12–1   CLASSIFICATION OF VOLTAGE-GATED CALCIUM CHANNELS

Property	L	T	N	P
Conductance (pS)	25	8 12–20	10–12	
Activation threshold	High	Low	High	Moderate
Permeation	$Ba^{2+} > Ca^{2+}$	$Ba^{2+} = Ca^{2+}$	$Ba^{2+} > Ca^{2+}$	$Ba^{2+} > Ca^{2+}$
Location	Widely distributed	Widely distributed	Neuronal only	Neuronal only
Function	E-C coupling cardio-vascular system, smooth muscle, endocrine cells, and some neurons	Cardiac sinoatrial node spiking, repetitive spike activity in neurons and endocrine cells	Neurotransmitter release	Neurotransmitter release
Ligand sensitivity				
1,4-dihydropyridine	Sensitive	Insensitive	Insensitive	Insensitive
w-Conotoxin	Insensitive	Insensitive	Sensitive	Insensitive
Octanol, amiloride	Insensitive	Sensitive	Insensitive	Insensitive
Agatoxin (funnel-web spider)	Insensitive	Insensitive	Insensitive	Sensitive

Modified from Triggle DJ. Cleve Clin J Med 1991;1991:23–5.

and possible prevention of central nervous system (CNS) ischemia.

CNS ischemia may affect the homeostasis of intracellular free calcium in several ways. When the supply of oxygen and glucose is insufficient, the amount of ATP synthesized cannot meet cellular demand for high-energy phosphates. As a consequence, the neurons depolarize, leading to opening of the voltage-gated calcium channels and widespread release of neurotransmitters (such as glutamate), which, in turn, may open the receptor-operated calcium channels (such as the N-methyl-D-aspartate [NMDA] receptor) and activate phosphatidylinositol (PI) turnover.[57] These events lead to an increase in free cytosolic calcium. Elevated intracellular Ca^{2+} results in the activation of lipases, proteases, endonucleases, and nitric oxide synthase and leads to alterations in receptor function, membrane channel integrity, and free radical production.[58] The voltage-gated calcium channels located in both presynaptic and postsynaptic neurons (usually N- and T-types) control the entry of Ca^{2+} across the surface membrane of neurons and involve glutamate-mediated neurotoxicity.[59]

There has been considerable focus in the past on the therapeutic potential of agents that block calcium influx into nerve cells via the NMDA receptors. Isradipine (PN200–110), a 1,4-dihydropyridine calcium antagonist, easily crosses the blood-brain barrier and is a promising agent for the control of neuronal calcium overload following ischemia.[60-62] Dihydropyridine calcium antagonists may reduce ischemic consequences in two ways:

1. By direct action on cerebral vessels, dihydropyridine calcium antagonists may increase the cerebral blood flow and, hence, the supply of oxygen and glucose to the brain, resulting in a higher rate of ATP synthesis.

2. By closing the voltage-gated calcium channels on the brain cells, dihydropyridine calcium antagonists may reduce the entry of calcium into the cytosol and thus decrease calcium overload.[57, 63]

The restoration of cerebral blood flow alone, however, although obviously necessary for brain survival, is not sufficient in itself to protect the brain following ischemia. Calcium channel antagonists prevent neuronal damage mainly by inhibiting calcium influx into neuronal cells through voltage-gated calcium channels.[64]

Flunarizine is the most extensively studied piperazine derivative and is of value experimentally in protecting the CNS from anoxic or ischemic insult.[64] Although its exact mechanisms of action are unknown, flunarizine is believed to block both L- and T-type calcium channels in isolated heart muscle.[65] Beneficial effects of intravenous calcium channel blockers have been obtained only when they are administered before or shortly after onset of cerebral ischemia, since postischemic treatment involving systemic administration of a calcium channel blocker more than 1 hour after ischemic insult has not increased focal cerebral blood flow (CBF) or resulted in reduction of infarct volume.[66, 67] Hosaka et al., however, found a significantly beneficial effect 3 hours after occlusion of the rat middle cerebral artery (MCA) by transvenous perfusion of the brain with verapamil.[68] We studied flunarizine in a baboon spinal cord ischemia model by administering it before aortic cross-clamping. We were unable to show any beneficial effects, however, either in preventing paraplegia or increasing spinal cord blood flow during ischemia.[28] Of interest was the finding that all the animals developed acute hemorrhagic gastritis.[69] The failure of flunarizine may have been related to its lack of effect on N- and P-type calcium channels in the spinal cord.

Amlodipine was the first calcium channel antagonist approved for clinical trial and treatment of patients with ischemic stroke and had been expected to be the most promising agent because of its higher lipid:water partition coefficient. This property enables amlodipine to penetrate brain tissue through the blood-brain barrier and underlies its higher apparent distribution volume in the brain and its cerebral selectivity.[70-72] In recent experimental studies, however, the neuroprotective effects of nimodipine have yielded conflicting, if not disappointing, results.[73-78] Possible explanations for such untoward results are that amlodipine has no effect on N- or P-type calcium channels, which are predominant in neuronal tissues; calcium influx is not blocked through receptor-operated calcium channels (NMDA receptor); ischemia-induced failure of calcium pump and intracellular calcium release mechanisms are not affected by nimodipine; and administration of the drug is started too late.[78] Therefore, because of the problems with many calcium channel blockers, calcium antagonists acting on intracellular calcium sequestering sites or on N- and P-type calcium channels or on both have attracted considerable attention and are under extensive investigation.[79, 80]

Intracellular calcium accumulation during hypoxia and ischemia plays a central role in neuronal injury and comes from multiple sources. Calcium can enter neurons through a variety of different channels and pathways either from on the surface of the membrane or from the intracellular stores. Currently available calcium antagonists only target certain types of voltage-gated calcium channels on the cellular membrane. Glutamate antagonists, on the other hand, decrease Ca^{2+} influx by blocking receptor-operated calcium channels, for example, the NMDA receptor-channel complex. Since elevated calcium itself may trigger various biological events in neurons such as the proteolysis of important cytoskeletal proteins, targeting calcium-activated proteolysis would be a useful therapeutic approach for preventing ischemic neuronal death.[81] Calpain, once activated by calcium, may proteolyze several proteins, including neurofilament, spectrin, and calmodulin.[82] A calpain inhibitor, Cbz-Val-Phe-H (MDL-28170), greatly improved the posthypoxic recovery of synaptic transmission in the neocortex by preserving those protein molecules.[81, 83]

Neurotransmitters

Depolarization and repolarization are caused by the change of ion concentrations across cell membranes. The maintenance of such ion concentrations and the chemical gradients requires energy. Of these ions, calcium has the largest gradient. Extracellularly the concentration of calcium is 1.25 to 1.35 mmol/L, and intracellularly it is approximately 1 nmol/L. With depolarization, calcium moves from the extracellular compartment to the intracellular compartment, releasing neurotransmitters. A theory that has gained increasing acceptance is that the excitatory amino acids, glutamate and aspartate, may be false transmitters that are neurotoxic during ischemia.[84] The mechanism is poorly understood, but it may be that the increased calcium conductance results in postsynaptic activation of the calcium-dependent enzyme phospholipase A_2.[6] The latter may then destroy cell membranes. The influx of ions into the cell draws water into the cell further, osmolytically damaging the cell and causing edema.[8]

Excitatory Amino Acids

The excitatory amino acids have been blamed for tissue damage in a variety of neurological disorders, including epilepsy, in neurodegenerative disorders, and in cerebral ischemia. Experimental evidence has shown that glutamate is excitotoxic in high extracellular concentrations, and raised extracellular concentrations of glutamate have been demonstrated following both global and focal ischemia.[12, 58, 85-87]

Considerable evidence supports a role of glutamate in the mediation of ischemic neuronal damage. Specific glutamate antagonists, however, have not been consistently protective in models of transient global ischemia, a finding suggesting that not only glutamate but also other neurotransmitter systems may be involved in ischemic neuronal damage. Imbalance between excitation and inhibition is important, since recent studies have demonstrated that neurotransmitters such as γ-aminobutyric acid (GABA) and glycine may also be involved in the ischemic process.[88] Glutamate plays an unexpectedly important role in neuroendocrine regulation in the hypothalamus and accounts for most of the excitatory synapses in the neuroendocrine hypothalamus.[89] Glutamate is believed to be the major excitatory neurotransmitter regulating neuroendocrine neurons, and amino acid neurotransmitters account for most of all presynaptic axons involved in neuroendocrine regulation, greatly outnumbering amines, peptides, or other neuroactive substances.[89]

The intracellular glutamate concentration in brain tissue is approximately 10 nmol/L,[90] in contrast to 0.6 μmol/L extracellular concentration,[91] because of the activity of glutamate transporters. During cerebral ischemia there is a substantial release of glutamate and aspartate in the hippocampus as well as in other brain tissue, ranging from 3.5 to 15 times normal as measured by microdialysis.[91-95] Cell culture studies have shown that exposure to concentrations of 100 μmol/L glutamate for more than 5 minutes is lethal.[96] Other studies have shown that substantial excitotoxic damage to cortical neurons or hippocampal neurons may occur when glutamate concentration reach 2 to 5 μmol/L.[97] Nonetheless, the excess extracellular accumulation of glutamate may be caused by impairment of presynaptic uptake; by leakage from postsynaptic neurons and astrocytes, for example, by reversal of the direction of transport; or by excessive exocytosis from presynaptic vesicles potentiated by glutamate itself[12, 85] (Fig. 12-1). Energy failure after ischemia disturbs ion homeostasis in the context of glutamate accumulation. Approximately 2 minutes after induction of ischemia or anoxia, extracellular K^+ levels rise steeply to 60 to 80 mmol/L, with an accompanying decrease in extracellular sodium and chloride. This drastic change of the K^+-Na^+

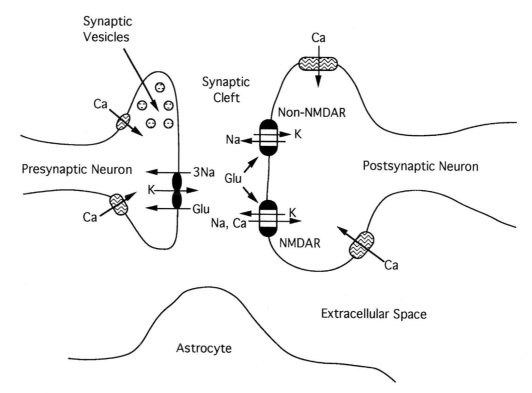

FIGURE 12–1 Mechanisms of extracellular glutamate accumulation. NMDAR, *N*-methyl-D-aspartate receptor; non-NMDAR, non-NMDA receptors including AMPA and kainate receptor; Glu, glutamate. There are some types of voltage-gated calcium channels on the presynaptic and postsynaptic neurons.

ratio reverses the glutamate uptake carriers in astrocytes and presynaptic terminals.[98]

A number of glutamate release inhibitors are effective in reducing ischemic brain injury in animal models[99-101] and may reduce undesirable side effects, such as excessive sedation or production of a psychotomimetic state by NMDA antagonists.[102, 103] Riluzole acts presynaptically to inhibit glutamate release, possibly by blocking sodium channels or interacting with G proteins.[104] The κ-opioid receptor agonist CI-977 is associated with presynaptic modulation of glutamate release.

Excitotoxin-induced cell death appears to be mediated through specific receptors. Two major subtypes of glutamate receptors have been recognized on the basis of their molecular cloning, electrophysiological properties, and pharmacological antagonism. These two categories are (1) **inotropic** receptors that are coupled directly to membrane ion channels and (2) **metabotropic** receptors that are coupled to G proteins and modulate intracellular second messengers such as inositol triphosphate, calcium, and cyclic nucleotides. The **metabotropic** type of glutamate receptor coupled to Phosphoinositol metabolism has been described.[105-106] A number of agonists to the metabotropic receptor have been developed; ibotenic and especially quisqualic acid are potent stimulators but not very selective. The endogenous agonist is supposed to be L-glutamate. A selective agonist $1_s,3_r$-ACPD (*trans*-1-aminocyclopentane-1,3-dicarboxylic acid) has the same potency as ibotenic acid.[107]

Only a few antagonists to the metabotropic receptor are known; for example, AP3 is a more useful antagonist than AP4. AP4 also acts on a presynaptic inhibitory L-AP4 glutamate receptor. It is not known whether the metabotropic receptor participates in neurotoxicity involving glutamate. The metabotropic receptors for other neurotransmitters have been known for some time, such as β-adrenergic, muscarinic cholinergic, and histaminergic receptors.

The **inotropic** receptors can be divided into three major types based on their selective agonists: **NMDA,** α-amino-3-hydroxy-5-methyl-4-isoxazole propionate (**AMPA**), and **kainate.** These selective receptor agonists resemble glutamate or aspartate but do not occur naturally.[85] The NMDA receptor-channel complex is a receptor-operated ion channel permeable to Na^+, K^+, and Ca^{2+}. The AMPA receptor is linked to a channel providing a nonselective conductance mechanism for monovalent cations, that is, Na^+ and K^+, whereas an NMDA subtype of glutamate receptor gates a channel permeable to both monovalent cations and calcium. There is coordination of information between these two subtypes of receptors. It is postulated, for example, that depolarization of AMPA receptor-linked channels by Na^+ influx triggers calcium influx via the NMDA-gated channel as well as through L- and T-type voltage-gated calcium channels. The latter are also located on the postsynaptic membrane.[58]

The **NMDA** receptor is stimulated by *N*-methyl-D-aspartate or glutamate. Glycine acts as a coagonist, potentiating

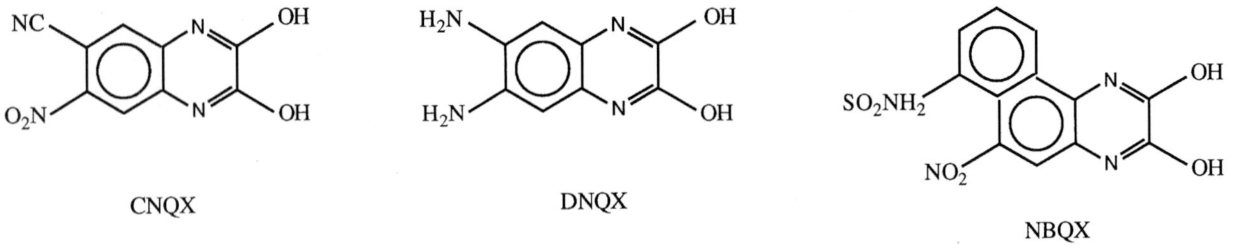

FIGURE 12–2   The structures of three quinoxaline dione non-NMDA receptor antagonists: CNQX, 6-cyano-7-nitroquinoxaline-2,3-dione; DNQX, 6,7-dinitroquinoxaline-2,3-dione; NBQX, 2,3-dehydroxy-6-nitro-7-sulfamoyl-benzo(F)quinoxaline.

the effect of NMDA by increasing channel opening frequency.[108] The modulatory effects of glycine are thought to be mediated by a strychnine-insensitive glycine receptor that can be antagonized by 1-hydroxy-3-aminopyrrolidone-2 (HA-966),[109, 110] 7-chlorokynurenic acid (7-CK),[111] and Felbamate.[112] Felbamate has been shown to ameliorate hypoxic-ischemic brain damage in animals.[113] More recent studies suggest that glycine may enhance the maximal activation of the NMDA receptor and play a central permissive role in NMDA-mediated neurotoxicity.[114]

NMDA receptor activation can be competitively inhibited at the glutamate recognition site by a number of agents. The classic competitive antagonists are phosphonates such as 2-amino-5-phosphonovalerate (APV)[115] and 2-amino-7-phosphonoheptanoate (APH). Newly developed compounds exhibit fewer polar properties and penetrate the blood-brain barrier more readily. These include 4-(-3-phosphonopropyl)-2-piperazine-2-carboxylic acid (CPP) or its unsaturated analogue CPP-ene and cis-4-(phosphonomethyl)-2-piperidine-carboxylic acid (CGS 19755, selfotel), cis-(±)-4-[(2H-tetrazol-5-yl)methyl]-piperidine-2-carboxylic acid (LY233053),[102] and (R)-4-oxo-5-phosphononorvaline (MDL-100,453).[116] We investigated the use of selfotel (CGS 19755) as a competitive antagonist to glutamate at the NMDA receptor site but found it did not protect against 60 minutes of descending thoracic aorta cross- clamping in our porcine model.

There are multiple modulatory sites that regulate the cation influx through the receptor-associated channel. The channel itself has binding sites for magnesium or various drugs such as dizocilpine (MK-801), phencyclidine (PCP), ketamine (interacts at the phencyclidine binding site too), and all are considered as NMDA noncompetitive antagonists, blocking the receptor-gated channel rather than the receptor itself.[117-123] The other noncompetitive NMDA antagonists are dextromethorphan (D-3-methoxy-N-methylmorphinan, DM), a widely used antitussive, and its O-demethylated metabolite, dextrorphan (DX),[124-126] CNS 1102 [N-(1-naphthyl)-N'-(3-ethylphenyl)-N'-methyl-guanidine hydrochloride].[127, 128] Both DM and DX are believed to block the NMDA receptor-channel complex by binding to the phencyclidine site, but the protective effect of DM and DX may not be related to their NMDA-antagonist properties.[126] They improve postischemic hypoperfusion by increasing collateral blood flow or by decreasing neuronal metabolic require-

ments.[126] In addition, DM and DX may also act on the voltage-gated calcium channels.[129] Although the exact mechanisms of action of DM and DX are not clear, it is of interest that Rokkas and Kouchoukos and colleagues[130] found that dextrorphan protects the spinal cord against ischemic injury. The other modulatory sites include a pH-sensitive region; a polyamine-binding site for spermine and spermidine; a zinc-binding site; and a redox site consisting of one or more thiol (sulfhydryl, SH) groups, which may react with an oxidized congener of nitric oxide to form an S-nitrosothiol (NO-S) and may facilitate disulfide-bond formation.[85, 131-133]

The **AMPA** receptor is activated by α-amino-3-hydroxy-5-methyl-4-isoxazole propionate, kainic acid, or glutamate but not by NMDA. A modulatory site for benzodiazepines affects the degree of desensitization of the channel, which may be permeated by sodium and possibly calcium. The 2,3-benzodiazepine GYKI 52466 acts at this site to inhibit non-NMDA receptor responses.[134, 135]

The **kainate** receptor is activated by kainic acid or glutamate but not by AMPA or NMDA. Both types of receptors are referred to as non-NMDA receptors. The discovery of the quinoxaline diones,[136] a series of potent and selective antagonists against the non-NMDA receptors, has greatly facilitated the study of the pharmacology of the quisqualate and kainate receptor subtypes. Three antagonists are 6-cyano-7-nitro-quinoxaline-2,3-dione (CNQX),[89] 2,3-dehydroxy-6-nitro-7-sulfamoyl-benzo(F)quinoxaline (NBQX),[137, 138] and 6,7-dinitroquinoxaline-2,3-dione (DNQX) (Fig. 12–2). Quisqualate was discovered to bind to the kainate site as well as to a metabotropic glutamate receptor.[12] Some nonspecific glutamate antagonists such as kynurenate and dipeptides such as DGG (γ-D-glutamylglycine) act on both AMPA- and NMDA-activated receptors.

Recent evidence in neuronal tissue culture strongly suggests that activation of the NMDA receptor by glutamate, with opening of its calcium channel, is the major mechanism of calcium-mediated neurotoxicity following ischemia.[115] Overstimulation of NMDA receptors is one mechanism for calcium overload in neurons; some variants of AMPA-kainate receptors are coupled to ion channels that are somewhat permeable to calcium and can thus contribute to excessive calcium entry.[85]

The activation of voltage-gated calcium channels through which calcium flows into neurons is also associated with ionotropic glutamate receptors.[59] Excessive elevation of intracellular calcium may activate a series of enzymes, including protein kinase C (PKC), phospholipase C (PLC), phospholipase A_2, endonucleases, and nitric oxide synthase (NOS). The stimulation of PLC leads to the formation of both IP_3 and diacylglycerol (DG), the latter leading to the activation and membrane translocation of PKC, which in turn triggers a cascade of events involving phosphorylation.[139-140] With phospholipase A_2 activated, arachidonic acid and its metabolites and platelet-activating factor (PAF, 1-o-alkyl-2-acetyl-sn-glycero-3-phosphorylcholine) are generated. PAF is involved in various pathologic processes and increases the neuronal calcium levels, apparently by stimulating the release of glutamate.[141, 142] Arachidonic acid potentiates NMDA-evoked currents[143] and inhibits reuptake of glutamate into astrocytes and neurons,[144] further exacerbating the cell damage. Oxygen free radicals can be formed during arachidonic acid metabolism,[145] leading to further phospholipase A_2 activation. Activation of endonucleases results in condensation of nuclear chromatin and ultimately DNA fragmentation and nuclear breakdown, a pathologic process known as programmed cell death (apoptosis).

In addition to glutamate and aspartate, some other excitatory amino acids may also be involved in the development of ischemic brain damage. Recently, the role of serotonin in ischemic neuronal injury in the setting of transient global forebrain ischemia has been explored, based on observations such as the existence of the $5\text{-}HT_2$ receptor in neuronal as well as vascular tissues and ischemia-induced serotonin release in the brain.[146] A few specific serotonin ($5\text{-}HT_2$) receptor antagonists have been tested in both global and focal ischemic animal models, with conflicting results. Ritanserin, which is the most frequently used serotonin antagonist, had a protective effect on hippocampal CA1 neurons in the transient global forebrain ischemia rat[146] but failed to reduce infarct volume in a permanent focal ischemia model of the rat.[147] Ketanserin, another $5\text{-}HT_2$ receptor antagonist, has been reported to increase the cerebral blood flow (CBF) in remote cortical brain regions after cortical thrombotic infarction.[148] (S)-Emopamil, having both calcium channel blocking and $5\text{-}HT_2$ receptor blocking properties, seems to be more effective than ritanserin in the permanent middle cerebral artery (MCA) occlusion rat model as well as in global ischemia.[149, 150]

It has been postulated that magnesium ions inhibit synaptic transmitter release and protect the cell.[151, 152] Reuptake of neurotransmitter amino acids is inhibited by arachidonic acid, and inhibition of uptake is countered by α-tocopherol or steroids.[16]

Free Fatty Acids and Prostaglandins

With neuronal ischemia, concentrations of free fatty acids (FFAs) and sodium in the cytosol increase.[153] FFAs in turn can release calcium from mitochondria, amplifying the effects of calcium. Clark and Roman[154] have demonstrated that FFA-stimulated release of calcium from mitochondria in the brain can be suppressed as much as 70% by magnesium

ions. Excessive intracellular calcium activates calcium-dependent phospholipase A_2 with further liberation of FFAs from the plasma membrane into the cytosol.[16] The released FFA, mostly arachidonic acid, is transformed by cyclooxygenase and lipoxygenase into prostaglandins.[6] Of the prostaglandins, thromboxane activates platelets, causing vasospasm and further accentuating ischemia. Indomethacin, a cyclooxygenase inhibitor, inhibits prostaglandin production, improves cerebral blood flow, and may aid in recovery.[155] Pentobarbital, after global ischemia or spinal cord ischemia, may also reduce arachidonic acid and FFA levels and thus may have an effect.[156]

Adenosine

Adenosine is a purine byproduct of ATP metabolism and has multiple beneficial effects in cerebrovascular neurological diseases. Cellular adenosine is generally extremely low under normal conditions, since most of it exists in the form of ATP. Adenosine accumulates only when ATP catabolism increases, as in seizure, ischemia, and trauma. In other words, adenosine levels rise in a parallel and reciprocal fashion to the depletion of ATP.[157] The elevated level of adenosine in metabolic stress may imply its neuroprotective participation. Functions of adenosine are numerous, including reduction in membrane permeability, attenuation of neurotransmitter release, vasodilation, and the regulation of hemodynamics and CBF.[158, 159] All these effects are now believed to be mediated by adenosine receptors which have at least two subtypes, namely A1 and A2.[160] The A1 receptor predominates in the CNS. The A2 receptor is mainly responsible for the peripheral effects of adenosine in the cardiovascular, neural, and immune systems.[161] It has been reported that the adenosine antagonist theophylline is enhanced, whereas agonist stimulation of adenosine receptors ameliorated the cellular damage following short periods of ischemia. Of interest, the up regulation of adenosine A1 receptors reducing ischemic neuronal damage has been demonstrated following long-term administration of the adenosine antagonist theophylline.[162, 163] Highly selective adenosine derivatives on the A1 receptor, such as N^6 cyclohexyladenosine (CHA) and N^6 cyclopentyladenosine (CPA), have been synthesized and are under active investigation.[157] Two enzymes, adenosine deaminase and xanthine oxidase, are involved in the catabolism of adenosine and generation of neurotoxic free radicals following ischemia (Fig. 12–3). Intracellular adenosine is metabolized to inosine and adenosine 5'-monophosphate (AMP), both of which are inactive at adenosine receptors but yield oxygen free radicals by the process per se. Deoxycoformycin, an adenosine deaminase inhibitor, and oxypurinol, a xanthine inhibitor, have been used in a gerbil forebrain ischemia model to demonstrate cerebroprotection.[159, 164, 165] Inhibitors of adenosine uptake such as dipyridamole and nitrobenzylthionosine (NBI) increase the levels of extracellular adenosine and its functional half-life. The adenosine neuromodulator systems can therefore be affected at both the receptor level by synthetic agonists and at the level of endogenous adenosine production

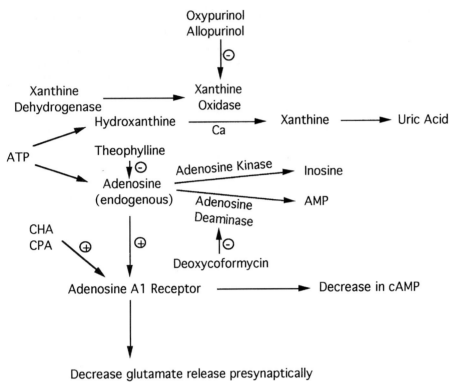

FIGURE 12–3 Pathways of adenosine metabolism and its pathophysiological roles in ischemic cellular damage. ATP, adenosine triphosphate; AMP, adenosine monophosphate; CBF, cerebral blood flow; CHA, N6-cyclohexyladenosine; CPA, N6-cyclopentyladenosine.

via inhibition of adenosine transport.[157] The roles of adenosine and its receptors are interwoven with oxygen free radicals and excitatory neurotransmitter release, implicating it in the pathophysiological processes of ischemic damage (Fig. 12–2). Of interest, Herold and colleagues[166] have shown in rabbit experiments that adenosine infusion with hypothermic saline into an occluded aorta prevents postoperative paraplegia.

DNA

At what stage of neuronal damage cellular recovery is impossible and cell death occurs has not been elucidated.

Cell death is an irreversible injury. Morphologically, there are two forms of cell death: necrosis and apoptosis. Necrosis or coagulation necrosis is a pathological process manifested by severe cell swelling or cell rupture, denaturation and coagulation of cytoplasmic proteins, breakdown of cell organelles, focal tissue destruction, and often is associated with serious systemic consequences. Apoptosis or programmed cell death (PCD), on the other hand, usually occurs in various physiological situations and may eliminate unwanted cell clusters, for example, during embryogenesis. It is initiated by an endonuclease and is characterized by DNA fragmentation into multiples of 180 to 200 base pairs. Apoptotic cells are ingested by macrophages without release of proteolytic enzymes or toxic oxygen free radicals.

Breakages in double-stranded DNA may be critical in irreversible ischemia because cellular repair processes fail. Decreased protein synthesis[167, 168] due to decreased RNA synthesis, probably because of DNA breakages, has been observed after both brain and kidney ischemia. One hour of normothermic ischemia to the kidney results in as much as 6% of the DNA being denatured to single-stranded moieties.[169] Furthermore, with an increased period of ischemia, this percentage increases.[169] Chromatin clumping occurs after 10 minutes of brain ischemia as a result of calcium-dependent nucleases' being activated by the increased concentrations of calcium, and this leads to DNA degradation.[16]

Certain brain regions and specific neuronal types are especially vulnerable to ischemic insults and cell death. Among the neurons that are particularly susceptible to transient ischemia are the CA1 pyramidal cells of the hippocampus. In the rat, more than 3 to 4 minutes of ischemia destroys the pyramidal cells.[170] One of the most studied brain regions is the hippocampal CA1 sector. In the hippocampal CA1 region, two types of neurons are mainly found: pyramidal neurons with typical spiny dendrites and interneurons, often with beaded processes.[12] NMDA receptors are numerous in the hippocampus, with the density especially high in the dendritic fields of CA1 as labeled with the noncompetitive ligand [³H]TCP. The hippocampal distribution of the AMPA receptor almost overlaps with that of the NMDA receptor with highest density corresponding to the dendritic fields of CA1. The kainate receptors, as labeled with [³H] kainic acid, are concentrated in the stratum lucidum of CA1, in the supragranular layer of the dentate fascia, and in the dentate hilus, which contains 2 or 3 cell types vulnerable to ischemia.[12]

REPERFUSION INJURY

Oxygen-derived Free Radicals and Scavengers

Free radicals are chemical species with one or more unpaired electrons in an outer orbit.[171] In such a state the radical is extremely reactive and unstable and enters into reactions with inorganic or organic chemicals—proteins, lipids, carbohydrates—particularly with key molecules in membranes and nucleic acids.[172]

When two radicals combine with each other, a stable molecule results. If the formed molecule is hydrogen peroxide (H_2O_2) from two hydroxyl radicals (OH[1]), however, it can still be harmful to tissue. The combination of a radical with a nonradical produces another free radical. Both molecules from such a reaction may damage tissue. An example is hydrogen peroxide and the free radical ion. The ability of free radicals to form bonds with other nonradicals enables them to produce chain reactions. Free radicals may, therefore, result in the peroxidation of unsaturated FFAs by molecular oxygen.[9] Peroxidation of fatty acids and lipids destroys both epithelial cell and endothelial cell membranes. Double-stranded DNA is broken. Radicals degrade hyaluronic acid and collagen within the cell membranes and basement membranes.[4] The net result is further loss of cellular integrity and increased permeability across cells including endothecal cells. The chain reaction set in motion by the free radicals' peroxidation of FFA is rapidly magnified by transitional metals, such as iron and copper, further increasing membrane destruction. Of interest, studies have shown that deferoxamine, an iron chelator, if administered during the first 15 minutes of reperfusion, can inhibit the reaction.[16] The basic pathways of inducing oxygen free radicals, metabolic enzymes involved, and specific inhibitors are shown in Fig. 12–4.

Oxygen free radicals are partially reduced toxic intermediates of oxygen that otherwise undergo a four-electron reduction to H_2O catalyzed by cytochrome oxidase. Reperfusion brings oxygen into the tissues or cells that previously were ischemic, resulting in generation of oxygen free radicals. Oxygen free radicals are considered to be a major factor in ischemia-reperfusion injury.[173, 174] Oxygen free radicals are produced by reduction of molecular oxygen through a variety of oxidative enzymes in the different sites of the cell—cytosol, mitochondria, lysosomes, peroxisomes,

FIGURE 12–4 The basic pathways of producing oxygen free radicals, metabolic enzymes as well as specific inhibitors. SOD, superoxide dismutase; oxidative enzymes include P-450 oxidase, reduced nicotine adenosine dinucleotide phosphate oxidase, oxidases from peroxisome, respiratory chain enzymes in mitochondria, and cytosolic enzymes.

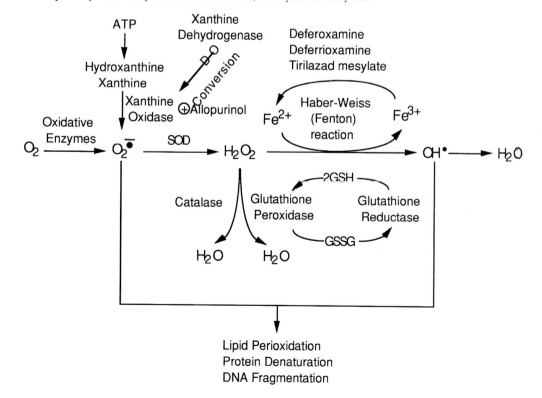

and plasma membrane. The three most important oxygen free radicals are superoxide ($O_2^{\bullet-}$), hydrogen peroxide, and hydroxyl ions ($OH^{\bullet}$). Two other radicals that may be produced from oxygen are the perhydroxyl radical, which is a stronger oxidant than superoxide,[175] and singlet oxygen, with histidine as a specific effective scavenger.[176]

Superoxide is a byproduct of normal cellular metabolism derived from mitochondrial, endoplasmic reticular, and nuclear membrane electron transport processes and of soluble proteins such as hemoglobin, aldehyde oxidase, and xanthine oxidase.[177] It is generated either directly during autooxidation in mitochondria or enzymatically by cytoplasmic enzymes, such as xanthine oxidase, cytochrome P-450, and other oxidases.[172] Once produced, superoxide can be inactivated spontaneously or, more rapidly, by the enzyme SOD, forming hydrogen peroxide. Catalase, in turn, breaks down hydrogen peroxide.

Because there is evidence that free radicals contribute to neural injury during reperfusion of ischemic tissue, attempts have been made at identifying the source of the radicals. Superoxide radicals are normally produced by the mitochondrial electron-transport chain, and some of these radicals may leak out during ischemia.[178] The major source of radicals, however, is the reaction caused by the enzyme xanthine oxidase.[5] This ubiquitous enzyme in the cellular matrix has been intensively studied. Xanthine oxidase is synthesized largely (90% of it) in the type D (dehydrogenase) form.[5] The D type reduces the nicotinamide adenine dinucleotide ion (NAD^+) to NADH but cannot transfer electrons to oxygen to form hydrogen peroxide or radicals. In ischemic tissues, however, type D xanthine oxidase is rapidly transformed into type O (oxidase) form. The importance of this is that once reperfusion occurs and oxygen is again available to the cell, the type O form uses oxygen instead of NAD^+ to produce hydrogen peroxide and radicals.[5] The role of calcium during ischemia is again apparent, since it catalyzes the conversion of type D to type O form. During ischemia, ATP levels fall and AMP accumulates. The AMP is catabolized to adenosine, inosine, and then hypoxanthine. Hypoxanthine and xanthine are substrates for xanthine dehydrogenase or oxidase reaction. Thus, when reperfusion occurs with oxygen in the presence of type O (xanthine oxidase), there is a burst of superoxide and peroxide production, resulting in tissue damage.[5]

Hydrogen peroxide is also produced directly by oxidases present in peroxisomes—the catalase-containing organelles present in many organs. Glutathione peroxidase and catalase are metabolic enzymes required to convert the hydrogen peroxide into water and carbon dioxide. Glutathione peroxidase enables reduced glutathione (GSH) to convert hydrogen in sulfhydryl to a hydroxyl radical or to hydrogen peroxide (Fig. 12–4). In a previous study we have used the level of glutathione as a marker of oxygen free radical release after aortic cross-clamping.[28] If glutathione peroxidase and catalase are not effective in eliminating hydrogen peroxide, hydroxyl radicals ($OH^{\bullet}$) are generated via the iron-catalyzed Haber-Weiss (Fenton) reaction.[179]

The hydroxyl radicals are the most potent and reactive species of the free radicals in biological systems and are probably responsible for most of the cellular damage done by free radicals.[180, 181] Iron plays a particularly important role in the Haber-Weiss reaction. Most free iron is in the ferric (Fe^{2+}) form and has to be reduced to the ferrous (Fe^{3+}) form to participate in the reaction. This reduction can be enhanced by superoxide, and thus sources of iron and superoxide are required for maximal oxidative cell damage.

Lipid Peroxidation

Lipid peroxidation underlies the pathogenesis of cell damage by oxygen free radicals. Cell membranes are composed of polyunsaturated fatty acids and phospholipid, which are most susceptible to peroxidatic damage, resulting in structural and functional alterations and disorders of membrane permeability.

Unsaturated fatty acids of membrane lipids possess double bonds between some of the carbon atoms. Such bonds are vulnerable to attack by oxygen-derived free radicals, particularly by hydroxyl radicals. The lipid-radical interactions yield peroxides, which are themselves reactive species, initiating the subsequent reduction of more fatty acids. Free radicals also promote sulfhydryl-mediated cross-linking of such labile amino acids as methionine, histidine, cystine, and lysine, as well as fragmentation of polypeptide chains. The reactions of free radicals with thymine in DNA produce single-stranded breaks in DNA, and such DNA damage has been implicated both in cell death and in possible malignant transformation of cells.[172] Lipid peroxidation also inhibits the synthesis of prostacyclin (prostaglandin I_2) and leads to vessel contraction and blood coagulation, resulting in "no reflow" and worsening cell damage. Exhaled ethane and conjugated dienes are biomarkers used to observe lipid peroxidation and measures of lipid damage caused by reperfusion.[182, 183] Malonyldialdehyde, an end-product of lipid hydroperoxides, can also be used as a marker of lipid peroxidation.[173]

Arachidonic acid produced from lipid peroxidation is converted by cyclooxygenase to prostaglandins thromboxane and prostacyclin. The latter chemicals have extensive effects on platelet function and vascular tone.[16] Hydroperoxide levels can be reduced by using glutathione peroxidase to remove them and thus reduce the activation of cyclooxygenase.[153, 184, 185] Glutathione peroxidase requires glutathione as a substrate; however, glutathione levels are decreased by ischemia followed by reperfusion.[186] In fact, we have measured glutathione levels in animals after reperfusion to see if free oxygen radicals were produced.[186, 187]

Arachidonic acid is also converted by lipoxygenase to leukotrienes (LTA_4, LTB_4, LTC_4, LTD_4). These leukotrienes influence leukocyte chemotaxis, vascular permeability, and smooth muscle tone in several tissues.[188] Indeed, LTD_4 is known to be a potent vasoconstrictor in rat,[189] gerbil,[190] and human cerebral arteries.[189] In fact, it may be responsible for the "no-reflow" phenomenon of secondary ischemia following reperfusion.

Production of Free Radicals

Several mechanisms of free radical production have been identified in biological systems. Oxygen free radicals are normally generated during oxidative metabolism but are well controlled by enzymatic and nonenzymatic systems. SOD and glutathione peroxidase are the major intracellular enzymatic defense systems against oxygen-derived free radicals. GSH is an important intracellular nonenzymatic defense against reactive oxygen metabolites.[191] Small amounts of free radicals may be produced physiologically from "leaky" sites in the mitochondrial electron transport chain.[192, 193]

In pathological situations, free radicals are derived from xanthine oxidase metabolism, activated neutrophils, catecholamine oxidation, endothelial cells, and prostaglandins. The mechanism of superoxide production during ischemia reperfusion has recently been reviewed extensively by Welbourn et al.[194] The enzyme xanthine oxidase is a major source of free radicals in postischemic tissue. Ischemia produces accumulation of metabolites including xanthine oxidase and its substrate hypoxanthine derived from AMP. Subsequent reperfusion brings molecular oxygen. The enzyme xanthine oxidase uses molecular oxygen to convert hypoxanthine to xanthine, releasing superoxide in the reaction.[5]

Transition Metals and Free Radicals

Superoxide and its immediate metabolite hydrogen peroxide are poorly reactive and do not damage tissues on their own.[195] In the presence of transition metals like iron, they are converted into more potent and reactive forms such as the hydroxyl radicals and other reactive iron-oxygen complexes that contribute to most of cell injury caused by free radicals. Hemoglobin-derived iron due to ischemic and hemorrhagic injury maintains a source of iron. Superoxide enhances the reduction of ferric iron to ferrous iron, which is the reactive form of iron for the Haber-Weiss reaction (Fig. 12–4). Thus, a considerable amount of iron may be available to catalyze the generation of hydroxyl radicals from hydrogen peroxide via the Haber-Weiss reaction.[196] The central nervous system (CNS) is especially vulnerable to iron-related free radical damage, since it is relatively poorly endowed with SOD, which would inhibit iron release from intracellular stores such as ferritin.[197]

The effect of iron on cell injury mediated by free radicals has been extensively studied.[198-200] When iron is injected directly into the brain in the form of ferric chloride, heme, or hemoglobin, it induces lipid peroxidation and inhibits the Na^+-K^+-ATPase of cell membranes. Deferoxamine is an iron chelator with a high affinity for ferric iron and may inhibit hydroxyl radical formation and reduce reperfusion or hemorrhagic brain injury.[201-203] The brain-protective effect by tirilazadmesylate—21-[4-(2,6-di-1-pyrrolidine-4-pyrimidinyl)-1-piperazinyl]-16-methylpregna-1,4,9 (11)-triene-3,20-dione, monomethane sulfonate—a 21-aminosteroid with potent antioxidant activity, was thought to be due to iron-dependent inhibition.[204-206] Tirilazad mesylate has been shown to inhibit arachidonic acid–induced breakdown of the blood-brain barrier[207] and to significantly reduce infarct volumes due to temporary focal ischemia but not those due to permanent ischemia.[208] Lasaroids, the inhibitors of iron-induced lipid peroxidation, attenuate postischemic cortical neuronal necrosis after 3-hour unilateral carotid occlusions.[209]

Protection against Free Radicals

A great effort has been made to seek pharmacological agents and antioxidants that block the initiation of free radical formation or that inactivate (e.g., scavenge) free radicals.[107, 209-213] These agents include enzymes (SOD), allopurinol, vitamin E, Coenzyme Q_{10}, sulfhydryl-containing compounds (cysteine and glutathione), and serum proteins (albumin, ceruloplasmin and transferrin). Scavenging or inhibiting production of oxygen free radicals offers a potential mechanism to reduce ischemic-reperfusion tissue injury. Endogenous scavengers are SOD, which converts superoxide to H_2O_2; catalase, which decomposes H_2O_2 into O_2 + H_2O; and glutathione peroxidase, which enables reduced glutathione (GSH) to convert hydrogen in sulfhydryl to a hydroxyl radical or to H_2O_2. Allopurinol is a xanthine oxidase inhibitor and is oxidized by xanthine oxidase to oxypurinol, which then binds tightly to reduced xanthine oxidase, completely inhibiting its ability to generate free radicals.[213] Ubiquinone (Coenzyme Q_{10}), a benzoquinone with a long isoprenoid side chain, may also function as a free radical scavenger and stabilize cell membranes by inhibiting phospholipase activity.[214] It has been shown to protect the brain against damage during cardiopulmonary bypass (CPB) and deep hypothermic circulatory arrest by improving cerebral metabolism and ultrastructure.[45, 214]

Allopurinol

In 1986, we used allopurinol to try to prevent paraplegia after aortic cross-clamping,[28] but it was ineffective. Allopurinol has been reported to be useful but only with long-term administration (at least 3 days) before the ischemic interval of aortic cross-clamping.[215] The same author reported only 25% recovery was provided by allopurinol with 3-day administration.[211] An additive protection by allopurinol and deferoxamine, both acting on independent pathways of the same pathologic process, was observed in the prevention of spinal cord injury caused by aortic cross-clamping.[212] Because of the absence of detectable levels of xanthine oxidase in rabbits, pigs, and human myocardium,[216-218] the protective effect of allopurinol in patients undergoing coronary artery bypass graft (CABG) is thought to be limited.[213] A number of other possible mechanisms of allopurinol protection have been proposed, including an increased efficiency of ATP salvage, facilitation of mitochondrial electron transfer, and direct activation of endogenously formed reactive substances, such as hydroxyl radicals or myeloperoxidase-derived hypochlorous acid.[212]

Superoxide Dismutase

Exogenous application of the enzymes in the metabolic pathways of free radicals is another alternative. SOD is able to dismutate superoxide anions to hydrogen peroxide, which can be converted into water and carbon dioxide by catalase or glutathione peroxidase. Studies on capillary permeability in the ileum in cats have shown that SOD provides nearly complete protection against the manifestation of tissue injury.[4] SOD is an enzyme that scavenges superoxide radicals by catalyzing the radicals by dismutation to hydrogen peroxide and oxygen.[219] These intracellular enzymes are ubiquitous in tissues. Allopurinol and SOD protect the small bowel[4] and the heart[220] after periods of ischemia followed by reperfusion. In previous nonhuman primate studies, we found that both SOD and allopurinol protected the stomach but not the spinal cord against reperfusion injury.[69, 221] Allopurinol inhibits xanthine oxidase,[4] and SOD scavenges the free radicals.[222] Other than our use of SOD and allopurinol to inhibit the effects of free radicals, sodium thiopental and corticosteroids have been reported to be protective.[9, 156, 223] In 1986, we reported[28] a disappointing result with SOD in preventing spinal cord injury after aortic cross-clamping. Despite strong theoretical support for the combined use of SOD and catalase, Myers and associates did not find any evidence of added protection with SOD in a canine model of regional ischemia and attributed the protective effect to catalase not SOD.[224] However, SOD may provide some degree of protection by itself without catalase or glutathione peroxidase.[225] Dimethylthiourea, dimethyl sulfoxide, and mercaptopropionyl glycine are all putative scavengers of the hydroxyl radical,[226, 227] and mannitol has been used clinically for its hydroxyl radical scavenging effects for many years.[228] Even hypothermia initiated after resuscitation can significantly inhibit the accumulation of lipid peroxidation products and decrease the consumption of free radical scavengers in the brain.[191]

Current Research

Although oxygen radicals have been widely recognized as contributing to tissue injury after reperfusion, their exact role in the pathogenesis of infarction after brain or spinal cord ischemia and reperfusion has not been clearly established, despite some recent findings regarding the use of pharmacological agents and antioxidants. This strategy of using protective pharmacological agents, however, creates problems that cannot be easily resolved: the hemodynamic, pharmacokinetic, and possibly toxic side effects of the drugs, as well as the problem of their blood-brain barrier permeability properties. An alternate and more direct method for the study of oxidative stress in ischemia and reperfusion injury is to use genetically modified animals that overexpress antioxidant enzymes. Transgenic (Tg) mice overexpressing human copper-zinc–superoxide dismutase (SOD-1) activity have been successfully developed and used as a unique model in the protection against ischemia and infarction.[229, 230]

This study demonstrates that Tg mice with a three times normal SOD-1 activity level are resistant to injury induced by cerebral ischemia and reperfusion both in infarct volume and neurological deficits and is believed to be the first to demonstrate that elevating the levels of endogenous antioxidant enzyme by molecular genetic manipulation can ameliorate reperfusion injury.[230]

A cautionary note is the finding by Rehncrona and colleagues[20] that brain injury was not associated with the generation of superoxide radicals. Nevertheless, there is also evidence that reperfusion pulmonary edema after lower torso ischemia is associated with LTB_4, thromboxane, and superoxide production.[231] Oxygen radicals also appear to be the mediators of further tissue injury after reperfusion of ischemic and damaged tissues associated with the crush syndrome.[27]

The interrelationship of chemical reactions on both ischemic injury and injury caused by reperfusion are only beginning to be understood. In fact, ischemia may play less of a role than reperfusion in the resulting injury, particularly if the period of ischemia is short. A delayed reperfusion injury would partially explain delayed neurological injury following stroke, cardiac arrest, head injury, deep hypothermia with circulatory arrest, and delayed paraplegia after thoracic aortic cross-clamping.

BLOOD FLOW AFTER ISCHEMIA AND NO-REFLOW PHENOMENON

Nitric Oxide

Nitric oxide (NO) has long been known to stimulate soluble guanylate cyclase and generate cyclic AMP (cAMP) from guanosine triphosphate (GTP).[232] The endothelium-derived relaxing factor (EDRF), initially described by Furchgott and Zawadzki,[233] appears to have pharmacological and chemical properties similar to those of nitric oxide, and is probably the same chemical. EDRF has been associated with a wide variety of biological effects both beneficial and detrimental.[234, 235] Nitric oxide is generated from L-arginine by at least three distinct isoforms of nitric oxide synthase in the brain, endothelium, and macrophage, respectively[236] (Table 12–2).

The major effect of nitric oxide is the modulation of vascular tone and regulation of local blood flow in different tissues including cerebral circulation.[237, 238] In addition, basal release of nitric oxide by constitutive nitric oxide synthase (NOS) in a physiological situation may protect cerebral endothelium by inhibiting aggregation of platelets and leukocytes.[29, 240] However, nitric oxide may participate in free radical reactions[241-243] and mediate glutamate-induced neurotoxicity, thus damaging tissues.[85, 236, 244, 245]

Nitric Oxide and the CNS

In general, normal release of nitric oxide mediates physiological vasodilation; however, excessive release may play a role in the pathogenesis of tissue damage and cell death.[246] Although a biological role for nitric oxide was first ascertained from studies in nonneuronal tissues, recent evidence suggests several important roles for this substance in the central and peripheral nervous systems, mainly because NOS is widely distributed in the nervous system and nitric oxide has been characterized as a neurotransmitter.[247] There appear to be several major neuronal sources of nitric oxide: neurons,[248] astrocytes,[249] and probably perivascular nerves that innervate cerebral blood vessels.[250] The existence of nitric oxide in the brain was first suggested by demonstrations that cerebellar neuronal cultures release a factor with properties resembling nitric oxide, as well as by observation of nitric oxide–forming activity in brain extracts and slices.[251, 252] Nitric oxide production in a variety of intact living systems, such as macrophages and cerebellar slices, has been inferred by measurement of nitrite (NO_{2-}), nitrate (NO_{3-}), and cyclic guanosine 3',5'-monophosphate (cGMP) in the absence and presence of potent and selective inhibitors of NOS.[253-255] Nitrite and nitrate are the major stable metabolites of nitric oxide under aerobic conditions, and nitric oxide acts as a messenger in the brain, where it can influence cGMP formation through activation of guanylyl cyclase.[232, 256]

NOS Types and Metabolism

NOS converts L-arginine into nitric oxide and L-citrulline, requiring NADPH and oxygen as cosubstrates in the reaction (Fig. 12–4). Three distinct isoforms of NOS (brain, endothelium, and macrophage) have been cloned.[236, 257-259]

These NOS isoforms generally fall into two categories: a constitutive form regulated by calcium-calmodulin and an inducible form regulated by cytokines and lipopolysaccharide (Table 12–2).[235, 257] The constitutive NOSs isolated from rat[260, 261] and porcine cerebellums[234] are cytosolic proteins (M_r = 150 to 160 kDa), and the inducible NOS purified from lipopolysaccharide- or interferon γ-treated murine macrophage RAW 264.7 cells is also a cytosolic protein with a M_r = 130 kDa.[262] The constitutive endothelial isoform from bovine aorta was found to be a membrane-associated protein with a M_r = 135 kDa.[263]

NO Action

NO is a potent dilator of cerebral blood vessels both in vitro and in vivo.[264, 265] In situ hybridization has demonstrated that messenger RNA for a constitutive form of NOS is present in cerebral endothelium.[266] After release by endothelium, nitric oxide stimulates soluble guanylate cyclase in smooth muscle, resulting in a rise in cGMP and relaxation. Nitrovasodilators such as sodium nitroprusside, papaverine, and nitroglycerin also increase formation of cGMP and relax cerebrovascular muscle. Nitroprusside and nitroglycerin also release NO. Papaverine has been used for the treatment of clinical and experimental vasospasm, especially cerebral vasospasm, by intravenous or intrathecal administration.[267] We have used intrathecal irrigation of papaverine to try to prevent paraplegia.[28] Methylene blue, which can inhibit soluble guanylate cyclase under some conditions, attenuates relaxation of cerebral vessels in response to nitric oxide and nitroprusside.[268-270] It has been shown that relaxation of blood vessels in response to acetylcholine, serotonin, bradykinin, substance P, and ATP also depends on formation of nitric oxide and will be abolished in blood vessels stripped of endothelium.[271-273] These mediators act on receptors on endothelial cells to trigger the release of an EDRF, which diffuses to adjacent smooth muscle cells to elicit relaxation.[246] Nitric oxide is also a messenger molecule that regulates macrophage killing of tumor cells and bacteria.[274]

Nitric oxide has been implicated in leukocyte–endothelial cell adhesion and vascular protein leakage associated with ischemia-reperfusion.[275] Enhanced superoxide production in postischemic tissues inactivates endothelial cell–derived nitric oxide, which in turn results in leukocyte–endothelial cell adhesion and vascular protein leakage.[276-279] This concept has led to the proposal that nitric oxide donors such as sodium nitroprusside may be useful in preventing or attenuating reperfusion-induced leukocyte–endothelial cell adhesion and vascular protein leakage. Kurose et al. demonstrated that plasma nitrate/nitrite levels in the superior mesenteric vein of rats were significantly reduced by ischemia and reperfusion and that microvascular dysfunction (albumin leakage) induced by ischemia and reperfusion is attenuated by nitric oxide.[280]

The role of nitric oxide in the mechanism of brain injury following ischemia and reperfusion is controversial and has not yet been completely elucidated. The neurotoxicity of

TABLE 12–2 CHARACTERISTICS OF TWO DIFFERENT FORMS OF NITRIC OXIDE SYNTHASE

Form	Constitutive	Inducible
Location	Brain and spinal cord Endothelium	Macrophage
Modulator	Ca^{2+}	Cytokines, lipopolysaccharides, glucocorticoids, Ca^{2+}

Activity	Physiology	Pathophysiology
Expression	Short	Hours
Posttranscription	Yes	Unknown
NO production	Basal	No basal, large amount upon stimulation
cGMP	Dependent	Independent

nitric oxide may involve nitric oxide itself or, more importantly, its combination with superoxide free radical to form peroxynitrite (ONOO⁻), which decomposes to form strong oxidant hydroxide free radical (OH•) and NO_2 free radical (NO_2•), which are substantially more reactive and toxic than nitric oxide, with a reactivity similar to that of hydroxyl radical.[281]

Thus the oxidation-reduction state of nitric oxide may determine whether nitric oxide is protective or destructive. Reduction of nitric oxide by superoxide is proposed to generate peroxynitrite ion; and oxidation of nitric oxide produces nitrosonium ion, which is believed to oxidize a critical sulfhydryl group in NMDA receptors, which might decrease calcium influx and thereby reduce NOS activity.[282] Excessive activation of NMDA receptors may mediate cellular damage and lead to further production of nitric oxide.[283] Stimulation of non-NMDA glutamate receptors is also thought to generate nitric oxide.[248, 255] This feedback reflects a protective mechanism halting excessive production of nitric oxide. On the other hand, nitric oxide, with subsequent Ca^{2+} fluxes, mediates presynaptic neurotransmitter release including norepinephrine and glutamate, and glutamate in turn activates NMDA receptors on postsynaptic neurons.[283]

The NADPH-dependent enzyme NOS is required for the formation of nitric oxide from L-arginine. Because nitric oxide has a short half-life, quantification of nitric oxide production is often difficult. Therefore many studies of the biological effects of nitric oxide have relied on studies of NOS and especially on the use of certain analogues of L-arginine that can be relatively specific enzyme inhibitors.[247] These inhibitors include N^G-nitro-L-arginine methyl ester (L-NAME), N^G-monomethyl-L-arginine (L-NMMA), and N^G-nitro-L-arginine (LNNA). Inhibitory effects by these agents can be reversed by L-arginine administration. The inhibitory effects are stereospecific, with the inactive optical isomers having no effect. This stereospecificity of the block and the reversibility of the weaker inhibitor suggest that the inhibitors do not act by a nonspecific, but rather by a specific blockade of NOS.[283]

Expression of NOS in the endothelial cells after middle cerebral artery (MCA) occlusion was rapidly upregulated in the cerebral microvasculature throughout the ischemic region as well as in the periphery of the area of necrosis in the cortices.[284] Overexpression of endothelial NOS in the microvessels may increase the synthesis of nitric oxide in order to dilate blood vessels and thereby to compensate for the reduction of cerebral blood flow.[284] Improvement of cerebral blood flow, however, seems not to provide protection during MCA occlusion. In fact, elevation of arterial pressure and blood flow promotion following inhibition of NOS would more likely be detrimental to neurological recovery, since parasympathetic denervation increased infarction volume after MCA occlusion.[285] Since only partial protection from injury in the caudate nucleus but not in the cerebral hemispheres was observed by intravenous administration of L-NAME, metabolic characteristics of different

tissues could not be excluded.[286, 287] Inhibition of NOS activity may not be protective in all types of ischemia.

Nitric oxide is thought to be a major cause of the hemodynamic alterations seen in sepsis, which is characterized by a high cardiac output, maldistribution of blood flow, and altered peripheral oxygen utilization, ultimately resulting in tissue hypoxia, organ failure, and death.[23] Endotoxin and several other cytokines induce a calcium-independent NOS, not only in endothelial cells but also in a variety of other tissues like macrophages and the smooth muscle cell.[235, 262] Thus, inhibition of NOS would reverse the increase in cardiac output and increase the systemic vascular resistance without changing oxygen consumption. In fact, NOS inhibitors have already been used in individual patients with sepsis[288] and may be a therapeutic option in the treatment of hyperdynamic states accompanied by sepsis when conventional therapy fails to maintain a minimum of cardiovascular performance.[289]

Others have found that NOS inhibition does not affect infarct volume after permanent focal ischemia. In spontaneously hypertensive rats (SHR), inhibition of NOS increases the degree of cortical injury after MCA occlusion.[290] It is assumed that genetic hypertension is associated with altered metabolism of L-arginine, increased susceptibility to brain injury following focal ischemia because of decreased ability to develop an adequate collateral circulation, and with an altered cAMP pathway in cerebral blood vessels.[291, 292]

Mechanisms proposed for nitric oxide neurotoxicity and as well as tumoricidal and bactericidal actions include mono–adenosine 5'-diphosphate (ADP)–ribosylation and S-nitrosylation of glyceraldehyde-3-phosphate dehydrogenase (GAPDH), inhibition of mitochondrial enzymes such as cis-aconitase, inhibition of the mitochondrial electron transport chain, inhibition of ribonucleotide reductase, and DNA damage, which activates PARS [poly (adenosine 5'-diphosphoribose) synthetase]. PARS is a nuclear enzyme that, when activated by DNA strand breaks, adds up to 100 adenosine 5'-diphosphoribose (ADP-ribose) units to nuclear proteins such as histones and PARS itself. This activation can lead to cell death through depletion of b-NAD (the source of ADP-ribose) and ATP.[293] Thus, nitric oxide triggers DNA damage, which in turn activates PARS, which ultimately depletes energy sources from the cell. Nitric oxide production and energy depletion are two major effects of glutamate neurotoxicity. In rat brain nuclear extracts, increase of PARS activity was associated with DNA and nitric oxide in a dosage-dependent manner and reduced by PARS inhibitors, such as 4-amino-1,8-naphthalimide and 1,5-dihydroxyisoquinoline.[293] Similarly, DNA that had been treated with 3-morpholinosydnonimine (SIN-1) and sodium nitroprusside, two nitric oxide donors, can stimulate poly-ADP-ribose synthesis, which was inhibited by benzamide, another PARS inhibitor. Neither sodium nitroprusside nor SIN-1 alone had an effect on PARS.[293]

Currently, little is known about nitric oxide production in the spinal cord during and after ischemia produced by aortic cross-clamping. However, it is interesting to speculate that the hyperemia of the spinal cord we noted after aortic cross-clamping, particularly in paraplegic baboons, was due to vasodilation caused by nitric oxide release.[28]

INTERRELATIONSHIPS OF BIOCHEMICAL EVENTS

Clearly, neuron damage and cell death can be caused by protein breakdown, DNA fragmentation, free radical formation, and lipid peroxidation.[85] However, nitric oxide–mediated glutamatergic neurotoxicity via NMDA receptors is considered to be one of the most important pathogeneses (Figs. 12–1 and 12–5). NOS is present in vascular endothelium, astrocytes, and neurons, including perivascular neurons,[287] and can be activated by calcium influx as a result of NMDA-receptor stimulation, leading to production of nitric

oxide.[244] Enhanced nitric oxide production during reperfusion may be attributable to persistent elevation of excitatory amino acids during reperfusion.[244] Using a porphysinic microsensor, Malinski et al. were able to present evidence for increased nitric oxide production in brain during transient focal ischemia.[295] Nitric oxide can either be protective or destructive, depending upon its oxidation or reduction state. Under reduction, nitric oxide (NO•) with one more free electrons interacts with superoxide anion, which is also produced during transient ischemia, to form peroxynitrite (ONOO), which may in turn decompose to form a strong oxidant with a reactivity similar to that of hydroxyl radical.[296] On the other hand, nitric oxide becomes nitrosonium ion (NO+) with one less electron under oxidation, and the latter binds to a redox modulatory site on the NMDA receptor, decreasing activity of NMDA receptors and affording protection from excessive stimulation.[297] Nitric oxide itself may accelerate glutamate release presynaptically, exert

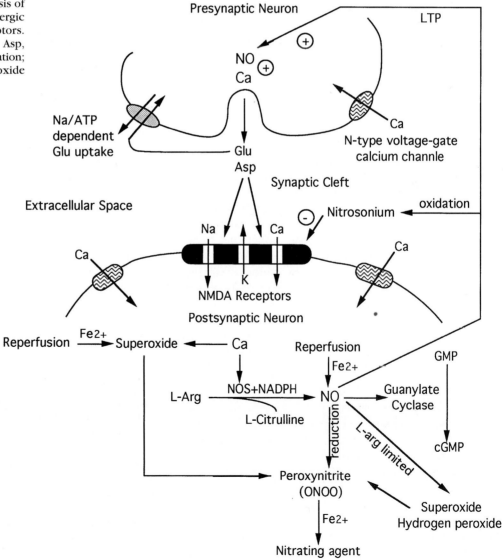

FIGURE 12–5 The pathogenesis of nitric oxide mediating glutamergic neurotoxicity via NMDA receptors. NO, nitric oxide; Glu, glutamate; Asp, aspartate; LTP, long-term potentiation; L-arg, L-arginine; NOS, nitric oxide synthase.

direct effects by forming nitrite (NO_{2-}) and nitrate (NO_{3-}) if overproduced, and produce free radicals such as superoxide and hydrogen peroxide if L-arginine is limited (Figs. 12–1 and 12–5).

The relationship between NMDA receptors and nitric oxide can be elucidated by long-term potentiation (LTP) of synaptic transmission. Although mechanisms underlying the induction and maintenance of LTP at CA1 hippocampal synapses are uncertain, it is clear that the activation of NMDA receptors[298, 299] and the influx of Ca^{2+} into postsynaptic neurons are critical to CA1 LTP activation.[300, 301] This has led to speculation that a retrograde messenger travels from the postsynaptic to the presynaptic cell during the induction of LTP.[302, 303] Experimental evidence suggests that nitric oxide liberated from postsynaptic neurons may travel back to presynaptic terminals to cause LTP expression, since the extracellular application or postsynaptic injection of two inhibitors of NOS, N-nitro-L-arginine or N^G-methyl-L-arginine, blocks LTP; extracellular application of hemoglobin, which binds nitric oxide, also attenuates LTP.[302, 304] In addition, NMDA evokes a Ca^{2+}-dependent release of nitric oxide; high concentrations of sodium nitroprusside, an agent that spontaneously releases nitric oxide, augment synaptic responses in the CA1 region of hippocampal slices; and perfusion of nitric oxide increases the frequency of spontaneous miniature excitatory synaptic current in cultured hippocampal neurons.

Hypothermia

Hypothermia had been introduced as an adjunct in cardiovascular surgery and neurosurgery in the late 1950s and early 1960s (see Chapter 13).[305-311] It is a simple and effective technique, with as little as 2 to 3° C reduction in cerebral temperature being protective.[312, 313] The neuroprotection of hypothermia is attributed to reduction in cellular metabolism. Recent studies, however, have shown that hypothermia may preserve ATP and other important metabolites, stabilize plasma membrane, inhibit the synthesis, release, and uptake of neurotransmitters, and reduce postischemic cerebral edema and generation of leukotrienes.[191, 312, 314, 315] Baiping et al. found that hypothermia initiated after resuscitation can significantly suppress the generation of oxygen free radicals and decrease the consumption of free radical scavengers in the brain.[191]

Gangliosides

Gangliosides, a class of glycosphingolipids present in the mammalian nervous system, are associated with nerve growth and repair.[316] A purified preparation of GM_1 has been used in stroke clinical trials by several groups.[317, 318] The experimental results are favorable on neurological outcome, and the authors conclude that GM_1 is safe and effective in decreasing neurological deficit and mortality in patients with acute anterior or MCA ischemic stroke. The protective mechanism of GM_1 is widely believed to be due to its inhibition of polymorphonuclear leukocyte adhesion,

which would otherwise mediate additional tissue injury by releasing oxygen free radicals and other toxic substances in the ischemic area.[319] In addition, the protective effect may also be due to GM_1's attenuation of excitotoxicity.[320] The reparative mechanism has also been postulated in a spinal cord injury clinical trial.[321]

Pentoxifylline

Pentoxifylline is a xanthine derivative and a potent vasodilator in both systemic and pulmonary circulation. Pentoxifylline also increases cerebral blood flow; however, this does not improve recovery of cerebral electrical activity and metabolic function after transient cerebral global ischemia.[322]

Anion Transport Inhibitor

L-644,711 {R(+)[(5,6-dichloro 9a-propyl 2,3,9,9a-tetrahydro 3-oxo-1H fluoren-7yl)oxylacetic acid} is an anion transport inhibitor that has been shown to reduce the infarct size by 80% and 51% in the normotensive and hypotensive cerebral ischemic rabbit, respectively. Two possible mechanisms of action for the beneficial effects of L-644,711 in these animal models were thought to be inhibition of astrocyte swelling and inhibition of neutrophil function.[323]

Arachidonic Acid and Metabolites

Arachidonic acid metabolites—prostacyclin (PGI_2), thromboxane A_2 (TXA_2), and leukotrienes (LTs)—have been implicated in the development of neuronal ischemia. TXA_2 in particular has been blamed for ischemic cell injury, since it causes platelet aggregation and vasoconstriction, leading to the reduction of microcirculatory blood flow in various organs.[324] TXA_2 is also a powerful chemoattractant that may enhance neutrophil adhesion to endothelium. Under physiological conditions the degree of platelet aggregation and vasoconstriction is controlled by relative amounts of TXA_2 and PGI_2, which was the first agent identified from endothelial cells with antiplatelet aggregation and vasodilatory properties.[325] Increased amounts of arachidonate metabolites including TXA_2 were found in cerebral ischemia-reperfusion conditions.[326] (+)-(5Z)-7-{3-Endo-[(phenylsulfonyl)amino] bicyclo [2.2.1]hept-2-exo-yl}heptanoic acid (S-1452) is a stable calcium salt of the (+)-isomer of S-145 that has been shown to be a potent and selective TXA_2 receptor antagonist.[327] In the transient MCA rat model, S-1452 significantly suppressed the elevation of water content in the cerebral cortex, improved infarct areas in the anterior parts of the cerebrum, and may have a protective effect on postischemic brain injury.[327] PGI_2 and its analogues may have therapeutic potential and provide protection against TXA_2.

Polyamines

Polyamines are a group of ornithine-derived molecules involving many cellular functions, such as cell growth and differentiation, protein synthesis, membrane integrity and transportation, and calcium mobilization.[328] Brain polyamines have been associated with posttraumatic vasogenic edema and blood-brain barrier breakdown in brain injury.[329] Ornithine decarboxylase (ODC), the rate-limiting enzyme for polyamine synthesis, is stimulated by cerebral ischemia. Increase in ODC activity was found to parallel the increase in polyamine activity as well as the cerebral infarct volume.[330] Difluoromethylornithine (DFMO), an inhibitor of ODC, has been shown to provide protective effect against blood-brain barrier breakdown and vasogenic edema development in a region subjected to ischemia.[329]

Leukocytes

It is now agreed that leukocytes play an important role in ischemia-reperfusion injury. Leukocyte adhesion to the endothelium is the critical initial step and may trigger a cascade of biological events including production of oxygen free radicals and release of nitric oxide and other chemical mediators.[331, 332] Thus the inhibition of leukocyte adherence may offer a potential way of preventing neuronal damage.

Doxycycline

Doxycycline, a member of the tetracycline family of antibiotics, was found to reduce significantly CNS ischemic injury in the rabbit spinal cord ischemia model, and is thought to be a safe and readily available clinical therapeutic agent.[333]

Ischemic Brain and Spinal Cord Injury

The biochemical mechanisms of brain and spinal cord injury after hypothermic circulatory arrest or aortic cross-clamping and possible interventional therapies have received limited attention for the past decades. Since lipid peroxidation of the cellular membrane caused by oxygen species occurs generally in all tissues, the pathogenesis of oxygen free radicals in ischemic spinal cord injury is conceivable. In fact, a significant fraction of the damage that can occur in cardiovascular surgery may represent injury caused by free radicals generated at reperfusion rather than by the ischemia itself.[183] The same authors, using exhaled ethane as a biomarker of lipid peroxidation, found approximately a two-fold transient increase in the ethane level at around 15 minutes after reperfusion in those patients whose aortas were cross-clamped for more than 18 minutes.[18] Theoretically, administration of free radical scavengers should benefit patients who undergo cardiovascular surgery with prolonged cardiac and circulatory arrest; however, several groups have yielded controversial and sometimes disappointing results.[28, 212, 213, 224, 334] Recently, the role of excitatory amino acids in ischemic spinal cord injury has drawn attention.[130, 315] Simpson et al. used microdialysis to investigate changes in the extracellular concentrations of amino acids in the spinal cord after aortic occlusion in the rabbit and found the concentrations of glutamate, glycine, and taurine were significantly higher during ischemia and reperfusion than in controls.[335] Dizocilpine (MK-801), a selective

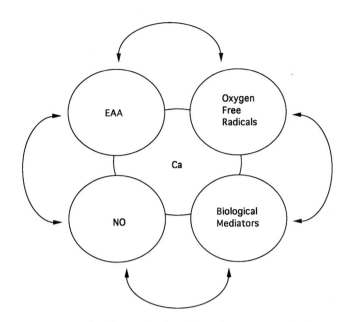

FIGURE 12–6 The pathophysiological processes of ischemia involving calcium, nitric oxide (NO), excitatory amino acids (EAA), oxygen free radicals, and some biological mediators such as PGI_2, thromboxane A_2, leukotriene B_4, platelet-activating factor, endothelin, and cytokines.

N-methyl-D-aspartate-glutamate receptor antagonist, has been shown to significantly improve the neurological outcome after trauma and neuroprotective capacity in prolonged periods of hypothermic circulatory arrest in animal experiments.[336, 337]

Since the constitutive isoform of nitric oxide synthase is also found in the spinal cord, the role of nitric oxide in spinal cord injury has been under intensive study. Bolt et al. used NOS inhibitor L-NAME to treat chronically stroke-prone spontaneously hypertensive rats (SPSHR) and found a higher incidence of infarction in the spinal cord and suggested that nitric oxide is a key factor in spinal cord arteriolar vasomotion and structure in rats.[338]

CONCLUSION

Ischemia, especially neuronal ischemia, covers a wide range of topics as we have discussed above. More than one single factor plays a role in the pathophysiological process of ischemia. With intracellular calcium being a central and final pathway, nitric oxide, oxygen free radicals, excitatory amino acids, arachidonic acid metabolites (prostacyclin, TXA_2, LTB_4), endothelin, PAF, cytokines, and complement all play a role in the consequences of ischemic injury and reperfusion (Fig. 12–6). As a result, no single approach has proven effective, and discrepancies among experimental data with any single agent seem to be plausible. It can be expected, however, that the further understanding of the pathogenesis and pathophysiological processes of ischemia and the combined uses of therapeutic agents would result in a practical and effective approach in the prevention of ischemia-induced injury in both the brain and spinal cord.

REFERENCES

1. Svensson LG, Crawford ES. Aortic dissection and aortic aneurysm surgery: clinical observations, experimental investigations, and statistical analyses. Part I. Curr Probl Surg 1992;29:819-912.
2. Svensson LG, Crawford ES. Aortic dissection and aortic aneurysm surgery: clinical observations, experimental investigations, and statistical analyses. Part II. Curr Probl Surg 1992;29:915-1057.
3. Svensson LG, Crawford ES. Aortic dissection and aortic aneurysm surgery: clinical observations, experimental investigations, and statistical analyses. Part III. Curr Probl Surg 1993;30:1-172.
4. Granger DN, Parks DA. Role of oxygen radicals in the pathogenesis of intestinal ischemia. Physiologist 1983;26:159-64.
5. McCord JM. Oxygen-derived free radicals in post-ischemic tissue injury. N Engl J Med 1985;312:159-63.
6. Siesjö BK. Cell damage in the brain: a speculative synthesis. J Cereb Blood Flow Metab 1981;1:155-85.
7. Siesjö BK, Bendek G, Koide T, et al. Influence of acidosis on lipid peroxidation in brain tissues in vitro. J Cereb Blood Flow Metab 1985;5:253-8.
8. Siesjö BK. Mechanisms of ischemic brain damage. Crit Care Med 1988;16:954-63.
9. Demopoulos HB, Flamm ES, Pietronigro DD, et al. The free radical pathology and the microcirculation in the major central nervous system disorders. Acta Physiol Scand Suppl 1980;492:91-119.
10. Kontos HA, Wei EP, Ellis EF, et al. Prostaglandins in physiological and in certain pathologic responses of the cerebral circulation. Fed Proc 1981;40:2326-30.
11. Diemer NH, Siemkowicz E. Regional neurone damage after cerebral ischemia in the normo- and hypoglycemic rat. Neuropathol Appl Neurobiol 1981;7:217-27.
12. Diemer NH, Valente E, Bruhn T, et al. Glutamate receptor transmission and ischemic nerve cell damage: evidence for involvement of excitotoxic mechanisms. Progr Brain Res 1993;96:105-23.
13. Pulsinelli W, Brierley J, Plum F. Temporal profile of neuronal damage in a model of transient forebrain ischemia. Ann Neurol 1982;11:491-8.
14. Szilagyi DE, Hageman JH, Smith RF, et al. Spinal cord damage in surgery of the abdominal aorta. Surgery 1978;83:38-56.
15. Lehninger AL. Generation of ATP in anaerobic cells. In: Bioenergetics, ed 2. Menlo Park, Calif: WA Benjamin;1971:53-71.
16. Krause GS, White BC, Aust SD, et al. Brain cell death following ischemia and reperfusion: a proposed biochemical sequence. Crit Care Med 1988;16:714-26.
17. Balentine JD, Spector M. Calcification of axons in experimental spinal cord trauma. Ann Neurol 1977;2:520-3.
18. Borgers M, Van Reempts J. The distribution of calcium in normal and ischemic brain tissue. Clin Res Rev 1984;4:70-1.
19. Meldrum BS. Metabolic effects of prolonged epileptic seizures and the causation of epileptic brain damage. In: Cliffor Rose S, ed: Metabolic Disorders of the Nervous System. London: Pitman;1981:175-87.
20. Rehncrona S, Siesjö BK, Smith DS. Reversible ischemia of the brain: biochemical factors influencing restitution. Acta Physiol Scand Suppl 1980;492:135-40.
21. Ljunggren B, Norberg K, Siesjö BK. Influence of tissue acidosis upon restitution of brain energy metabolism following total ischemia. Brain Res 1974;77:173-86.
22. Siemkowicz E, Hansen AJ. Clinical restitution following cerebral ischemia in hypo-, normo-, and hyperglycemic rats. Acta Neurol Scand 1978;58:1.
23. Kubler W, Katz AM. Mechanism of early pump failure of the ischemic heart: possible role of ATP depletion and inorganic H_2PO_4 accumulation. Am J Cardiol 1977;40:467.
24. Van Reempts J, Borgers M. Morphological assessment of pharmacological brain protection. In: Wauquier A, Borgers M, Amery W, eds: Protection of Tissues Against Hypoxia. Amsterdam: Elsevier Biomedical Press;1982:263-74.
25. Happel RD, Smith KP, Banik NL, et al. Ca^{2+} accumulation in experimental spinal cord trauma. Brain Res 1981;211:476-9.
26. Cheung JY, Bonventre JV, Malis CD, Leaf A. Calcium and ischemic injury. N Engl J Med 1986;314:1670-6.
27. Obeh M. The rate of reperfusion-induced injury in the pathogenesis of the crush syndrome. N Engl J Med 1991;324:1417-22.
28. Svensson LG, Von Ritter CM, Groeneveld HT, et al. Cross-clamping of the thoracic aorta: influence of aortic shunts, laminectomy, papaverine, calcium channel blocker, allopurinol, and superoxide dismutase on spinal cord blood flow and paraplegia in baboons. Ann Surg 1986;204:38-47.
29. Campbell AK. Intracellular Calcium: Its Universal Role as Regulator. New York: J. Wiley & Sons, Inc; 1983.
30. Janis RA, Silver P, Triggle DJ. Drug action and cellular calcium regulation. Adv Drug Res 1987;16:309-591.
31. Triggle DJ. Calcium, calcium channels, and calcium antagonists. In: Drugs in Development. ed. Branford, Conn: Neva Press; 1993:3-13.
32. Williamson JR, Monck JR. Hormone effects on cellular Ca^{2+} fluxes. Ann Rev Physiol 1989;51:107-24.
33. Carafoli E. The regulation of intracellular calcium. Adv Exp Med Biol 1982;151:461-72.
34. Miller RJ. Multiple calcium channels and neuronal function. Science 1987;235:46-52.
35. Augustine GJ, Charlton MP. Calcium action in synaptic transmitter release. Ann Rev Neurosci 1987;10:633-93.
36. Trimble WA, Linial M, Scheller RH. Cellular and molecular biology of the presynaptic nerve terminal. Ann Rev Neurosci 1991;14:93-122.
37. Miller RJ. Calcium signalling in neurons. TINS 1988;11:415-9.
38. Schanne FAX, Kane AB, Young EE, Farber JL. Calcium dependence of toxic cell death: a final common pathway. Science 1979;206:701-2.
39. Catterall WA. Structure and function of voltage-sensitive ion channels. Science 1988;242:50-61.
40. Tsien RW, Lipscombe D, Madison DV, Bley KR, Fox AP. Multiple types of neuronal calcium channels and their selective modulation. TINS 1988;11:431-7.
41. Bean BP CoccivcARP53-3 1989. Classes of calcium channels in vertebrate cells. Ann Rev Physiol 1989;51:367-84.
42. Hess P. Calcium channels in vertebrate cells. Ann Rev Neurosci 1990;13:337-56.
43. Catterall WA. Functional subunit structure of voltage-gated calcium channels. Science 1991;255:1499-1500.
44. Catterall WA. Structure and function of voltage-gated ion channels. TINS 1993;16:500-6.
45. Baker EJ, Ayton V, Smith MA, et al. Magnetic resonance imaging of coarctation of the aorta in infants: use of a high field strength. Br Heart J 1989;62:97-101.
46. Perney TM, Hiroring LD, Leeman SE, Miller RJ. Multiple neurotransmitter release from peripheral neurons. Proc Natl Acad Sci USA 1986;83:6655-9.
47. Murphy TH, Worley PF, Baraban JM. L-type voltage-sensitive calcium channels mediate synaptic activation of immediate early genes. Neuron 1991;7:625-35.
48. Johnston D, Williams S, Jaffe D, Gray R. NMDA-receptor independent long-term potentiation. Ann Rev Physiol 1992;54:489-505.
49. Tang CM, Presses F, Morad M. Amiloride selectively blocks the low threshold (T) calcium channel. Science 1988;240:213-5.
50. Scott RH, Wootton JF, Dolphin AC. Modulation of neuronal T-type calcium channel currents by photoactivation of intracellular guanosine 5'-o (3-THIO) triphosphate. Neuroscience 1990;38:285-94.
51. Hirning LD, Fox AP, McCleskey EW, et al. Dominant role of N-type Ca^{2+} channels in evoked release of norepinephrine from sympathetic neurons. Science 1988;239:57-61.
52. Turner TJ, Adams ME, Dunlap K. Calcium channels coupled to glutamate release identified by w-Aga-IVA. Science 1992;258:310-3.
53. Triggle DJ. Calcium channel antagonists: mechanisms of action, vascular selectivities and their clinical relevance. Cleve Clin J Med 1991;1991:23-5.
54. McCleskey EW, Fox AP, Feldman DH, et al. w-Conotoxin: direct and persistent blockade of specific types of calcium channels in neurons but not muscle. Proc Natl Acad Sci USA 1987;84:4327-31.
55. Llinas R, Sugimori M, Lin J-W, Cherksey B. Blocking and isolation of a calcium channel from neurons in mammals and cephalopods utilizing a toxin fraction (FTX) from funnel-web spider poison. Proc Natl Acad Sci USA 1989;86:1689-93.
56. Olivera BM, Rivier J, Scott JK, et al. Conotoxins. J Biol Chem 1991;266:22067-70.
57. Sauter A, Rudin M. Prevention of stroke and brain damage with calcium antagonists in animals. Am J Hypertension 1991;4:121S-7S.

58. Siesjö BK, Memezawa H, Smith ML. Neurocytotoxicity: pharmacological implications. Fundam Clin Pharmacol 1991;5(9):755-67.

59. Sucher NJ, Lei SZ, Lipton 5A. Calcium channel antagonists attenuate NMDA receptor-mediated neurotoxicity of retinal ganglion cells in culture. Brain Res 1991;551:297-302.

60. Hof RP, Hof A, Scholtysik G, Menninger K. Effects of a new calcium antagonist PN200-110 on the myocardium and the regional peripheral circulation in anaesthetized cats and dogs. J Cardiovasc Pharmacol 1984;6:407-16.

61. Supavilai P, Karobath M. The interaction of [H³] PY108-068 and of [H³]PN200-110 with calcium channel binding sites in rat brain. J Neurol Transm 1984;60:149-67.

62. Sauter A, Rudin M. Calcium antagonists for reduction of brain damage in stroke. J Cardiovasc Pharmacol 1990;15(Suppl):S43-S7.

63. Ohta S, Smith M-L, Siesjö BK. The effect of a dihydropyridine calcium antagonist (isradipine) on selective neuronal necrosis. J Neurol Sci 1991;103:109-15.

64. Cohan SL. Pharmacology of calcium antagonists: clinical relevance in neurology. Eur Neurol 1990;30(Suppl 2):28-30.

65. Tygat J, Vereecke J, Carmeliet E. Differential effects of verapamil and flunarizine on cardiac L-type and T-type Ca channels. Naunyn-Schmiedebergs Arch Pharmacol 1988;337:690-2.

66. Date H, Hossmann KA. Effect of vasodilating drugs on intracortical and extracortical vascular resistance following middle cerebral artery occlusion in cats. Ann Neurol 1984;16:330-6.

67. Kobayashi S, Obana W, Andrews BT, et al. Lack of effect of nimodipine in experimental regional cerebral ischemia (abstract). Stroke 1988;19:147.

68. Hosaka T, Yamamoto YL, Diksic M. Efficacy of retrograde perfusion of the cerebral vein with verapamil after focal ischemia in rat brain. Stroke 1991;22:1562-6.

69. Svensson LG, Von Ritter C, Oosthuizen MM, et al. Prevention of gastric mucosal lesions following aortic cross-clamping. Br J Surg 1987;74:282-5.

70. Kazda S, Towart R. Nimodipine: a new calcium antagonistic drug with a preferential cerebrovascular action. Acta Neurochir (Wien) 1982;63:259-65.

71. Scriabine A, Schuurman T, Traber J. Pharmacological basis for the use of nimodipine in central nervous system disorders. FASEB J 1989;3:1799-806.

72. Mason RP, Rhode DG, Herbette LG. Reevaluating equilibrium and kinetic binding parameters for lipophilic drugs based on a structural model for drug interaction with biological membranes. J Med Chem 1991;34:869-77.

73. Gelmer HJ, Gorter K, de Weerdt CJ, Wiezer HJA. A controlled trial of nimodipine in acute ischemic stroke. N Engl J Med 1988;18:203-7.

74. Paci A, Ottaviano P, Trenta A, et al. Nimodipine in acute ischemic stroke: a double-blind controlled study. Acta Neurol Scand 1989; 80:282-6.

75. Martinez-Vila E, Guillén F, Villanueva JA, et al. Placebo-controlled trial of nimodipine in the treatment of acute ischemic cerebral infarction. Stroke 1990;21:1023-8.

76. Horning CR, Kaps M, Hacke W, et al. Nimodipine in acute ischemic stroke: results of the Nimodipine German Austrian Stoke Trial. Stroke 1991;22:153.

77. The American Nimodipine Study Group. Clinical trial of nimodipine in acute ischemic stroke. Stroke 1992;23:3-8.

78. Kaste M, Fogelholm R, Erila T, et al. A randomized, double-blind, placebo-controlled trial of nimodipine in acute ischemic hemispheric stroke. Stroke 1994;25:1348-53.

79. McBurney RN, Daly D, Fischer JB, et al. New CNS-specific calcium antagonists. J Neurotrauma 1992;2(9 Suppl):S531-43.

80. Ohtaki M, Tranmer B. Pretreatment of transient focal cerebral ischemia in rats with the calcium antagonist AT877. Stroke 1994;25: 1234-40.

81. Hiramatsu K-I, Kassell NF, Lee KS. Improved posthypoxic recovery of synaptic transmission in gerbil neocortical slices treated with a calpain inhibitor. Stroke 1993;24:1725-8.

82. Seubert P, Lee K, Lynch G. Ischemia triggers NMDA receptor-linked cytoskeletal proteolysis in hippocampus. Brain Res 1989;492:366-70.

83. Mehdi S. Cell-penetrating inhibitors of calpain. Trends Biochem Sci 1991;16:150-3.

84. Rothman S. Synaptic activity mediates death of hypoxic neurons. Science 1983;226:850.

85. Lipton SA, Rosenberg PA. Excitatory amino acids as a final common pathway for neurologic disorders. Mechanisms Dis 1994;330:613-22.

86. Rothman SM, Olney JW. Glutamate and the pathophysiology of hypoxic-ischemic brain damage. Ann Neurol 1986;19:105-11.

87. Benveniste H. The excitotoxin hypothesis in relation to cerebral ischemia. Cerebrovasc Brain Metab Rev 1991;3:213-45.

88. Globus M-T, Busto R, Martinez E, et al. Comparative effect of transient global ischemia on extracellular levels of glutamate, glycine, and γ-aminobutyric acid in vulnerable and nonvulnerable brain regions in the rat. J Neurochem 1991;57:470-8.

89. van den Pol AN, Wuarin JP, Dudek FE. Glutamate, the dominant excitatory transmitter in neuroendocrine regulation. Science 1990;250:1276-8.

90. Kvamme E, Schousboe A, Hertz L, Torgner IA, G. S. Developmental change of endogenous glutamate and gamma-glutamyl transferase in cultured cerebral cortical interneurons and cerebellar granule cells, and in mouse cerebral cortex and cerebellum in vivo. Neurochem Res 1985;10:993-1008.

91. Benveniste H, Drejer J, Schousboe A, Diemer NH. Elevation of extracellular concentrations of glutamate and aspartate in rat hippocampus during transient cerebral ischemia monitored by intracerebral microdialysis. J Neurochem 1984;43:1369-74.

92. Benveniste H, Jorgensen MB, Sandberg M, et al. Ischemic damage in hippocampal CA1 is dependent on glutamate-release and intact innervation from CA3. J Cereb Blood Flow Metab 1989;9:629-39.

93. Hagberg H, Lehmann A, Sandberg M, Hyström B, Jacobson I, Hamberger A. Ischemia-induced shift of inhibitory and excitatory amino acids from intra- to extracellular compartments. J Cereb Blood Flow Metab 1985;5:413-9.

94. Korf J, Klein HC, Venema K, Postema F. Increases in striatal and hippocampal impedance and extracellular levels of amino acids by cardiac arrest in freely moving rats. J Neurochem 1988;50:1087-96.

95. Chreistensen T, Bruhn T, Diemer NH, Schousboe A. Effect of phenylsuccinate on potassium- and ischemia-induced release of glutamate in rat hippocampus monitored by microdialysis. Neurosci Lett 1991; 134:71-4.

96. Choi DW, Maulucci-Gedde M, Kriegstein AR. Glutamate neurotoxicity in cortical cell culture. J Neurosci 1987;7:357-68.

97. Rosenberg PA, Amin S, Leitner M. Glutamate uptake disguises neurotoxic potency of glutamate agonists in cerebral cortex in dissociated cell culture. J Neurosci 1992;12:56-61.

98. Hansen AJ. Effect of anoxia on ion distribution in the brain. Physiol Rev 1985;65:101-48.

99. Johnston GA, Hailstone MN, Freeman CG. Baclofen: stereoselective inhibition of excitant amino acid release. J Pharm Pharmacol 1980;32:230-1.

100. Meldrum B. Protection against ischemic neuronal damage by drugs acting on excitatory neurotransmission. Cerebrovasc Brain Metab Rev 1990;2:25-57.

101. Leach MJ, Swan JH, Eisenthal D, et al. BW619C89, a glutamate release inhibitor, protects against focal cerebral ischemic damage. Stroke 1993;24:1063-7.

102. Madden KP, Clark WM, Kochhar A, Zivin JA. Efficacy of LY 233053, a competitive glutamate antagonist, in experimental central nervous system ischemia. J Neurosurg 1992;76:106-110.

103. Olney JW, Labruyere J, Wang G, et al. NMDA antagonist neurotoxicity: mechanism and prevention. Science 1991;254:1515-8.

104. Bensimon G, Lacomblez, Meininger V, ALS/Riluzole Study Group. A controlled trial of Riluzole in amyotrophic lateral sclerosis. N Engl J Med 1994;330:585-91.

105. Sugiyama H, Ito I, Hirono C. A new type of glutamate receptor linked to inositol phospholipid metabolism. Nature 1987;325:531-3.

106. Sladeczek F, Recasens M, Bockaert J. A new mechanism for glutamate receptor action: phosphoinositide hydrolysis. Trends Neurosci 1988;11:545-9.

107. Palmer E, Monaghan DT, Cotman CW. Trans-ACPD, a selective agonist of the phosphoinositide-coupled excitatory amino acid receptors. Eur J Pharmacol 1989;166:585-7.

108. Johnson JW, Ascher P. Glycine potentiates the NMDA response in cultured mouse brain neurons. Nature 1987;325:529-31.

109. Fletcher EJ, Lodge D. Glycine reverses antagonism of N-methyl-D-aspartate (NMDA) by 1-hydroxy-3-aminopyrrolidone-2 (HA-966) but not by D-2-amino-5-phosphonovalerate (D-AP5) on rat cortical slices. Eur J Pharmacol 1988;151:161-2.

110. Keith RA, Mangano TJ, Meiners BA, et al. HA-966 acts at a modulatory glycine site to inhibit N-methyl-D-aspartate–evoked neurotransmitter release. Eur J Pharmacol 1989;166:393–400.

111. Kemp JA, Foster AC, Leeson PD, et al. 7-chlorokynurenic acid is a selective antagonist at the glycine modulatory site of N-methyl-D-aspartate receptor complex. Proc Natl Acad Sci USA 1988;85:6547–50.

112. McCabe RT, Wasterlain CG, Kucharczyk N, et al. Evidence for anticonvulsant and neuroprotectant action of felbamate mediated by strychnine-insensitive glycine receptors. J Pharmacol Exp Ther 1993;264:1248–52.

113. Wasterlain CG, Adams LM, Hattori H, Schwartz PH. Felbamate reduces hypoxic-ischemic brain damage in vivo. Eur J Pharmacol 1992;212:275–8.

114. Patel J, Zinkand WC, Thompson C, et al. Role of glycine in the N-methyl-D-aspartate-mediated neuronal cytotoxicity. J Neurochem 1990;54:849–54.

115. Choi DW. Calcium-mediated neurotoxicity: relationship to specific channel types and roles in ischemic damage. Trends Neurosci 1988;11:465–69.

116. Hasegawa Y, Fisher M, Baron BM, Metcalf G. The competitive NMDA antagonist MDL-100,453 reduces infarct size after experimental stroke. Stroke 1994;25:1241–6.

117. Gill A, Foster AC, Woodruff GN. Systemic administration of MK-801 protects against ischemia-induced hippocampal neurodegeneration in the gerbil. J Neurosci 1987;7:3343–9.

118. Rothman SM, Thurston JH, Hauhart RE, Clark CD, Solomon JS. Ketamine protects hippocampal neurons from anoxia in vitro. Neurosci 1987;21:673–8.

119. Choi DW, Koh J-Y, Peters S. Pharmacology of glutamate neurotoxicity in cortical cell culture: attenuation by NMDA antagonists. J Neurosci 1988;8:185–96.

120. Park CK, Nehls DG, Graham Dl, Teasdale GM, McCulloch J. The glutamate antagonist MK-801 reduces focal ischemic brain damage in the rat. Ann Neurol 1988;24:543–51.

121. Reynolds IJ, Miller RJ. Multiple sites for the regulation of the NMDA receptor. Mol Pharmacol 1988;33:581–4.

122. Mies G, Kohno K, Hossmann KA. MK-801, a glutamate antagonist, lowers flow threshold for inhibition of protein synthesis after middle cerebral artery occlusion of rat. Neurosci Lett 1993;155:65–8.

123. Shapira Y, Lam AM, Eng CC, et al. Therapeutic time window and dose response of the beneficial effects of ketamine in experimental head injury. Stroke 1994;25:1637–43.

124. Church J, Lodge D, Berry SC. Differential effects of dextrorphan and levorphanol on the excitation of rat spinal neurons by amino acids. Eur J Pharmacol 1985;111:185–90.

125. Choi DW. Dextrorphan and dextromethorphan attenuate glutamate neurotoxicity. Brain Res 1987;403:333–6.

126. Steinberg G, Saleh J, Kunis D, DeLaPaz R, Zarnegar S. Protective effect of N-methyl-D-aspartate antagonists after focal cerebral ischemia in rabbits. Stroke 1989;20(9):1247–1252.

127. Minematsu K, Fisher M, Li L, et al. Effects of a novel NMDA antagonist on experimental stroke rapidly and quantitatively assessed by diffusion-weighted MRI. Neurology 1993;43:397–403.

128. Minematsu K, Fisher M, Li L, Sotak CH. Diffusion and perfusion magnetic resonance imaging studies to evaluate a noncompetitive N-methyl-D-aspartate antagonist and reperfusion in experimental stroke in rats. Stroke 1993;24:2074–81.

129. Carpenter CL, Marks SS, Watson DL, Greenberg DA. Detromethorphan and dextrorphan as calcium channel antagonists. Brain Res 1988;439:372–75.

130. Rokkas CK, Helfrich LA, Lobner DC, et al. Dextrorphan inhibits the release of excitatory amino acids during spinal cord ischemia. Ann Thorac Surg 1994;58:312–20.

131. Watkins JC, Olvermann HJ. Agonists and antagonists for excitatory amino acid receptors. Trends Neurosci 1987;10:265–72.

132. Choi DW. Methods for antagonizing glutamate neurotoxicity. Cerebrovasc Brain Metabol Rev 1990;2:105–47.

133. Lodge D, Collingridge G. Les agents provocateurs: a series on the pharmacology of excitatory amino acids. Trends Pharmacol Sci 1990;11:22–4.

134. Donevan SD, Rogawski MA. GYKI 52446, a 2,3-benzodiazepine, is a highly selective, noncompetitive antagonist of AMPA/kainate receptor responses. Neuron 1993;10:51–9.

135. Zorumski CF, Yamada KA, Price MT, Olney JW. A benzodiazepine

136. Honoré T, Davis SN, Drejer J, et al. Quinoxaline diones: potent competitive non-NMDA glutamate receptor antagonists. Science 1988;241:701–3.

137. Sheardown MJ, Nielsen EO, Hansen AJ, et al. 2,3-dihydroxy-6-nitro-7-sulfamoyl-benzo(F)quinoxaline: a neuroprotectant for cerebral ischemia. Science 1990;247:571–4.

138. Nellgard B, Wieloch T. Differential protection by 2,3-dihydro-6-nitro-7-sulfamoyl-benzo(F)quinoxaline (NBQX) and dizocilpine (MK-801) following complete ischemia and insulin-induced hypoglycemia in the rat. J Cereb Blood Flow Metab 1992;12:2–11.

139. Nishizuka Y. The role of protein kinase C in cell surface signal transduction and tumor promotion. Nature 1984;308:693–8.

140. Nishizuka Y. Studies and perspectives of protein kinase C. Science 1986;233:305–12.

141. Bito H, Nakamura M, Honda Z, et al. Platelet-activating factor (PAF) receptor in rat brain: PAF mobilizes intracellular Ca^{2+} in hippocampal neurons. Neuron 1992;9:285–94.

142. Clark WM, Calcagno FA, Gabler WL, et al. Reduction of central nervous system reperfusion injury in rabbits using doxycycline treatment. Stroke 1994;25:1411–6.

143. Miller B, Sarantis M, Traynelis SF, Attwell D. Potentiation of NMDA receptor currents by arachidonic acid. Nature 1992;355:722–5.

144. Volterra A, Trotti D, Cassutti P, et al. High sensitivity of glutamate uptake to extracellular free arachidonic acid levels in rat cortical synaptosomes and astrocytes. J Neurochem 1992;59:600–6.

145. Lafon-Cazal M, Pietri S, Culcasi M, Bockaert J. NMDA-dependent superoxide production and neurotoxicity. Nature 1993;364:535–7.

146. Globus M-T, Wester P, Busto R, Dietrich WD. Ischemia-induced extracellular release of serotonin plays a role in CA1 neuronal cell death. Stroke 1992;23:1595–601.

147. LeMay DR, Neal S, Neal S, et al. Paraplegia in the rat induced by aortic cross-clamping: model characterization and glucose exacerbation of neurologic deficit. J Vasc Surg 1987;6:383–90.

148. Dietrich WD, Busto R, Ginsberg MD. Effect on the serotonin antagonist ketanserin on the hemodynamic and morphological consequences of thrombotic infarction. J Cereb Blood Flow Metab 1989;9:812–20.

149. Lin B, Dietrich WD, Busto R, Ginsberg MD. (S)-Emopamil protects against global ischemic brain injury in rats. Stroke 1990;21:1734–9.

150. Morikawa E, Ginsberg MD, Dietrich WD, et al. Postichemic (S)-emopamil therapy ameliorates focal ischemic brain injury in rats. Stroke 1991;22:355–60.

151. Ames A III. Earliest reversible changes during ischemia. Am J Emerg Med 1983;2:139–46.

152. Drejer J, Benveniste H, Diemer NH, Schousboe A. Cellular origin of ischemia-induced glutamate release from brain tissue in vivo and in vitro. J Neurochem 1985;45:145–51.

153. Cook HW, Lands WE. Mechanism for suppression of cellular biosynthesis of prostaglandins. Nature 1976;260-2:630.

154. Clark AF, Roman IJ. Mg^{2+} inhibition of Na^+ stimulated Ca^{2+} release from brain mitochondria. J Biol Chem 1980;255:6556–8.

155. Hallenbeck JM, Furlow TW. Prostaglandin I_2 and indomethacin prevent impairment of post-ischemic brain reperfusion in the dog. Stroke 1979;10:629–37.

156. Nylander WA, Plunkett RJ, Hammon JW, et al. Thiopental modification of ischemic spinal cord injury in the dog. Ann Thoracic Surg 1982;33:64–8.

157. Marangos PJ, von Lubitz D, Daval J-L, Deckert J. Adenosine: its relevance to the treatment of brain ischemia and trauma. In: Current and Future Trends in Anticonvulsant, Anxiety, and Stroke Therapy. New York: Wiley-Liss, Inc; 1990:331–49.

158. Van Wylen DGL, Park TS, Rubio R, Berne RM. Increases in cerebral interstitial fluid adenosine concentration during hypoxia, local potassium infusion, and ischemia. J Cereb Blood Flow Metab 1986;6:522–8.

159. Lin Y, Phillis JW. Deoxycoformycin and oxypurinol: protection against focal ischemic brain injury in the rat. Brain Res 1992;571:272–80.

160. Marangos PJ, Boulenger JP. Basic and clinical aspects of adenosinergic neuromodulation. Neurosci Biobehav Rev 1985;9:421–30.

161. Hamilton HW, Taylor MD, Steffen RP, Haleen SJ, Braun RF. Correlation of adenosine receptor affinities and cardiovascular activity. Life Sci 1987;41:2295–302.

162. Rudolphi KA, Keil M, Hinze HJ. Effect of theophylline on ischemically induced hippocampal damage in mongolian gerbils: a behavioral and histopathological study. J Cereb Blood Flow Metab 1987;7(74-81).

163. Rudolphi KA, Keil M, Fastbom J, Fredholm BB. Ischemic damage in gerbil hippocampus is reduced following upregulation of adenosine (A1) receptors by caffeine treatment. Neurosci Lett 1989;103: 275-80.

164. Phillis JW, O'Regan MH. Deoxycoformycin antagonizes ischemia-induced neuronal degeneration. Brain Res Bull 1989;22:537-40.

165. Phillis JW. Oxypurinol attenuates ischemia-induced hippocampal damage in the gerbil. Brain Res Bull 1989;23:467-70.

166. Herold JA, Kron IL, Langenburg SE, et al. Complete prevention of postischemic spinal cord injury by means of regional infusion with hypothermic saline and adenosine. J Thorac Cardiovasc Surg 1994; 107:536-41.

167. Hossman K-A, Paschen W, Csiba L. Relationship between calcium accumulation and recovery of cat brain after prolonged cerebral ischemia. J Cereb Blood Flow Metab 1983;3:346-53.

168. Lazarus HM. Ischemic effects on kidney nuclear RNA synthesis. Life Sci 1970;9:721-7.

169. Warnick CW, Dierenfeld SM, Lazarus HM. A description of the damaged DNA produced during tissue injury. Exp Mol Pathol 1984;41:397.

170. Johansen FF, Jorgensen MB, von Lubits DKJE, Diemer NH. Selective dendrite damage in hippocampal CA1 stratum radiatum with unchanged axon ultrastructure and glutamate uptake after transient cerebral ischemia in the rat. Brain Res 1984;291:373-7.

171. Halliwell B. Free radicals, reactive oxygen species and human disease: a critical evaluation with special reference to atherosclerosis. Br J Exp Pathol 1989;70:737-57.

172. Robbins SL. Cellular injury and cellular death. In: Robbins SL, ed. Pathologic Basis of Disease. 5th ed. Philadelphia: W. B. Saunders Co; 1994:1-34.

173. Slater TF. Free radical mechanisms in tissue injury. Biochem 1984;222:1-15.

174. Traystman RJ, Kirsch JR, Koehler RC. Oxygen radical mechanisms of brain injury following ischemia and reperfusion. J Appl Physiol 1991;71:1185-95.

175. Kukreja RC, Hess ML. The oxygen free radical system: from equations through membrane protein interactions to cardiovascular injury and protection. Cardiovasc Res 1992;26:641-55.

176. Loesser KE, Qian Y-Z, Wei EP. In vivo protection of ischemia reperfusion injury by histidine, a singlet oxygen scavenger. FASEB J 1992;6(A1342).

177. Chance B, Sies H, Boveris A. Hydroperoxide metabolism in mammalian organs. Physiol Rev 1979;59:527-605.

178. Turrens JF, Freeman BA, Levitt JG, et al. The effect of hyperoxia on superoxide production by lung submitochondrial particles. Arch Biochem Biophys 1982;217:401-10.

179. Halliwell B. Oxidants and human disease: some new concepts. FASEB J 1987;1:358-64.

180. Weiss SJ. Oxygen, ischaemia and inflammation. Acta Physiol Scand Suppl 1986;548:9-37.

181. Perry MO. Skeletal muscle ischemia and revascularization injury. In: Bernhard VM, Towne JB, eds. Complications in Vascular Surgery. St Louis, MO: Quality Medical Publishing; 1991:330-5.

182. Kazui M, Andreoni KA, Norris EJ, et al. Breath ethane: a specific indicator of free radical mediated lipid peroxidation following reperfusion of the ischemic liver. Free Radic Biol Med 1992;13:509-15.

183. Kazui M, Andreoni KA, Williams M, et al. Visceral lipid peroxidation occurs at reperfusion after supraceliac aortic cross-clamping. J Vasc Surg 1994;19:473-77.

184. Lands WEM, Lee R, Smith M. Factors regulating the biosynthesis of various prostaglandins. Ann NY Acad Sci 1971;180:107.

185. Smith WL, Lands WE. Oxygenation of polyunsaturated fatty acids during prostaglandin biosynthesis by sheep vesicular gland. Biochemistry 1972;11:3276-85.

186. Svensson LG, Ritter CV, Oosthuizen MMJ, et al. Prevention of gastric mucosal lesions following aortic cross-clamping. Br J Surg 1987; 74:282-5.

187. Svensson LG. Facteurs étiologiques et prevention de la paraplegia après champage de l'aorte thoracique. In: Kieffer E, ed. Chirugie de l'aorte thoracique descendante et thoracoabdominale. Paris: Expansion Scientifique Française; 1986:99-103.

188. Piper PJ. Pharmacology of leukotrienes. Br Med Bull 1983;39:255-9.

189. Tagari P, Boullin DJ, Du Boulay GH, et al. Vasoconstrictor and vasodilator effects of leukotriene D_4, and FPL 55712 on human and rat cerebral arteries. Adv Prostaglandin Thromboxane Leukot Res 1983;12:357-64.

190. Moskowitz MA, Kiwak KJ, Hekimian K, Levine L. Synthesis of compounds with properties of leukotrienes C_4 and D_4 in gerbil brains after ischemia and reperfusion. Science 1984;224:886-9.

191. Baiping L, Xiujuan T, Hongwei C, Qiming X, Quling G. Effect of moderate hypothermia on lipid peroxidation in canine brain tissue after cardiac arrest and resuscitation. Stroke 1994;25:147-52.

192. Boveris A. Mitochondrial production of superoxide radical and hydrogen peroxide. Adv Exp Med Biol 1977;78:67-82.

193. Turrens JF, Freeman BA, Levitt JG, Crapo JD. The effect of hyperoxia on superoxide production by lung submitochondrial particles. Arch Biochem Biophys 1982;217:401-10.

194. Welbourn CRB, Goldman G, Paterson IS, et al. Pathophysiology of ischaemia-reperfusion injury: central role of the neutrophil. Br J Surg 1991;78:651-5.

195. Halliwell B, Gutteridge JMC. Oxygen toxicity, oxygen radicals, transition metals and disease. Biochem J 1984;219:1-14.

196. Rosen GM, Freeman BA. Detection of superoxide generated by endothelial cells. Proc Natl Acad Sci USA 1984;81:7269-73.

197. Davalos A, Fernandez-Real JM, Ricart W, et al. Iron-related damage in acute ischemic stroke. Stroke 1994;25:1543-6.

198. Sadrzadeh SMH, Anderson DK, Panter SS, et al. Hemoglobin potentiates central nervous system damage. J Clin Invest 1979;79:662-4.

199. Sadrzadeh SMH, Eaton JW. Hemoglobin-induced oxidant damage to the central nervous system requires endogenous ascorbate. J Clin Invest 1988;82:1510-5.

200. Ciuffi M, Gentilini G, Franchi-Micheli S, Zilletti L. Lipid peroxidation induced 'in vivo' by iron-carbohydrate complex in the rat brain cortex. Neurochem Res 1991;16:43-9.

201. Gutteridge JMC, Richmond R, Halliwell B. Inhibition of iron-catalysed formation of hydroxyl radicals from superoxide and of lipid peroxidation by desferrioxamine. Biochem J 1979;184:469-72.

202. Aust DS, White BC. Iron chelation prevents tissue injury following ischemia. Adv Free Rad Biol Med 1985;1:1-17.

203. Hernandez LA, Grisham MB, Granger DN. A role for iron in oxidant-mediated ischemic injury to intestinal microvasculature. Am J Physiol 1986;253:G49-53.

204. Braughler JM, Pregenzer JF, Chase RL, et al. Novel 21-amino steroids as potent inhibitors of iron-dependent lipid peroxidation. J Biol Chem 1987;262:10438-40.

205. Braughler JM, Pregenzer JF. The 21-aminosteroid inhibitors of lipid peroxidation: reactions with lipid peroxyl and phenoxy radicals. Free Rad Biol Med 1989;7:125-30.

206. Takeshima R, Kirsh JR, Koehler RC, Traystman RJ. Tirilazad treatment does not decrease early brain injury after transient focal ischemia in cats. Stroke 1994;25:670-6.

207. Hall ED, Travis MA. Inhibition of arachidonic acid-induced vasogenic brain edema by the non-glucocorticoid 21-aminosteroid U74006F. Brain Res 1988;451:350-2.

208. Xue D, Sliuka A, Buchan AM. Tirilazad reduces cortical infarction after transient but not permanent focal cerebral ischemia in rats. Stroke 1992;23:894-9.

209. Chan PH, Longar S, Fishman RA. Protective effects of liposome-entrapped superoxide dismutase on post-traumatic brain edema. Ann Neurol 1987;21:540-7.

210. Imaizumi S, Woolworth V, Fishman RA, Chan PH. Liposome-entrapped superoxide dismutase reduces cerebral infarction in cerebral ischemia in rat. Stroke 1990;21:1312-7.

211. Qayumi AK, Janusz MT, Eric Jamieson WR, Lyster DM. Pharmacologic interventions for prevention of spinal cord injury caused by aortic crossclamping. J Thor Cardiovasc Surg 1992;104:256-61.

212. Qayumi AK, Janusz MT, Dorovini-Zis K, et al. Additive effect of allopurinol and deferoxamine in the prevention of spinal cord injury caused by aortic crossclamping. J Thor Cardiovasc Surg 1994;107:1203-9.

213. Coghlan JG, Flitter WD, Glutton SM, et al. Allopurinol pretreatment improves postoperative recovery and reduces lipid peroxidation in patients undergoing coronary artery bypass grafting. J Thorac Cardiovasc Surg 1994;107(1):248-56.

214. Zhen R, Wenxiang D, Zhaokang S, et al. Mechanisms of brain injury

with deep hypothermic circulatory arrest and protective effects of coenzyme Q_{10}. J Thor Cardiovasc Surg 1993;108:126–33.

215. Qayumi AK, Jamieson WRE, Godin DV, et al. Response to allopurinol pretreatment in a swine model of heart-lung transplantation. J Invest Surg 1990;3:331–40.

216. Eddy LJ, Stewart JR, Jones HP, et al. Free radical-producing enzyme, xanthine oxidase, is undetectable in human hearts. Am J Physiol 1987;253:H709–11.

217. Muxfeldt M, Schaper W. The activity of xanthine oxidase in the hearts of pigs, guinea pigs, rabbits, rats and humans. Bas Res Cardiol 1987;82:486–92.

218. Grum CM, Gallagher KP, Kirsh MM, Shlafer M. Absence of detectable xanthine oxidase in human myocardium. J Mol Cell Cardiol 1989;21:263–7.

219. Michelson AM, Puget K. Cell penetration by exogenous superoxide dismutase. Acta Physiol Scand Suppl 1980;492:67–80.

220. Shlafer M, Kane PF, Kirsch MM. Superoxide dismutase plus catalase enhance the efficacy of hypothermia cardioplegia to protect the globally ischemic, reperfused heart. J Thorac Cardiovasc Surg 1982; 83:830–9.

221. Svensson LG, Von Ritter CM, Groenveld HT, et al. Cross-clamping of the thoracic aorta: influence of aortic shunts, laminectomy, papaverine, calcium channel blockers, allopurinol, and superoxide dismutase on spinal cord blood flow and paraplegia in baboons. Ann Surg 1986;204:38–47.

222. Fridovich I. The biology of oxygen radicals. Science 1978;201: 875–80.

223. Laschinger JC, Cunningham JN, Cooper MM, et al. Prevention of ischemic spinal cord injury following aortic cross-clamping: use of corticosteroids. Ann Thorac Surg 1984;38:500–7.

224. Myers CL, Weiss SJ, Kirsh MM, et al. Effects of supplementing hypothermic crystalloid cardioplegic solution with catalase, superoxide dismutase, allopurinol, or deferoxamine on functional recovery of globally ischemic and reperfused isolated hearts. J Thorac Cardiovasc Surg 1986;91:281–9.

225. Menasche P, Piwnica A. Free radicals and myocardial protection: a surgical viewpoint. Ann Thorac Surg 1989;47:939–45.

226. Bagchi D, Prasad A, Das DK. Direct scavenging of free radicals by captopril, an angiotensin converting enzyme inhibitor. Biochem Biophys Res Commun 1989;158:52–7.

227. Parks DA, Bulkley GB, Granger DN. Role of oxygen-derived free radicals in digestive tract disease. Surgery 1983;94:15–22.

228. Freeman BA, Crapo JD. Biology of disease, free radicals and tissue injury. Lab Invest 1982;47:412–26.

229. Epstein CJ, Avraham KB, Lovett M, et al. Transgenic mice with increased Cu/Zn-superoxide dismutase activity: animal model of dosage effects in Down syndrome. Proc Natl Acad Sci USA 1987; 84:8044–8.

230. Yang G, Chan PH, Chen J, et al. Human copper-zinc superoxide dismutase transgenic mice are highly resistant to reperfusion injury after focal cerebral ischemia. Stroke 1994;25:165–70.

231. Klausner JM, Paterson IS, Mannick JA, et al. Reperfusion pulmonary edema. JAMA 1989;261:1030–5.

232. Arnold WP, Mittal CK, Katsuki S, Murad F. Nitric oxide activates guanulate cyclase and increases guanosine 3':5'-cyclic monophosphate levels in various tissue preparations. Proc Natl Acad Sci USA 1977;74:3023–7.

233. Furchgott RF, Zawadzki JV. The obligatory role of endothelial cells in the relaxation of arterial smooth muscle by acetylcholine. Nature 1980;288:373–6.

234. Myers PR, Minor RL, Guerra R, et al. Vasorelaxant properties of the endothelium-derived relaxing factor more closely resemble S-nitrosocysteine than nitric oxide. Nature 1990;(161–4).

235. Moncada S, Palmer RMJ, Higgs EA. Nitric oxide: physiology, pathophysiology, and pharmacology. Pharmacol Rev 1991;43:109–42.

236. Bredt DS, Snyder SH. Nitric oxide, a novel neuronal messenger. Neuron 1992;8:3–11.

237. Rees DD, Palmer RM, Hodson HF, Moncada S. A specific inhibitor of nitric oxide formation from L-arginine attenuates endothelium-dependent relaxation. Br J Pharmacol 1989;96:418–24.

238. Persson MG, Wiklund NP, Gustafsson LE. Nitric oxide requirement for vasomotor nerve-induced vasodilatation and modulation of resting blood flow in muscle microcirculation. Acta Physiol Scand 1991;141:49–56.

239. Nishimura H, Rosenblum WI, Nelson GH, Boynton S. Agents that modify EDRF formation alter antiplatelet properties of brain arteriolar endothelium in vivo. Am J Physiol 1991;261:H15–21.

240. Rosenblum WI, Nishimura H, Ellis EF, Nelson GH. The endothelium-dependent effects of thimerosal on mouse pial arterioles in vivo: evidence for control of microvascular events by EDRF as well as prostaglandins. J Cereb Blood Flow Metab 1992;12:703–6.

241. Heinzel B, John M, Klatt P, et al. Ca^{2+}/calmodulin-dependent formation of hydrogen peroxide by brain nitric oxide synthase. Biochem J 1992;281:627–30.

242. Pou S, Pou WS, Bredt DS, et al. Generation of superoxide by purified brain nitric oxide synthase. J Biol Chem 1992;267: 24173–6.

243. Klatt P, Schmidt K, Uray G, Mayer B. Multiple catalytic functions of brain nitric oxide synthase. J Biol Chem 1993;268:14781–7.

244. Dawson VL, Dawson TM, London ED, et al. Nitric oxide mediates glutamate neurotoxicity in primary cortical cultures. Proc Natl Acad Sci USA 1991;88:6368–71.

245. Reif DW. Delayed production of nitric oxide contributes to NMDA-mediated neuronal damage. Neuroreport 1993;4:566–8.

246. Snyder SH. Nitric oxide: first in a new class of neurotransmitters. Science 1992;257:494–6.

247. Faraci FM, Brian JE. Nitric oxide and the cerebral circulation. Stroke 1994;25:692–703.

248. Garthwaite J, Garthwaite G, Palmer RMJ, Moncada S. NMDA receptor activation induces nitric oxide synthesis from arginine in rat brain slices. Eur J Pharmacol 1989;172:413–6.

249. Murphy S, Minor R. R, Welk G, Harrison DG. Evidence for an astrocyte-derived vasorelaxing factor with properties similar to nitric oxide. J Neurochem 1990;55:349–51.

250. Toda N, Okamura T. Mechanism underlying the response to vasodilator nerve stimulation in isolated dog and monkey cerebral arteries. Am J Physiol 1990;259:H 1511–7.

251. Bredt DS, Snyder SH. Nitric oxide mediates glutamate-linked enhancement of cGMP levels in the cerebellum. Proc Natl Acad Sci USA 1989;86:9030–3.

252. Radomski MW, Palmer RM, Mocada S. An L-arginine/nitric oxide pathway present in human platelets regulates aggregation. Proc Natl Acad Sci USA 1990;87:5193–7.

253. Marletta MA. Nitric oxide: biosynthesis and biological significance. Trends Biol Sci 1989;14:488–92.

254. East SJ, Garthwaite J. NMDA receptor activation in rat hippocampus induces cyclic GMP formation through the L-arginine-nitric oxide pathway. Neurosci Lett 1991;123:17–9.

255. Southam E, East SJ, Garthwaite J. Excitatory amino acid receptors coupled to the nitric oxide/cyclic GMP pathway in rat cerebellum during development. J Neurochem 1991;56:2072–81.

256. Miki N, Kawabe Y, Kuriyama K. Activation of cerebral guanylate cyclase by nitric oxide. Biochem Biophys Res Commun 1977;75: 851–6.

257. Förstermann U, Schmidt HHHW, Pollack JS, et al. Isoforms of nitric oxide synthase. Biochem Pharmacol 1991;42:1849–57.

258. Geller D, Lowenstein C, Shapiro R, et al. Molecular coning and expression of inducible nitric oxide synthase from human hepatocytes. Proc Natl Acad Sci USA 1993;90:3491–5.

259. Sessa WC, Harrison JK, Luthin DR, et al. Genomic analysis and expression patterns reveal distinct genes for endothelial and brain nitric oxide synthase. Hypertension 1993;21:934–8.

260. Bredt DS, Hwang PM, Snyder SH. Localization of nitric oxide synthase indicating a neural role for nitric oxide. Nature 1990;347: 768–770.

261. Schimdt HHHW, Lohmann SM, Walter U. The nitric oxide and cGMP signal transduction system: regulation and mechanism of action. Biochim Biophys Acta 1993;1178:153–5.

262. Stuehr DJ, Griffith OW. Mammalian nitric oxide synthases. Adv Enzymol Relat Areas Mole Biol 1992;65:287–346.

263. Pollock JS, Förstermann U, Mitchell JA, et al. Purification and characterization of particular endothelium-derived relaxing factor synthase from cultured and native bovine aortic endothelial cells. Proc Natl Acad Sci USA 1991;88:10480–4.

264. Marshall JJ, Wei EP, Kontos HA. Independent blockade of cerebral vasodilation from acetylcholine and nitric oxide. Am J Physiol 1988;255:H847–54.

265. Yang ST, Mayhan WG, Faraci FM, Heistad DD. Endothelium-dependent responses of cerebral vessels during chronic hypertension. Hypertension 1991;17:612–8.

266. Marsden PA, Schappert KT, Chen HS, et al. Molecular cloning and characterization of human endothelial nitric oxide synthase. FEBS Lett 1992;307:287-93.

267. Kuku Y, Yonekawa Y, Tsukahara T, Kazekawa K. Superselective intra-arterial infusion of papaverine for the treatment of cerebral vasospasm after subarachnoid hemorrhage. J Neurosurg 1992;77:842-7.

268. Watanabe M, Rosenblum W, Nelson GH. In vivo effect of emthylene blue on endothelium-dependent and endothelium-independent dilations of brain microvessels in mice. Circ Res 1988;62:86-90.

269. Katusic ZS, Marshall JJ, Kontos HA, Vanhoutte PM. Similar responsiveness of smooth muscle of the canine basilar artery to EDRF and nitric oxide. Am J Physiol 1989;257:H1235-9.

270. Kim P, Schini VB, Sundt TM, Vanhoutte PM. Reduced production of cGMP underlies the loss of endothelium-dependent relaxations in the canine basilar artery after subarachnoid hemorrhage. Circ Res 1992;70:248-56.

271. Faraci FM. Role of endothelium-derived relaxing factor in cerebral circulation: large arteries vs. microcirculation. Am J Physiol 1991;261:H1038-42.

272. Bauknight GC, Faraci FM, Heistad DD. Endothelium-derived relaxing factor modulates noradrenergic constriction of cerebral arterioles in rabbits. Stroke 1992;23:1522-6.

273. Wei EP, Kukreja R, Kontos HA. Effects of inhibition of nitric oxide synthesis on cerebral vasodilation and endothelium-derived relaxing factor from acetylcholine. Stroke 1992;23:1623-9.

274. Nathan CF, Hibbs JB Jr. Role of nitric oxide synthesis in macrophage antimicrobial activity. Curr Opin Immunol 1991;3:65-70.

275. Ma X-L, Weyrich AS, Lefer DJ, Lefer AM. Diminished basal nitric oxide release after myocardial ischemia and reperfusion promotes neurophil adherence to coronary endothelium. Circ Res 1993;72:403-12.

276. Hutcheson IR, Whittle BJR, Boughton-Smith NK. Role of nitric oxide in maintaining vascular integrity in endotoxin-induced acute intestinal madage in the rat. Br J Pharmacol 1990;101:815-20.

277. Kubes P, Suzuki M, Granger DN. Nitric oxide: an endogenous modulator of leukocyte adhesion. Proc Natl Acad Sci USA 1991;88:4651-5.

278. Kubes P, Granger DN. Nitric oxide modulates microvascular permeability. Am J Physiol 1992;262:H611-5.

279. Filep JG, Foldes-Filep E, Sirois P. Nitric oxide modulates vascular permeability in the rat coronary circulation. Br J Pharmacol 1993;108:323-6.

280. Kurose I, Wolf R, Grisham MB, Granger DN. Modulation of ischemia/reperfusion-induced microvascular dysfunction by nitric oxide. Cir Res 1994;74:376-82.

281. Beckman JS, Beckman TW, Chen J, et al. Apparent hydroxyl radical production by peroxynitrite: implications for endothelial injury from nitric oxide and superoxide. Proc Natl Acad Sci USA 1990;87:1620-4.

282. Kader A, Frazzini VI, Solomon RA, Trifiletti RR. Nitric oxide production during focal cerebral ischemia in rats. Stroke 1993;24:1709-16.

283. Montague PR, Gancayco CD, Winn MJ, et al. Role of NO production in NMDA receptor-mediated neurotransmitter release in cerebral cortex. Science 1994;263:973-7.

284. Zhang ZG, Chopp M, Zaloga C, et al. Cerebral endothelial nitric oxide synthase expression after focal cerebral ischemia in rats. Stroke 1993;24:2016-22.

285. Kano M, Moskowitz MA, Yokota M. Parasympathetic denervation of rat pial vessels significantly increases infarction volume following middle cerebral artery occlusion. J Cereb Blood Flow Metab 1991;11:628-37.

286. Nishikawa T, Kirsh JR, Koehler RC, et al. Effect of nitric oxide synthase inhibition on cerebral blood flow and injury volume during focal ischemia in cats. Stroke 1993;24:1717-24.

287. Nishikawa T, Kirsh JR, Koehler RC, et al. Nitric oxide synthase inhibition reduces caudate injury following transient focal ischemia in cats. Stroke 1994;25:877-85.

288. Petros A, Bennett D, Vallance P. Effect of nitric oxide synthase inhibitors on hypotension in patients with septic shock. Lancet 1991;338:1557-8.

289. Meyer J, Lentz CW, Stothert JC, et al. Effects of nitric oxide synthesis inhibition in hyperdynamic endotoxemia. Crit Care Med 1994;22:306-12.

290. Yamamoto S, Golanov EV, Berger SB, Reis DJ. Inhibition of nitric oxide synthesis increases focal ischemic infarction in rat. J Cereb Blood Flow Metab 1992;12:717-26.

291. Coyle P. Different susceptibilities to cerebral infarction in spontaneously hypertensive (SHR) and normotensive Sprague-Dawley rats. Stroke 1986;17:520-25.

292. Mourlon-Le Grand MC, Benessiano J, Levy BI. cGMP pathway and mechanical properties of carotid artery wall in WKY rats and SHR: role of endothelium. Am J Physiol 1992;263:H61-7.

293. Zhang J, Dawson VL, Dawson TM, Snyder SH. Nitric oxide activation of poly(ADP-ribose) synthetase in neurotoxicity. Science 1994;263:687-9.

294. Baker AJ, Zornow MH, Scheller MS, et al. Changes in extracellular concentration glutamate, aspartate, glycine, dopamine, serotonin, and dopamine metabolites after transient global ischemia in the rabbit brain. J Neurochem 1991;57:1370-9.

295. Malinski T, Bailey F, Zhang ZG, Chopp M. Nitric oxide measured by a porphysinic microsensor in rat brain after transient middle cerebral artery occlusion. J Cereb Blood Flow Metab 1993;13:355-8.

296. Lipton SA, Choi Y-B, Pan Z-H, et al. A redox-based mechanism for the neuroprotective and neurodestructive effects of nitric oxide and related nitroso-compounds. Nature 1993;364:626-32.

297. Robles A, Vaughan M, Lau JK, et al. Long-term assessment of aortic valve replacement with autologous pulmonary valve. Ann Thorac Surg 1985;39:238-42.

298. Collingridge GL, Kehl SJ, McLannan H. Excitatory amino acids in synaptic transmission in the Schaffer collateral-commissural pathway of the rat hippocampus. J Physiol (Lond) 1983;334:33-46.

299. Errington ML, Lynch MA, Bliss TV. Long-term potentiation in the dentate gyrus: induction and increased glutamate release are blocked by D(-)aminophosphonovalerate. Neurosci 1987;20:279-84.

300. Lynch G, Larson J, Kelso S, et al. Intracellular injections of EGTA block induction of hippocampal long-term potentiation. Nature 1983;305:719-21.

301. Malenka RC. Postsynaptic factors control the duration of synaptic enhancement in area CA1 of the hippocampus. Neuron 1991;6:53-60.

302. Schuman EM, Madison DV. A requirement for the intercellular messenger nitric oxide in long-term potentiation. Science 1991;254:1503-6.

303. Izumi Y, Clifford DB, Zorumski CF. Inhibition of long-term potentiation by NMDA-mediated nitric oxide release. Science 1992;257:1273-6.

304. Haley JE, Wilcox, Chapman PF. The role of nitric oxide in hippocampal long-term potentiation. Neuron 1992;8:211-6.

305. Bigelow WG, Callaghan JC, Hoops JA. General hypothermia for experimental intracardiac surgery. Ann Surg 1950;132:531-9.

306. Bigelow WG, Lindsay WK, Greenwood WF. Hypothermia—Its possible role in cardiac surgery: an investigation of factors governing survival in dogs at low body temperatures. Ann Surg 1950;132:849-66.

307. Bigelow WG, McBirnie JE. Further experiences with hypothermia for intracardiac surgery in monkeys and groundhogs. Ann Surg 1953;137:361-8.

308. Bjork VO, Hultquist G. Brain damage in children after deep hypothermia for open heart surgery. Thorax 1960;15:284-91.

309. Barnard CN, Schire V. The surgical treatment of acquired aneurysms of the thoracic aorta. Thorax 1963;18:101-5.

310. Silverberg GD, Reitz BA, Ream AK. Hypothermia and cardiac arrest in the treatment of giant aneurysms of the cerebral circulation and hemangioblastoma of the medulla. J Neurosurg 1981;55:337-46.

311. Tan PS, Aveling W, Pugsley WB, et al. Experience with circulatory arrest and hypothermia to facilitate thoracic aortic surgery. Ann R Col Surg Engl 1989;71:81-6.

312. Busto R, Dietrich WD, Globus MYT, et al. Small differences in intraischemic brain temperature critically determine the extent of ischemic neuronal injury. J Cereb Blood Flow Metab 1987;7:729-38.

313. Busto R, Globus MYT, Dietrich WD, et al. Effect of mild hypothermia on ischemia induced release of neurotransmitters and free fatty acids in rat brain. Stroke 1989;20:904-10.

314. Welsh FA, Sims RE, Harris VA. Mild hypothermia prevents ischemia in gerbil hippocampus. J Cereb Blood Flow Metab 1990;10:557-63.

315. Allen BT, Davis CG, Osborne D, Karl I. Spinal cord ischemia and

reperfusion metabolism: the effect of hypothermia. J Vasc Surg 1994;19(2):332–340.

316. Carolei A, Fieschi C, Bruno R, Toffano G. Monosialoganglioside GM$_1$ in cerebral ischemia. Cerebrovasc Brain Metab Rev 1991;3:134–57.

317. The SASS investigators. Ganglioside GM$_1$ in acute ischemic stroke: the SASS trial. Stroke 1994;25:1141–8.

318. Lenzi GL, Grigoletto F, Gent M, et al. Early treatment of stroke with monosialoganglioside GM-1: Efficacy and safety results of the early stroke trial. Stroke 1994;25:1552–8.

319. Kochawek PM, Hallenback JM. Polymorphonuclear leukocytes and monocytes/macrophages in the pathogenesis of cerebral ischemia and stroke. Stroke 1992;23:1367–79.

320. Vaccarino F, Guidotti A, Costa E. Ganglioside inhibition of gluta-mate-mediated protein kinase C translocation in primary cultures of cerebral neurons. Proc Natl Acad Sci USA 1987;84:8707–11.

321. Geisler FH, Dorsey FC, Coleman WP. Correction: recovery of motor function after spinal-cord injury—a randomized, placebo-controlled trial with GM-1 ganglioside. N Engl J Med 1991;325:1659–60.

322. Toung TJK, Kirsch JR, Maruki Y, Traystman RJ. Effects of pentoxi-fylline on cerebral blood flow, metabolism, and evoked response after total cerebral ischemia in dogs. Crit Care Med 1994;22:273–81.

323. Kohut JJ, Bednar MM, Kimelberg HK, et al. Reduction in ischemic brain injury in rabbits by the anion transport inhibitor L-644,711. Stroke 1992;23:93–7.

324. Hamberg M, Svensson J, Sammuelsson B. Thromboxanes: a new group of biologically active compounds derived from prostaglandin endoperoxides. Proc Natl Acad Sci USA 1975;72:2994–8.

325. Grace PAI-riBJS86-6 1994. Ischaemia-reperfusion injury. Br J Surg 1994;81:637–47.

326. Shohami E, Rosenthal J, Lavy S. The effect of incomplete cerebral ischemia on prostaglandin levels in rat brain. Stroke 1982;13:494–9.

327. Matsuo Y, Izumiyama M, Onodera H, et al. Effect of a novel throm-boxane A$_2$ receptor antagonist, S-1452, on postischemic brain injury in rats. Stroke 1993;24:2059–65.

328. Pegg AE, McCann. Polyamine metabolism and function. Am J Physi-ol 1982;243:C211–21.

329. Schmitz MP, Combs DJ, Dempsey RJ. Difluoromethylornithine decreases postischemic brain edema and blood-brain barrier break-down. Neurosurg 1993;33:882–8.

330. Dempsey RJ, Roy MW, Meyer K, et al. Polyamine and prostaglandin markers in focal cerebral ischemia. Neurosurg 1985;17:635–40.

331. Hallenbeck J, Dutka A. Background review and current concepts of reperfusion injury. Arch Neurol 1990;47:1245–54.

332. Granger DN, Kvietys PR, Perry MA. Leukocyte-endothelial cell adhe-sion induced by ischemia and reperfusion. Can J Physiol Pharmacol 1993;71:67–75.

333. Clark GD, Happel LT, Zorumski CF, Bazan NG. Enhancement of hip-pocampal excitatory synaptic transmission by platelet-activating fac-tor. Neuron 1992;9:1211–6.

334. Menasche P, Grousset C, Gouduely M, Piwnica A. Prevention of hydroxyl radical formation: a critical concept for improving cardio-plegia. Circulation 1987;76:V2–180.

335. Simpson RK Jr, Robertson CS, Goodman JC. Spinal cord ischemia-induced elevation of amino acids: extracellular measurement with microdialysis. Neurochem Res 1990;15:635–9.

336. Faden AI, Simon RP. A potential role for excitotoxins in the patho-physiology of spinal cord injury. Ann Neurol 1988;23:623–6.

337. Redmond JM, Gillinov AM, Zehr KJ, et al. Glutamate excitotoxicity: a mechanism of neurologic injury associated with hypothermic cir-culatory arrest. J Thorac Cardiovasc Surg 1994;107:776–87.

338. Bolt S, Arnal J-F, Xu Y, et al. Spinal cord infarcts during long-term inhibition of nitric oxide synthase in rats. Stroke 1994;25:1666–73.

Deep Hypothermia with Circulatory Arrest and Retrograde Brain Perfusion

HISTORY

Early research with deep hypothermia and circulatory arrest, but without the use of cardiopulmonary bypass, was performed by Bigelow and associates[1, 2] in animals. Subsequently Lewis and Taufic[3] used deep hypothermia to repair an atrial septal defect with use of venous inflow occlusion. The development of the technique of cardiopulmonary bypass for cardiovascular operations must surely be counted as one of the great achievements of modern medicine. Gibbon[4] first tested the technique in animals and later used it in patients.[5] Bjork's[6] and Senning's[7] early research led to removal of an atrial myxoma by the technique.[8] In 1963, on the basis of research by Terblanche,[9] Barnard and Schire[10] used cardiopulmonary bypass with deep hypothermia and circulatory arrest in patients with aortic aneurysm disease and aortic dissection. In the same report, Barnard introduced moderate hypothermia to 32° C with atriofemoral bypass for descending aortic operations.

pH CONTROL OF PERFUSATE

Despite many years of use of deep hypothermia with circulatory arrest, controversy continues as to how best to manage pH and $Paco_2$. From our experience[11] with 656 patients undergoing circulatory arrest, we are of the opinion that the alpha-stat is safe; however, in recent publications it has been reported that pH-stat may be better for infants.[12] For alpha-stat, perfusate pH and $Paco_2$ (at normal temperature, uncorrected for hypothermia) are kept at approximately pH 7.4 and $Paco_2$ at 30 to 40 mm Hg by relative hyperventilation.[13] The net result is that the pH is elevated and alkalotic (approximately pH 7.6) when measured at the lower temperature.

Similarly, $Paco_2$ is approximately 14 to 24 mm Hg at 20° C (respiratory alkalosis). For pH-stat, $Paco_2$ during hypothermia, corrected for temperature, is at 30 to 40 mm Hg and pH at 7.4. This is done by adding CO_2, resulting in res-

piratory acidosis when measured at normal temperature. Table 13-1 shows the differences.

The reason for using hypothermia during circulatory arrest is that it slows metabolic activity, thus reducing the rate of use of substrates, including oxygen. The rate of metabolic activity is related in Arrhenius' equation, which relates temperature to the rate constant of a chemical reaction. The equation does not, however, account for the metabolism that continues during hypothermia. Evidence from the work of Govier and colleagues[14] suggests that oxygen consumption may continue because autoregulation is maintained despite lower pressures and flow rates. There is some controversy over the actual measured oxygen consumption. Fox and associates[15, 16] found that oxygen demand is only slightly diminished at a temperature of 20° C. Oxygen consumption may be uncoupled from metabolic activity at a lower temperature, but it rapidly returns on rewarming. Cooling below 10° C, however, may be hazardous.[13, 17, 18]

Critical to the function of metabolic pathways and the function of enzymes is the presence of high-energy phosphate stores. Obviously, during normothermia, high-energy phosphates are rapidly depleted by normal metabolic activity if they are not replenished during ischemia. Norwood

TABLE 13-1   DIFFERENCES IN ALPHA-STAT AND PH-STAT AT 37° AND 20° C

	Alpha-stat	pH stat
Measured at 37° C		
pH	7.4	7.2
$Paco_2$ (mm Hg)	35.4	45
Measured at 20° C		
pH	7.6	7.4
$Paco_2$ (mm Hg)	18	35
	Constant H^+/OH^-	Constant H^+

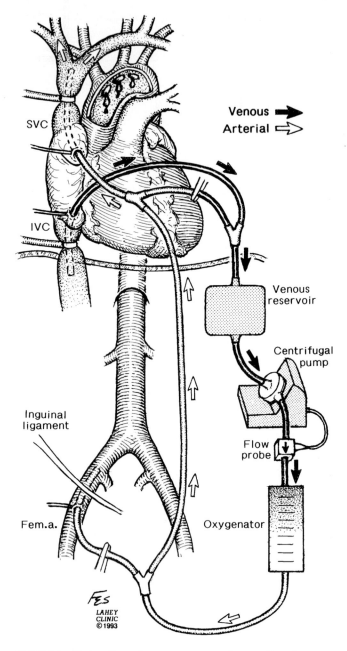

lactic acid production, which would cause a decrease in pH with the risk of causing neural tissue injury (see detailed discussion of neural ischemia in Chapter 12).[13]

Because of the risks associated with intracellular acidosis, we have favored the alpha-stat method of pH control in the belief that this may reduce the risk of intracellular acidosis. However, one of the reasons that the pH-stat method has been advocated is that adding CO_2 dilates the cerebral vasculature, thus increasing blood flow and also allowing the increasingly stiffer red cells at hypothermia to traverse the capillaries.[13] This viewpoint does not however, take into account the effect of hemodilution on blood viscosity during cardiopulmonary bypass. Cooley and associates[21] showed that it was safe to add crystalloid as the prime for cardiopulmonary bypass and that a lower hematocrit is well tolerated. Furthermore, Murkin and colleagues[22] have shown that with the pH-stat method of pH control, autoregulation by metabolic demands of the brain is uncoupled, resulting in a relative hyperperfusion of the brain, which may have harmful effects.

The method by which electrochemical neutrality in cells is maintained was first described by Rahn and coworkers.[23] Critical to this process was the balance between H^+ and OH^- on the alpha-imidazole groups of the histidine molecule. When the alpha-stat method is used, a constant charge is kept to maintain electrochemical neutrality; thus the ratio of the alpha-imidazole H^+ to OH^- is kept constant. In contradistinction, with the pH-stat method the concentration of H^+ is kept constant. A further advantage of the alpha-stat method is that histidine is still able to buffer any possible acid build-up during prolonged periods of circulatory arrest. In summary, with the alpha-stat method of pH control, CO_2 levels are adjusted so that pH and Pa_{CO_2} measured (uncorrected) at 37° C are within normal range.[11, 13]

ELECTROENCEPHALOGRAM MONITORING AND TEMPERATURE MEASUREMENT

For deep hypothermia with circulatory arrest to be used for longer periods, it is essential that electrical silence of the entire brain, not just of the cerebral cortex, be established. The reason for this is that neuronal activity uses up most of the oxygen and ATP requirement of the brain. To establish when electrical silence has occurred electroencephalograms (EEGs) are obtained during cooling. Early in the research of deep hypothermia, Woodhall and colleagues[24, 25] and others[9, 10] found this technique to be useful and showed that electrical silence usually occurred at a brain temperature of less than 20° C. Although Connally[11] has routinely monitored brain temperature during deep hypothermia, we have relied on temperatures measured at other sites. The reason for doing this, however, is the finding by Coselli from our group[26] that in humans temperatures measured at any specific site, such as the esophagus, rectum, or naso-

FIGURE 13–1 Cannula arrangement for cardiopulmonary bypass with deep hypothermic circulatory arrest and retrograde brain perfusion. Note the Y connection of the arterial line to the superior vena cava cannula and the tape around the superior vena cava.

and colleagues[19] have shown, however, that the stores of adenosine triphosphate (ATP) and phosphocreatine are not depleted during hypothermia in conjunction with ischemia (circulatory arrest) and that during reperfusion any depleted stores are restored. Swain and colleagues[20] have shown that high-energy phosphate stores may even be regenerated during deep hypothermic arrest. Norwood and associates[19] have shown that normal intracellular pH must be preserved so that high-energy phosphates are not depleted. Critical to preserving intracellular pH is the prevention of pharynx, do not correlate well with electrical silence as determined by EEG. To obviate this problem, patients are cooled until all measured temperatures are below 20° C and electrical silence has occurred at a sensitivity of 2 µV; then we cool for a further 5 minutes to allow temperature gradients to equilibrate. The circulation is only then arrested. Another reason for further cooling is the evidence that subcortical wave activity continues after cortical activity has disappeared.[13, 27] This continued activity can be monitored by somatosensory-evoked potentials.[13, 27]

ANCILLARY MEASURES

Barbiturates

Traditionally, barbiturates have been advocated as being protective for the brain. However, much of this research was performed during normothermia in animals or patients. Furthermore, during deep hypothermia, barbiturates have been reported to be protective if electrical silence has not been attained.[28, 29] We formerly used thiopental at a dosage of 20 mg/kg. However, because of the marked myocardial depressant effects and delayed awakening of patients with this high dosage, we have reduced the dose to 5 mg/kg.[11] This has resulted in patients' being considerably more alert the morning after the operation. A further reason for reducing the dosage is the recent finding by Swain's group[30] that thiopental may be harmful to the brain during deep hypothermia. Of note, hyperglycemia[31] may also be harmful, as has been shown after aortic cross-clamping and also in stroke victims.[13]

Membrane Stabilizers

Lidocaine in high doses suppresses metabolic activity by inhibiting the Na-K membrane pump and is reported to have an additive effect to hypothermia.[28] Furthermore, in a porcine spinal cord ischemia model using aortic cross-clamping, we[32] were able to reduce spinal cord injury by combining lidocaine with a cold solution at 5° C. Dilantin and etomidate are also reported to be protective.[33, 34] In the past we used high-dosage methylprednisolone sodium succinate (Solu-Medrol) for both brain and spinal cord protection during aortic operations. We found, however, that patients were more prone to sepsis and multiple organ failure with these steroids. Since we abandoned the use of steroids, the sepsis rate has declined and there has been no increase in neurological complications. It has also been reported that patients who are given steroids for traumatic spinal cord injuries have an increased rate of infections and complications and that hospitalization is prolonged, with an increase in expense.[35] Because calcium influx into cells and lipid peroxidation appear to occur during reperfusion, we use liberal amounts of mannitol to reduce the possible generation of oxygen free radicals (see Chapter 12).[11, 36]

RETROGRADE PERFUSION OF THE BRAIN

Retrograde flushing out of the cerebral circulation via the venous system during cardiopulmonary bypass in patients with air embolism was reported by Mills and Ochsner.[37] Subsequently, Lemole and associates[38] reported using the technique during antegrade arterial circulatory arrest for aortic arch operations. However, the method was popularized only when Japanese authors, among them Ueda and colleagues, noted the method's safety and protective effect. We reported our experience with more than 50 patients,[11] of whom a subgroup were analyzed in detail,[39] with only one postoperative stroke related to an embolus from the descending thoracic aorta. Lytle and colleagues[40] reported on 43 patients who had retrograde brain perfusion, with four postoperative deaths and three transient neurologic complications, and they also concluded that the technique was a useful adjunct. We continue to find that there is marked improvement in the patient's postoperative mental status, the incidence of stroke is lower, and the technique has caused no complications in our patients.

Currently retrograde perfusion via the superior vena cava (Fig. 13-1) is performed at a flow rate of 500 ml/min because this has been shown to be adequate to meet the oxygen and metabolic requirements of the brain during hypothermia when antegrade flow is used. Clearly, however, retrograde perfusion is not as effective as antegrade perfusion in delivering nutrients to the brain. The central (superior vena cava) pressure is maintained below 30 mm Hg.

The possible beneficial effects include flushing out of arterial embolic material, delivery of oxygen and metabolic substrate to the brain, removal of the products of metabolism, better pH control by the removal of lactic acid, maintenance of more uniform brain temperatures, and prevention of rewarming of the brain during circulatory arrest.[11] We prefer to use the term retrograde brain perfusion since this implies that the entire brain is perfused, as compared to the term retrograde cerebral perfusion. The latter term implies by anatomical definition that only the cerebral hemispheres are perfused. The term retrograde brain perfusion also has significance because recent research indicates that blood via Batson's vein plexus and the azygous system predominantly perfuses the medulla oblongata, pons, and brain stem, and less so, if at all, the cerebral hemispheres.

RESULTS

In our initial experience with 615 patients, the incidence of neurological complications was dependent on the length of the circulatory arrest period. Of 72 patients who had circulatory arrest for less than 15 minutes, none developed a neurological deficit. With 15 minutes of circulatory arrest, the risk increased to 5%, after 45 minutes it increased to 10%, and after 90 minutes to 20%. In a more detailed study of 656 patients,[11] it was found that the safe period of circulatory arrest was approximately 40 minutes for stroke and that after 65 minutes of circulatory arrest the mortality rate increased markedly. With the increasing use of retrograde perfusion of the brain, however, it would appear that longer periods of circulatory arrest may be better tolerated. Ergin and colleagues[41] analyzed their experience with hypothermic arrest in 200 patients and found similar results. Their mortality rate was 15%; 19% of their patients developed temporary neurologic deficits and 11% had embolic strokes. They found by multivariate analysis that older age and duration of circulatory arrest were predictors of temporary deficits and that older age and arch or descending aortic operations were predictors of embolic stroke.

Although hypothermic circulatory arrest with retrograde brain perfusion is safe for shorter periods of circulatory arrest, technical and pharmacological innovations are still required to make this technique safer for circulatory arrest periods longer than 60 minutes.

REFERENCES

1. Bigelow WG, Callaghan JC, Hoops JA. General hypothermia for experimental intracardiac surgery. Ann Surg 1950;132:531-9.
2. Bigelow WG, McBirnie JE. Further experiences with hypothermia for intracardiac surgery in monkeys and groundhogs. Ann Surg 1953;137:361-8.
3. Lewis FJ, Tauffic M. Closure of atrial septal defects with the aid of hypothermia: experimental accomplishments and the report of one successful case. Surgery 1953;33:52-8.
4. Gibbon JH Jr. The maintenance of life during experimental occlusion of the pulmonary artery followed by survival. Surg Gynecol Obstet 1939;69:602-14.
5. Gibbon JH Jr. Application of a mechanical heart and lung apparatus to cardiac surgery. Minn Med 1954;37:171-80.
6. Bjork VO. Brain perfusions in dogs with artificially oxygenated blood. Acta Chir Scand 1948;96(Supp 137):I-122.
7. Senning A. Ventricular fibrillation during extracorporeal circulation: used as a method to prevent air-embolisms and to facilitate intracardiac operations. Acta Chir Scand 1952;171:1.
8. Craaford C, Norberg B, Senning A. Clinical studies in extracorporeal circulation with a heart-lung machine. Acta Chir Scand 1957;112:200.
9. Terblanche J, Barnard CN. Profound hypothermia using extracorporeal circulation without an artificial oxygenator. S Afr Med J 1960;34:1003-8.
10. Barnard CN, Schire V. The surgical treatment of acquired aneurysms of the thoracic aorta. Thorax 1963;18:101-5.
11. Svensson LG, Crawford ES, Hess KR, et al. Deep hypothermia with circulatory arrest: determinants of stroke and early mortality in 656 patients. J Thorac Cardiovasc Surg 1992;106:19-31.
12. Newburger JW, Jonas RA, Wernovsky G, et al. A comparison of the perioperative neurologic effects of hypothermic circulatory arrest versus low-flow cardiopulmonary bypass in infant heart surgery. N Engl J Med 1993;329:1057-64.
13. Svensson LG, Crawford ES. Aortic dissection and aortic aneurysm surgery: clinical observations, experimental investigations and statistical analyses. Part I. Curr Probl Surg 1992;29:819-912.
14. Govier AV, Reves JG, McKay RD, et al. Factors and their influence on regional cerebral blood flow during nonpulsatile cardiopulmonary bypass. Ann Thorac Surg 1984;38:592-600.
15. Fox LS, Blackstone EH, Kirklin JW, et al. Relationship of whole body oxygen consumption to perfusion flow rate during hypothermic cardiopulmonary bypass. J Thorac Cardiovasc Surg 1982;83:239-48.
16. Fox LS, Blackston EH, Kirklin JW, et al. Relationship of brain blood flow and oxygen consumption to perfusion flow rate during profoundly hypothermic cardiopulmonary bypass. J Thorac Cardiovasc Surg 1984;87:658-64.
17. Bjork VO, Hultquist G. Brain damage in children after deep hypothermia for open heart surgery. Thorax 1960;15:284-91.
18. Bjork VO, Hultquist G. Contraindications to profound hypothermia in open heart surgery. J Thorac Cardiovasc Surg 1962;44:1-13.
19. Norwood WI, Norwood CR, Ingwall JS, et al. Hypothermic circulatory arrest: 31-phosphorus nuclear magnetic resonance of isolated perfused neonatal rat brain. J Thorac Cardiovasc Surg 1979;78:823-30.
20. Swain JA, McDonald TJ Jr, Balaban RS, et al. Metabolism of the heart and brain during hypothermic cardiopulmonary bypass. Ann Thorac Surg 1991;51:105-9.
21. Cooley DA, Beall AC Jr, Grondin P. Open heart operations using disposable oxygenators, five percent dextrose prime, and normothermia. Surgery 1962;52:713-9.
22. Murkin JM, Farrar JK, Tweed WA. Acid-base management during hypothermic cardiopulmonary bypass profoundly influences cerebral blood flow and cerebral auto-regulation (abstract). Anesthesiology 1986;65:A320.
23. Rahn H, Reeves RB, Howell BJ. Hydrogen ion regulation, temperature and evolution. In: Rahn H, Prakash O, eds: Acid-Base Regulation and Body Temperature. Boston: Nijhoff, 1985:55-80.
24. Woodhall B, Reynolds DH, Mahaley S Jr, et al. The physiological and pathological effects of localized cerebral hypothermia. Ann Surg 1958;147:673.
25. Woodhall B. Experimental and clinical studies in localized cerebral perfusion. Ann Surg 1959;150:640
26. Coselli JS, Crawford ES, Beall ACJ, et al. Determination of brain temperatures for safe circulatory arrest during cardiovascular operation. Ann Thorac Surg 1988;45:638-42.
27. Guerit JM, Soveges L, Baele P, et al. Median nerve somatosensory evoked potentials in profound hypothermia for ascending aorta repair. Electroencephalogr Clin Neurophysiol 1990;77:163-73.
28. Astrup J, Sorenson PM, Sorenson HR. Inhibition of cerebral oxygen and glucose consumption in the dog by hypothermia, pentobarbital, and lidocaine. Anesthesiology 1981;55:263-8.
29. Steen PA, Newberg L, Milde JH, et al. Hypothermia and barbiturates: individual and combined effects on canine cerebral oxygen consumption. Anesthesiology 1983;58:527-32.
30. Siegman MG, Anderson RV, Balaban RS, et al. Barbiturates impair cerebral metabolism during hypothermic circulatory arrest. Ann Thorac Surg 1992;54:1131-6.
31. Anderson RV, Siegmen MG, Balaban RS, et al. Hyperglycemia increases cerebral intracellular acidosis during circulatory arrest. Ann Thorac Surg 1992;54:1126-30.
32. Svensson LG, Crawford ES, Patel V, et al. Spinal cord oxygenation, intraoperative blood supply localization, cooling and function with aortic clamping. Ann Thorac Surg 1992;54:74-9.
33. Govier AV. Central nervous system complications after cardiopulmonary bypass. In: Tinker JH, ed. Cardiopulmonary Bypass: Current Concepts and Controversies. Philadelphia: WB Saunders, 1989:41-68.
34. Nussmeier NA, Arlund C, Slogoff S. Neuropsychiatric complications after cardiopulmonary bypass: cerebral protection by a barbiturate. Anesthesiology 1986;64:165-70.
35. Galandiuk S, Raque G, Appel S, Polk HCJ. The two-edged sword of large-dose steroids for spinal cord trauma. Ann Surg 1993;218:419-27.
36. Magovern GJ, Bolling SF, Casale AS, et al. The mechanism of mannitol in reducing ischemic injury: hyperosmolarity or hydroxyl scavenger. Circulation 1984;70(Supp):I-91.
37. Mills NL, Ochsner JL. Massive air embolism during cardiopulmonary bypass. J Thorac Cardiovasc Surg 1980;80:708-17.
38. Lemole GM, Strong MD, Spagna PM, Karmilowicz NP. Improved results for dissecting aneurysms: intraluminal sutureless prosthesis. J Thorac Cardiovasc Surg 1982;83:249-55.
39. Safi HJ, Brien HW, Winter JN, et al. Brain protection via cerebral retrograde perfusion during aortic arch aneurysm repair. Ann Thorac Surg 1993;56:270-6.
40. Lytle BW, McCarthy PM, Meaney KM, et al. Systemic hypothermia and circulatory arrest combined with arterial perfusion of the superior vena cava: effective intraoperative cerebral protection. J Thorac Cardiovasc Surg 1995;109:738-43.
41. Ergin MA, Galla JD, Lansman SL, et al. Hypothermic circulatory arrest in operations on the thoracic aorta: determinants of operative mortality and neurologic outcome. J Thorac Cardiovasc Surg 1994;107:788-99.

14

Myocardial Protection

PREOPERATIVE CONSIDERATIONS

The successful outcome of cardiovascular and vascular operations on the aorta is dependent on preservation of myocardial function during and after the operations. Thus myocardial function should be optimized whenever possible before an operation. For patients undergoing cardiopulmonary bypass, this will usually entail ensuring that preoperative myocardial ischemia, if present as a result of coronary artery disease, is minimized. Afterload reduction in patients with valvular disease, particularly aortic valve incompetence, is of some value. In patients who are not undergoing cardiopulmonary bypass and who therefore are not candidates for coronary artery bypass for coronary artery disease or valve replacement for valvular disease, cardiac function has to be carefully evaluated and treated if not adequate. In particular, coronary artery disease amenable to therapy must be detected, as is discussed in Chapter 2.

Patients who are taking preoperative medications for cardiac disease will have to continue these until the operative procedure. In particular, patients who are taking beta-blockers should continue to do so, because sudden cessation of these agents may precipitate severe hemodynamic problems and rhythm disturbances.[1] Aspirin should be discontinued if possible at least 5 days before elective surgery to allow platelet function to recover and reduce the risk of bleeding complications. Preoperative monitoring by Holter examination has clearly shown that cardiac ischemia is not an infrequent event in the preoperative period and that this correlates with an increased risk of postoperative cardiac complications.[2]

For patients undergoing cardiac or noncardiac operations, the prevention of myocardial stress with the use of narcotic anesthesia is important. Thereafter, the priority should be to optimize cardiac function by the use of inotropes, afterload reduction with the use of nitroglycerin, and fluid loading to optimize myocardial contractility.[3, 4]

CARDIAC FIBRILLATION AND CARDIOPLEGIA DURING CARDIOPULMONARY BYPASS

Fibrillation

For most patients undergoing cardiovascular operations on the aorta, the heart must be arrested to protect it from ischemia and sometimes to permit coronary artery bypasses

to be performed on a dormant heart. However, for patients who are undergoing deep hypothermia with circulatory arrest through the left side of the chest, this is not feasible. Furthermore, for patients who are having aortic arch procedures alone performed through a mediastinotomy, cardioplegia is not essential. Nevertheless, with the ease of retrograde cardioplegia administration while the aortic arch is being operated upon, we would advise cardioplegia while one is working on the aortic arch, particularly if circulatory arrest may be prolonged and the heart may rewarm from exposure to the environment. Although we do use topical hypothermia, we would caution against the use of ice and prolonged exposure to the cold solution in the pericardial cavity, since the risk of phrenic nerve damage appears to be increased when cardioplegia is combined with deep hypothermia. Irrespective of the operation, either with or without cardioplegia, the left ventricle must not be allowed to distend once the heart fibrillates from core cooling, because severe subendocardial ischemia can occur from distention. In patients with severe aortic incompetence (for example, due to aortic dissection) the risk of left ventricular distention can be a problem. To prevent distention, a left ventricular sump drain should be inserted through the right superior pulmonary vein to decompress the left ventricle. A cautionary note, however, is that if the aortic regurgitation is particularly severe, then most of the arterial inflow via the femoral artery will be sucked into the left ventricle without perfusion of the rest of the body. In essence, what happens is that blood is pumped via the femoral artery into the left ventricle and back again to the venous reservoir and pump. Thus, sump drainage should not be too vigorous; indeed, intermittent squeezing of the heart to empty the left ventricle will relieve some of the distention and still allow systemic perfusion while deep hypothermia is being established. Clearly, this is not a problem when only the ascending aorta is being repaired and the aorta can be cross-clamped.[3]

If, for example, distal coronary artery anastomoses are going to be performed while the heart is fibrillating during cooling for circulatory arrest (without the use of cardioplegia) or because of a calcified aorta, three rules should be followed: (1) The left ventricle must be vented; (2) hypothermia of the heart should be established by cooling the blood from the cardiopulmonary bypass pump; and (3) a high arterial perfusion pressure must be maintained during fibrillation.

At 20° C, fibrillation of the heart is minimal and coronary artery bypass anastomoses can be performed. For the circumflex and obtuse marginal arteries, distention should be carefully avoided. If this should occur, it is better to perform the coronary artery anastomoses after the aorta has been repaired, when the aortic graft can be cross-clamped and cardioplegia can be administered. Obviously, cross-clamping the aorta and infusing cardioplegia into a diseased aorta may be hazardous, since atherosclerotic and thrombotic material may embolize to the coronary arteries or other end organs.[3]

Cardioplegia

Buckberg and others[5-14] have done extensive research on the use and administration of cardioplegic solutions. The interested reader is referred to their work and to more extensive reviews of the subject.[15] This chapter briefly discusses the use of cardioplegia in conjunction with aortic operations.

For most patients undergoing operations in the ascending aorta, the aortic arch, or both, the heart must be arrested and protected during aortic cross-clamping. To do this effectively, electromechanical work must be stopped and hypothermia established. Melrose[16] first found that for cardiac procedures cardiac arrest was easily established with the use of potassium, which continues to be the key element of cardioplegic solutions, albeit at a lower concentration (10 to 20 mEq/L).[3]

The importance of cardiac arrest and hypothermia is illustrated by oxygen requirements of the heart. A normothermic beating heart needs 5.2 ml/100 g of oxygen per minute.[7] A fibrillating heart consumes 2 to 3 ml/100 g per minute versus 0.3 ml/100 g per minute for the arrested heart at 20° C.[5, 6]

Although potassium and hypothermia have been the standard and essential components of cardioplegia, acidosis produced by lactic acid during ischemia should be buffered and the myocardial cell membranes should be stabilized. Buffering of acid is attained with sodium bicarbonate, phosphate, or, in Buckberg's solution, with tris(hydroxymethyl)-aminomethane (THAM).[17] Stabilization of cellular membranes has been more difficult to achieve, partly because the mechanisms are less clearly understood. Medications that have been used include low-calcium solutions and the addition of magnesium, procaine, or calcium channel blockers. The addition of procaine may also reduce the incidence of arrhythmias.[11, 18] The situation is further complicated by the finding that the infant or neonate heart responds differently to low-calcium solution. After a period of cardiac ischemia, substrates of the Embden-Meyerhof pathway need to be reestablished for the production of high-energy phosphate stores. Buckberg[17] recommends the addition of glucose, aspartate, and glutamate together with oxygen. Particularly with long periods of aortic cross-clamping, myocardial edema may be a problem, and this may be reduced by the addition of albumin or mannitol. Despite the investigation of methods to reduce the production of free oxygen radicals, scavengers have not proved to be effective in further improving myocardial function after a period of reperfusion (see Chapter 12).[3, 17]

Whether or not oxygen should be included in cardioplegic solutions has been controversial, but the use of oxygenated solutions is increasing.[6, 9] Oxygen can be added to crystalloid cardioplegic solutions,[9] blood,[6, 9, 14] fluorocarbons,[19] and stroma-free hemoglobin.[5] The techniques and methods developed by Buckberg and his colleagues[6, 14] for the delivery of oxygenated blood solution are currently popular. The advantages are that the heart is kept oxygenated as reoxygenation occurs with each repeated administration of cardioplegia, reperfusion injury may be reduced, blood acts as a buffer for any acid produced, blood improves oncotic pressure, and hemodilution is reduced. Possible disadvantages are that the oxygen disassociation curve is shifted to the left by the cold solution and less oxygen is available for use, the white cells in the blood may generate free oxygen radicals, the higher viscosity of the blood may result in sludging (particularly since red cell pliability is reduced), and there is a possibility of distribution problems beyond coronary stenoses.[3, 6]

Antegrade perfusion of coronary arteries with stenoses greater than 50% narrowing can result in maldistribution of cardioplegia to the myocardium distally. We observed 143 patients undergoing coronary surgery and analyzed the multivariate factors associated with failure to adequately reduce myocardial temperatures in the distribution of the left anterior descending, right, and circumflex coronary arteries after 1000 ml of cold cardioplegia. Factors associated with failure or reduced rate of cooling were severity of coronary stenoses, particularly of the left anterior descending coronary artery and circumflex coronary artery; male gender; emergency surgery; and blood cardioplegia. Raised temperatures in the circumflex artery distribution were associated with postoperative elevations of the cardiac enzymes and electrocardiographic evidence of myocardial ischemia.[3]

Because of the problems of administering antegrade cardioplegia in patients with severe coronary artery disease and aortic valve regurgitation, we frequently use retrograde cardioplegia in association with antegrade cardioplegia. Retrograde cardioplegia is particularly useful and easy to establish during periods of systemic circulatory arrest, since this can be controlled by the perfusionist. Furthermore, it is easy to do this at the same time that retrograde perfusion of the brain is performed. Once the period of brain circulatory arrest is over, antegrade cardioplegia into the coronary ostia can be administered if a further period of cardiac arrest is needed. Although retrograde cardioplegia is clearly effective,[10] because of the problems of distribution and retrograde blood to the right ventricle, antegrade cardioplegia should be used if more complex procedures, such as insertion of a composite valve graft, are necessary. Continuous retrograde cold cardioplegia maintains arrest, cools the heart, buffers lactic acid, washes out metabolites, replenishes ATP levels, restores substrate, and prevents edema.[6] We have not used warm cardioplegia because of the frequent need to use deep hypothermia with circulatory arrest.

The reintroduction of this method by some groups will require further evaluation, particularly because of concerns about mechanical pump failure requiring repair and end-organ failure.[20]

REFERENCES

1. Acar C, Partington MT, Buckberg GD. Studies of controlled reperfusion after ischemia. XX. Reperfusate composition: detrimental effects of initial asanguineous cardioplegic washout after acute coronary occlusion. J Thorac Cardiovasc Surg 1991;101:294-302.

2. Mangano DT, Hollenberg M, Fegert G, et al. Perioperative myocardial ischemia in patients undergoing noncardiac surgery. I. incidence and severity during the four day perioperative period. J Am Coll Cardiol 1991;17:843-50.

3. Svensson LG, Crawford ES. Aortic dissection and aortic aneurysm surgery: clinical observations, experimental investigations and statistical analyses. Part I. Curr Probl Surg 1992;29:819-912.

4. Whittmore AD, Clowes AW, Hectman HB, et al. Aortic aneurysm repair: reduced operation mortality associated with maintenance of optimal cardiac performance. Ann Surg 1980;193:414-21.

5. Buckberg GD. A proposed "solution" to the cardioplegia controversy. J Thorac Cardiovasc Surg 1979;77:803-15.

6. Buckberg GD. Strategies and logic of cardioplegic delivery to prevent, avoid, and reverse ischemic and perfusion damage. J Thorac Cardiovasc Surg 1987;93:127-39.

7. Chitwood WR, Sink JD, Hill RC, et al. The effects of hypothermia on myocardial oxygen consumption and transmural coronary blood flow in the potassium-arrested heart. Ann Surg 1979;190:106-16.

8. Chitwood WC. Myocardial Preservation. State of the Art Reviews, Vol 2, No 2. Philadelphia: Hanley & Belfus, 1987.

9. Daggett WM, Randolph JD, Jacobs ML, et al. The superiority of cold oxygenated diluted blood cardioplegia. Ann Thorac Surg 1987;43:397-402.

10. Drinkwater DC, Laks H, Buckberg GD. A new simplified method of optimizing cardioplegia delivery without right heart isolation: antegrade/retrograde blood cardioplegia. J Thorac Cardiovasc Surg 1990;100:56-64.

11. Hearse DJ, O'Brien K, Braimbridge MV. Protection of the myocardium during ischemic arrest: dose-response curves for procaine and lignocaine in cardioplegia solutions. J Thorac Cardiovasc Surg 1981;81:873-9.

12. Heitmiller RF, DeBoer LWV, Geffin GA, et al. Comparison of myocardial recovery following hypothermic arrest with oxygenated crystalloid and blood cardioplegia: the role of calcium. Circulation 1985;72(Supp II):241-52.

13. Matsuda H, Maeda S, Hirose H, et al. Optimum dose of cold potassium cardioplegia for patients with chronic aortic valve disease: determination by left ventricular mass. Ann Thorac Surg 1986;31:22-6.

14. Rosenkranz ER, Okamoto F, Buckberg GD, et al. The safety of prolonged aortic clamping with blood cardioplegia. II. Glutamate enrichment in energy-depleted hearts. J Thorac Cardiovasc Surg 1984;88:402-10.

15. Chitwood WRJ. Update in myocardial protection. Ann Thorac Surg 1995;59:253-4.

16. Melrose DG. Elective cardiac arrest: historical perspectives. In: Longmone D, ed. Modern Cardiac Surgery. Baltimore: University Park Press, 1978:271-5.

17. McCann RL, Clements FM. Silent myocardial ischemia in patients undergoing peripheral vascular surgery: incidence and association with perioperative cardiac morbidity and mortality. J Vasc Surg 1989;9:583-7.

18. Vercillo AP, Squier RC, Chawla S, et al. Procaine versus magnesium in cardioplegia solution. Conn Med 1987;51:74-6.

19. Novick RJ, Stefaniszyn HJ, Michel RP, et al. Protection of the hypertrophied pig myocardium: a comparison of crystalloid, blood, and Fluosal-DA cardioplegia during prolonged aortic clamping. J Thorac Cardiovasc Surg 1985;89:547-66.

20. Salermo TA, Christakis GT, Abel J, et al. Technique and pitfalls of retrograde continuous warm blood cardioplegia. Ann Thorac Surg 1991;51:102-5.

Pathophysiology of Aortic Cross-clamping and Influence of Spinal Cord Anatomy

CARDIOVASCULAR AND HEMODYNAMIC ALTERATIONS

Aortic cross-clamping has profound effects on normal hemodynamics and the risks of end-organ ischemia to sensitive tissues. For patients undergoing repairs of the ascending aorta, the aortic arch, or both, the risks are related predominantly to cardiac ischemia and brain perfusion. Protection of the heart and brain is discussed in the chapters on cardioplegia and deep hypothermia. This chapter discusses the consequences of cross-clamping of the descending thoracic aorta.

Several hemodynamic changes occur with cross-clamping of the descending thoracic aorta. The blood pressure proximal to the aortic clamp immediately rises and the blood pressure distal to it concomitantly falls precipitously to approximately 10 to 20 mm Hg (Fig. 15–1). With the sudden increase in cardiac afterload, left ventricular strain increases and cardiac preload increases. The increased preload is reflected by an increase in central venous pressure and right heart pressures (Fig. 15–2). The rise in central venous pressure, in turn, results in back-pressure in the veins and a rise in the cerebrospinal fluid (CSF) pressure. Besides the direct consequences of aortic cross-clamping, organs beyond the clamp are deprived of their blood supply and, therefore, of oxygen and metabolic substrates (Fig. 15–2).

The spinal cord is precipitously balanced between its available blood supply and metabolic requirements. Spinal cord blood flow provides both the oxygen and substrate requirements for energy production by the cord and removes waste products. Factors that influence spinal cord blood flow include the following:

1. Arterial pressure. Under normal circumstances, the spinal cord autoregulates between perfusion pressures of 60 and 160 mm Hg, whereas below 60 mm Hg the blood flow falls in proportion to the perfusion pressure.[1] At perfusion pressures higher than 160 mm Hg, increasing hydrostatic pressure causes disruption of the blood brain barrier.[2]

Feedback loops interact to preserve normal function of the spinal cord. During aortic cross-clamping, many of these feedback loops cannot function and spinal cord hypoxia or ischemia may occur, leading to loss of ion homeostasis and cytotoxicity as described previously (see Chapter 12). A "no-reflow" phenomenon may follow ischemia; that is, there may be arrest of perfusion, possibly related to vasospasm, platelet aggregation, or pericapillary edema. Because of aortic cross-clamping, blood supply to the spinal cord is dependent on flow through collateral vessels. Thus arterial pressure is important in maintaining an adequate pressure head to perfuse the collaterals. The anatomical arrangement of the spinal cord blood supply is also critical in being able to supply the spinal cord with blood. Spinal cord anatomy and the relationship to hemodynamic alterations with cross-clamping will be discussed later.[2]

2. Increase in CSF Pressure. An increase in the CSF pressure during aortic cross-clamping may reduce perfusion of the spinal cord.[3] The possible effects of an elevated CSF pressure will be included in our discussion below of the hemodynamic consequences of distal aortic cross-clamping.

RENAL BLOOD FLOW

Suprarenal or more proximal aortic cross-clamping results in reduced distal organ perfusion, including renal ischemia with the potential risk of acute renal failure developing (Fig. 15–2).[4-22] It is postulated that acute renal failure after ischemia is caused by three progressive mechanisms: (1) intraluminal obstruction of the proximal renal tubule by sequestrated necrotic cellular debris[18, 19]; (2) transtubular back-leakage of the tubular ultrafiltrate into the renal interstitium[16, 19]; and (3) alterations in renal hemodynamics.[16, 19] The alterations in renal hemodynamics appear to be associated mainly with either preglomerular afferent arteriolar sphincter constriction[16] or efferent arteriolar spasm causing proximal tubular cell ischemia. It is believed that there are certain metabolic consequences of ischemia, many of which are similar to those postulated to occur in brain ischemia. Some of these theories have encompassed the hypothesis that renin–angiotensin activation induces renal precapillary

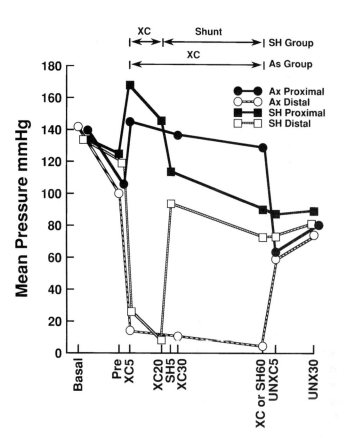

FIGURE 15–1 Changes in mean aortic pressure with aortic cross-clamping *(XC)* and insertion of an aortic shunt *(SH)* in two sets of experiments of animals operated on with either cross-clamping alone *(Ax)* or also with a shunt *(SH)*. Pre-XC5, five minutes before clamping; *XC,* time since cross-clamping; *SH,* time since shunt was opened; *UNXC,* time since unclamping. Note the marked fall in distal aortic pressure with cross-clamping and the rise in proximal pressure. This is reversed by insertion of an effective shunt. (From Svensson LG, Rickards E, Coull A, et al. J Thorac Cardiovasc Surg 1986;91:71–8.)

arteriolar sphincter spasm, possibly associated with the effects of prostaglandins.[7, 18] This, in turn, leads to the release of either adenosine[9] or circulating catecholamines, provoking further renal vasoconstriction,[22] and damage by free oxygen radicals released from reperfused ischemic tissue.[10, 20] Calcium may also be an important mediator of renal injury.[2, 23]

Because of the consequences of ischemia on end organs (Fig. 15–2), various methods have been used in attempts to prevent organ ischemia, particularly of the spinal cord and kidneys. Methods of protection have included shunts, cardiopulmonary bypass, hypothermia, and atriofemoral bypass.[2, 21, 24–38]

RESEARCH INTO HEMODYNAMIC CHANGES AND SPINAL CORD BLOOD FLOW

Because of the controversies concerning the use of distal aortic perfusion techniques, we[34] evaluated the effects of aortic cross-clamping for 60 minutes in normothermic chacma baboons *(Papio ursinus)*. These animals were chosen because of the very similar anatomy of the nonhuman primates and man.[39] Using this animal model, we wished to determine whether an aortoaortic shunt increases distal spinal cord blood flow and how shunted blood flow to the distal aorta related to the arteria radicularis magna (ARM), also known as the artery of Adamikiewicz, and the anterior spinal artery (ASA). In groups treated with cross-clamping alone and in groups treated with shunting, proximal aortic hypertension developed during aortic cross-clamping, while the distal aortic pressure fell precipitously (Fig. 15–1). After the shunts were inserted and opened, the proximal aortic pressure decreased and the distal aortic pressure increased. Immediately after unclamping, the mean proximal pressure, distal aortic pressure, and total peripheral resistance were lower in the group of baboons with cross-clamping alone than in the shunted group. Nevertheless, 5

FIGURE 15–2 Influence of aortic cross-clamping alone *(cross-clamp)* or funarizine, a calcium channel blocker, on blood flow to various organs, measured at a basal level, after 60 minutes of aortic cross-clamping, and after recovery (30 minutes after unclamping). Note the marked hyperemia seen with flunarizine, which was associated with extensive hemorrhagic stress ulceration in the stomach.

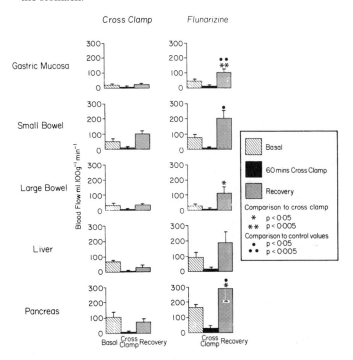

minutes after the aorta was unclamped, there was no significant difference in the pressures between the two groups. There was no significant difference in any of the hemodynamic parameters (mean proximal and distal pressures, cardiac index, total peripheral resistance, and rate pressure product) between the nonshunted and shunted groups 30 minutes after unclamping.[34] There was no significant difference in the left ventricular end diastolic pressures between the group with cross-clamping alone and the shunted group. Roberts and associates[21] also noted no left ventricular hemodynamic advantages in shunted animals. Although we have been unable to show that the incidence of postoperative cardiac complications is reduced by atriofemoral bypass, the blood pressure management of patients who have had atriofemoral bypass is considerably easier after aortic unclamping. In subsequent evaluations of patients undergoing aortic cross-clamping alone, it is of interest that hemodynamic and pressure alterations were similar to those noted in the animal experiments, although these alterations were somewhat attenuated by pharmacological manipulations during anesthesia (Fig. 15–3).[2, 37]

Blood flow in the animal experiments was determined in segmental sections of the spinal cord with the use of radioactive microspheres. In the animals that had cross-clamping alone, without the insertion of shunts, blood flow decreased progressively down the length of the spinal cord so that the distal lumbar spinal cord was the most ischemic during cross-clamping.[34] The decrease in blood flow down the length of the spinal cord we subsequently found was associated, as expected, with a greater amount of deoxygenation as measured by oxygen sensors on the spinal cord (Fig. 15–4A and B).[38] Gelman and associates[40] have shown that, when the proximal hypertension is decreased with sodium nitroprusside, distal aortic perfusion of tissues also decreases, further corroborating dependence of the spinal cord blood flow on the proximal aortic pressure head. We also observed an increased spinal cord blood flow below the level of clamping with reperfusion of the spinal cord after aortic unclamping as compared to blood flow measured before aortic cross-clamping. Of considerable interest was the finding that this hyperemic response 30 minutes after aortic unclamping was most marked in the lumbar spinal cord in paralyzed animals.[41] It is speculative whether this hyperemia may have been caused by vasodilation after severe tissue ischemia during cross-clamping or by oxygen-derived free radicals damaging the endothelial cells during the period of reperfusion. Nitric oxide is also clearly a factor (see Chapter 12). In more recent experiments examining this phenomenon of hyperemia, we[38] have noted that the hyperemic response is associated with hyperoxygenation of

FIGURE 15–3 Hemodynamic and CSF alterations with various stages of aortic surgery in patients. *MAP,* mean arterial pressure; *CVP,* central venous pressure; *CSFP,* cerebrospinal fluid pressure; *SVR,* systemic vascular resistance; *CI,* cardiac index. P-values indicate significant changes. (From Svensson LG, Grum DF, Bednarski M, et al. J Vasc Surg 1990;11:423–9.)

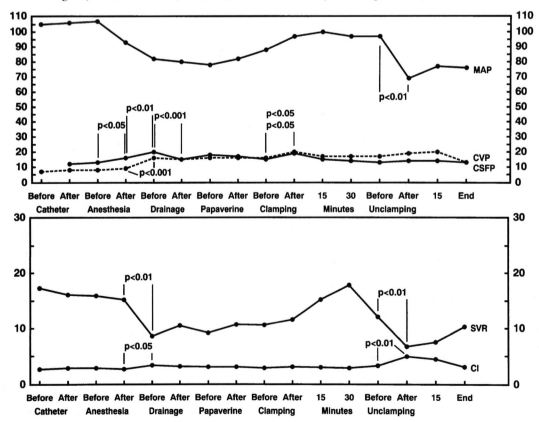

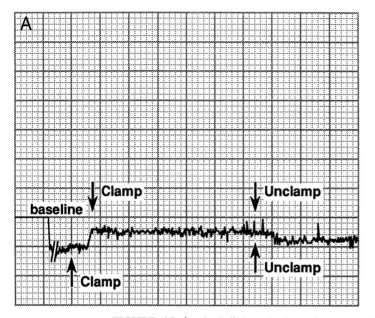

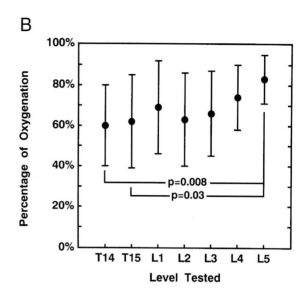

FIGURE 15–4 **A,** Fall in spinal cord oxygenation with aortic cross-clamping (upward deflection) and return of oxygenation with unclamping of the aorta. Note that the fall in oxygenation is rapid. **B,** Influence of the level of aortic cross-clamping on the degree of deoxygenation of the spinal cord in pigs. Note that with cross-clamping at the lower levels (e.g., L5), the fall is significantly less than that at T14. (**B** reprinted with permission from the Society of Thoracic Surgeons. From Svensson LG, Crawford ES, Patel V, et al. Ann Thorac Surg 1992;54:74–9.)

the spinal cord as measured by oxygen concentrations on the spinal cord, which suggests that it may be associated with a reperfusion injury (Fig. 15–5).[2]

On examination of the spinal cord segments and the measured radioactive blood flow rates, it was noted that the lower thoracic spinal cord blood flow in the shunted group did not increase once the shunt was opened (Fig. 15–6). However, a highly significant increase in lumbar spinal cord blood flow was observed.[34, 42] These findings corroborated the anatomical findings that blood would be preferentially shunted to the lumbar spinal cord but not to the thoracic

spinal cord because of the hairpin bend in the ARM forcing blood down the length of the spinal cord from the ARM level of entry. Distal perfusion of the aorta, therefore, provides adequate lumbar spinal cord protection, but the arrangement of the vascular anatomy leaves the lower thoracic spinal cord at risk from ischemia. Thus the lower thoracic spinal cord seems to be mainly dependent on blood flowing down the ASA from the cervical and upper thoracic spinal segments for its oxygen supply (Fig. 15–4). There is a caveat, however, to this finding. If the radicular arteries above the ARM are perfused, blood can flow both up and

FIGURE 15–5 Influence of cross-clamp time on spinal cord deoxygenation in a pig model and on hyperoxygenation, possibly related to free oxygen radicals, with unclamping of the aorta and reperfusion of the spinal cord. (Reprinted with permission from the Society of Thoracic Surgeons. From Svensson LG, Crawford ES, Patel V, et al. Ann Thorac Surg 1992;54:74-9.)

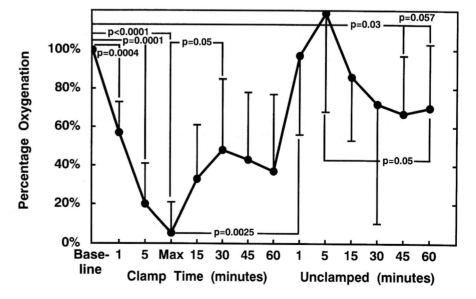

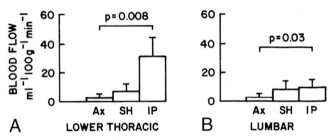

FIGURE 15–6   Influence of aortic cross-clamping alone *(Ax)*, shunts *(SH)*, and intrathecal papaverine *(IP)* on spinal cord blood flow in nonhuman primates in the lower thoracic spinal cord **(A)** and lumbar spinal cord **(B)** after 60 minutes of aortic cross-clamping. Note that IP resulted in a significantly better blood flow. (From Svensson LG, Von Ritter CM, Groeneveld HT, et al. Ann Surg 1986;204:38-47.)

down the length of the spinal cord via the ASA. The reason for this is that, in contradistinction to the ARM, the other thoracic radicular arteries (and also the iliolumbar radicular artery), do not have a hairpin bend and therefore blood can flow both up and down the spinal cord from these radicular arteries.[43]

An unknown parameter is the amount of pressure that is required in the aorta to perfuse the spinal cord. From our[38, 44] experience with injecting hydrogen solutions into aortic aneurysms and determining whether the solution reaches the spinal cord, it would appear that a pressure of at least 100 mm Hg is desirable. However, these pressures are difficult to reach with shunts to the distal aorta. In our nonhuman primate studies flow through the shunts accounted for 77% of the cardiac output, and the mean gradient across the shunts was 18 mm Hg. Since this is approximately the proportion of blood that normally flows to the lower torso, it would be reasonable to assume that the flow rate through the shunts was adequate. In clinical practice this proportion of blood flowing through the shunt may not be achieved, as a relatively smaller shunt has to be used, usually 7.5 or 9 mm in internal diameter. In comparison, a shunt equivalent in size to that used in the animal experiments would need to be at least 25 mm. This discrepancy between shunted animals and the clinical situation in which there is usually a significant gradient between the proximal and distal aortas may account for the poorer flow rates achieved in humans with shunts. Laschinger and colleagues,[30] have come to the conclusion that a distal perfusion pressure of at least 40 mm Hg appears to be needed to perfuse critical arteries supplying the spinal cord. We[45, 46] and others have reported that in humans distal perfusion techniques do not always protect against paraplegia.[26, 31, 32, 47] This is because of the anatomical problems with spinal cord perfusion described above and also the fact that the cause of postoperative neurologic injury is multifactorial. Nevertheless, there is increasing evidence that distal aortic perfusion by shunt as espoused by Verdant and associates,[48, 49] and atriofemoral bypass for descending aortic aneurysms as reported by us[50] and by Borst[51] are significantly protective to both the spinal cord

and kidneys. Furthermore, it would appear that for thoraco-abdominal aneurysms, sequential segmental repair of the aneurysms are associated with a lower risk of paraplegia.[52] Verdant (personal communication, June, 1995) now no longer uses a shunt but, rather, uses atriofemoral bypass for distal perfusion. These various methods will be considered in detail in our discussion of the prevention of postoperative complications. As noted in our animal studies,[41] we[45] also observed in humans a close relationship between the flow rate with atriofemoral bypass and distal aortic pressures. Furthermore, we have also noted that the larger the peripheral vascular bed that is perfused, the higher the flow rates that can be achieved or have to be reached to maintain adequate distal aortic pressures.[43] Clearly, the driving proximal blood pressure for blood flow, produced either by the heart or by a pump, is an important factor in supplying blood to the spinal cord.[34, 41, 42] Thus it is of interest that several papers have shown that the use of nitroprusside to reduce proximal hypertension during aortic cross-clamping may increase the risk of spinal cord injury[53] (see also Comments[53]). Another factor in this adverse effect may be the biochemical effects of nitroprusside and the relationship of nitroprusside to nitric oxide (see Chapter 12 on the biochemistry of ischemia).

CEROBROSPINAL FLUID PRESSURE CHANGES

We prospectively evaluated the alterations in cerebrospinal fluid pressure in patients undergoing intrathecal injection of papaverine and CSF drainage, including changes in CSF, pH, and pO_2.[36, 37, 54] We[37] found that during the course of the aortic operation the CSF pressure progressively and significantly increased (Fig. 15-3) during induction of general anesthesia and intubation, during the period between induction of anesthesia and CSF drainage, and immediately after aortic cross-clamping. As would be expected, however, CSF pressure was significantly reduced by CSF drainage before aortic cross-clamping.[43]

Concurrent with the progressive increase in CSF pressure, there was also a progressive increase in central venous pressure (CVP) during the period from the induction of general anesthesia to aortic cross-clamping. There were no consistent changes in cardiac index or systemic vascular resistance with aortic cross-clamping. However, our impression is that systemic vascular resistance proximal to the aortic cross-clamp increases markedly because of the increased afterload, although there is some compensatory vasodilatation of other perfused arteries. The cardiac output also decreases because of the increased afterload. Beyond the aortic cross-clamp, the vascular resistance probably decreases during aortic cross-clamping as a result of the accumulation of the products of metabolism. Furthermore, it is clear that, with aortic unclamping, the peripheral vascular resistance is very low. However, during the period between induction of anesthesia and aspiration of CSF, the cardiac index was increased and systemic vascular resistance was decreased by pharmacological manipulation and administration of intravenous solutions, including mannitol. The significant increase in the CVP during this period probably reflects the administration of fluid, including mannitol. As expected, mean arterial pressure fell significantly with aortic unclamping, as did systemic vascular resistance, and cardiac index significantly increased (Fig. 15–3). Although not as marked, similar hemodynamic changes have been noted with infrarenal abdominal aortic operations and may, in part, be related to the production of thromboxane (TXA$_2$) from the ischemic tissues of the lower torso.[43, 55]

The cause of the increase in the CSF pressure during aortic operations, particularly with aortic cross-clamping, is of interest. We[37] have speculated that reasons may include the following: (1) The higher proximal mean arterial pressure (MAP) may cause either dilatation of intracranial arteries or expansion of nervous tissue volume; (2) there may be increased CSF secretion, possibly related to increased blood flow to the brain; and (3) the rise in CVP results in back pressure in the intracranial veins, Batson's plexus, venous sinuses, and other veins surrounding the spinal cord. We tend to favor the third postulate, namely, that the increase in CVP causes the increase in CSF pressure by back pressure on veins that increase CSF pressure. The classic Monro-Kellie hypothesis that the total cranial and spinal column volumes remain constant within the enclosed space occupied by the brain and spinal cord is generally relevant for this discussion. Any volume increase of the components (nervous tissue volume, blood volume, CSF volume) must therefore be at the expense of the other components. Normal CSF pressure will thus be maintained only until the compensatory mechanisms are exceeded, as venous volume increases within the confines of the central nervous system.[37] However, with aortic cross-clamping, the one compensatory mechanism, namely, compression of venous capacitance vessels (loss of blood volume vis-à-vis above), fails. Rather than compensating for any increases in the intracranial components, the venous capacitance vessels are the more likely cause of the increase in CSF pressure. Hence our hypothesis that intracranial venous engorgement and back pressure on the CSF might more logically account for the increased CSF pressure noted during induction of anesthesia and aortic cross-clamping.[37] Blaisdell and Cooley[56] noted in their dog experiments that CSF pressure increased with both anesthetic induction and cross-clamping, and in our own animal experiments and those by others[57, 58] it has been noted that the CVP increases with aortic cross-clamping.[43] Maughan and colleagues[59] used exsanguination during aortic cross-clamping and noted that CSF pressure was significantly lower, confirming our theory that the rise in CSF pressure with aortic cross-clamping is due to venous engorgement from back pressure and that if this is reduced, as in the study by Maughan, by reducing the preload, CSF pressure rise is not as great. Similarly, in a study that we performed[46, 60] on patients who had been given intrathecal papaverine during aortic cross-clamping, we

noted that infusion of mannitol before aortic cross-clamping resulted in a rise in the CVP and a concurrent rise in the CSF pressure. Although Maughan and colleagues found that nitroprusside reduced the calculated spinal cord perfusion pressure in animals, we[46, 60] were not able to show a significant effect in patients. However, the calculated spinal cord perfusion pressure tended to be reduced. Gelman[40, 61] has found that, on the basis of animal research, the increase in CVP may be related to blood from the heart being pumped predominantly to the upper torso with an increase in upper body blood volume. This shunting of blood to the upper torso would be in keeping with the operative technique that we sometimes use, in which the distal aorta is not cross-clamped when a single proximal clamp alone is used. Under these circumstances, venous drainage from the lower torso returns blood to the upper torso, but blood does not get back to the lower torso; thus all the lower torso blood volume is in the upper torso, with the noted increase in CVP.

It is clear from our animal research in nonhuman primates and porcine experiments that CSF pressure measured in the cisterna magna may not accurately reflect the CSF pressure alterations in the vicinity of the lumbar spinal cord. Thus any extrapolation of pressures measured in the lumbar spinal cord to those in the cranium are suspect. Of further note is the finding by Killen and colleagues[28] that the distal aortic pressure does not reflect the spinal cord arteriolar (or capillary) blood pressure but that the higher segmental intercostal or lumbar artery end pressures are a closer approximation. By implication, therefore, the double assumption of Miyamoto and associates[58] that "relative spinal cord perfusion pressure" is equal to distal aortic pressure minus the cisterna magna pressure may not hold true (perfusion pressure = distal map – CSF presssure). Clearly, both measured spinal cord blood flow in animals, despite a low distal aortic pressure,[34] and the low incidence of paraplegia in humans, even when the distal aorta is left unclamped and totally decompressed during aortic replacements by our technique,[62, 63] contradict this concept. Moreover, Griffiths and colleagues[1] have shown that perfusion pressure is a far greater determinant of blood flow than the possible effect of an elevated CSF pressure reducing spinal cord blood flow. Griffiths and colleagues[1] concluded that "spinal cord blood flow can accommodate any fluctuations in CSFP." There are even reports of increased cerebral blood flow with an increased intracranial pressure.[37] Of further note is the finding that the resistance to reabsorption of CSF is 17 times greater in dogs than in humans, and thus any increases in CSF pressure may be more quickly compensated for in humans.[37] Killen and associates[28] were unable to show a protective effect by draining CSF from the cisterna magna in dogs. Similarly, in the study by Wadouh and colleagues,[59] using a pig model, and in our own nonhuman primate model, CSF drainage by a limited lumbar laminectomy failed to reduce the incidence of paraplegia.[41] Whether CSF drainage alone would reduce the incidence of paraplegia after aortic cross-clamping in humans remained an unanswered question until our recent prospective randomized trial[25] showed that

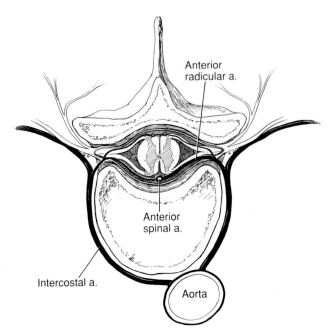

FIGURE 15–7   Illustration of the course of the intercostal arteries from the aorta around the vertebral bodies, after which anterior and posterior radicular arteries are given off to the anterior spinal artery and the two posterolateral spinal arteries. (Reprinted with permission from the Society of Thoracic Surgeons. From Svensson LG, Patel V, Coselli JS, Crawford ES. Ann Thorac Surg 1990;49:528–35.)

CSF drainage had no effect on the postoperative incidence of neurological dysfunction of the lower limb in any subgroup of patients. This study will be described in detail in our discussion of prevention of paraplegia after distal aortic surgery.[43]

BLOOD SUPPLY OF THE SPINAL CORD

To understand the possible causes of paralysis after aortic surgery, a review of the spinal cord vascular anatomy is required. We[39, 44] dissected out the spinal cords of a total of 64 adult male baboons, 20 pigs, 2 dogs, and 8 adult male human cadavers in an attempt to evaluate the influence of spinal cord vascular anatomy on neurologic injuries after aortic operations. In addition, the anatomy of the spinal cord has been studied by other authors.[57, 64-77] From these studies, an understanding of the vascular anatomy of the spinal cord has been achieved and is discussed below.[2]

Feeney and Watterson[69] stated: "There exists a very close relationship between the metabolic requirements of the nervous tissue and the final distribution of intraneural vessels in the adult, a relationship which functions in such a way as to provide the nervous system with a blood supply just adequate for its minimal needs." To this can be added Woollam and Millen's[75] corollary: "To put it in somewhat crude evolutionary terms, man has just as much nervous system as he can supply with oxygen and no more." Clearly,

the spinal cord is very finely balanced between an adequate blood supply and the occurrence of ischemia and thus is vulnerable to any alterations in the delivery of blood to the cord by arteries. This very delicate balance is the result of involution of excessive radicular arteries found in the embryo and neonate. The human neonate has the greatest abundance of blood vessels. Dommisse[67] has found that, weight for weight, neonates have a sixfold advantage over adults in the spinal cord in response to metabolic demands. As a child grows and matures, however, the paired radicular arteries at each vertebral level involute, and the adult is left with only a few radicular arteries that supply the spinal cord. Furthermore, as atheroma, atherosclerosis, or thrombus occludes the origins of segmental intercostal or lumbar arteries within aneurysms, the remaining radicular arteries are deprived of the native source of blood supply and then require collateral pathways to maintain spinal cord viability. Indeed, in our studies with hydrogen to determine the origin of spinal cord blood supply and in our postoperative evaluation with highly selective angiography, it has been interesting to note that some patients with occluded segemental arteries have entirely collateral sources of blood supply to the spinal cord (see below).[44]

The blood supply of the spinal cord can be thought of as three centripetal divisions of arterial pathways. These are the primary division, consisting of the segmental arteries; an intermediate division of radicular arteries; and a terminal division in the spinal cord itself (Fig. 15-7). The primary division consists of vertebral, costocervical, intercostal, and lumbar arteries (Fig. 15-8). The intermediate division of sparse radicular arteries in the adult is a result of involution. Although initially the spinal cord receives paired radicular arteries, these disappear, leaving one or two cervical, two or three thoracic, and one or two lumbar arteries. The largest of these has a characteristic hairpin bend, and this radicular artery is referred to as the arteria radicularis magna (ARM) (Fig. 15-9). The ARM is also known as the artery of Adamkiewicz.[39] The spinal cord has a unique feature in that there are longitudinal arteries linking the radicular arteries together. These arteries are the anterior spinal artery (ASA) and the posterolateral spinal arteries. In fact, cross-sectioning of the spinal cord has shown that 75% of the blood supply is derived from the central end arteries arising from the ASA.[78]

Caudal to the basilar artery are the two vertebral arteries that join to form the basilar artery. Immediately before the two vertebral arteries unite to form the basilar artery, they each give off a branch that turns caudally. These two caudally directed branches unite to form the origin of the ASA. The two vessels from either side, one from each vertebral artery, unite between the levels of C1 and C6. The single arterial channel runs in the anterior median sulcus and is a continuous artery in humans, nonhuman primates, pigs, and dogs.[44, 79] The ASA may be duplicated proximally as far as C6 but seldom further. This is because of persistence of the embryonic vessels, which are longitudinal links between the segmental arteries of the developing neural tube.[66, 67]

There are spinal arteries on the posterior aspect of the spinal cord similar to those of the ASA. These are smaller in size and show more variation in position. There is usually a rich network of arborizing smaller arteries and arterioles interlinking these arteries across the midline of the posterior spinal cord. The posterior spinal arteries originate from the posterior inferior cerebellar artery. They tend to be duplicated throughout the course of the spinal cord as they proceed distally as the posterolateral spinal artery. These continuous vessels extend from the medulla oblongata to the conus medullaris, weaving between the posterior nerve roots. Although there is extensive linking between the two arteries, there is scanty communication between the posterolateral trunks and the ASA by means of small arteries and arterioles. There is, however, a constant cruciate anastomosis at the conus medullaris.[67] Between the junction of the ARM and the origin of these communicating branches of the cruciate anastomosis to the ASA, the ASA remains of uniform caliber in spite of the number of branches joining

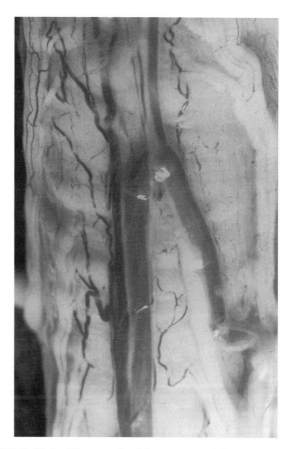

FIGURE 15–9   Photograph of the junction of the ARM with the anterior spinal artery on a human spinal cord. Note the acute hairpin bend the ARM takes in joining the anterior spinal artery and then running caudally down the spinal cord. (From Svensson LG, Loop FD. In: Bergan JJ, Yao JST, eds. Arterial Surgery: New Diagnostic and Operative Techniques. New York, NY: Grune & Stratton; 1988:273-85.)

FIGURE 15–8   Summary of findings in eight human cadaver dissections. **C,** cervical level; **T,** thoracic; **L,** lumbar; **ARM,** arteria radicularis magna. The sizes are the mean sizes for these arteries when distended under pressure with blood. The level of origin of the arteries may vary in any one person, however, the diagram summarizes the most commonly identified sites of origin. Note the large iliolumbar artery, in this diagram shown as arising from L2. (From Svensson LG, Klepp P, Hinder AA. S Afr J Surg 1986;24: 32-4.)

it, even where the particularly large iliolumbar radicular artery joins the ASA.[67] The latter radicular artery is found in approximately 80% of human cadavers and most likely can act as a useful adjunct to the blood supply to the lumbar spinal cord if the ARM is sacrificed.

Similar to the arterial longitudinal arterial system on the spinal cord, but less well defined on the posterior aspect of the spinal cord, are the anterior and posterior longitudinal venous trunks. Anteriorly, a single vein courses deep to the ASA in the anterior median sulcus, and into it drain the pial perforating and central perforating veins.[67] Posteriorly, the veins are often replaced by ramifying vessels. These longitudinal trunks, in turn, drain into Batson's plexus surrounding the theca of the spinal cord within the spinal canal. This plexus is also known as the "extradural vertebral venous plexus."[67]

Segmental arteries of the vertebral column, the most important being the intercostal arteries, supply the radicular arteries with blood flow (Fig. 15-7). In the thoracic and lumbar regions, the segmental arteries are known as the intercostal and lumbar arteries. These arteries arise in pairs from the posterolateral aspect of the aorta. In the cervical region of the spinal cord, they arise from branches of the

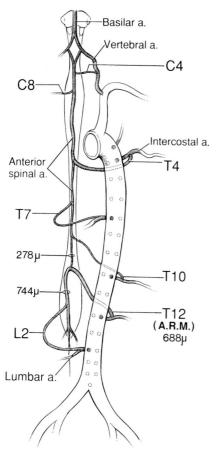

subclavian or vertebral arteries. In the sacral area, they arise from the lateral sacral arteries with some contribution from the middle sacral, iliolumbar, and lower lumbar arteries. It is interesting that in animals such as baboons, dogs, and pigs the contribution of the middle sacral artery is considerably greater than in humans, possibly related to the tail that is present in these animals. The segmental arteries course around the vertebral bodies and then proceed to the intervertebral foramen appropriate to their level, where they divide into the terminal branches and radicular branches. The largest radicular artery with the characteristic hairpin bend is the ARM (Fig. 15-9). Most commonly, the ARM arises at T10 (Kadyi, 1889, quoted by Dommisse[67]). Dommisse[67] found that the position varied from T7 to L4. Kadyi, Dommisse, and we[39] noted that this artery most commonly arises from the left segmental intercostal or lumbar artery. Dommisse found that in only 17% of cadavers did it arise from the right segmental artery of the pair. Our dissections confirmed this.[39] The arterial outflow from the longitudinal vessels is mostly through the central arteries but also through the sulcal and pial perforating vessels. The central arteries in the cervical and lumbar regions are of larger caliber and density than those in the thoracic region.[74] The terminal arterioles do not interconnect but give rise to interlocking capillary networks, particularly in the gray matter.

Spinal Cord Blood Flow During Aortic Cross-clamping and Shunting

An important feature of spinal cord vascular anatomy is the continuous ASA, which supplies the entire length of the spinal cord in all the animals and the humans we[39, 44] studied. This is corroborated by the findings of Dommisse in 42 human specimens[66] and by the findings of others.[57, 76, 80] The ASAs in the pigs and dogs, however, were relatively smaller. Thus one cannot agree with the speculative claims, unsubstantiated by anatomical dissections, that the lack of a continuous ASA is the cause of paraplegia in humans. The difficulty in seeing the ASA on injection of radiopaque contrast medium into the aorta without dissection of the spinal cord and then studying radiographs may account for previous reports that the ASA was not continuous. Although dye was injected solely into the occluded descending aorta segment in our studies,[39, 52, 79] the entire length of the ASA from the cervical to the lumbar spinal cord, with the joining radicular arteries, was stained with dye and contrast when the spinal cord was dissected out. The finding of a continuous ASA and also of the posterolateral arteries forming a further longitudinal pathway for possible blood flow constitutes an important factor in maintaining an adequate blood supply to the distal spinal cord during thoracic aortic cross-clamping when the distal aorta is not perfused. The hypertension that occurs proximal to a descending thoracic aortic clamp is the driving force for the supply of blood by collaterals to the distal spinal cord. The most important pathways are through the vertebral arteries, the cervical radicular arteries, and any thoracic radicular arteries that remain perfused

proximal to an aortic clamp and, in turn, supply the ASA. Thus, if these collateral pathways are well developed, paraplegia is less likely to occur as, for example, with coarctation of the aorta.[81, 82] This collateral pathway is probably well developed in patients with atherosclerosis or thrombotic occlusion of segmental arteries that normally supply the radicular arteries, including the ARM. Hence the lower incidence of paraplegia in patients undergoing surgery for atherosclerotic disease of the aorta compared with procedures for traumatic rupture of the thoracic aorta or acute aortic dissection (Fig. 15-10). We therefore speculated that if the ASA could be dilated at the narrow point immediately above the junction with the ARM, then blood flow down the ASA could be increased, thus increasing protection of the distal spinal cord during a longer period of aortic cross-clamping. Our research in animals showed that intrathecal papaverine increased spinal cord blood flow, dilated the anterior spinal artery, and prevented paralysis (Fig. 15-6).[51]

Of importance in improving distal spinal cord blood flow was the discrepancy between the diameter of the ASA above and below the junction of the ARM found in both nonhuman and human primates. This is because to supply the distal (lumbar) spinal cord with blood from distal aortic perfusion, blood has to reach the spinal cord predominantly via the ARM, since the latter is the largest radicular artery (Fig. 15-9). In humans we have reported the mean diameter of the distended human ASA to be 0.231 mm (SEM 0.04 mm) above and 0.941 mm (SEM 0.07 mm) below the ARM junction ($p = 0.0057$). The mean ARM diameter was 0.871 mm (SEM 0.04 mm) (Fig. 15-9).[39]

The importance of these findings is that resistance to blood flow is inversely proportional to the fourth power of the radius (Poiseuille's equation). Thus the resistance to flow up the ASA as opposed to downward is calculated to be 51.7 times greater. In humans, with a larger ASA radius, the resistance is even more marked, being 278 times greater. Our hypothesis is that if a distal aortic perfusion method is used to perfuse the aorta beyond an occluded segment of the descending aorta that is being operated on, blood will preferentially flow through the ARM and then turn down the hairpin bend at the ASA to perfuse the lumbar spinal cord. Our subsequent experimental studies confirmed that blood shunted to the distal aorta preferentially perfuses the lumbar spinal cord (Fig. 15-6). In contrast, blood flow to the lower thoracic spinal cord, referred to by Dommisse[66] as "the critical zone of the spinal cord," is not increased in spite of distal aortic perfusion and hence is prone to be inadequate, causing a neurologic injury. The inference from these observations is that paraplegia may still occur, in spite of perfusion of the distal aorta, because of lower thoracic spinal cord ischemia above the ARM. A caveat should be added, however, that if in the clinical situation a thoracic radicular artery above the ARM is perfused, then, because the thoracic radicular arteries do not have a hairpin bend at their junction with the ASA, blood can flow both up and down the ASA, thus protecting the spinal cord. This would be a likely reason for the appearance of improved

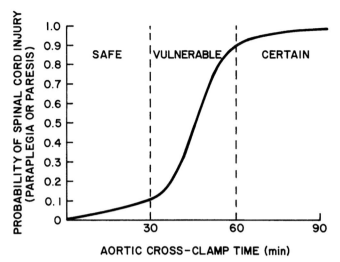

FIGURE 15–10 Influence of aortic cross-clamp time on the risk of spinal cord injury. Note the transition of the sigmoid curve from a safe period, to a vulnerable period, to an area of virtual certainty. This curve would apply to traumatic ruptures of the aorta and acute aortic dissection repairs without any protective adjuncts for the spinal cord. The curve is shifted to the right by protective measures such as cooling, distal aortic perfusion, intrathecal papaverine, and lower-risk aneurysms that have more extensive collateral vessels such as medial degenerative (nondissection) aneurysms, Crawford type III or IV thoracoabdominal aneurysms, or coarctation of the aorta. (From Svensson LG, Loop FD. In: Bergan JJ, Yao JST, eds. Arterial Surgery: New Diagnostic and Operative Techniques. New York, NY: Grune & Stratton; 1988:273-85.)

protection of the spinal cord in our experience when sequential segmental repair of thoracoabdominal aneurysms is performed.

Of importance during descending and thoracoabdominal repairs when the ARM and thoracic radicular arteries have not been identified is the site from which the ARM most likely would arise. The importance of this is that the segment of aorta that has the origin of the spinal cord blood supply should be reattached at the time of operation. In our study,[39] the ARM originated from the T9-T12 intercostal arteries in 7 of the 8 humans. One arose from T7. The ARM arose from the T9-L1 segment in most baboons. Studies with larger sample sizes have shown that the ARM in humans arises from the T5-T8 segment in 15%, T9-T12 in 75%, L1-L2 in 10%, L3 in 1.4%, and L4-L5 in 0.2% (Fig. 15-11).[71, 73] Knowledge of the level of origin of the ARM and the other large radicular arteries is critical in the prevention of paraplegia for the following reasons:

1. If the ARM arises above the aortic clamps, spinal ischemia is less likely to occur since the spinal cord is partially perfused during aortic cross-clamping.

2. If the ARM or other major radicular arteries arise from the occluded segment of the aorta, then perfusion of the distal aorta beyond the lower clamp is unlikely to have a protective effect unless a large iliolumbar artery can provide adequate blood supply to the lumbar spinal cord.

3. If the descending or thoracoabdominal aorta is replaced with a tubular graft, then reimplantation of the intercostal or lumbar arteries supplying the spinal cord, including the ARM, is important to maintain perfusion of the lumbar spinal cord. This aspect will be discussed in greater detail in subsequent chapters.

4. If the ARM arises below the clamps, distal aortic perfusion may have some protective effect on the lumbar spinal cord, provided that perfusion pressures are adequate. Paraplegia may still occur, even if the ARM is perfused and preserved, because higher or lower critical radicular arteries are not perfused or preserved, although the risks would probably be lower.

The spinal cord diverse and complex anatomy in both animals and humans thus creates a major problem in determining which of the 13 or more pairs of segmental arteries (intercostal or lumbar) arising from the aorta supply the spinal radicular arteries. Angiography has been used for preoperative localization of the segmental arteries that give off radicular arteries that supply the spinal cord. However, there have been problems with this method of preoperative localization. Di Chiro and associates[65] have described a technique of doing a "flush aortogram" while compressing the abdomen or using adrenaline to demonstrate the ARM and the ASA. In Di Chiro's[65] study, paraplegia developed in two of the 33 monkeys after angiography. A similar technique has been advocated in humans.[66] However, Szilagyi[80] has collected a series of patients who developed paraplegia after aortography. Kieffer and colleagues[77] and Williams and associates[83] have advocated preoperative highly selective angiography and have had a measure of success with this technique. Because of the problems of preoperative localization and intraoperative identification of exactly which artery was shown to supply the spinal cord, we developed a research technique of intraoperatively identifying the spinal

FIGURE 15–11 Percentage of times the ARM is found at various thoracic (T) and lumbar (L) levels in humans. (Reprinted with permission from the Society of Thoracic Surgeons. From Svensson LG, Patel V, Coselli JS, Crawford ES. Ann Thorac Surg 1990; 49:528-35.)

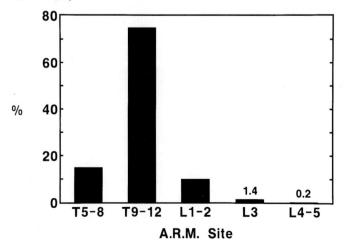

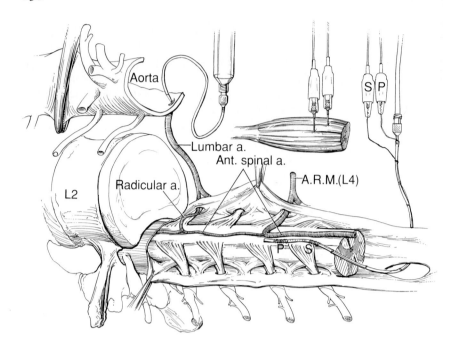

FIGURE 15–12   Illustration of how hydrogen in solution with a syringe is injected into a segmental artery, in this case L2, and how it reaches the spinal cord via a radicular artery and then travels down the anterior spinal artery to produce a current in the platinum electrode *(P)*. *ARM,* arteria radicularis magna; *S,* stainless steel electrode. (Reprinted with permission from the Society of Thoracic Surgeons. From Svensson LG, Patel V, Coselli JS, Crawford ES. Ann Thorac Surg 1990;49:528–35.)

cord blood supply, which we have used in both porcine experiments and in humans (Figs. 15–12 to 15–20).[44, 79] The advantage of this technique is that the surgeon can determine which segmental arteries can be safely oversewn during aortic operations and which arteries should be reanastomosed to the aortic graft to avoid depriving the spinal cord of its vital blood supply.

The method we developed is based on the fact that hydrogen dissolved in solution produces a weak current when in contact with platinum. This weak current can be measured by a sensitive ammeter. We hypothesized that, since hydrogen readily crosses tissue membranes, if it was injected into a radicular artery supplying the spinal cord then it would reach the anterior spinal artery, cross the membranes and

Text continued on page 243

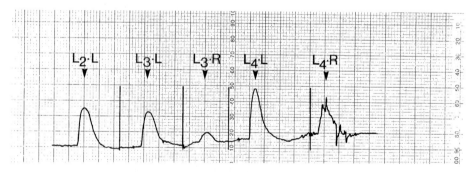

FIGURE 15–13   Example of the hydrogen-induced current impulses produced after segmental injection of the aorta with hydrogen in a porcine model. (Reprinted with permission from the Society of Thoracic Surgeons. From Svensson LG, Patel V, Coselli JS, Crawford ES. Ann Thorac Surg 1990;49:528–35.)

FIGURE 15–14   Correlation between current strength and size of radicular arteries that supply the spinal cord by hydrogen testing. (Reprinted with permission from the Society of Thoracic Surgeons. From Svensson LG, Patel V, Coselli JS, Crawford ES. Ann Thorac Surg 1990;49:528–35.)

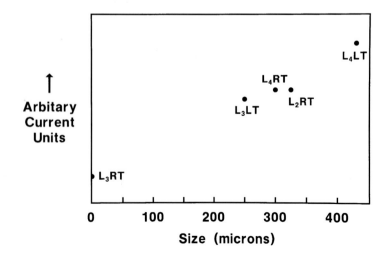

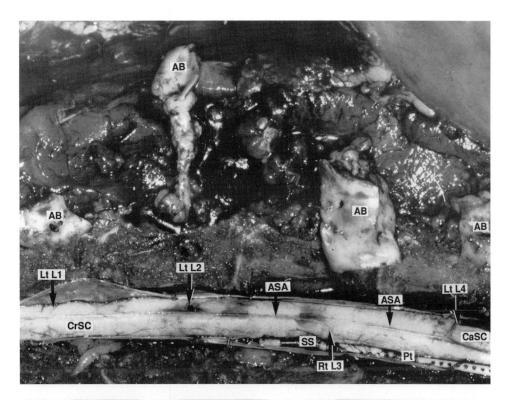

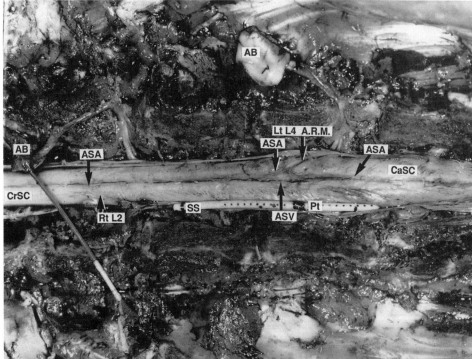

FIGURE 15–15 Postmortem dissections of porcine spinal cords after the use of hydrogen to identify levels at which blood vessels supplied the spinal cord and confirmation with methylene blue that the correct arteries were identified. *AB,* aortic button; *C,* catheter; *ASA,* anterior spinal artery; *Lt,* left; *L,* lumbar level; *CrSC,* cranial spinal cord; *CaSC,* caudal spinal cord; *SS,* stainless steel electrode for spinal motor evoked potentials; *Pt,* platinum electrode; *ARM,* arteria radicularis magna; *Rt,* right; *LA,* lumbar artery; *ASV,* anterior spinal vein. (Reprinted with permission from the Society of Thoracic Surgeons. From Svensson LG, Patel V, Coselli JS, Crawford ES. Ann Thorac Surg 1990;49:528–35.)

Illustration continued on following page

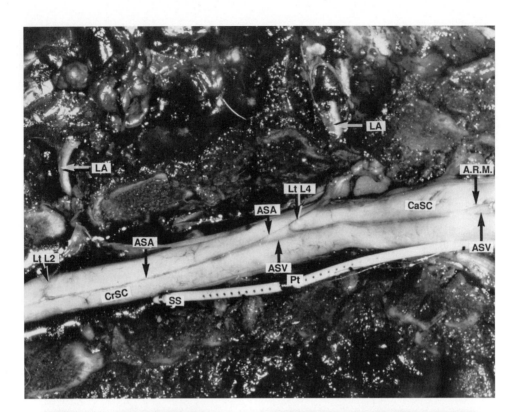

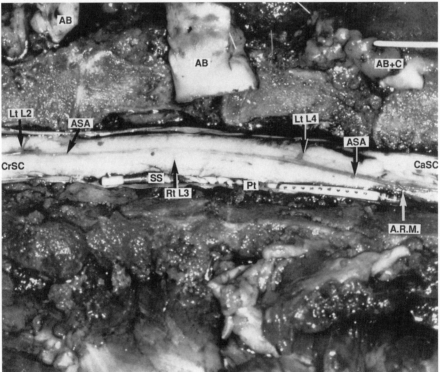

FIGURE 15–15 *Continued* Postmortem dissections of porcine spinal cords after the use of hydrogen to identify levels at which blood vessels supplied the spinal cord and confirmation with methylene blue that the correct arteries were identified. *AB,* aortic button; *C,* catheter; *ASA,* anterior spinal artery; *Lt,* left; *L,* lumbar level; *CrSC,* cranial spinal cord; *CaSC,* caudal spinal cord; *SS,* stainless steel electrode for spinal motor evoked potentials; *Pt,* platinum electrode; *ARM,* arteria radicularis magna; *Rt,* right; *LA,* lumbar artery; *ASV,* anterior spinal vein. (Reprinted with permission from the Society of Thoracic Surgeons. From Svensson LG, Patel V, Coselli JS, Crawford ES. Ann Thorac Surg 1990;49:528–35.)

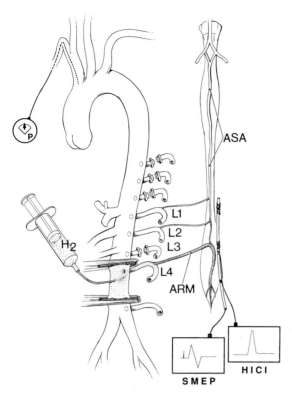

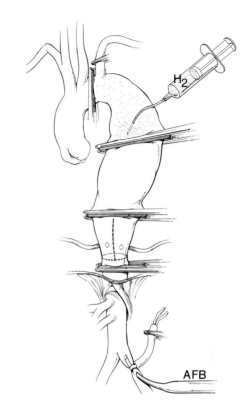

FIGURE 15–16 Experimental testing with hydrogen for arteries that supply the spinal cord in pigs. The arteries that supplied the spinal cord were preserved, and those did not were then divided and the spinal motor evoked potentials and postoperative result were then noted. The animals with preserved arteries were significantly protected against paraplegia compared with those in which the arteries identified as supplying the spinal cord were divided. (From Svensson LG, Patel V, Robinson MF, et al. J Vasc Surg 1991;13:355–65.)

FIGURE 15–17 Segmental repair of descending aortic aneurysm with hydrogen testing of segments that may supply the spinal cord. Note that hydrogen is also inserted into the atriofemoral bypass pump to determine whether distal aortic perfusion supplies the spinal cord with blood, even when the distal clamps are removed while the proximal anastomosis is performed. When multiple intercostal arteries were present in a segment that showed a response, individual arteries were then tested by injecting directly into the intercostal artery ostia.

FIGURE 15–18 **A,** Patient with pseudocoarctation of the aorta and poststenotic aneurysm (see Chapter 8 on congenital lesions for intraoperative photographs). Testing revealed that hydrogen inserted into the artriofemoral bypass pump reached the spinal cord and therefore indicating that intercostal arteries below the level of the distal clamp should be preserved. However, those vessels above the level of T9 did not supply the spinal cord. **B** and **C,** Postoperative arteriograms shown in the tracings revealed that predominantly arteries at levels T9 and T10 supplied the spinal cord with blood. (From Svensson LG, Patel V, Robinson MF, et al. J Vasc Surg 1991;13:355–65.)

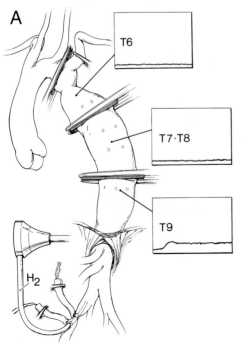

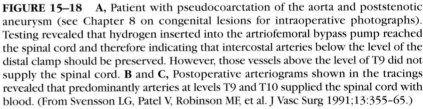

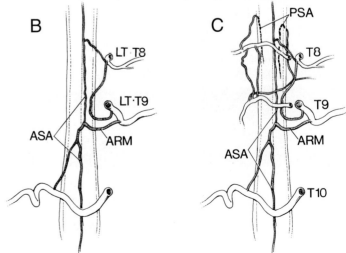

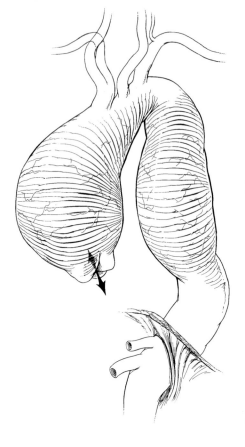

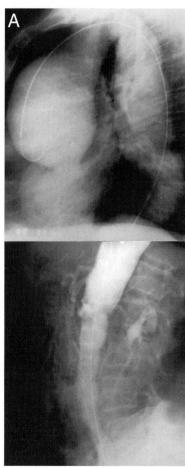

FIGURE 15–19 **A,** Patient who presented with ascending, aortic arch, and thoracoabdominal aortic aneurysm with aortic valve regurgitation. **B,** Arrows indicating platinum electrode *(top arrow),* course of the catheter alongside the spinal cord *(middle arrow),* and exit from the spinal canal onto the skin *(lower arrow).* **C,** After the patient underwent an initial stage one elephant trunk procedure, she returned for the second stage elephant trunk operation. Placement of aortic cross-clamps for intraoperative testing with hydrogen for possible intercostal arteries supplying the spinal cord. The upper window indicated no response, and the lower window indicated the presence of arteries supplying the spinal cord. On opening of the aorta, only one artery was patent, and this artery was reattached.

Illustration continued on following page

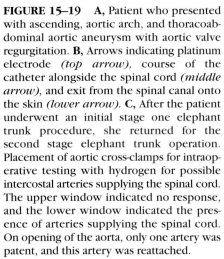

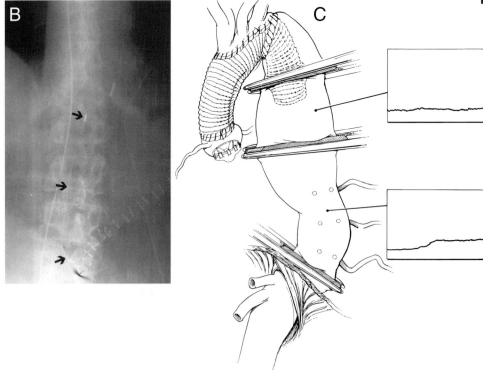

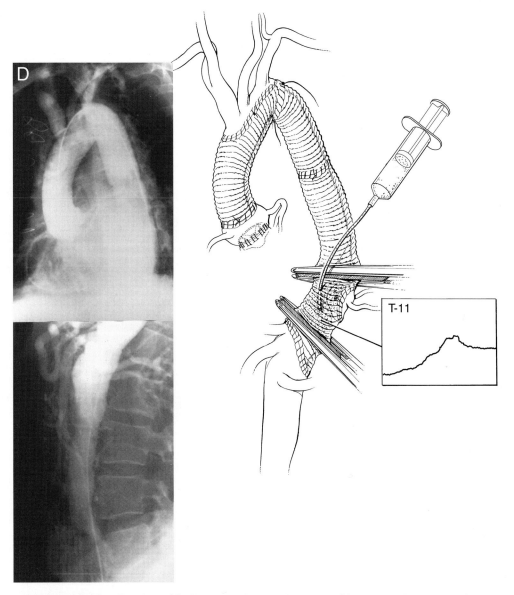

FIGURE 15–19 *Continued* **D,** Postoperative arteriogram and intraoperative testing of reattached arteries indicating preserved blood supply to the spinal cord. (From Svensson LG, Patel V, Robinson MF, et al. J Vasc Surg 1991;13:355-65.)

Illustration continued on following page

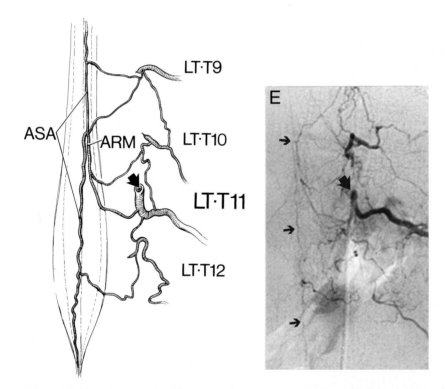

FIGURE 15–19 *Continued* **E,** The artery that was reattached supplied the arteria radicularis magna *(ARM)* and also, through collateral arteries, the other radicular arteries above and below this level (left T11) as seen on the postoperative highly selective arteriogram. *ASA,* Anterior spinal artery.

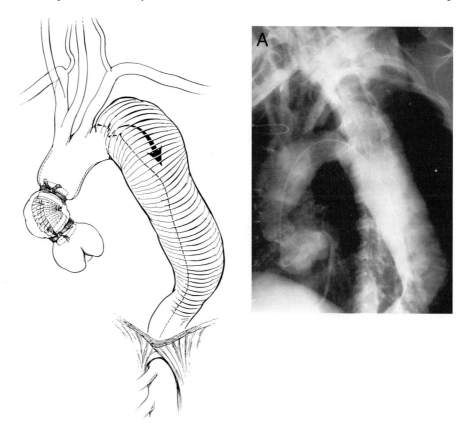

FIGURE 15–20 A, Patient with previous ascending aorta repair with intraluminal graft done elsewhere for a type III aortic dissection. B, Intraoperative testing of the aortic segments. Note that the lowest segment indicated that there were blood vessels supplying the spinal cord.

Illustration continued on following page

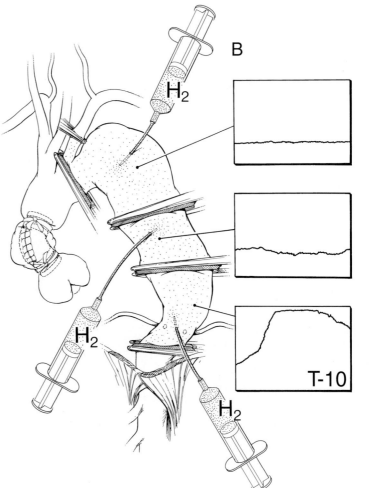

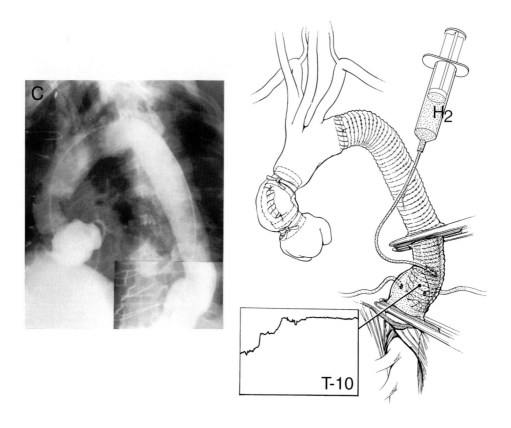

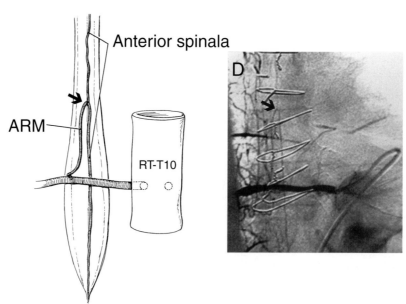

FIGURE 15–20 *Continued* **C,** Intraoperative testing revealed that the reattached vessels at T10 had preserved the spinal cord blood supply. Two 20 ml boluses were used, and thus the window indicates two peaks. **D,** Postoperative highly selective angiography confirmed that the right intercostal at T10 level supplied the ARM and hence the anterior spinal artery. (From Svensson LG, Patel V, Robinson MF, et al. J Vasc Surg 1991;13:355–65.)

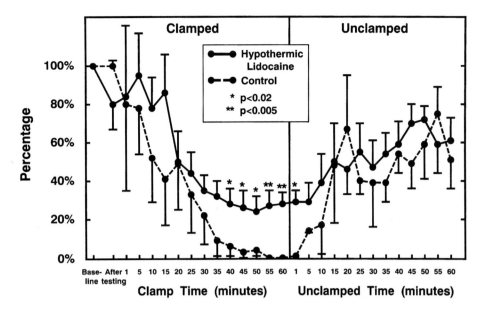

FIGURE 15–21 Effect of hypothermic lidocaine "spinoplegia" on spinal motor evoked potentials as compared with a control group during 1 hour of aortic cross-clamping. (Reprinted with permission from the Society of Thoracic Surgeons. From Svensson LG, Crawford ES, Patel V, et al. Ann Thorac Surg 1992;54:74–9.

arterial wall, and be detected by a platinum electrode lying intrathecally alongside the spinal cord[79] (Figs. 15-12 to 15-20). This technique was found to be accurate in both animals[44, 79] and humans.[44] The influence of preservation, division, or perfusion of the arteries identified as supplying the spinal cord during aortic cross-clamping will be discussed subsequently. In both animals and humans failure to reanastomose the correct segmental arteries can be detected after aortic unclamping by the failure of spinal motor evoked potentials to return to normal after a period of reperfusion (Fig. 15-21).[38]

REFERENCES

1. Griffiths IR, Pitts LH, Crawford RA, et al. Spinal cord compression and blood flow. 1. The effect of raised cerebrospinal fluid pressure on spinal cord blood flow. Neurology 1978;28:1145–51.
2. Svensson LG, Crawford ES. Aortic dissection and aortic aneurysm surgery: clinical observations, experimental investigations and statistical analyses. Part I. Curr Probl Surg 1992;29:819–912.
3. Berendes JN, Bredee JJ, Schipperheyn JJ, et al. Mechanism of spinal cord injury after cross clamping of the descending thoracic aorta. Circulation 1972;66(Supp 1):112–6.
4. Svensson LG, Von Ritter C, Oosthuizen MM, et al. Prevention of gastric mucosal lesions following aortic cross-clamping. Br J Surg 1987; 74:282–5.
5. Abbott WM, Cooper JD, Austen WG. The effect of aortic clamping and declamping on renal blood flow distribution. J Surg Res 1973; 14:385–92.
6. Carlson DA, Karp RB, Kouchoukos NT. Surgical treatment of aneurysms of the descending thoracic aorta: an analysis of 85 patients. Ann Thorac Surg 1983;35:58–69.
7. Conger J, Schrier R. Renal hemodynamics in acute renal failure. Annu Rev Physiol 1980;42:603–14.
8. Flamenbaum W. Pathophysiology of acute renal failure. Arch Intern Med 1983;131:911–28.
9. Frank RS, Moursi MM, Podrazik RM, et al. Renal vasocontriction and transient declamp hypotension after infrarenal aortic occlusion:

10. role of plasma purine degradation products. J Vasc Surg 1988;7: 515–23.
10. Hannson R, Jonsson O, Lundstrum S, et al. Effects of free radical scavengers on renal circulation after ischemia in the rabbit. Clin Sci 1983;65:605–10.
11. Hickey PR, Buckley MJ, Philbin DM. Pulsatile and nonpulsatile cardiopulmonary bypass: review of a counterproductive controversy. Ann Thorac Surg 1983;36:720–36.
12. Joob AW, Harman PK, Kaiser DL, Kron DL. The effect of renin/angiotensin system blockage on visceral blood flow during and after thoracic aortic cross-clamping. J Thorac Cardiovasc Surg 1986; 91:411–8.
13. Joob AW, Dunn C, Miller E, et al. Effect of left atrial to left femoral artery bypass and renin-angiotensin system blockage on renal blood flow and function during and after thoracic aortic occlusion. J Vasc Surg 1987;5:329–35.
14. Livesay JJ, Coolley DA, Ventemiglia RA, et al. Surgical experience in descending thoracic aneurysmectomy with and without adjuncts to avoid ischemia. Ann Surg 1985;39:37–44.
15. Miller DC, Myers BD. Pathophysiology and prevention of acute renal failure associated with thoracoabdominal or abdominal surgery. J Vasc Surg 1987;5:518–23.
16. Moran SM, Myers BD. Pathophysiology of protracted acute renal failure in man. J Clin Invest 1985;76:1440–8.
17. Myers BD, Miller DC, Mihigan JT, et al. Nature of the renal injury following total renal ischemia in man. J Clin Invest 1984;73:329–41.
18. Myers BD, Moran SM. Hemodynamically mediated acute renal failure. N Engl J Med 1986;314:97–105.
19. Oliver J, MacDowell M, Tracy A. Pathogenesis of acute renal failure associated with traumatic and toxic injury: renal ischemia, nephrotoxic damage, and the ischemuric episode. J Clin Invest 1951;30: 1305–51.
20. Paller MS, Hoidal JR, Ferris TF. Oxygen free radicals in ischemic acute renal failure in the rat. J Clin Invest 1984;74:1156–64.
21. Roberts AJ, Nora JD, Hughes WA, et al. Cardiac and renal responses to cross-clamping of the descending thoracic aorta. J Thorac Cardiovasc Surg 1983;86:732–41.
22. Symbas P, Pfaender L, Drucker M, et al. Cross-clamping of the descending aorta. J Thorac Cardiovasc Surg 1983;85:300–5.
23. Svensson LG, Coselli JS, Safi HJ, et al. Appraisal of adjuncts to prevent acute renal failure after surgery on the thoracic or thoracoabdominal aorta. J Vasc Med 1989;10:230–9.

24. Applebaum A, Karp RB, Kirklin JW. Ascending vs. descending aortic dissections. Ann Surg 1976;183:296-300.

25. Crawford ES, Svensson LG, Hess KR, et al. A prospective randomized study of cerebrospinal fluid drainage to prevent paraplegia after high-risk surgery on the thoracoabdominal aorta. J Vasc Surg 1991;13:36-45.

26. DeBakey ME, McCollum CH, Graham JM. Surgical treatment of aneurysms of the descending thoracic aorta. J Cardiovasc Surg 1978;19:571-6.

27. Fosburg RG, Brewer LA III. Arterial vascular injury to the spinal cord. Handbook Clin Neurol 1976;26:63-79.

28. Killen DA, Edwards RH, Tinsley EA, Boehm FH. Effect of low molecular weight dextran, heparin, urea, cerebrospinal fluid drainage, and hypothermia on ischemic injury of the spinal cord secondary to mobilization of the thoracic aorta from the posterior parietes. J Thorac Cardiovasc Surg 1965;50:882-7.

29. Krieger KH, Spencer FC. Is paraplegia after repair of coarctation of the aorta due principally to distal hypotension during aortic cross-clamping? Surgery 1985;97:2-6.

30. Laschinger JC, Cunningham JN, Nathan IM, et al. Experimental and clinical assessment of the adequacy of partial bypass in maintenance of spinal cord flow during operations on the thoracic aorta. Ann Thorac Surg 1983;36:417-26.

31. Molina JE, Cogordan J, Einzig S, et al. Adequacy of ascending aorta-descending aorta shunt during cross-clamping of the thoracic aorta for prevention of spinal cord injury. J Thorac Cardiovasc Surg 1985;90:126-36.

32. Najafi H, Javid H, Hushang J, et al. Descending aortic aneurysmectomy without adjuncts to avoid ischemia. Ann Thorac Surg 1980; 30:326-35.

33. Normann NA, Taylor AA, Crawford ES, et al. Catecholamine release during and after cross-clamping of the descending thoracic aorta. J Surg Res 1983;85:457-63.

34. Svensson LG, Rickards E, Coull A, et al. Relationship of spinal cord blood flow to vascular anatomy during thoracic aortic cross-clamping and shunting. J Thorac Cardiovasc Surg 1986;91:71-8.

35. Svensson LG, Stewart RW, Cosgrove DM, et al. Preliminary results and rationale for the use of intrathecal papaverine for the prevention of paraplegia after aortic surgery. S Afr J Surg 1988;26:153-60.

36. Svensson LG, Stewart RW, Cosgrove DM, et al. Intrathecal papaverine for the prevention of paraplegia after operation on the thoracic or thoracoabdominal aorta. J Thorac Cardiovasc Surg 1988;96:823-9.

37. Svensson LG, Grum DF, Bednarski M, et al. Appraisal of cerebrospinal fluid alterations during aortic surgery with intrathecal papaverine administration and cerebrospinal fluid drainage. J Vasc Surg 1990;11:423-9.

38. Svensson LG, Crawford ES, Patel V, et al. Spinal cord oxygenation, intraoperative blood supply localization, cooling and function with aortic clamping. Ann Thorac Surg 1992;54:74-9.

39. Svensson LG, Klepp P, Hinder RA. Spinal cord anatomy of the baboon: comparison with man and implications on spinal cord blood flow during thoracic aortic cross-clamping. S Afr J Surg 1986; 24:32-4.

40. Gelman S, Reves JG, Fowler K, et al. Regional blood flow during cross-clamping of the thoracic aorta and infusion of sodium nitroprusside. J Thorac Cardiovasc Surg 1983;85:287-91.

41. Svensson LG, Von Ritter CM, Groeneveld HT, et al. Cross-clamping of the thoracic aorta: influence of aortic shunts, laminectomy, papaverine, calcium channel blocker, allopurinol, and superoxide dismutase on spinal cord blood flow and paraplegia in baboons. Ann Surg 1986;204:38-47.

42. Svensson LG, Hinder RA. Hemodynamics of aortic cross-clamping: experimental observations and clinical applications. Surg Annu 1987;19:41-65.

43. Svensson LG, Crawford ES. Aortic dissection and aortic aneurysm surgery: clinical observations, experimental investigations, and statistical analyses. Part II. Curr Probl Surg 1992;29:915-1057.

44. Svensson LG, Patel V, Robinson MF, et al. Influence of preservation or perfusion of intraoperatively identified spinal cord blood supply on spinal motor evoked potentials and paraplegia after aortic surgery. J Vasc Surg 1991;13:355-65.

45. Crawford ES, Walker HSJ III, Salch SA, et al. Recent advances in management of complex aortic aneurysms: In: Bergan JJ, Yao JST, eds. Arterial Surgery: New Diagnostic and Operative Techniques. New York: Grune & Stratton, 1988;299-321.

46. Svensson LG, Grum DF, Cosgrove DM, et al. Appraisal of cerebrospinal fluid alterations during aortic surgery with intrathecal papaverine administration and cerebrospinal fluid drainage. J Vasc Surg 1990;11:423-9.

47. Applebaum A, Karp RB, Kirklin JW. Surgical treatment for closed thoracic aortic injuries. J Thorac Cardiovasc Surg 1976;71:458-60.

48. Verdant A, Page A, Cossette R, et al. Surgery of the descending thoracic aorta: spinal cord protection with the Gott shunt. Ann Thorac Surg 1988;46:147-54.

49. Verdant A, Cossette R, Page A, et al. Aneurysms of the descending thoracic aorta: three hundred sixty-six consecutive cases resected without paraplegia. J Vasc Surg 1995;21:385-91.

50. Svensson LG, Crawford ES, Hess KR, et al. Variables predictive of outcome in 832 patients undergoing repairs of the descending thoracic aorta. Chest 1993;104:1248-53.

51. Borst HG, Jurmann M, Buhner B, Laas J. Risk of replacement of descending aorta with a standardized left heart bypass technique. J Thorac Cardiovasc Surg 1994;107:126-33.

52. Svensson LG, Crawford ES, Hess KR, et al. Experience with 1509 patients undergoing thoracoabdominal aortic operations. J Vasc Surg 1993;17:357-70.

53. Cernaiau AC, Olah A, Cilley JH, et al. Effect of sodium nitroprusside on paraplegia during cross-clamping of the thoracic aorta. Ann Thorac Surg 1993;56:1035-8.

54. Svensson LG, Stewart RW, Cosgrove DM, et al. Preliminary results and rationale for the use of intrathecal papaverine for the prevention of paraplegia after aortic surgery. S Afr J Surg 1988;26:153-60.

55. Paterson IS, Klausner JM, Pugatch R, et al. Noncardiogenic pulmonary edema after abdominal aortic aneurysm surgery. Ann Surg 1989;209:231-6.

56. Blaisdell FW, Cooley DA. The mechanism of paraplegia after temporary thoracic aortic occlusion and its relationship to spinal fluid pressure. Surgery 1962;51:351-5.

57. Wadouh F, Lindemann EM, Arndt CF, et al. The arteria radicularis magna anterior as a decisive factor influencing spinal cord damage during aortic occlusion. J Thorac Cardiovasc Surg 1984;88:1-10.

58. Miyamoto K, Keno A, Wada T, et al. A new and simple method of preventing spinal cord damage following temporary occlusion of the thoracic aorta by draining the cerebrospinal fluid. J Cardiovasc Surg 1960;16:188-99.

59. Maughan RE, Mohan C, Levy R, et al. Effects of exsanguination and sodium nitroprusside on compliance of the spinal canal during aortic occlusion. J Surg Research 1992;52:571-6.

60. Grum DF, Svensson LG. Changes in cerebrospinal fluid pressure and spinal cord perfusion pressure prior to cross-clamping of the thoracic aorta in humans. J Cardiothorac Vasc Anesth 1991;5:331-6.

61. Gelman S. The pathophysiology of aortic cross-clamping and unclamping. Anesthesiology 1995;82:1026-60.

62. Crawford ES, Crawford JL, Safi HJ, et al. Thoracoabdominal aortic aneurysms: preoperative and intraoperative factors determining immediate and long-term results of operation in 605 patients. J Vasc Surg 1986;3:389-404.

63. Svensson LG, Crawford ES, Hess KR, et al. Dissection of the aorta and dissecting aortic aneurysms: improving early and long-term surgical results. Circulation 1990;82(5 Suppl):IV 24-38.

64. Di Chiro G, Doppman JL. Paraplegia after resection of aneurysm (letter to the editor). N Engl J Med 1969;281:799.

65. Di Chiro G, Fried LC, Doppman JL. Experimental spinal cord angiography. Br J Radiology 1970;43:19-30.

66. Dommisse GF. The blood supply of the spinal cord. J Bone Joint Surg (Br) 1974;56:225-35.

67. Dommisse GF. The Arteries and Veins of the Human Spinal Cord From Birth. Edinburgh: Churchill Livingstone, 1975.

68. Doppman JL, DiChiro G, Ommaya AK. Selective Arteriography of the Spinal Cord. St. Louis: Warren H. Green, Inc., 1969.

69. Feeney JF Jr, Watterson RL. The development of the vascular pattern within the walls of the central nervous system of the chick embryo. J Morphol 1946;78:231.

70. Fereschetian A, Kadir S, Kaufman SL, et al. Digital subtraction spinal cord angiography in patients undergoing thoracic aneurysm surgery. Cardiovasc Intervent Radiol 1989;12:7-9.

71. Jellinger K. Zur orthologie und pathologie der ruckenmarksdur lutung. Wien: Springer-Verlag, 1966:8-41, 55-9.

72. Patten BM. How much blood makes the cerebrospinal fluid bloody? JAMA 1968;206:378.

73. Piscol K. Die Blutversorgung des Ruckenmarkes und ihre klinis-chem relevanz. Berlin: Springer-Verlag, 1972:1-77.

74. Turnbull IM. Microvasculature of the human spinal cord. J Neuro-surg 1971;35:141-7.

75. Woollam DHM, Millen JW. In discussion on vascular disease of the spinal cord. Proc R Soc Med 1958;51:540.

76. Zuber WF, Gaspar MR, Rothschild PD. The anterior spinal artery syndrome—a complication of abdominal aortic surgery. Ann Surg 1970;172:909-15.

77. Kieffer E, Richard T, Chiras J, et al. Preoperative spinal cord arteri-ography in aneurysmal disease of the descending thoracic and tho-racoabdominal aorta: preliminary results in 45 patients. Ann Vasc Surg 1989;3:34-46.

78. Cunningham JN, Laschinger JC, Merkin HA, et al. Measurement of spinal cord ischemia during operations. Ann Surg 1982;196:285-96.

79. Svensson LG, Patel V, Coselli JS, Crawford ES. Preliminary report of localization of spinal cord blood supply by hydrogen during aortic operations. Ann Thorac Surg 1990;49:528-36.

80. Szilagyi DE, Hageman JH, Smith RF, et al. Spinal cord damage in surgery of the abdominal aorta. Surgery 1978;83:38-56.

81. Svensson LG, Hinder RA. Hemodynamics of aortic cross-clamping: experimental observations and clinical applications. Surg Annu 1987;19:41-65.

82. Svensson LG, Loop FD. Prevention of spinal cord ischemia in aortic surgery. In: Bergan JJ, Yao JST, eds. Arterial Surgery: New Diagnostic and Operative Techniques. New York; Grune & Stratton, 1988: 273-85.

83. Williams GM, Perler BA, Burdick JF, et al. Angiographic localization of spinal cord blood supply and its relationship to postoperative paraplegia. J Vasc Surg 1991;13:23-33.

16

Anesthesia and Perfusion Management

MONITORING

The successful outcome of aortic operations is dependent on careful monitoring of cardiovascular hemodynamics and other organ function. Early detection of problems arising in the vital organs can prevent the serious development of life-threatening complications. Thus monitoring of cardiac pre-load, myocardial contractility, afterload, oxygenation, blood pressures, urine output, and coagulation are critical to the prevention of intraoperative and postoperative complications related to cardiac dysfunction, renal failure, paraplegia, respiratory failure, stroke, and hemorrhage.[1-26]

To monitor the patient during aortic surgery, we routinely insert a femoral and radial arterial line for monitoring arterial pressures, a central venous pressure line, a Swan-Ganz catheter with oxygen-saturation monitoring, a subclavian line, and peripheral intravenous lines. The electrocardiograph is monitored continuously for two leads. Cardiac output, cardiac index, and systemic peripheral resistance are monitored and adjusted to optimal levels with cardiac inotropes and peripheral dilators, particularly nitroglycerin. Exhaled carbon dioxide and peripheral oxygen saturation are also routinely monitored. A Foley catheter with thermistor probe to measure bladder temperature is placed in each patient. Bladder temperature is partially influenced by the rate of urine flow to the bladder. In addition, therefore, in those patients undergoing ascending aorta and aortic arch surgery, particularly with deep hypothermia and circulatory arrest, temperature is monitored from the esophagus (approximates aortic temperature), nasopharynx (approximates brain temperature), tympanic membrane (approximates brain temperature), and rectum (an approximation of core temperature).[26]

In patients undergoing operations on the ascending aorta, the aortic arch, or both, or aortic dissection repairs, bilateral radial arterial catheters are inserted. The reason for this is that if an aortic dissection septum occludes the aorta during retrograde flow, then this lack of perfusion of the head vessels or a dissection lumen during cardiopulmonary bypass will be detected. In patients in whom atriofemoral bypass is going to be used for distal aortic perfusion, it is essential to place a femoral artery catheter for monitoring of distal aortic pressure. In patients having ascending thoracic or arch repairs for aortic dissection, the femoral arteri-

al pressure catheter is usually placed in the left groin since in 70% to 80% of patients this is the false lumen,[27] as determined by aortography. The right groin, which usually is perfused by the true lumen, should be used for aortic arterial inflow perfusion. In patients in whom atriofemoral bypass will be used during distal aortic surgery, the catheter is usually placed in the right femoral artery because the left femoral artery is more accessible for later femoral artery cannulation.[26]

Cardiac output is commonly monitored by means of Swan-Ganz catheters and therefore, by extrapolation, the cardiac contractility. This method, however, does not eliminate the effect of preload and afterload. In the laboratory we have used the measurement of dP/dt in the left ventricle in an effort to better monitor cardiac contractility but have found inconsistent results with aortic cross-clamping and unclamping. Because of the problems of monitoring cardiac contractility and the great stress placed on the heart during aortic cross-clamping, transesophageal echocardiography (TEE) is increasingly being advocated. The role of TEE has yet to be determined and will probably remain limited to high-risk patients with cardiac disease. It is, however, useful for aortic dissection operations, second-stage elephant trunk procedures, Ross procedures, and placement of right atrial venous catheters during fem-fem bypass. The plotting of volume pressure loops is one of the more accurate methods of determining myocardial contractility and is fairly independent of preload and afterload. With this method, however, it takes time to plot the volume pressure loops, and in the setting of rapidly changing parameters with aortic surgery the technique currently has little application for clinical monitoring.[26]

INTRATHECAL PRESSURE MONITORING AND CSF DRAINAGE

For patients undergoing descending thoracic or thoraco-abdominal repairs, intrathecal catheters provide a useful route for injecting medications, monitoring of cerebrospinal fluid (CSF) pressure, drainage of CSF, and spinal cord cooling. Other uses are postoperative pain control, localization of the spinal cord blood supply, monitoring of spinal cord oxygen saturation, and evoking directly from the spinal

248

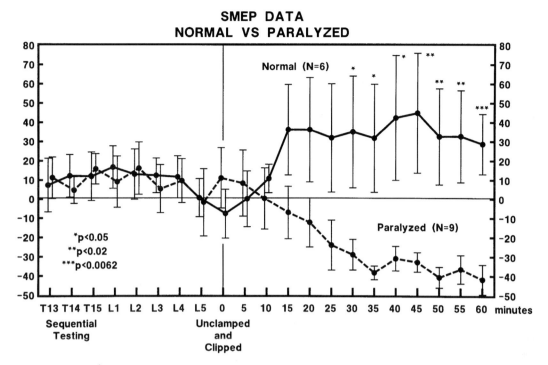

FIGURE 16–1 Spinal motor evoked potentials (SMEP) of animals that had arteries divided or preserved according to whether they supplied the spinal cord by hydrogen testing. Note that 30 minutes after division of the arteries, there was a significant difference in the SMEPs between normal and paralyzed animals. (From Svensson LG, Patel V, Robinson MF, et al. J Vasc Surg 1991;13:355–65.)

cord of spinal motor evoked potentials (SMEPs).[25, 28–31] We[31] have used SMEP monitoring to detect evidence of spinal cord dysfunction in both animals and humans. In the animal studies it was accurate for detecting paraplegia (Fig. 16–1), whereas in a large clinical study we[9] have found somatosensory evoked potentials (SSEP) to be inaccurate.[26]

Our method of inserting an intrathecal catheter is the standard technique for inserting spinal catheters except that we place the tip farther in than usual (Figs. 16–2 to 16–4). We do this to ensure that for intrathecal papaverine, when used, and for hydrogen monitoring, the catheter tip is at about the level of T10. At this level, the spinal cord segment is at approximately T12. The subarachnoid catheter is placed, with the aid of local anesthesia, via L3–4 or L4–5 intervertebral spaces and advanced approximately 25 to 30 cm from the skin so that the tip lies between vertebrae T10 and L1. An appropriate intervertebral space where the spinal processes are well apart is selected. The latter is ensured by placing the patient on his or her right side and flexing the back as much as possible. Local anesthetic is liberally injected at the site and down to the dura, with care being taken not to perforate the dura. A size 14 G Tuohy needle is used so that the catheter can be directed cranially. This is aided by placing a soft guidewire in the soft silicone catheter to allow better steering of the tip. The catheter can be advanced gently and cautiously, provided that no resistance is encountered or the patient has neither discomfort nor paresthesia. Once inserted, the silicone catheter is connected to

an arterial line type of extension tubing and strapped to the patient's back below the level of the spinal processes up to the neck so that it is not in the operative field and is accessible to the anesthesiologist for either pressure monitoring or injection of papaverine. In patients undergoing intraoperative spinal cord blood supply localization, a radiograph is taken to check the position of the catheter tip. When the pleural cavity is opened in patients in whom intrathecal papaverine has been inserted, 20 ml of CSF is withdrawn. Ten minutes before aortic cross-clamping, 3 ml (30 mg) of a specially prepared 1% preservative-free papaverine hydrochloride in 10% dextrose water solution is instilled over a 5-minute interval to allow complete solubilization of the papaverine in the CSF. The solution should be injected at body temperature. After injection of the papaverine, the catheter is slowly flushed of remaining papaverine solution over a 5-minute interval with 2 ml of either normal saline solution or CSF. This is done to prevent the occurrence of hypotension from sympathetic vasodilatation, which can follow the injection of any intrathecal medication. The patient is then placed in a slight Trendelenburg position to allow the solution of papaverine, which is denser than CSF, to gravitate downward alongside the spinal cord. During aortic cross-clamping, CSF is allowed to drain freely. More recently, however, in the prospective randomized study of CSF drainage that we[32] conducted, CSF pressure was kept between 5 and 10 mm Hg and the total volume of CSF drained was kept to 50 ml. Limiting the volume drained

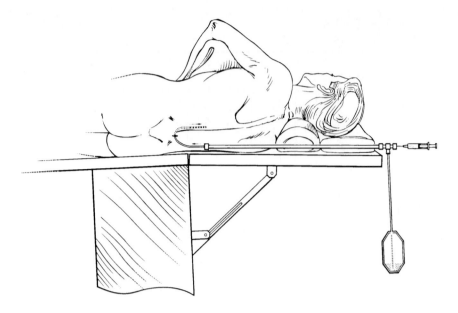

FIGURE 16–2 Positioning for intrathecal catheter with the ability to monitor pressure or inject intrathecal papaverine. Note that the catheter is placed below the spinal processes on the skine so that it does not interfere with the thoracic incision.

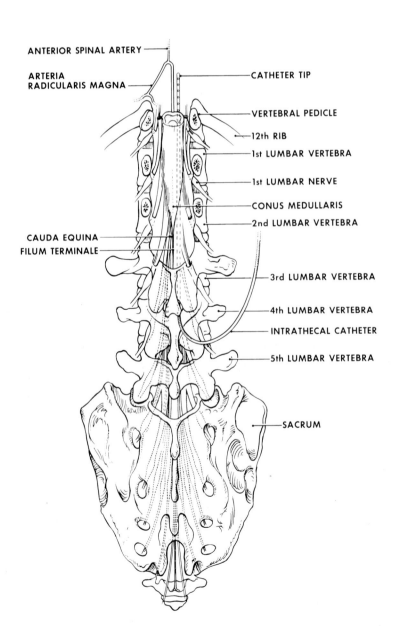

FIGURE 16–3 Course of the catheter into the intrathecal space between the third and fourth lumbar vertebrae. Note that the conus medullaris ends usually at the lower level of L2 and that the catheter tip is placed around T10 to T11, near the arteria radicularis magna, allowing for delivery of intrathecal papaverine in the critical area of the spinal cord.

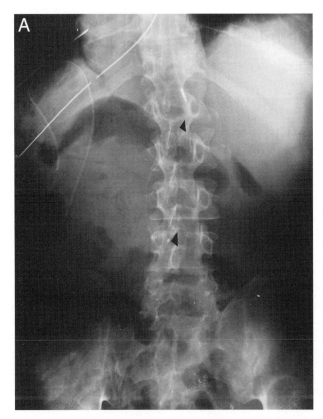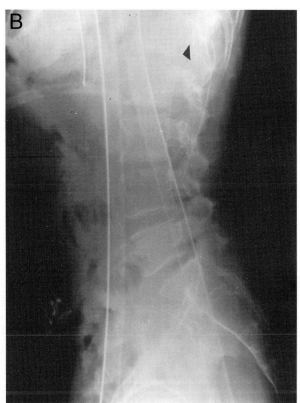

FIGURE 16–4 **A,** Intrathecal catheter on abdominal radiograph. The *upper arrow* indicates the tip and the *lower arrow* the site of entry through the skin. **B,** Lateral radiograph with the *arrow* indicating the tip of the catheter.

may reduce the risk of herniation of the brain stem. In the prospective randomized study that we conducted in 99 patients, there were no complications that could be associated with the use of CSF drainage and insertion of intrathecal catheters.[26]

INTRAVENOUS CATHETERS

During aortic operations, particularly on the descending thoracic and thoracoabdominal aorta, large volumes of blood can be lost in a very short time with the exsanguination of the patient. It must be possible to rapidly reinfuse this blood to prevent serious complications. Thus large-bore venous catheters for administration of fluid are important. Because of this, we liberally insert intravenous lines into the internal jugular vein together with the Swan-Ganz catheter, into the subclavian vein, and size 16G catheters in both arms. In patients who undergo descending thoracic or thoracoabdominal aneurysm surgery, bilateral saphenous vein size 16G catheters can also be inserted at the ankles. In addition, in those patients expected to have large volume losses, such as those undergoing first- or second-stage elephant trunk repairs or aortic dissection repairs of the thoracoabdominal aorta, a dialysis type of subclavian cannula is inserted. Two autotransfusion devices are also used in these patients and also in patients who are undergoing atriofemoral bypass. If

available, it is wise to have two autotransfusion devices working for descending thoracic and thoracoabdominal aneurysms, since a single device often has to be stopped because of excessive blood in the reservoir, a clot blocking the line, or pump malfunction. We avoid using the femoral vein for the administration of fluids because we have found that infection and thrombosis are prone to occur, whereas femoral artery catheters rarely cause problems. The subclavian catheter is usually connected directly to the autotransfusion device so that any collected blood can be rapidly reinfused. A blood warmer is also included in the reinfusion circuit. These devices for rewarming blood and rapidly reinfusing it can be purchased or a heart-lung machine can be set up to perform the same function. If bleeding is excessive and the patient is hypotensive, collected blood can be reinfused directly without being washed. Since this is heparinized blood, the patient will require protamine to reverse the effects of heparin.[26]

PROCEDURES WITHOUT CARDIOPULMONARY BYPASS

For patients undergoing descending thoracic, thoracoabdominal, and abdominal operations, optimization of preload, cardiac contractility, and afterload is important to reduce the risk of complications. To achieve this, preoperative hydration is imperative, particularly in patients with renal dysfunction. If severe cardiac dysfunction also is present, then hydration is preferably done overnight in the intensive care unit with Swan-Ganz monitoring before surgery. The aim is to achieve a cardiac index of at least 2.5 L/m² and a systemic vascular resistance of 800 to 1200 dynes/sec/cm.[5] Before aortic unclamping it is even more important that the patient be well hydrated. We rely more on the pulmonary mean arterial pressure than on the pulmonary wedge pressure because of the inaccuracy of the latter when the left side of the chest is open and the patient is lying on the right side. The left lung is also usually collapsed for thoracic aortic surgery. A further hazard that we[15] have reported is the complication of balloon inflation causing pulmonary artery rupture and hemoptysis, sometimes leading to death.[26]

Physiological Aspects

The physiological parameters that affect cardiac function are reviewed, with particular emphasis on the importance of fluid management in aortic operations. Cardiac output and cardiac index (cardiac output divided by body surface area) are directly related to the stroke volume and heart rate (CO = SV • HR). Stroke volume is a function of myocardial muscle fiber length. The total muscle length of all the constituent fibers is determined by the volume-load that stretches the fibers, namely, the preload. As the cardiac muscle is stretched by increasing the preload volume, the muscle tension generated increases to a maximum and then declines as defined by Starling's law, whereby the energy of contraction is proportional to the initial length of the cardiac muscle fiber before contraction. The preload determines the end diastolic volume, which in turn is determined by ventricular compliance (stiffness). Intramyocardial wall tension generated during contraction is thus determined by the end diastolic pressure (preload) and radius of the ventricle.[26]

The afterload is the resistance against which the blood must be expelled. The afterload is determined by the resistance or impedance and is proportional to the aortic valve and peripheral vascular resistance. Myocardial contractility is influenced by circulating inotropes and cardiac sympathetic innervation. The oxygen demand of the heart for the work that it performs is, in turn, determined by the intramyocardial wall tension, contractile state, and heart rate. Of lesser importance for the oxygen requirements are the external work performed, activation energy, and basal oxygen demands. Performance curves constructed to relate left atrial pressure (pulmonary capillary wedge pressure) to cardiac output show that, with increasing preload, cardiac performance improves to a maximum and thereafter declines. These curves, however, have limited usefulness in aortic surgery because of the time it takes to construct them, changing contractility due to ischemia, preload, and the frequent inaccuracy of wedge pressures. Furthermore, it is our impression that in patients undergoing descending or thoracoabdominal aortic surgery, cardiac performance declines with time during aortic cross-clamping, diastolic compli-

ance deteriorates, and increasing preload is required to achieve the same performance. Because of the increased wall tension produced by the increased afterload with aortic cross-clamping, oxygen demand is further increased. If afterload is not reduced, then the following cardiac problems can arise: electrocardiographic (ECG) evidence of subendocardial ischemia; arrhythmias, especially bradycardia and ventricular arrhythmias such as bigeminy; and left ventricular failure as evidenced by ventricular dilatation. The latter is particularly likely to occur when preoperative cardiac dysfunction is present, particularly if it is of valvular or ischemic origin. Thus, to prevent myocardial dysfunction, afterload has to be reduced with the use of vasodilators. Nitroglycerin is preferable since this agent also dilates the coronary arteries,[1, 33] whereas sodium nitroprusside may reduce coronary blood flow[24] by lowering the blood perfusion pressure and may also have deleterious effects on the spinal cord (see Chapter 15 on hemodynamics). When nitroglycerin is used, however, there are two consequences that must be guarded against: (1) further decrease in cardiac output induced by excessively reduced preload, which leads to tachycardia and systemic hypotension with reduced coronary blood flow, especially across any coronary stenoses; (2) hypoperfusion of other organs and the spinal cord as a result of a reduced pressure head. Cardiac output (CO = stroke volume • heart rate) can be increased by increasing the heart rate with a pacemaker or by positive chronotropes. For example, dopamine has both inotropic and chronotropic effects. This is not desirable, however, in those patients who are undergoing aortic surgery without coronary bypasses, because oxygen demand may exceed the supply available from coronary blood flow. Furthermore, coronary blood flow occurs during diastole; thus the higher the heart rate, the shorter the diastolic period for coronary perfusion. Clearly this results in reduced blood flow to the myocardium which may not be sufficient to meet the increased oxygen demands.[26]

Because of the stress that will be imposed on the heart during aortic surgery, particularly for descending thoracic and thoracoabdominal aortic operations, both adequate fluid loading and the use of vasodilators are critical for the optimal preparation of patients before aortic cross-clamping. The two most beneficial effects of these measures are the improvement of cardiac performance and optimizing of oxygen demand. The importance of fluid loading is that a reservoir of fluid is stored in the venous capacitance vessels and, under the stress of aortic cross-clamping or massive fluid loss, can be drawn on by reducing the level of nitroglycerin infusion. Fluid loading may also reduce the risk of hypotension occurring because of mesenteric traction during infrarenal aortic surgery. This type of hypotension may be caused by the release of prostacyclin.[11] Both Bush and associates[3, 4] and Whittmore and colleagues[34] have shown that when fluid loading is used during aortic surgery, the risks of cardiac complications are significantly reduced. Harpole and colleagues[12] have shown that the stress on the heart that results in cardiac adaptations is largely due to changes in the afterload during cardiac surgery. Of interest, therefore, is the finding that in patients undergoing infrarenal aortic operations aortic cross-clamping is less detrimental to the heart in patients with aortoiliac occlusive disease than in those with infrarenal aortic aneurysms.[10] The reason for this is believed to be that the patients with aortoiliac disease have extensive networks of collateral vessels and thus the increase in afterload in these patients with aortic cross-clamping is not as great.[10] These collateral arteries that reduce the afterload by offering less resistance to aortic outflow during aortic cross-clamping would be similar to those found in patients with coarctation of the aorta. In patients with coarctation of the aorta, cross-clamping of the aorta does not have as marked an effect on cardiac function and hemodynamics as, for example, a patient with a traumatic rupture of the aorta.[26]

The volume of fluid that is required in each individual patient will vary according to the operative procedure, the use of cardiopulmonary bypass or atriofemoral bypass, responses of the patient, blood loss, and intrinsic cardiac function. As a reasonable guide to fluid administration, although it must be borne in mind that each patient varies considerably, we recommend that fluid be given to patients undergoing infrarenal aortic surgery until the pulmonary artery mean pressure reaches 10 to 15 mm Hg. For thoracic aortic procedures a pressure of greater than 20 mm Hg is usually needed to maintain hemodynamic stability. However, patients who have poor ventricular compliance with diastolic dysfunction, usually from scarring from prior myocardial infarcts, require greater filling pressures, even as high as 35 mm Hg. Furthermore, if the period of aortic cross-clamping of the descending thoracic aorta has been long for patients undergoing thoracic aortic procedures, higher filling pressures may be required because of left ventricular dysfunction, particularly if a distal perfusion technique has not been used. It is extremely important to maintain a finely tuned balance between preload and excessive fluid administration in patients with poor heart function, since an excessive fluid preload may result in heart failure. With experience and patience, the point of maximal performance can be achieved, particularly in the postoperative period when large volumes of fluid loss do not, as a rule, suddenly occur, making it easier to optimize intravascular blood volume and preload.[26]

During aortic operations it is essential that the anesthesiologist and the surgeon remain in communication as the operation progresses or as problems occur. Before the application of aortic clamps in patients undergoing distal aortic surgery, the surgeon should notify the anesthesiologist that the clamps are about to be applied. In patients undergoing infrarenal aortic operations, the anesthesiologist can then observe hemodynamic alterations, particularly if the blood pressure increases excessively and requires adjustment. In patients in whom the thoracic aorta is being cross-clamped, this gives the anesthesiologist time to increase the rate of nitroprusside infusion and, if preload is adequate, to increase the rate of nitroglycerin. However, excessive nitro-

prusside or any other strong vasodilator should be used with caution in case the blood pressure drops excessively and results in decreased perfusion of the spinal cord.[35, 36] At the same time, a continuous infusion of sodium bicarbonate should be commenced and the rate of fluid administration increased in preparation for aortic unclamping. Blood collected by the autotransfusion device should also be reinfused. Similarly, the anesthesiologist should be notified 5 minutes before unclamping. At this time it is recommended that the rate of crystalloid fluid administration be increased and, for thoracoabdominal aortic aneurysms in particular, blood and blood products are infused so that by the time the clamps are removed the pulmonary artery mean pressure is at least 20 mm Hg. At the same time, the infusion of nitroprusside and nitroglycerin must be stopped or decreased. The clamps should be gradually removed, allowing a few beats at a time to send blood flowing through the graft, until the patient's blood pressure is at a sufficient level to permit complete removal of the clamps. Calcium chloride and additional sodium bicarbonate are useful in improving cardiac performance, particularly if acidosis is still present. Preload, contractility, and afterload will need to be optimized once again as the patient stabilizes and bleeding is controlled. High filling pressures (preload) and dopamine at 3 μg/kg per minute, if the latter has not already been commenced, improve renal blood flow and possibly reduce the risk of postoperative renal failure.[13, 37] We also intravenously administer indigo carmine, which appears in the urine shortly after unclamping of the aorta. We have found that the time taken for indigo carmine to reappear in the urine correlates with the postoperative risk of acute renal failure.[37] Of particular concern is whether the time taken for dye to appear exceeds 30 minutes. If this should occur, then the left renal artery should be palpated and examined with a sterile intraoperative duplex study if the latter is available. If renal perfusion is still of concern, the incision can be closed, the patient taken to the angiography suite, and the renal arteries checked for patency.[26]

CARDIOPULMONARY BYPASS

Operations on the ascending aorta, the aortic arch, and the heart require control of heart function and hemodynamics during the operation. This is best achieved with cardiopulmonary bypass, cardioplegia for cardiac arrest and protection, and, if necessary, deep hypothermia with circulatory arrest for protection of the brain (see Chapter 15 on Deep Hypothermia with Circulatory Arrest and Retrograde Brain Perfusion). The preferred method of cardiopulmonary bypass cannulation is venous drainage from the two venae cavae through the right atrium and arterial inflow through the femoral artery (Figs. 16-5 and 16-6).[27, 38] The cavae are looped by umbilical tape to ensure cardiac isolation from venous blood flow, and ventricular distention is prevented by the insertion of a right superior pulmonary vein cannula extending through the left atrium into the left ventricle. A

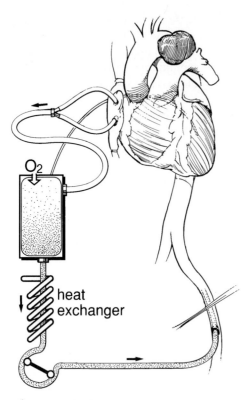

In patients in whom cardiopulmonary bypass is necessary because of distal aortic arch, descending thoracic, or thoracoabdominal aortic aneurysms, cannulation techniques are different because the right side of the heart is not as accessible during the operation through the left thoracotomy.[39] Nevertheless, we have used a two-stage cannula through the right atrial auricle to place patients on cardiopulmonary bypass. The technique is illustrated in Figures 16-7 and 16-8. If deep hypothermia and circulatory arrest are planned in addition because, for example, control of the proximal aorta is a problem or the aorta needs to be replaced from the distal ascending aorta throughout its entire course along the chest to the abdomen, then femorofemoral bypass is the best choice (Fig. 16-7).[39] If cardiac distention is noted dur-

FIGURE 16–6   Cannulation setup for deep hypothermic arrest with retrograde brain perfusion. Note that a Y arm off the arterial line is connected to the superior vena cava cannula for retrograde brain perfusion. The superior vena cava cannula is also ensnared with an umbilical tape tourniquet.

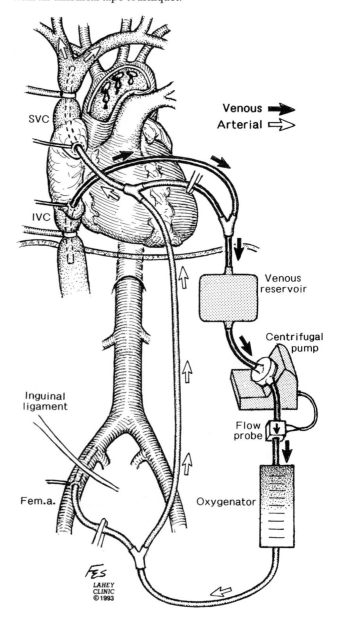

FIGURE 16–5   Standard cannulation technique for most aortic aneurysm repairs through the mediastinum. The superior and inferior venae cavae are cannulated for venous drainage and the femoral artery for arterial inflow. A cannula is also placed through the superior right pulmonary vein into the left ventricle. (From Svensson LG, Crawford ES. Curr Probl Surg 1992;29:819–912.)

two-stage venous cannula through the right atrial appendage can be used, although this is not recommended in most cases. There are several reasons for this: the heart is not completely isolated; dissection in the angle between the aorta and the atrium to obtain a proximal anastomosis at the aortic value sometimes results in the atrium being inadvertently opened, with air being sucked into the right atrium and thus the venous cannula; and the cannula tends to get in the way during the operation. For reoperations, it is necessary for both the femoral artery and the femoral vein to be identified and ensnared before the chest is opened (Fig. 16-7). The right subclavian artery can also be used for arterial cannulation in patients with distal atheromatous disease or complex aortic dissections. If a pseudoaneurysm or the posterior sternum is involved, then the patients are placed electively on femorofemoral (artery and vein) bypass, cooled, and deep hypothermia with circulatory arrest is established before the sternum is opened. If this approach is adopted for the more complex sternal entry cases, inadvertent opening of the aortic aneurysm during reentry entails a lower risk of fatal complications since both the heart and the brain are protected while intrathoracic control is established. Once the chest is successfully opened, the patient is again placed on cardiopulmonary bypass until the aortic repair is performed.[26]

ing bypass or after the heart fibrillates, then the left ventricle can be sumped through a left ventriculotomy or through the left auricle. Another method is to obtain venous drainage through the pulmonary artery by placing a cannula through the pulmonary valve into the right ventricle. Using this approach alone without drainage of the inferior vena cava via the femoral vein is less desirable because of warming of the right side of the heart. If atriofemoral bypass (namely, without oxygenator) is in use when a decision is made to institute full cardiopulmonary bypass, then the "venous" drainage from the left atrium can be supplemented by draining blood from the femoral vein or from the pulmonary artery or right atrium with a two-stage cannula to establish drainage to achieve adequate flow rates for complete cardiopulmonary bypass.[26]

Myocardial and brain protection during cardiopulmonary bypass has been discussed in previous chapters. A detailed review of cardiopulmonary bypass techniques, complications, and hematological alterations is beyond the scope of

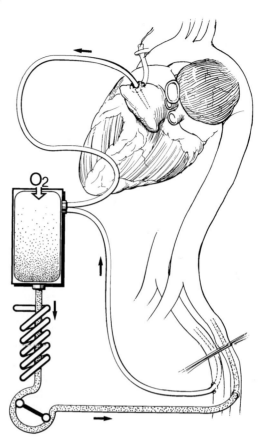

FIGURE 16–8 Cannulation sites for repair of a distal aortic arch aneurysm with deep hypothermic arrest through the left side of the chest. Note that the femoral artery and vein are cannulated for cardiopulmonary bypass. The femoral vein cannula should be inserted so that the tip is in the right atrium. To confirm its positioning, we have used TEE to check where the tip is. If venous drainage is inadequate, then a left atrial cannula, as shown, can be added, or a cannula can be placed in the pulmonary artery and gently guided into the right ventricle through the pulmonary valve, or a two-stage cannula can be inserted through the right atrial appendage without too much difficulty. (From Svensson LG, Crawford ES. Curr Probl Surg 1992;29:819–912.)

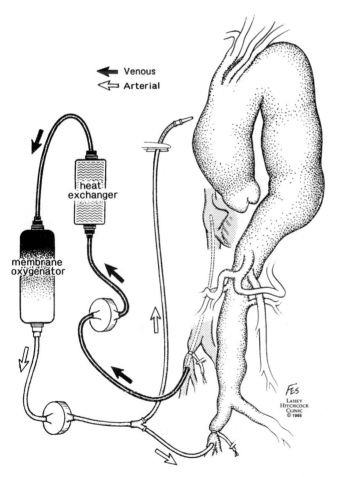

FIGURE 16–7 Cannulation setup for reoperations through the mediastium or an extensive repair of the aorta through the left side of the chest. Note that the venous cannula tip is placed in the right atrium with the aid of intraoperative transesophageal echocardiography and connected to a centrifugal pump on the venous line to aid venous drainage. A Y off the arterial line is available for insertion into a side graft coming off the new aortic graft so that arterial blood flow can initially be reestablished antegrade to the brain.

this book. Briefly, we attempt to maintain an optimal perfusion pressure above 50 mm Hg without the manipulation of vasoconstrictors. Particularly in the case of elderly patients, it is advisable to add blood to the pump to increase viscosity and systemic resistance, thus improving perfusion pressures. This also results in better venous drainage with the net outcome that higher flow rates can be achieved. In patients with known carotid artery stenoses we maintain the perfusion pressure at approximately 70 mm Hg.[26]

Discontinuation of cardiopulmonary bypass in patients who have had aortic operations is similar to that after routine coronary artery bypass. The process can be conveniently summarized by an alphabetical checklist of ten steps during and after discontinuing bypass[26]:

1. Anastomoses. Active bleeding other than oozing from the anastomoses should be obtained as much as possible before bypass is discontinued since this is easier without an ejecting heart and ultimate blood loss is less. Relying only on clotting factors to stop hemorrhage is not usually sufficient to obtain hemostasis. Oozing of blood from an inadequately baked graft or a collagen-impregnated graft, however, can be controlled only by rapid transfusion of clotting factors, including fresh frozen plasma, platelets, and cryoprecipitate.

2. Beat. Both heart rhythm and ECG of the beating heart must be checked. We routinely use both atrial and ventricular wires in patients undergoing aortic surgery, since heart block may occur postoperatively and malignant ventricular arrhythmias are not infrequent. Furthermore, atrial pacing can be used to improve cardiac output in patients with poor left ventricular function. If difficulty is experienced in pacing the heart with the atrial leads, placement of a lead on the inner aspect of the superior vena caval junction with the atrium near the sinoatrial node may be successful. Accumulated blood around either the atrial leads or the ventricular leads where they make contact with the heart may also short-circuit the leads, resulting in inadequate conduction. In patients with mild degrees of aortic valve regurgitation in whom the aortic valve has not been replaced, pacing at a higher rate can overcome much of the regurgitation.

3. Contractility. If inspection of the left ventricle reveals inadequate contractility, then appropriate inotropes can be promptly administered before bypass is discontinued. If the right ventricle is dysfunctional, the possibility of air in the right coronary artery should be considered, particularly if a composite valve graft has been inserted. If a Cabrol type of composite valve graft has been inserted, then the possibility of kinking of the graft to the right coronary ostium should be considered. Alternatively, if the clamp time has been prolonged and retrograde cardioplegia has been used, right-sided heart protection may have been inadequate.

4. Degree of temperature. In contrast to those patients undergoing coronary bypass surgery, patients who undergo aortic surgery should be rewarmed to a higher body temperature. The reason for this is that more time may be necessary to ensure adequate hemostasis after discontinuation of bypass without the patient becoming hypothermic.

5. Electrolytes, hematocrit, and arterial blood gases. Potassium levels may be very high if a considerable amount of cardioplegia has been used, particularly by the retrograde continuous cardioplegia technique, and thus furosemide or insulin may be needed for excretion of excessive amounts of these electrolytes. For the same reason, the serum levels of glucose should also be checked, since hyperglycemia may be present. Checking of blood gases ensures that the patient is well oxygenated before being taken off bypass.

6. Flow. Cardiopulmonary bypass flow rates are adjusted according to preload, contractility, and afterload while the patient is weaned from bypass. Most patients will require a mean pulmonary arterial pressure of more than 20 mm Hg to maintain an adequate preload to ensure hemodynamic stability, particularly for the first 10 to 12 hours after surgery. During weaning from bypass, the right ventricle is carefully observed to see whether it is collapsing, and the respiratory variation of the systolic peak blood pressure is observed to be sure that it is not more than approximately 7 mm Hg. If

either of these are present, then further blood and fluid can be administered from the pump. The pulmonary artery pressures and the position of the Swan-Ganz catheter are checked by gentle digital palpation of the pulmonary artery.

7. Gases. Arterial blood gases are checked again after discontinuing bypass to ensure that the patient is being adequately ventilated. Similarly, if the patient is acidotic from a prolonged cardiopulmonary bypass time, this will need correction with sodium bicarbonate.

8. Hypotensives. If pulmonary pressures become excessively high, nitroglycerine is administered, allowing all blood from the bypass pump, including the first flush of the pump, to be administered to the patient. If the patient is hypertensive, a vasodilator, usually nitroprusside, is commenced by intravenous infusion to reduce afterload and improve cardiac performance.

9. Index and Inotropes. If the cardiac index does not exceed 2.2 L/m^2 per minute after it has been visually ascertained that contractility is adequate and fluid loading is maximal, and after administration of hypotensives has begun, then further inotropes (particularly epinephrine, which is the most effective agent) must be added. Intraaortic balloon pumps are avoided but occasionally are used as a last resort,[27, 38] and rarely a left ventricular assist device is inserted. In fact, in our experience, on five occasions when left ventricular assist devices (centrifugal pumps) were used, four of the patients survived and were able to leave the hospital. This may be because cardiac ischemia may be too prolonged with extensive aortic repairs or that barbiturates, which are used to prevent cerebral injury, also depress the myocardial contractility. When the left ventricular devices are removed it is probably a good policy to swing an omental flap up into the chest to cover exposed aortic grafts and also fill the dead space left after resection of the aneurysm. We have used this technique, and postoperative mediastinal infection has not developed.

10. Juice. For lack of a better term, *juice* refers to frequent checking of urine output during bypass and after. If the total volume of urine output is inadequate, then the necessary steps should be taken to eliminate correctable causes of renal failure. For example, renal function may be compromised by preoperative renal failure, embolization of atheromatous material from the aorta into the renal arteries, or failure of adequate perfusion of the kidneys because of aortic dissection. If right-sided heart pressures have been excessively high during bypass, this could increase the risk of renal failure, particularly if it is associated with abdominal distension.[26]

ATRIOFEMORAL BYPASS

Increasingly it is becoming clear, from our recent review of our own 832 patients who had descending aortic repairs,[40] our series of 1508 thoracoabdominal aortic repairs,[41] the reports by Lawrie,[42] Borst,[43] Verdant and associates,[44] and the updated report by Najafi,[45] that perfusion of the distal aorta, particularly when carefully regulated and maximally used atriofemoral bypass is instituted, protects the kidneys and spinal cord. Initially, in our earlier reports[46] on smaller series, this protective effect was not obvious. However, with more statistical power in a study of 832 patients undergoing descending thoracic repairs (Fig. 16-9), 1508 thoracoabdominal repairs, and a prospective study of thoracoabdominal repairs, it is clear that atriofemoral bypass is protective[31, 40, 41] for prolonged aortic clamp times and when sequential segmental aortic repairs are performed. The use of the atriofemoral bypass reduces the need for vasodilators during cross-clamping and decreases the risk of hypotension with aortic unclamping. Furthermore, sodium bicarbonate is not required in the same volumes to correct acidosis after unclamping of the aorta.[26]

Atriofemoral bypass for distal aortic perfusion is established by cannulating the left atrium through a pledgeted pursestring suture placed as much as possible on the outside of the left atrial auricle. For this we use 3-0 Prolene suture material rather than silk or polyester because the latter two are more likely to tear the auricle when tightened. Alternatively, particularly in patients who have had previous cardiac surgery, the pulmonary veins can be used. When repairing the veins after decannulation, however, care should be taken that the veins are not narrowed. Narrowed veins can result in venous stasis and lung infarction. The

FIGURE 16–9   A, Influence of aortic cross-clamp time on the risk of spinal cord injury in 832 patients with descending aortic repairs of various extents. **B,** Influence of atriofemoral bypass on the risk of injury in patients having proximal repairs, distal repairs **(C)**, and repair of the entire descending aorta **(D)**. (From Svensson LG, Crawford ES, Hess KR, et al. Chest 1993;104: 1248-53.)

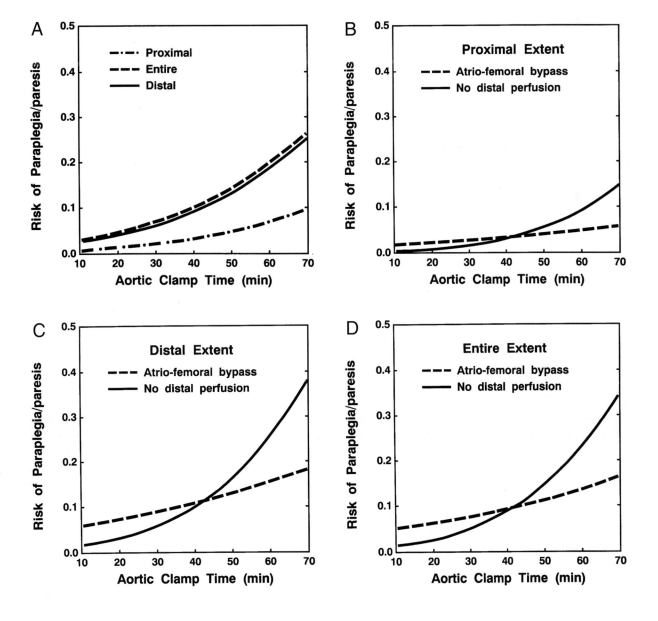

oxygenated blood that is drained from the atrium is pumped into the femoral artery with a centrifugal pump. The left femoral artery is used because it is more easily accessible for insertion of the arterial cannula. A transverse incision is made in the artery, the largest cannula up to 24FG is inserted, and then the umbilical tape around the artery is tightened around the cannula. The distal artery is occluded with an angled DeBakey clamp. Heparinization is optional. The pump is started immediately when the circuit is completed. An attempt should be made to perfuse the distal aorta for the entire period of aortic cross-clamping if possible and to segmentally repair the aneurysm. Use of atriofemoral bypass only for the proximal anatomosis, as used to be our practice, has a limited protective effect since this time period may be only one-fourth of the total aortic cross-clamp time.[26]

During atriofemoral bypass the pulmonary artery mean pressure should be maintained above 20 mm Hg. If this is not done, excessive blood is likely to be pumped from the atrium to the distal aorta, resulting in inadequate perfusion of the aorta proximal to the aortic clamp and hypotension with potential risk of brain ischemia. A low total fluid volume will also aggravate large swings in distal and proximal aortic pressures during pumping when blood loss is excessive.

AUTOTRANSFUSION AND MANAGEMENT OF COAGULATION

With the risk of life-threatening viral diseases being transmitted by blood and blood products during transfusions for major aortic operations, minimizing the use of blood and blood products is an enviable goal. Homologous blood has been used in large volumes to replace operative blood loss and drainage after operations. Homologous blood products in particular have traditionally been used to obtain hemostasis after cardiovascular and vascular operations on the aorta, exposing patients to multiple donors. The problem of minimizing blood use has been complicated by the volume of blood loss during many of these operations,[47-50] the use of cardiopulmonary bypass,[51-53] and antecedent clotting defects in these patients, because of either aneurysms or medications such as aspirin and Coumadin.[52] The problem of uncontrolled bleeding is illustrated by reports that up to one third of postoperative deaths after aortic surgery, particularly thoracic operations with bypass pumps and heparin, are due to hemorrhage.[54, 55] This problem of uncontrolled bleeding is further exacerbated by the not infrequent occurrence of preoperative disseminated intravascular coagulation (DIC) in patients undergoing aortic operations.[56]

In 1818 Blundell[57] reported the first human-to-human blood transfusion. To minimize the use of donor blood, the obvious course would be to use the patient's own blood. This was done in 1886 by Duncan,[58] who collected blood for later reinfusion during the amputation of a patient's limb after a railway accident. Early techniques entailed the use of collection reservoirs, after which blood was transfused into the patient. Later, heparin or citrate-phosphate-dextrose

(CPD) was added to the aspirated blood to keep it from clotting, and the blood was filtered before reinfusion. Because of the risk of disease transmission, alternative strategies such as autotransfusion devices were developed. Subsequent studies have shown the usefulness and effectiveness of autotransfusion by various techniques for various types of procedures.[47, 49, 51, 53, 59-63] Most of the modern collection devices suction blood into a reservoir from an external source outside the operating room. Heparin or citrate is mixed with the blood as it enters the suction nozzle, preventing clotting of the blood. From the reservoir, the patient's blood is pumped by a roller pump into a centrifuge, which is used to wash the red cells and separate out the red cells from the other blood constituents or debris. The red cells are then pumped into a transfusion plastic bag with saline solution, from which they can be pumped under pressure into the patient. Newer autotransfusion devices also have air-detection safety features that automatically shut off blood transfusion if air is detected beyond the in-line filters. In addition, a rapid reinfusion machine or a roller pump with appropriate warming coils can be used for warming the infused blood or blood products to reduce the risk of severe hypothermia. The hematocrit of the transfused red cells should be between 40% and 60%, depending on the centrifugation technique and device being used. Of note, most of the heparin, blood products, free hemoglobin, fat, platelets, coagulation factors, complement, and, to a lesser extent, bacteria are eliminated by this technique.[59, 61, 64, 65] Of course, not all the red cells are salvaged by this technique since some break down with centrifugation or are lost in blood clots. The time required to prepare a unit of blood is approximately 2 to 4 minutes with the Baylor Rapid Auto Transfuser (BRAT). If particularly uncontrolled bleeding occurs, then washing of the red cells does not have to be done and the heparinized blood is reinfused directly. The activated clotting time is then used as a guide for the administration of protamine.[48] The use of heparin for descending thoracic, thoracoabdominal, and abdominal aortic surgery is not essential unless cardiopulmonary bypass is instituted. We believe that this approach does not significantly increase the risk of thrombosis; furthermore, this avoids the risks involved with heparinization, including an increased mortality rate.[26, 55, 66]

With autotransfusion for ascending, aortic arch, descending thoracic, and infrarenal aneurysms repairs, these operations can fairly often be accomplished with less use of blood. In our experience with autotransfusion devices, a median of 4 units of blood was required intraoperatively for ascending aortic repairs (Fig. 16–10), 6 units for arch repairs, 6 units for descending aortic repairs, 7 units for thoracoabdominal aortic repairs, and 2 units for infrarenal aortic repairs. The median number of units of "saved red cells" autotransfused were similar, with 5, 6, 7, 8, and 3 units, respectively, being reinfused per patient. The average number of units of fresh frozen plasma being required for these operations were 11, 14, 12, 16, and 4, respectively. The median use of platelets was 20 units for all types of surgery with the exception of infrarenal aneurysms, for which the median was 10 units. In those patients undergoing either ascending aortic or ascending plus aortic arch repairs, the median use of cryoprecipitate was 6.5 and 10 units, respectively.[26] For patients undergoing aortic repairs that require deep hypothermic arrest, the intraoperative blood transfusion amounts required have been 6 units of packed red blood cells, 16 of fresh frozen plasma, 20 of platelets, and 20 of cryoprecipitate.[67] More recently one of us (L.G.S.), whenever possible using preoperative autologous blood donation, autotransfusion devices, intraoperative plasmapheresis, meticulous surgery, and postoperative reinfusion of blood shed from chest tubes, found that the amount of homologous blood transfused for ascending or aortic arch operations has been reduced until 87% of patients have no intraoperative homologous blood transfusions and 69% of patients are discharged from the hospital without ever having had a transfusion of homologous blood or blood products.[67] By stepwise logistic regression analysis, the independent predictors that a patient would require an in-hospital homologous blood transfusion were ($p < 0.05$), older age, cardiopulmonary bypass time, and postoperative amount of blood loss from chest tube drainage. Many of these patients underwent complex operations, including elephant trunk repairs, composite valve graft insertions, reoperations, and additional cardiac procedures. Maximizing the use of blood-conservation techniques does not appear to have affected the survival rate, since the 30-day survival rate was 98.6%.[67]

After the operative repair of the aorta is completed, hemostasis at the anastoses has to be assured when the aortic clamps are removed. For patients on cardiopulmonary bypass, this can conveniently be done during rewarming. For all patients an attempt should be made to ensure hemostasis as much as possible with the use of pledgeted sutures immediately after unclamping of the aorta. Thereafter, after

discontinuation of bypass for proximal procedures, protamine, autologous blood (if available), plasmapheresis, collected blood, and blood from the pump are administered. The hematocrit, platelet count, prothrombin time (PT), partial thromboplastin time (PTT), fibrinogen, and fibrin split products are checked. Thereafter, except in patients who have had infrarenal aneurysm repairs, these studies are repeated at 20-minute intervals, especially if bleeding continues. Laboratory results should be available within 15 to 20 minutes. This further helps in making a rapid decision, often with help from a hematologist, as to whether products or other agents should be administered. All blood products and blood should be filtered with a 40 μm filter. Stored bank packed red blood cell units should also be filtered with a white cell filter (7 μm) if a large volume blood transfusion is envisioned.[26]

For patients who have undergone aortic surgery, a hemoglobin level of 10 mg/dl or a hematocrit value of 30% is desirable, since a level below this can result in increased hemorrhage. The incidence of multiple organ failure may also be lower with a higher hemoglobin level and a greater amount of oxygen delivery to peripheral tissues. Young patients who have had coronary artery bypass surgery, however, are allowed to drop to a hematocrit value of 18%. As a result of the platelet dysfunction that occurs in patients who have undergone cardiopulmonary bypass, atriofemoral bypass and aortic surgery, or thoracoabdominal aortic repairs, platelet counts are corrected to a count of at least 150,000/mm³, which is also higher than that for coronary surgery. At the same time, DDAVP (1-deamino- (8-D-arginine)- vasopressin; desmopressin) at a dosage of 3 μg per kg is administered over a 15- to 20-minute interval to increase von Willebrand's factor and improve platelet adhesion to damaged endothelium. It may also increase factor VIII levels. If the PT is greater than 13 seconds, then fresh frozen

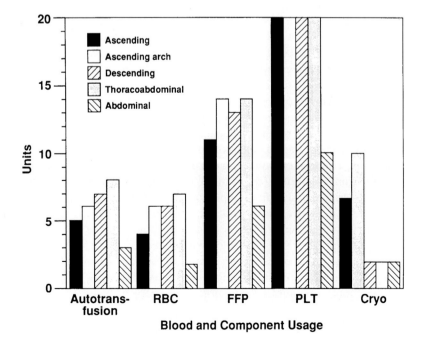

FIGURE 16–10 Average blood and blood product usage for various types of operation. (From Svensson LG, Crawford ES. Curr Probl Surg 1992;29:819–912.) With the use of blood-conservation techniques, many of these operations can now be done without homologous blood.[67]

plasma is administered in four-unit packs until the PT is corrected back to normal. Fresh frozen plasma is used because it contains all the necessary coagulation factors, including the labile factors V and VII, and complement. An elevated PTT is treated by further administration of protamine, particularly if the activated clotting time (ACT) is abnormal. In our experience, rarely does the use of protamine cause coagulation problems. Additional fresh frozen plasma and cryoprecipitate may also be needed to correct factor deficiencies. If the fibrinogen count is less than 100 µg/ml, then 10 units of cryoprecipitate are given, and this may have to be repeated to achieve a level of at least 200 µg/ml, particularly if there is evidence of fibrinolysis. If the latter occurs, where increased levels of fibrin split or degradation products are observed, then epsilon-aminocaproic acid (EACA, Amicar, 5 g intravenously) or tranexamic acid (Cyklokapron) is administered and repeated if bleeding appears to recur.

The use of aprotonin in the United States is still being debated, although it has been widely accepted in Europe. The cautionary prospective randomized study by Cosgrove and colleagues[68] from the Cleveland Clinic, showing a higher myocardial infarction rate and a trend toward a higher incidence of vein graft closure, should be noted.[68] Furthermore, Sundt and colleagues[69] found that one third (32%) of their patients who had deep hypothermia with circulatory arrest and who were given aprotonin died postoperatively with multiple organ failure and evidence of microvasculature thrombosis. It may be that obstruction of the capillary beds occurs with aprotonin and this leads to organ failure. Clearly, not all patients require that their coagulation studies be corrected to normal if they are not bleeding.[26]

We have found topical agents that we have used by themselves to be rather ineffective in preventing or treating hemorrhage. These have included Surgicel, Gelfoam, thrombin, Tisseel, Avitene, Resorcinon glue, and mixtures of these with blood products. Surgicel has a propensity to swell after surgery and can cause localized cardiac tamponade or superior vena caval obstruction in the pericardial cavity. Three instances of Surgicel causing paraplegia have been reported.[70] The paraplegia associated with Surgicel occurred after thoracic surgery, when the Surgicel was packed between the ribs to prevent bleeding and it migrated into the spinal canal, causing spinal cord compression. When Avitene (bovine microfibrillar collagen) is used, the autotransfusion device should be discontinued, since autotransfusion may result in embolization of collagen to the lungs. On occasion, a mixture of thrombin and Amicar may be useful to irrigate and soak the operative field. One of the more useful maneuvers is to pack the operative field with 4 × 4 inch sponges, laparotomy sponges, and some pieces of Surgicel. A period of hypotension will often aid clotting, although this should be used with great caution, particularly in patients who are undergoing either descending thoracic or thoracoabdominal aortic surgery, as paraplegia may result.[26]

True DIC after aortic operations is uncommon, and the failure of hemostasis to occur because of a lack of clot formation is usually due to dilution of clotting factors. We manage patients with DIC in a way similar to that described above and do not resort to heparin anticoagulation. With good secure anastomoses and prevention of graft oozing, bleeding should rarely be an insurmountable problem resulting in operative or postoperative death. The anastomoses should be done with generous and deep bites of the aorta and aortic graft, without undue tension. If an anastomosis needs to be tailored to make up for discrepancies in size, then less widely spaced, but still deep bites should be taken on the smaller lumen. More widely spaced sutures should not be placed on the larger lumen to tailor the anastomosis. After the anastomoses are completed, the graft should be firmly manipulated in different directions to check for hemostasis and allow the Prolene suture to adjust tension evenly along the suture line. This also exposes any potential leak sites, which are then oversewn. Exceptions to this are patients with acute aortic dissection and patients with Marfan syndrome, in which greater care and gentle handling of the anastomoses are required. If the patient's blood pressure is elevated, this aids in detecting leaks which could appear later if the patient were to become hypertensive in the intensive care unit. To prevent oozing, the graft should be baked in 25% albumin for 3 to 5 minutes by flash sterilization in an autoclave. Composite valve grafts, such as the St. Jude's valve graft that we use, can be painted while being held in a vertical position with the valve superiorly and then autoclaved in an upright position. This prevents the valve mechanism from jamming, which would happen if albumin seeped into the leaflet hinges. The grafts should not be so overbaked that they flake; nor should they still be wet. Other blood products that can be used for baking the graft are platelets, cryoprecipitate, or heparinized blood.[26]

REFERENCES

1. Brown BG, Bolson E, Petersen RB, et al. The mechanisms of nitroglycerin action: stenosis vasodilatation as a major component of the drug response. Circulation 1981;64:1089-97.
2. Bunt TJ, Manczuk M, Varley KV. Nitroglycerin-induced volume loading. Surgery 1988;103:513-9.
3. Bush HL Jr, LoGerfo FW, Weisel RD, et al. Assessment of myocardial performance and optimal volume loading during elective abdominal aortic aneurysm resection. Arch Surg 1977;112:1301-6.
4. Bush HL Jr, Huse JB, Johnson WC, et al. Prevention of renal insufficiency after abdominal aortic aneurysm resection by optimal volume loading. Arch Surg 1981;116:1517-24.
5. Cohn LH, Powell MR, Weidlizt L, et al. Fluid requirements and shifts after reconstruction of the aorta. Am J Surg 1970;120:182.
6. Colon R, Frazier OH, Cooley DA, McAllister HA. Hypothermic regional perfusion for protection of the spinal cord during periods of ischemia. Ann Thorac Surg 1987;43:639-43.
7. Coselli JS, Crawford ES. Femoral artery perfusion for cardiopulmonary bypass in patients with aortoiliac artery obstruction. Ann Thorac Surg 1987;43:437-9.
8. Crawford ES, Fenstermacher JM, Richardson MD, et al. Reappraisal of adjuncts to avoid ischemia in the treatment of thoracic aortic aneurysms. Surgery 1970;67:182-96.
9. Crawford ES, Mizrahi EM, Hess KR, et al. The impact of distal aortic perfusion and somatosensory evoked potential monitoring on pre-

vention of paraplegia after aortic aneurysm operation. J Thorac Cardiovasc Surg 1988;95:357-67.

10. Cunningham AJ, O'Toole DP, McDonald N, et al. The influence of collateral vascularisation on haemodynamic performance during abdominal aortic surgery. Can J Anaesth 1989;36:44-50.

11. Gottlieb A, Skrinska VA, O'Hara P, et al. The role of prostaglandin in the mesenteric traction syndrome during anesthesia of abdominal aortic reconstructive surgery. Ann Surg 1989;209:363-7.

12. Harpole DH, Clements FM, Quill T, et al. Right and left ventricular performance during and after abdominal aortic aneurysm repair. Ann Surg 1989;209:356-62.

13. Hesdorffer CS, Milne JF, Meyers AM, et al. The value of Swan-Ganz catheterization and volume loading in preventing renal failure in patients undergoing abdominal aneurysmectomy. Clin Nephrol 1987;28:272-6.

14. Kalman PG, Wellwood MR, Weisel RD, et al. Cardiac dysfunction during abdominal aortic operation: the limitations of pulmonary wedge pressures. J Vasc Surg 1986;3:773-81.

15. Kelly TF Jr, Morris GC Jr, Crawford ES, et al. Perforation of the pulmonary artery with Swan-Ganz catheters: diagnosis and surgical management. Ann Surg 1981;193:686-92.

16. Laschinger JC, Owen J, Rosenbloom M, et al. Direct noninvasive monitoring of spinal cord motor function during thoracic aortic occlusion: use of motor evoked potentials. J Vasc Surg 1988;7:161-71.

17. Levy WJ, York DH, McCaffrey M, et al. Motor evoked potentials from transcranial stimulation of the motor cortex in humans. Neurosurgery 1984;15:287-302.

18. McCloskey G. Intraoperative detection of ischemia in patients with coronary artery disease. Heart Failure 1990;6:89-97.

19. Miller RR, Olsa HG, Amsterdam EA, et al. Propranolol withdrawal rebound phenomenon exacerbation of coronary events after abrupt cessation of antianginal therapy. N Engl J Med 1975;293:416.

20. Mizrahi EM, Crawford ES. Somatosensory evoked potentials during reversible spinal cord ischemia in man. Electroencephalogr Clin Neurophysiol 1984;58:120-6.

21. Saleh SA. Anesthesia and monitoring for aortic aneurysm surgery. World J Surg 1980;4:689-92.

22. Shenaq SA, Chelly JE, Karlberg H, et al. Use of nitroprusside during surgery for thoracoabdominal aortic aneurysm. Circulation 1985;70 (Supp I):17-110.

23. Shenaq SA, Casar G, Chelly JE, et al. Continuous monitoring of mixed venous oxygen saturation during aortic surgery. Chest 1987; 92:796-9.

24. Stinson EB, Holloway EL, Derby GC, et al. Control of myocardial performance early after open-heart operations by vasodilator treatment. J Thorac Cardiovasc Surg 1977;73:523-30.

25. Tamaki T, Noguchi T, Takano H, et al. Spinal cord monitoring as a clinical utilization of the spinal cord evoked potential. Clin Orthop 1983;184:58-64.

26. Svensson LG, Crawford ES. Aortic dissection and aortic aneurysm surgery: clinical observations, experimental investigations and statistical analyses. Part I. Curr Probl Surg 1992;29:819-912.

27. Svensson LG, Crawford ES, Hess KR, et al. Dissection of the aorta and dissecting aortic aneurysms: improving early and long-term surgical results. Circulation 1990;82(5 Supp):IV 24-38.

28. Svensson LG, Stewart RW, Cosgrove DM, et al. Preliminary results and rationale for the use of intrathecal papaverine for the prevention of paraplegia after aortic surgery. S Afr J Surg 1988;26:153-60.

29. Svensson LG, Stewart RW, Cosgrove DM 3rd, et al. Intrathecal papaverine for the prevention of paraplegia after operation on the thoracic or thoracoabdominal aorta. J Thorac Cardiovasc Surg 1988; 96:823-9.

30. Svensson LG, Grum DF, Bednarski M, et al. Appraisal of cerebrospinal fluid alterations during aortic surgery with intrathecal papaverine administration and cerebrospinal fluid drainage. J Vasc Surg 1990;11:423-9.

31. Svensson LG, Patel V, Robinson MF, et al. Influence of preservation or perfusion of intraoperatively identified spinal cord blood supply on spinal motor evoked potentials and paraplegia after aortic surgery. J Vasc Surg 1991;13:355-65.

32. Crawford ES, Svensson LG, Hess KR, et al. A prospective randomized study of cerebrospinal fluid drainage to prevent paraplegia after high-risk surgery on the thoracoabdominal aorta. J Vasc Surg 1991;13:36-45.

33. Molina JE, Cogordan J, Einzig S, et al. Adequacy of ascending aorta-descending aorta shunt during cross-clamping of the thoracic aorta for prevention of spinal cord injury. J Thorac Cardiovasc Surg 1985; 90:126-36.

34. Whittmore AD, Clowes AW, Hectman HB, et al. Aortic aneurysm repair: reduced operation mortality associated with maintenance of optimal cardiac performance. Ann Surg 1980;193:414-21.

35. Svensson LG. Commentary on Cernaiau AC, Olah A, Cilley JH, et al. Effect of sodium nitroprusside on paraplegia during cross-clamping of the thoracic aorta. Ann Thorac Surg 1993;56:1035-8.

36. Cernaiau AC, Olah A, Cilley JH, et al. Effect of sodium nitroprusside on paraplegia during cross-clamping of the thoracic aorta. Ann Thorac Surg 1993;56:1035-8.

37. Svensson LG, Coselli JS, Safi HJ, et al. Appraisal of adjuncts to prevent acute renal failure after surgery on the thoracic or thoracoabdominal aorta. J Vasc Med 1989;10:230-9.

38. Crawford ES, Svensson LG, Coselli JS, et al. Surgical treatment of aneurysm and/or dissection of the ascending aorta, transverse aortic arch, and ascending aorta and transverse aortic arch: factors influencing survival in 717 patients. J Thorac Cardiovasc Surg 1989; 98:659-73.

39. Crawford ES, Coselli JS, Safi HJ. Partial cardiopulmonary bypass, hypothermic circulatory arrest, and posterolateral exposure for thoracic aortic aneurysm operation. J Thorac Cardiovasc Surg 1987;94: 824-7.

40. Svensson LG, Crawford ES, Hess KR, et al. Variables predictive of outcome in 832 patients undergoing repairs of the descending thoracic aorta. Chest 1993;104:1248-53.

41. Svensson LG, Crawford ES, Hess KR, et al. Experience with 1509 patients undergoing thoracoabdominal aortic operations. J Vasc Surg 1993;17:357-70.

42. Lawrie GM, Earle N, DeBakey ME. Evolution of surgical techniques for aneurysms of the descending thoracic aorta: twenty-nine years experience with 659 patients. J Cardiac Surg 1994;9:648-61.

43. Borst HG, Jurmann M, Buhner B, Laas J. Risk of replacement of descending aorta with a standardized left heart bypass technique. J Thorac Cardiovasc Surg 1994;107:126-33.

44. Verdant A, Cossette R, Page A, et al. Aneurysms of the descending thoracic aorta: three hundred sixty-six consecutive cases resected without paraplegia. J Vasc Surg 1995;21:385-91.

45. Najafi H. Descending aortic aneurysmectomy without adjuncts to avoid ischemia: 1993 update. Ann Thorac Surg 1993;55:1042-5.

46. Crawford ES, Mizrahi EM, Hess KR, et al. The impact of distal aortic perfusion and somatosensory evoked potential monitoring on prevention of paraplegia after aortic aneurysm operation. J Thorac Cardiovasc Surg 1988;95:357-67. (Published erratum appears in J Thorac Cardiovasc Surg 1989;97:665.)

47. Mattox KL, Beall AC Jr. Autotransfusion: use in penetrating trauma. Texas Med 1975;71:69-77.

48. Mattox KL, Guinn GA, Rubio PA, Beall AC Jr. Use of activated coagulation time in the intraoperative heparin reversal for cardiopulmonary surgery. Ann Thorac Surg 1975;19:634-8.

49. Mattox KL. Comparison of techniques of autotransfusion. Surgery 1978;84:700-2.

50. Hallett JW Jr, Popovsky M, Ilstrup D. Minimizing blood transfusions during abdominal aortic surgery: recent advances in rapid autotransfusion. J Vasc Surg 1987;5:601-6.

51. Cosgrove DM, Thurer RL, Lytle BW, et al. Blood conservation during myocardial revascularization. Ann Thorac Surg 1979;28:184-9.

52. Jones JW, Rawitscher RE, McLcan TR, ct al. Benefit from combining blood conservation measures in cardiac operations. Ann Thorac Surg 1991;51:541-6.

53. Thurer RL, Haver JM. Autotransfusion and blood conservation. Curr Probl Surg 1982;19:97-156.

54. Jex RK, Schaff HV, Piehler JM, et al. Early and late results following repair dissections of the descending thoracic aorta. J Vasc Surg 1986;3:226-37.

55. Svensson LG, Loop FD. Prevention of spinal cord ischemia in aortic surgery. In: Bergan JJ, Yao JST, eds: Arterial Surgery: New Diagnostic and Operative Techniques. New York: Grune & Stratton 1988: 2273-85.

56. Fisher DF Jr, Yawn DH, Crawford ES. Preoperative disseminated intravascular coagulation associated with aortic aneurysms: a prospective study of 76 cases. Arch Surg 1983;94:781-91.

57. Blundell J. Experiments on the transfusion of blood. Med Chir Trans 1818;9:56.

58. Duncan J. On reinfusion of blood in primary and other amputations. Br Med J 1886;1:192.

59. Boudreau JP, Bornside GH, Cohn I Jr. Emergency autotransfusion: partial cleansing of bacteria-laden blood by cell washing. J Trauma 1983;23:31-5.

60. Brewster DC, Ambrosino JJ, Darling RC, et al. Intraoperative autotransfusion in major vascular surgery. Am J Surg 1979;137:507-14.

61. Glover JL, Broadie TA. Intraoperative autotransfusion. World J Surg 1987;2:60-4.

62. McKenzie FN, Heimbecker RO, Wall W, et al. Intraoperative autotransfusion in elective and emergency vascular surgery. Surgery 1978;83:470-5.

63. Tawes RL Jr, Scribner RG, Duval TB, et al. The cell-saver and autologous transfusion: an underutilized resource in vascular surgery. Am J Surg 1986;152:105-9.

64. Andrews NJ, Bloor K. Autologous blood collection in abdominal vascular surgery: assessment of a low pressure blood salvage system with particular reference to the preservation of cellular elements, triglyceride, complement and bacterial content in the collected blood. Clin Lab Haematol 1983;5:361-70.

65. Orr M. Autotransfusion: the use of washed red cells as an adjunct to component therapy. Surgery 1978;84:728-32.

66. Svensson LG, Antunes MDJ, Kinsley RH. Traumatic rupture of the thoracic aorta: a report of 14 cases and a review of the literature. S Afr J Med 1985;67:853-7.

67. Svensson LG, Sun J, Nadolny E, Kimmel WA. Prospective evaluation of minimal blood use for ascending aorta and aortic arch operations. Ann Thorac Surg 1995;59:1501-8.

68. Cosgrove DMI, Heric B, Lytle BW, et al. Aprotinin therapy for reoperative myocardial revascularization: a placebo-controlled study. Ann Thorac Surg 1992;54:1031-8.

69. Sundt TMI, Kouchoukos NT, Saffitz JE, et al. Renal dysfunction and intravascular coagulation with aprotinin and hypothermic circulatory arrest. Ann Thorac Surg 1993;55:1418-24.

70. Walker WE. Paraplegia associated with thoracotomy. Ann Thorac Surg 1990;50:178.

17

Techniques for Medial Degenerative Aneurysms of the Proximal Aorta

OPERATIVE STRATEGY

This chapter and those that follow review the technical aspects of proximal aortic repairs. As defined previously by us, proximal repairs refer to those that involve the aorta proximal to the left subclavian artery.[1-4] The practical reason for using this definition is that repairs involving the proximal aorta will usually require a mediastinal incision for exposure of the aorta and the use of cardiopulmonary bypass. Those distal to the left subclavian artery (distal repairs) will usually require a left thoracotomy or left thoracoabdominal incision. There is clearly some overlap, since the descending aorta can be replaced through a mediastinal incision to the mid-descending aorta or the distal ascending aorta and aortic arch can be replaced through a left thoracotomy. These approaches, however, should be used only under special circumstances as illustrated in both Chapter 16 and Chapter 24 on Replacement of the Entire Aorta.

Earlier chapters have covered the preoperative studies usually performed in patients undergoing aortic repairs. For those patients undergoing proximal aortic repairs, these may include computed tomography (CT), or magnetic resonance imaging (MRI) scans or transesophogeal echocardiography (TEE) for diagnosis, pulmonary function tests with arterial blood gas analysis, 24-Holter examination, echocardiography, noninvasive carotid studies, cardiac catheterization, and aortography.

The decision as to which operative procedure is best in patients with degenerative aneurysms is based mainly on the preoperative studies, although certain intraoperative findings may require a change in the operative strategy. The two principles that guide the operative approach to the proximal and distal anastomoses are (1) whether the sinotubular ridge is preserved and (2) whether most of the aortic arch is aneurysmal.

For the proximal anastomosis, if the sinotubular ridge is preserved, then an end-to-end tube graft can be sutured into place above the aortic valve commissures. If the aortic valve is also diseased, typically by aortic stenosis, then the aortic valve is also replaced as a separate valve replacement in a standard manner. If the sinotubular ridge is not preserved and the aortic root is enlarged (for example, in Marfan syndrome), then usually a composite valve graft must be inserted. In selected elderly patients without Marfan syndrome, it may be appropriate to insert a separate aortic valve and tube graft if the aortic root is not too large (greater than approximately 4 cm), particularly if the Wheat procedure is used.

For the distal anastomosis, if the distal ascending aorta narrows down to a relatively normal size or a slight dilatation at the innominate artery, then an end-to-end anastomosis to the proximal aortic arch can be performed with an aortic clamp angled into the aortic arch. If most of the aortic arch is aneurysmal, however, then it should be replaced with the use of deep hypothermic circulatory arrest and retrograde brain perfusion (see Chapter 13 on hypothermic arrest). To replace the aortic arch, a decision has to be made as to whether the greater vessels should be reattached as a separate island. If the proximal descending aorta is dilated or if a two-stage elephant trunk procedure is required (see below), then the greater vessels should be reattached as a separate island. If, however, the dilatation ends at about the left subclavian artery, a beveled tube graft or a tongue of a tube graft can be sutured to the distal aorta, with the edges of the graft sutured behind and anterior to the greater vessels, ending the anastomosis at the innominate artery.

Normal Size of the Aorta

In making the decision as to which operative procedure is best used, the normal size of the aorta plays an important role, since aneurysmal segments must be resected and the anastomoses performed to the normal-sized aorta. The sizes of the aorta are summarized in Table 17–1 for an adult of 5 feet 6 inches to 5 feet 10 inches.

ASCENDING AORTIC TUBULAR GRAFT INSERTION

The methods of repairing the ascending aorta in patients who have degenerative aneurysms or aortic dissection are similar except that the adjunct of deep hypothermia with circulatory arrest is usually required for acute dissection, irrespective of whether the aortic arch is aneurysmal.[1-3, 5-8]

TABLE 17-1 NORMAL SIZES OF AORTA FOR ADULTS 5 FEET 6 INCHES TO 5 FEET 10 INCHES TALL

Segment	Transverse diameter (mm)
Root	31
Ascending	32
Proximal arch	32
Proximal descending	28
Mid descending	27
Distal descending at SMA	26
Proximal infrarenal	19
Distal infrarenal	17
Common iliac	9
Common femoral	7

For a patient taller than 6 feet or shorter than 5 feet, add or subtract 6 mm from each value. For the iliac artery 4 mm should be used and for the femoral artery 3 mm should be used. The length of the segments can be summarized as multiples of 5 cm. Thus the ascending aorta is 5 cm, the arch is 5 cm, the descending thoracic aorta to the SMA is 25 cm, SMA to the aortic bifurcation is 15 cm, and the aortic bifurcation to the femoral profunda artery is 20 cm.

If, however, the aorta shows evidence of atherosclerosis, then deep hypothermia plus circulatory arrest without clamping of the aorta should be used.[8] During insertion of the graft it is crucial that the surgeon pay particular attention to meticulous care in transection of the aorta both above the aortic valve commissures and proximal to the aortic clamp on the proximal aortic arch (Fig. 17-1). The reason for this concern is that it is easier to control bleeding from the anastomoses if the aorta has been transected. Furthermore, transection of the aorta reduces the risk of false aneurysm formation. A soft woven Dacron tube graft is selected to match the size of the aorta and is beveled distally to accommodate the proximal arch anastomosis just proximal to the aortic clamp. The distal anastomosis is performed first with a single layer of 3-0 Prolene starting posteriorly; first the posterior wall is done forehand, then the anterior wall from the outside is done forehand, and finally the proximal anastomosis is completed. Of note, Teflon strips are not included in the anastomosis. The patient is then placed in a Trendelenburg position and air is evacuated from the graft, hemostasis is obtained, and the patient is weaned from cardiopulmonary bypass.[4]

INSERTION OF AN AORTIC VALVE AND SEPARATE ASCENDING AORTIC GRAFT

The methods of inserting an aortic valve and a separate ascending aortic graft are optimally used in patients who have aortic valve disease associated with an ascending aortic aneurysm without marked annular dilatation (Fig. 17-2). When annular dilatation is more marked, particularly in elderly patients, the procedure first described by Wheat and associates[9] can be used (Fig. 17-3). In brief, the aortic valve is excised and the valve prosthesis is seated in a rou-

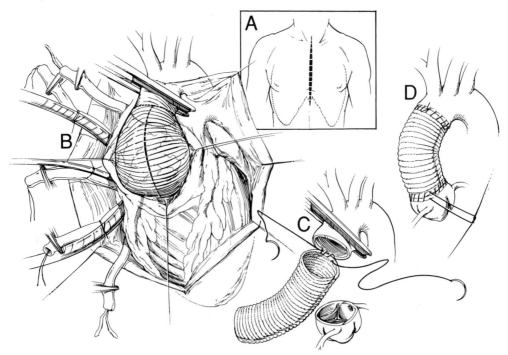

FIGURE 17–1 Steps in the repair of an ascending aortic aneurysm. Through a midline incision **(A),** the aneurysm **(B)** is incised, and the aorta is transected both proximally and distally. The selected tube graft is then sutured into position distally **(C),** and the proximal anastomosis is completed thereafter **(D).** (From Svensson LG, Crawford ES. Curr Probl Surg 1993;30:1–172.)

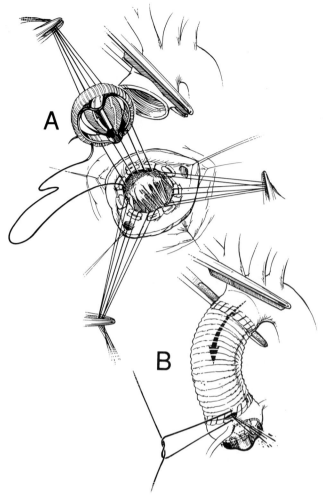

FIGURE 17–2 Steps for replacement of the aortic valve and insertion of a separate tube graft for the ascending aorta. First the aortic valve is excised **(A),** valve annular sutures are placed, and the valve prosthesis is seated. The tube graft is then inserted. The aortic clamp is removed with the final suture untied **(B),** so that the aorta can be flushed of any possible debris and also is de-aired. (From Svensson LG, Crawford ES. Curr Probl Surg 1993;30:1–172.)

tine manner with interrupted pledgeted sutures (Fig. 17–4). The aortic wall is then excised as far down as the coronary ostia and to just above the aortic valve prosthesis. Next the aortic graft is tailored to incorporate and circumvent the coronary ostia. The proximal anastomosis is then performed with a running Prolene suture. To strengthen the anastomosis, sutures can be taken through the aortic valve prosthesis sewing ring and the aortic tubular graft. When the Wheat procedure is used, it is usually easier to do the proximal anastomosis first, followed by the distal anastomosis to the transected aorta.[4]

Occasionally, the aortic valve can be preserved with the reimplantation of the valve in a tube graft, with or without reimplantation of the coronary arteries as advocated by David and Feindel.[10] Our experience, however, is too limited for us to comment on the technique, and long-term follow-up will be of interest, particularly in those patients with Marfan syndrome who have myxomatous involvement of the valves. Another procedure that is occasionally used is aortoplasty in conjunction with aortic valve replacement. During this procedure, favored by Robicsek and Thubrikar,[11] the narrowed-down ascending aorta is supported by an external graft to prevent late aneurysm formation (Fig. 17–5). Barnett and colleagues[12] reported performing annuloplasties without external graft support.

COMPOSITE VALVE GRAFT INSERTION

A composite valve graft is usually required in patients who have enlargement of the aortic annulus and sinotubular ridge or the sinuses of Valsalva. Thus such a procedure is frequently performed in patients with Marfan syndrome.[13, 14] The two well-known methods are the Bentall (Fig. 17–6) and button (Fig. 17–7) techniques.[15] In our experience, the Bentall technique, by which the coronary ostia are anastomosed

FIGURE 17–3 **A,** Preoperative diagram and arteriogram of a patient with an ascending aortic aneurysm and aortic valve regurgitation. **B,** Postoperative illustrations after insertion of an aortic valve and replacement of the ascending aorta with a tube graft by the Wheat procedure.

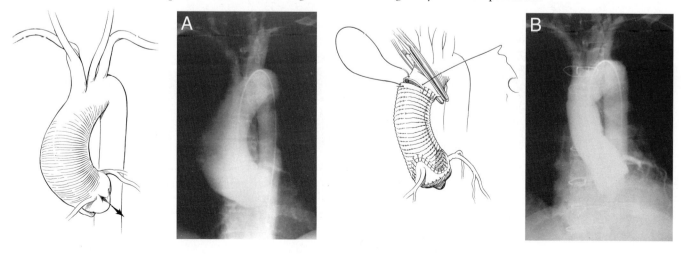

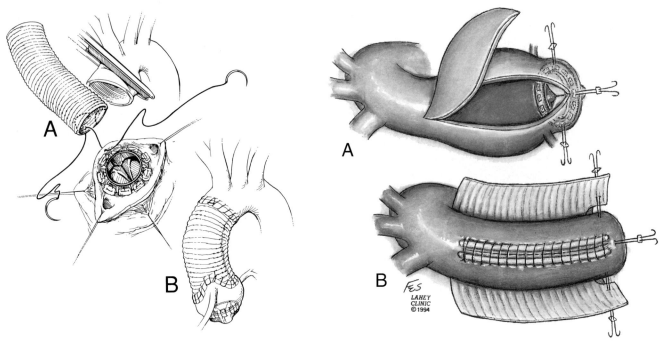

FIGURE 17–4   Wheat procedure. **A,** After excision of the aortic valve and placement of the new aortic valve, a graft that has been cut to fit around the coronary artery ostia is sutured into position. **B,** Distal repair completed and the graft sutured around the coronary artery ostia. (From Svensson LG, Crawford ES. Curr Probl Surg 1993;30:1–172.)

FIGURE 17–5   Aortoplasty with ascending aortic wrap of the repair. **A,** The aortic valve is seated and the commissure sutures are brought through the aortic wall to the outside and passed through pledgets. A piece of the aorta is excised to narrow down the aorta to the appropriate size. **B,** After the aorta is repaired with Teflon strips, an appropriately cut graft is wrapped around the aorta and the commissure sutures are passed through the graft and tied down. The graft is then sutured closed to complete the repair. The indications for the this type of repair are limited, but long-term results appear to be good according to Robicsek.[11]

FIGURE 17–6   Steps in the classic technique of composite valve graft insertion by the Bentall method. **A,** Seating of the composite valve graft. **B,** Excision of holes in the graft opposite the coronary ostia. **C,** Anastomosis of the ostia to the graft. Note that if the gap is large, tension at the anastomoses may result. **D,** Completion of the operation. Wrapping of the graft has been shown to be associated with a higher incidence of false aneurysm formation. (From Svensson LG, Crawford ES. Curr Probl Surg 1993;30:1–172.)

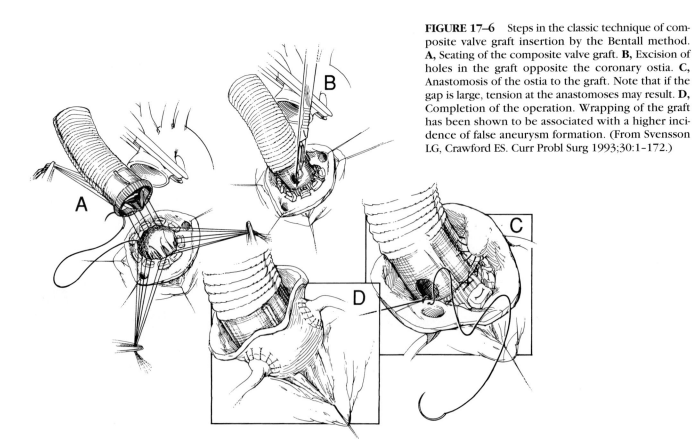

directly to the aortic graft, while fairly simple to perform, has a higher early and late reoperation rate because of bleeding and false aneurysm formation. We are fairly frequently called upon to correct this problem, particularly in patients with Marfan syndrome[14, 15] (Fig. 17-8). The reason appears to be the tension exerted on the anastomoses used to bridge the gap between the aneurysmal wall and the tubular graft, especially when the coronary ostia are too close to the annulus. To obviate this problem, excision of ostial buttons has been advocated, with mobilization of the proximal coronary arteries and then reattachment of these ostia to the composite graft. This allows for an increased length of artery, which would usually bridge the gap between the aneurysm wall and the graft with minimal tension on the anastomosis. The drawbacks of this technique are the time required to

dissect out the ostia, particularly for the left coronary artery, and the risk of damage or occlusion of the left main coronary artery, the circumflex artery, or the first septal perforator. Moreover, with acute aortic dissection, it may not be possible to use this technique. Furthermore, if bleeding should occur at the anastomosis between the left coronary ostium and the graft, as with the Bentall technique, obtaining hemostasis by adding sutures to the anastomosis can be difficult because the anastomosis is on the posterior aspect of the composite graft. Although this procedure is slightly more demanding, it has excellent long-term results, although left main stenosis and calcification may occur at the left coronary ostium.[13, 15-18] The third most commonly used technique is that described by Cabrol,[15, 19, 20] which involves placement of tube grafts, either 8 mm or 10 mm, to each

FIGURE 17–7 Insertion of a composite graft by the button technique. The aorta is incised (**A**) and the coronary ostia are mobilized (**B**) and the composite graft is seated (**C**). The coronary buttons with Teflon doughnut-shaped collars are sutured to the graft (**D**) to complete the repair. (From Svensson LG, Crawford ES. Curr Probl Surg 1993;30:1-172.)

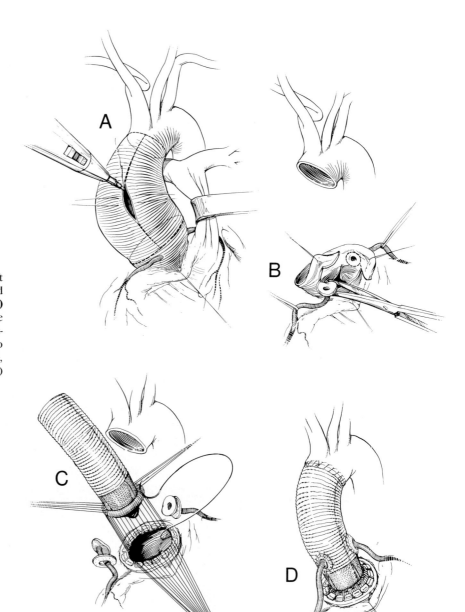

coronary ostium (Figs. 17-9 to 17-12). Initially, Cabrol described placement of the curved part of the tube graft connecting the two ostia anterior to the composite graft, although this was later modified and now it is placed behind the composite tube graft.[15, 19-21]

The usual methods for reattachment of the coronary ostia to the ascending aortic conduit have several disadvantages and potential complications. The Bentall, aortic button, and Cabrol techniques are the three standard methods for the insertion of composite valve grafts and the reattachment of

the coronary artery ostia.[1, 13-16, 20] The Bentall technique can lead to tension on the anastomoses and later false aneurysm formation (Fig. 17-8).[1, 14, 15] Furthermore, intraoperative bleeding is difficult to control because of the inaccessible anastomoses. With the aortic button technique, the potential risks include damage to the left main coronary artery, the circumflex coronary artery, the septal perforators, or the pulmonary artery during mobilization of the left main coronary artery. The Cabrol approach allows for easier access to the anastomoses for the purpose of obtaining hemostasis at the

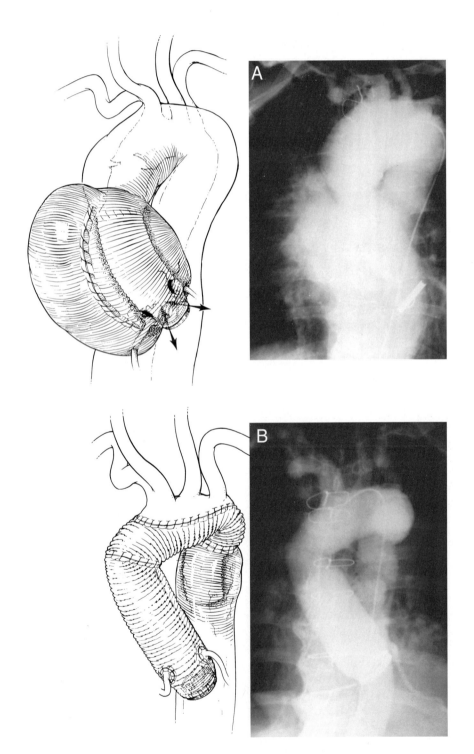

FIGURE 17-8 **A,** Diagram and angiogram showing the not uncommon complication of a false aneurysm developing after the classic Bentall procedure with direct reimplantation of the coronary ostia into the tube graft and wrapping of the aortic wall around the graft. **B,** Postoperative illustrations after reimplantation of the coronary ostia as aortic buttons and replacement of the aortic arch by the elephant trunk procedure.[15] (From Svensson LG, Crawford ES. Curr Probl Surg 1993; 30:1-172.)

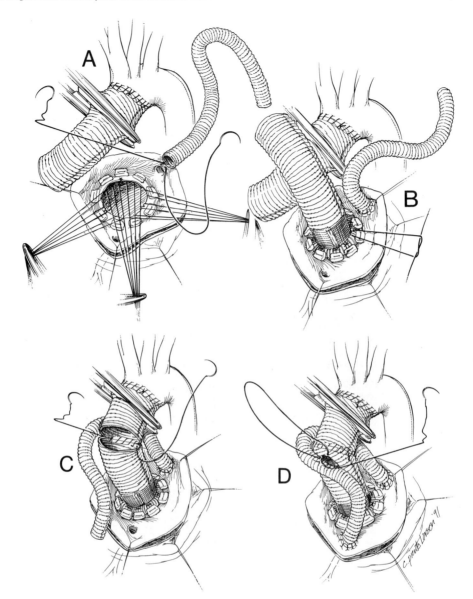

FIGURE 17–9 Insertion of a composite valve graft by the Cabrol technique. **A,** First the aortic arch part of the repair is performed if necessary. The valve annular sutures are then placed and the tube graft is sutured to the left main ostium. These latter two steps are interchangeable. However, if the valve sutures are placed after the tube graft to the left main ostium, the valve should be sized early so that the tube graft can be baked before insertion if a collagen-impregnated graft is not being used. **B,** The tube graft is seated and tied into position. **C,** The tube graft to the left main ostium is brought behind the composite graft and then the composite graft is sutured to either the aortic arch or the graft that has been used to repair the aortic arch. **D,** Finally, the coronary interposition graft is sutured to the right coronary artery ostium and the side-to-side anastomosis is performed. (From Svensson LG, Crawford ES. Curr Probl Surg 1993; 30:1–172.)

suture lines, including the aortic valve annulus and the coronary ostial anastomoses. The problems with this technique are that if the intercoronary ostial tube graft loop is placed to the left of the ascending aortic graft, as originally described, the limb to the left coronary artery tends to kink. Similarly, with placement of the 8 mm tube graft to the right of the ascending aortic graft, the preferred method, the side-to-side anastomosis has to be placed high on the aortic graft and in a left anterolateral position so that the graft to the right coronary artery does not kink. Even when this is being done, the left limb can kink from excessive tension over its long course at the tethered side-to-side anastomosis, the right limb can still be dysfunctional, or it can occlude because of the angle at which the 8 mm tube graft to the right coronary artery ostium has to be performed, including the ostium having to be rotated through 90 degrees for the anastomosis. During long-term follow-up it has also been noted that the limb to the right coronary artery can occlude.[4, 15, 22]

An easy-to-perform alternative approach that one of us (L.G.S.) has described[15, 22] involves insertion of an interposition graft to the left main coronary ostium and reattachment of the right coronary artery ostium as a button[22] (Fig. 17–13). This novel adaptation makes possible inspection of all the anastomoses and does not involve the associated high risk of thrombosis of the graft to the right coronary artery, as observed with the Cabrol procedure.[4, 15, 22]

The technique that evolved takes advantage of the attributes of the three types of operations described above but avoids the disadvantages and simplifies the insertion of the composite valve graft. The described procedure allows for all the anastomoses to be visualized so that hemostasis can be attained if bleeding should occur. In addition, the method enables the circumferential transection of the aorta to be performed as recommended by Kouchoukos and colleagues[16] without the need for wrapping the aortic graft to obtain hemostasis, thus reducing the risk of late false aneurysms forming at the anastomoses.[15, 22, 23]

After the patient has been placed on cardiopulmonary bypass, followed by clamping of the aorta and arrest of the heart, the distal ascending aorta is circumferentially transected to allow accurate and full-thickness suturing of the aorta, easier access to bleeding sites, and reduction of the

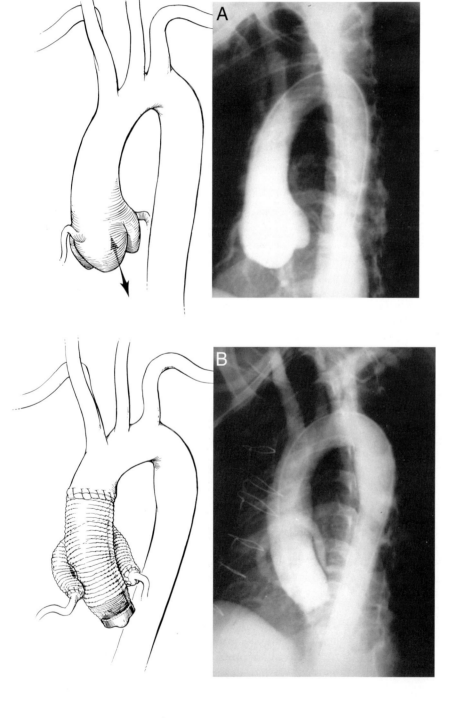

FIGURE 17–10 **A,** Example of a patient with aortic valve regurgitation and predominantly sinus of Valsalva dilatation. **B,** Postoperative angiogram after insertion of a composite valve graft by the Cabrol technique. Note the sharp angle between the tube graft and the right coronary artery.

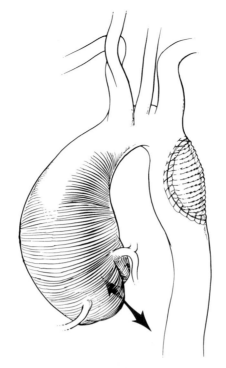

FIGURE 17–11 Example of a patient with more advanced dilatation of the ascending aorta with valve regurgitation and previous repair of a descending aorta saccular aneurysm.

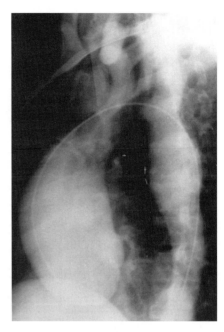

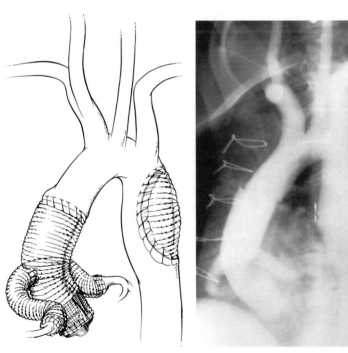

FIGURE 17–12 Postoperative angiogram and diagram after insertion of a composite graft by the Cabrol technique.

risk of late false aneurysm formation. The aortic valve cusps are then excised, leaving a 1 to 2 mm rim of annulus, the commissure sutures are placed, the valve annulus is sized, and the appropriate composite valve is selected.[4, 15, 22]

A previously baked 8 to 10 mm Dacron interposition tube graft is beveled at one end and then sutured end-to-end to the left coronary artery ostium with a running 4-0 prolene suture starting at the toe (Fig. 17–13, step A, panels 1 and 2). The sutures should be placed deep in the aorta but not through the coronary artery. This is so that no bleeding

occurs at the anastomosis and the graft does not tear loose, resulting in a false aneurysm. The remaining pledgeted 2-0 Ticron sutures are placed around the annulus, approximately five or six sutures per cusp, with care taken to make sure that the horizontal mattress sutures are close to each other, no more than 0.5 to 1.0 mm apart (Fig. 17–13, panel B). The previously prepared composite valve graft is then seated in the annulus after the annular valve sutures have been passed through the rim of the suturing ring. Again, the horizontal mattress sutures should be placed close together

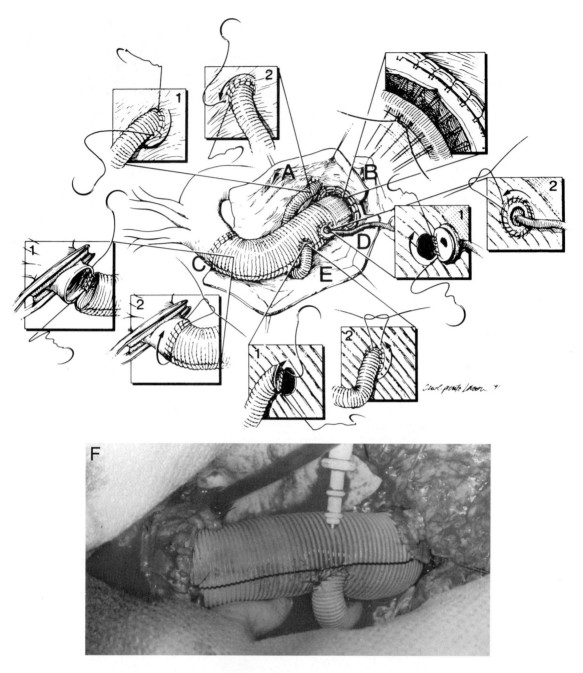

FIGURE 17–13 Insertion of a composite graft with use of an interposition graft to the left main artery and an aortic button for the right coronary artery. **A,** First the 10 mm tube graft is sutured to the left main coronary artery ostium with 4-0 Prolene while the composite graft is being prepared for insertion after the annulus has been sized. It is convenient to start at the 1 or 2 o'clock position and to run the right side forehand to the heel. Next **(A2)** the left side is run forehand. **B,** The composite valve graft is then seated and the mid-cusp sections tied down so that the valve is well seated in the annulus. **C,** The distal anastomosis is then performed with either 3-0 or 4-0 Prolene sutures; first, the posterior layer is done forehand from the inside, followed by the anterior layer done forehand from the outside. **D,** Next the mobilized right coronary artery ostial button is threaded through the center of a Teflon doughnut and sutured to the graft with a running 4-0 Prolene suture, from the inside forehand for the inferior margin **(1).** The suture is continued forehand from the outside to the superior margin. **D2,** The suture is tightened and then run forehand up to the other side and tied down. Through a hole in the ascending graft, where the left main graft will be anastomosed, the right coronary artery is probed to check for patency. The left main graft is then stretched so that there is approximately 1 to 1.5 cm of extra length to allow for when the graft is distended with blood and the ostia retract. The beveled graft is then sutured to the ascending aortic graft, first on the left side **(E1)** followed by forehand suturing of the inferior margin with 4-0 Prolene. For illustrative purposes, the 10 mm graft is shown longer than in reality. An intraoperative photograph is shown in **F.**[22]

and as near to the valve housing as possible to allow a maximum contact area between the valve suturing rim and the native annulus, thus preventing leaks at the anastomosis (Fig. 17–13, step B). The sutures at the midpoint between the commissures are tied first so that the valve will be seated deep in the annulus and thus further increase the contact area between the annulus and the valve rim.[4, 15, 22]

Next the distal aortic end-to-end anastomosis is performed with 3-0 Prolene sutures (4-0 Prolene for patients with acute dissection or Marfan syndrome).[1, 14, 24] (Fig. 17–13, step C, panels 1 and 2). Thereafter, the aortic clamp is gently released, allowing blood to briefly fill the conduit and distend it so that the site for the interposition tube graft and right coronary artery anastomoses can be determined and marked. Next the interposition tube graft lying behind the conduit is wrapped around the back of the conduit and divided approximately 1.0 cm to 1.5 cm more than the measured length. The reason for the additional length is to compensate for possible tension on the left coronary artery ostium because when the heart is filled and beating, the left coronary artery ostium tends to move further away from the graft. An oval hole that matches the beveled interposition tube graft is made at the site of the proposed anastomosis for the interposition graft to the ascending aorta. Similarly, a hole is made in the conduit opposite the right coronary artery ostium so that there will be no undue tension on the coronary artery. A generous aortic button (approximately 1.5 cm in diameter) containing the right coronary artery ostium is excised and the proximal coronary artery is freed from surrounding tissue, with care taken to preserve any major conal arterial branches of Vieussens. If the aorta is friable (for example, in patients with acute dissection or Marfan syndrome), then a circular patch (doughnut) of Teflon, with a central opening to accommodate the coronary artery, is threaded over the aortic button. Next the button is fastened to the conduit with a running 4-0 Prolene suture (Fig. 17–13, step D, panels 1 and 2). Patency of the anastomosis can be inspected by gently passing a probe through the opening for the left coronary tube graft into the proximal right coronary artery. The interposition tube graft is sutured to the conduit starting at the heel (Fig. 17–13, step E, panels 1 and 2). The patient is then placed in a head-down position while soft clamps are gently placed across both the right coronary artery and the interposition tube graft. The left ventricular sump is stopped, air is evacuated from the conduit graft and left ventricle, and then the aortic clamp is released. After all air has been evacuated from the ascending aorta, the clamps for the right and left coronary arteries are released, reestablishing blood flow to the heart. All the anastomoses are visible to the surgeon, and thus any bleeding points can be controlled before cardiopulmonary bypass is discontinued.[4, 15, 22]

The advantages of this technique are that the low-lying or distant left main coronary ostium can be easily reattached to the ascending conduit without undue tension (Fig. 17–13). A low-lying left main coronary artery ostium can be reattached without difficulty to the interposition graft, and

the position of the anastomosis for the interposition graft to the aortic conduit is easily determined. If there should be any mismatch between the level of the hole in the aortic conduit and the left main coronary artery, this is accommodated for by the interposition graft. The right coronary artery button can be rapidly mobilized, and the length obtained from dissecting the coronary artery free is sufficient to bridge the gap between the aneurysmal wall and the aortic graft. The shortened interposition graft without any kinks reduces the risk of neointimal buildup or thrombosis in the interposition graft. Neointimal proliferation has been minimal in the graft to the high-flow left main coronary artery in previous Cabrol repairs in patients taking warfarin. The problems of graft kinks forming at the side-to-side anastomosis with the Cabrol technique or of graft occlusion occurring at the angle of the right coronary artery ostium are avoided because the graft is not tethered by a side-to-side anastomosis. Because all the anastomoses are visible to the surgeon, hemostasis can be assured while the patient is still on cardiopulmonary bypass. This reduces the risk of blood transfusions being required and of the late development of false aneurysms at the anastomoses because the graft does not need to be wrapped to ensure hemostasis.[4, 15, 22]

The foregoing procedure has been used in 47 patients without any complications or problems related to the technique and no deaths within 30 days. Routine TEE, or angiography in selected patients (Fig. 17–14), has confirmed patent anastomoses, good coronary blood flow, the preservation of myocardial contractility, and the absence of false aneurysms. Approximately two thirds of these operations can be performed without homologous blood transfusion, and in 24 elective operations only one patient required an operative transfusion.[25]

AORTIC ROOT REPLACEMENT WITH A HOMOGRAFT OR PULMONARY AUTOGRAFT

The insertion of a homograft for replacement of the aortic valve and ascending aorta is similar to the button technique. The coronary ostia are mobilized, and then the left coronary artery is attached to the homograft, which has been seated in the aortic annulus with interrupted sutures. The distal anastomosis is then performed, and next the right coronary artery is anastomosed. This method is particularly useful when an aortoventricular repair has to be performed in those patients (Fig. 17–15) who have typically undergone previous procedures for congenital aortic valve stenosis or who require aortic outflow enlargement.[26] If an aortic homograft is being inserted, then the mitral leaflet can be used for repair of the septum by rotation of the graft. Alternatively, if a pulmonary homograft is the method of choice because of less likelihood of calcification,[27] then a polytetrafluoroethylene (PTFE) patch is used to repair the septum. A PTFE patch is also used to repair the right ventricular outflow tract. Aortic homograft valves in children and young adults are reported to have a 79% 10-year survival rate.[28] Homograft replacements, first unsuccessfully tried as a subcoronary aortic valve by Bigelow but successfully achieved by Ross,[29] have been followed for more than three decades by Belcher and Ross.[30] Long-term results have been good although initial mortality may be as high as 33% in those patients who have homografts inserted because of prosthetic valve endocarditis. Kirklin and colleagues[31]

FIGURE 17–14   **A,** CT scan of a patient with compression of the trachea and bronchi from a large aneurysms causing respiratory failure. The patient was intubated to obtain a CT of the chest in an effort to identify the cause of the respiratory failure. **B,** Preoperative angiogram of the ascending aorta obtained at the same time. **C,** Postoperative angiogram of the aortic root showing the composite valve graft that was inserted with a tube graft to the left main coronary artery, with a later phase **(D)** showing the coronary arteries and a saphenous vein bypass graft to the right coronary artery. The ascending aorta, arch, and thoracoabdominal aorta were all replaced during one operative procedure (see chapter on Replacement of the Entire Aorta).

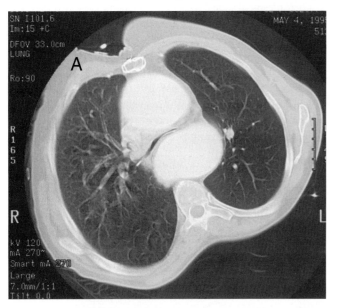

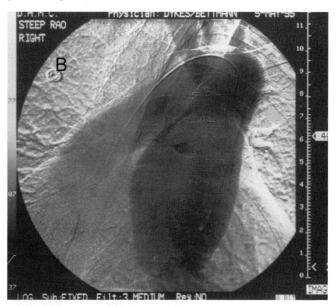

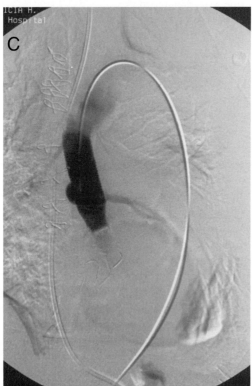

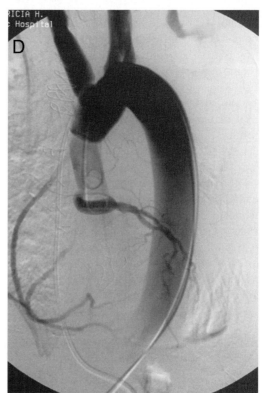

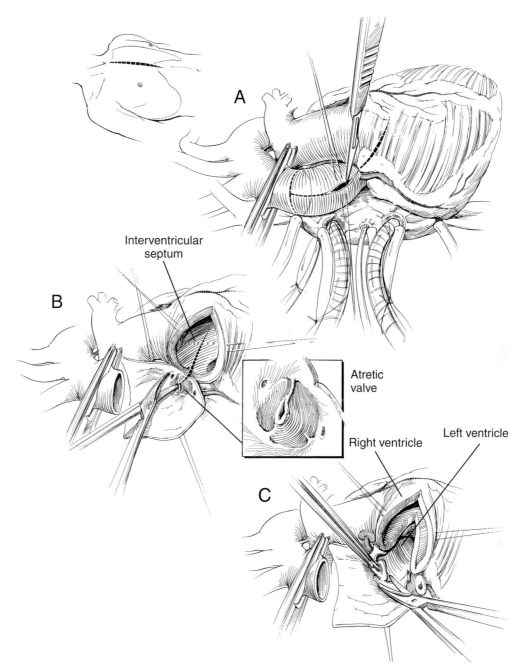

FIGURE 17–15 Illustrations of an aortoventriculoplasty with use of a pulmonary homograft and PTFE patch. The operation is typically used for patients with a small aortic root or with congenital aortic atresia that has previously been treated with surgery or balloon valve dilatation. **A,** The aorta is cross-clamped, and then the aorta and pulmonary outflow tract are opened along the dotted lines. Note that two venous cannulae and retrograde cardioplegia are used. **B,** The valve is cut with a pair of scissors, and the incision is extended along the interventricular septum, keeping close and parallel to the inferior margin of the pulmonary valve. This will reduce the risk of postoperative heart block. **C,** The coronary artery ostia are mobilized as buttons, and as much as possible of the old valve is excised.

Illustration continued on following page

reported on 178 patients who underwent insertion of homografts (155 freehand, 23 ascending root) with an 85% 8-year survival rate and freedom of explantation or 3+ or 4+ aortic regurgitation of 85% at 8 years. Among the patients who underwent root replacements, 12 of the 23 died (52%) and 11 were late survivors. The reasons for the original operations in the patients who died included endocarditis in four, acute dissection in three, previous composite graft insertion in one, ascending aortic aneurysms with New York Heart Association (NYHA) IV heart failure in two, and Konno procedure in one. On multivariate analysis of the deaths, NYHA IV class and ascending aortic repairs were identified risk factors. Among the patients who initially had totally competent valves, 20% had moderate incompetence 5 years later, resulting in more than 30% with moderate or more incompetence. The long-term results in these patients will be of interest.

The method of preservation does not appear to be critical for free root homografts.[30] In a series of 534 patients,

however, O'Brien and colleagues[32] found that antibiotic viable cryopreserved homografts (allografts) performed better, had a greater long-term survival rate, a lower incidence of structural deterioration, and a lower risk of reoperation being required. Of concern is the study by Jones and colleagues[33] of a series of 80 patients, 46 with infracoronary insertions and 34 with complete root replacements. The mortality rate was 6.3% (all infracoronary); 46% of infracoronary implants and 17% of root implants had progressed on late follow-up to grade 2 or greater aortic

FIGURE 17–15 *Continued* **D,** The posterior valve sutures are placed with the pledgets on top of the annulus, and the valve sutures are passed through the pulmonary homograft. **E,** A PTFE patch is cut to the appropriate size, and the remaining valve sutures are passed through the homograft, this time with the pledgets on the homograft exterior, and then through the PTFE patch. Note that they are not cut but are gathered together in a clamp. **F,** The patch is then sewn to the ventricular septum with interrupted valve sutures. The inset window illustrates the course of the sutures between the two pledgets. A running suture can be used, but it is more likely to leak.

Illustration continued on following page

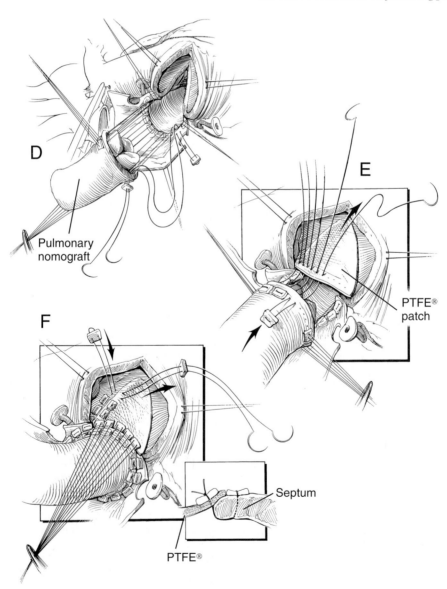

valve insufficiency, and nine (eight infracoronary) had required explantation. They concluded that infracoronary insertions should be abandoned and that the high incidence of late valve insufficiency of root replacements in 17% of patients who initially had no early insufficiency is a cause for concern. Daicoff and colleagues[34] have also reported better long-term results with mini-root replacements than with the freehand technique. As in the case of homografts used elsewhere in the aorta, if a long segment is replaced, there is the long-term risk of calcification and aneurysm

formation, as found by DeBakey (personal communication) in the follow-up of his patients. In spite of the initial popularity of aortic homograft replacements for aortic aneurysms in the late 1940s and early 1950s,[35-42] there have been few publications of long-term studies of patients who had these types of repairs.[43]

If the infracoronary freehand technique is used, important points are to undersize the homograft by 3 mm (compared to sizing of the annulus preoperatively by TEE), rotate the graft through 120 degrees, hold the graft with a clamp,

FIGURE 17–15 *Continued* **G,** The coronary ostia are reattached next, with a Teflon doughnut ring if necessary. A continuous distal anastomosis is then performed. **H,** Another PTFE patch is selected and cut to the appropriate size to repair the right ventricular outflow tract. The gathered previously placed anterior valve sutures are then passed through the patch and tied **(I).** The pulmonary outflow tract is sutured with a running continuous suture, and the repair is completed **(J).** (From Svensson LG, Crawford ES. Curr Probl Surg 1993;30:1–172.)

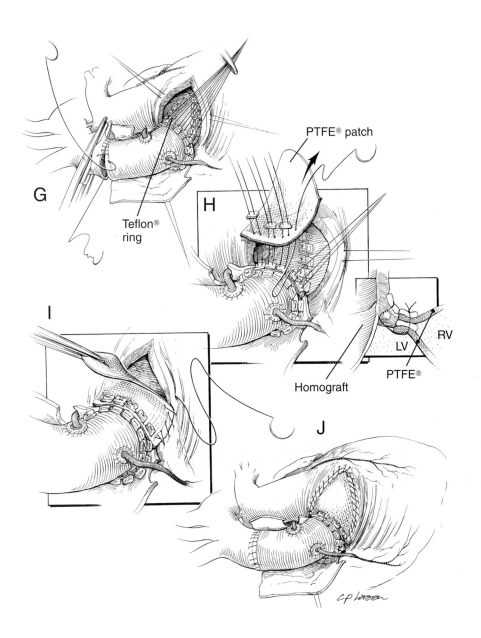

place three 4-0 PTFE sutures in the middle of the excised cusps below the old valve ridge, and then to make a more U-shaped distal suture line in the sinuses rather than a V-shaped suture line, starting in the mid-cusp area.

Insertion of a pulmonary autograft is one of the more complex yet gratifying aortic procedures if successfully performed (Fig. 17-16). This procedure should be considered in children, young adult patients, and particularly female patients who plan to have children. The basic technique that we have most often used consists of meticulous mobilization of both the pulmonary artery and the pulmonary valve with careful preservation of the left coronary artery and the septal perforators (Fig. 17-16). The ascending aorta and the aortic valve are excised and the coronary ostia are mobilized as aortic buttons. In contrast to the method described by Ross, who repaired the pulmonary artery before insertion of the pulmonary autograft in the aortic position, we put in the pulmonary autograft first.[27, 44] The original technique described by Ross and colleagues[27, 44]

also involved sewing interrupted sutures with a Teflon strip around the circumference of the annulus. The pulmonary outflow tract is then repaired with a homograft. The advantage of repairing the pulmonary outflow tract last is that it can be completed with the aorta unclamped and with reperfusion of the heart. The operation can be combined with a Konno procedure if necessary. We do not recommend the operation for patients with Marfan syndrome, and both Kouchoukos and Elkins also have commented that the procedure is not indicated in these patients. In a series of 200 patients, Elkins has used the pulmonary graft as a tube in 20 patients with annular aortic ectasia. In these latter patients, he has reduced the size of the annulus by using a ring of a piece of Dacron tube graft or by running a suture around the annulus as an annuloplasty. He has also described wedging the native aorta and suturing it around the graft without using an external Dacron graft to support the repair. We have used pledgeted horizontal mattress sutures at the annulus to reduce a large annulus in size so that a

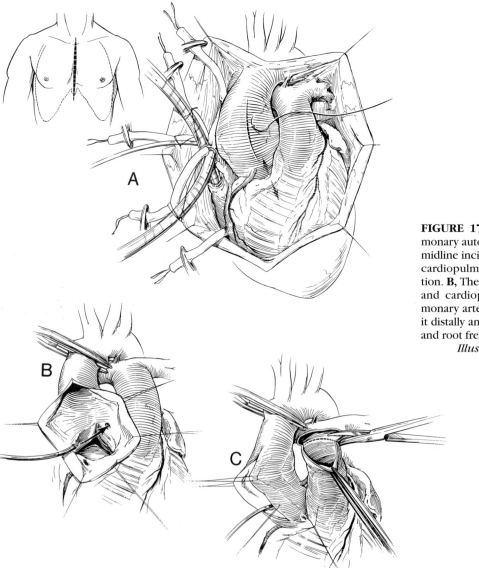

FIGURE 17–16 Steps for insertion of a pulmonary autograft in the aortic position. **A,** After a midline incision is made, the patient is placed on cardiopulmonary bypass with bicaval cannulation. **B,** The aorta is opened between stay sutures and cardioplegia is administered. **C,** The pulmonary artery is then mobilized by first dividing it distally and then dissecting the left main artery and root free **(D).**

Illustration continued on following page

pulmonary graft can be inserted. Each suture at a commissure reduces the annulus size by approximately 3 mm. Thus, using this method, we have reduced an annulus from 33 mm to 25 mm by placing a mattress suture at each commissure. In patients with aneurysms of the aorta, typically in association with a bicuspid valve, we have placed a Dacron tube graft between the pulmonary graft and the distal normal-size aorta.

In a remarkable report, Ross and associates[45] described their experience with 339 patients operated upon since 1967, when Ross first described the procedure. The mortality rate was 7.4%, with only one death since 1976, and the 20-year survival rate was 80%. Pulmonary valve autografts have been reported by Ross's group to have an event-free survival rate of 73% at 14 years postoperatively[44] and 70% at 20 years.[45] In 37 children, Elkins' group[46] have reported a 3% mortality rate, improvement in left ventricular architecture, and growth of the pulmonary autograft in the aortic position. Eighteen percent of their patients had moderate neo "aortic" valve regurgitation on follow-up. Long-term function of pulmonary homografts in the pulmonary position to replace the explanted pulmonary autograft remains a concern, although the risk of stenosis or calcification appears to be small and regurgitation is well tolerated.[4, 47] In a series of patients reported by Kouchoukos and colleagues,[48] there were no deaths and no serious complications: this shows the excellent results that can be achieved with this operation in young patients. The long-term results of the operation will be of future interest to ourselves and those patients who need this type of

FIGURE 17–16 *Continued* **D,** The dissection continues down to the muscle, and care is taken not to damage the first septal perforator in the muscle at about the 9 or 10 o'clock position. **E,** The sinuses of the pulmonary artery, the valve leaflets, and the lower extent of the valve leaflets are identified and inspected, and the pulmonary outflow tract is divided immediately below (approximately 3 to 4 mm) the valve cusps. A right-angled clamp in the pulmonary aids in determining the lower limit of the valve cusps. **F,** The conduit is excised for the aortic repair. We believe it is important to test the autograft to ensure the valve is competent. This can be done with saline irrigation after clamping the distal end with a vascular clamp. Alternatively, a needle with a pressure line can be inserted through a purse string suture into the autograft and the autograft distended. Based on testing, we have on one occasion reversed the repair because of a severe leaflet prolapse that was not detected on preoperative echocardiography and right heart angiography. **G,** The coronary artery ostia are mobilized, and the aortic valve is excised **(H). I,** The pulmonary autograft is next seated in the aortic annulus with interrupted simple sutures, although pledgeted sutures can also be used. Care is taken to ensure that the valve is properly seated, since the pulmonary valve does not have the differences in valve cusp edge lengths that the aortic valve has.

Illustration continued on following page

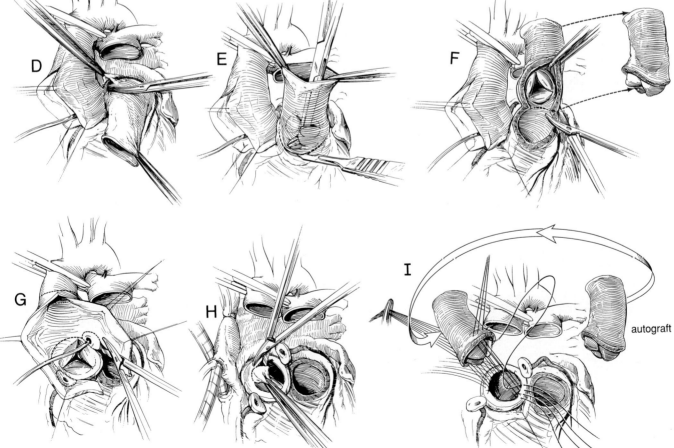

operation. The role of this procedure for aortic root dilatation in patients with Marfan syndrome is limited, because of the risk of dilatation of the aortic root that we and others have noted. In the unpublished findings from Elkins'

series of 200 patients presented at the American College of Surgeons Postgraduate Course in 1995, the 8-year freedom from reoperation was 84%, similar to that with a St Jude's valve, although with the additional benefits of a

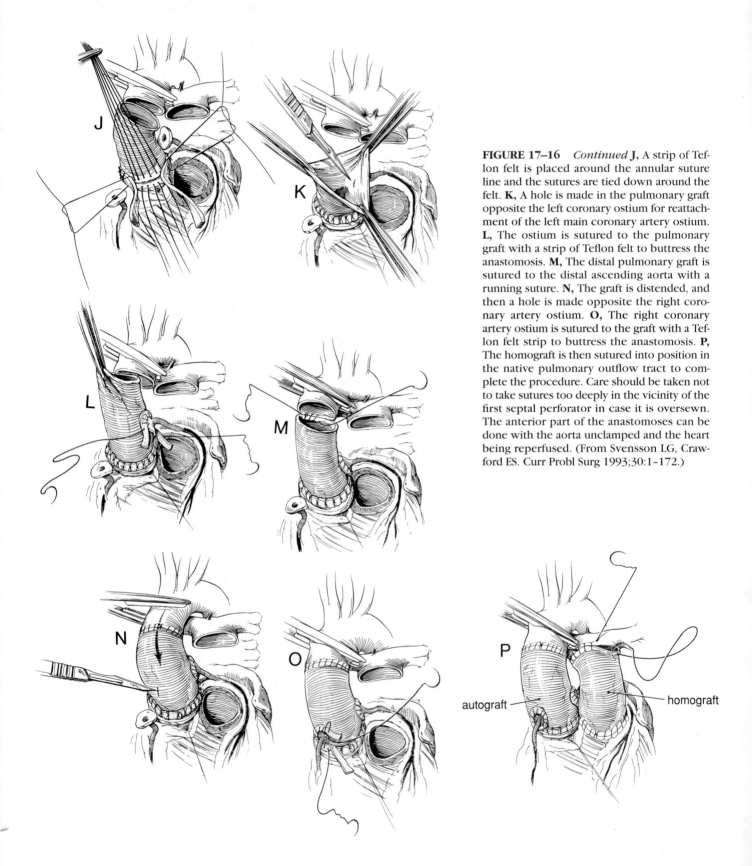

FIGURE 17–16 *Continued* **J,** A strip of Teflon felt is placed around the annular suture line and the sutures are tied down around the felt. **K,** A hole is made in the pulmonary graft opposite the left coronary ostium for reattachment of the left main coronary artery ostium. **L,** The ostium is sutured to the pulmonary graft with a strip of Teflon felt to buttress the anastomosis. **M,** The distal pulmonary graft is sutured to the distal ascending aorta with a running suture. **N,** The graft is distended, and then a hole is made opposite the right coronary artery ostium. **O,** The right coronary artery ostium is sutured to the graft with a Teflon felt strip to buttress the anastomosis. **P,** The homograft is then sutured into position in the native pulmonary outflow tract to complete the procedure. Care should be taken not to take sutures too deeply in the vicinity of the first septal perforator in case it is oversewn. The anterior part of the anastomoses can be done with the aorta unclamped and the heart being reperfused. (From Svensson LG, Crawford ES. Curr Probl Surg 1993;30:1–172.)

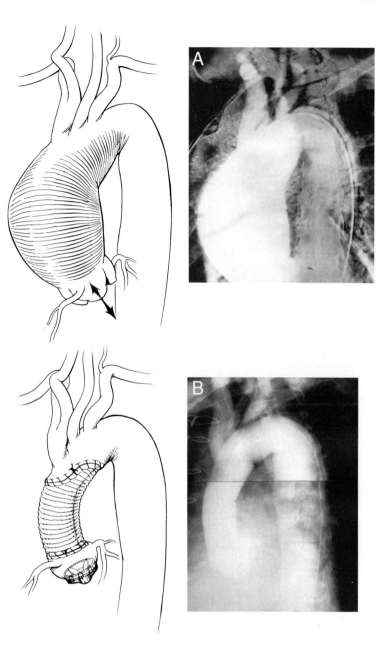

FIGURE 17–17   **A,** Patient with ascending and aortic arch aneurysm without annular dilatation and aortic valve regurgitation. **B,** Postoperative repair with a tongue of graft tissue behind the greater vessels. The tongue can be extended onto the descending aorta if necessary, with the anastomosis being kept closer to the origin of the greater vessels.

lower risk of both endocarditis and Coumadin associated hemorrhage.

REPLACEMENT OF THE AORTIC ARCH

The most critical step in the successful repair of extensively diseased aortas is replacement of the aortic arch. Aortic arch replacement with use of antegrade brain perfusion was first described by DeBakey and colleagues in 1957.[49] Subsequently, in 1963, Barnard and Schire[50] described the first series of replacements of the aortic arch for aortic dissection and degenerative disease with the use of deep hypothermia and circulatory arrest. Later, Griepp and colleagues[51] popularized the routine use of deep hypothermia and circulatory arrest for the repair of aortic arch repairs. Nonethe-

less, replacement of varying extents of the aorta from the coronary artery ostia to below the mid-descending aorta remained a difficult problem. To overcome this, Borst and associates[52, 53] described a two-stage technique by which the ascending aorta and aortic arch were replaced first, leaving a segment of distal tubular graft in the descending thoracic aorta. They termed this procedure the *elephant trunk technique.* At a second stage, the distal aorta was repaired beyond the subclavian artery. Subsequently, we[1, 7, 54] modified this technique as described below to simplify the operation and make it safer by inverting the tube graft on itself for the distal anastomosis.

The aortic arch can be replaced by several procedures. These include partial repair with a beveled anastomosis, a tongue of graft replacing all but the section beyond the left subclavian artery (Fig. 17-17), reattachment of the arch

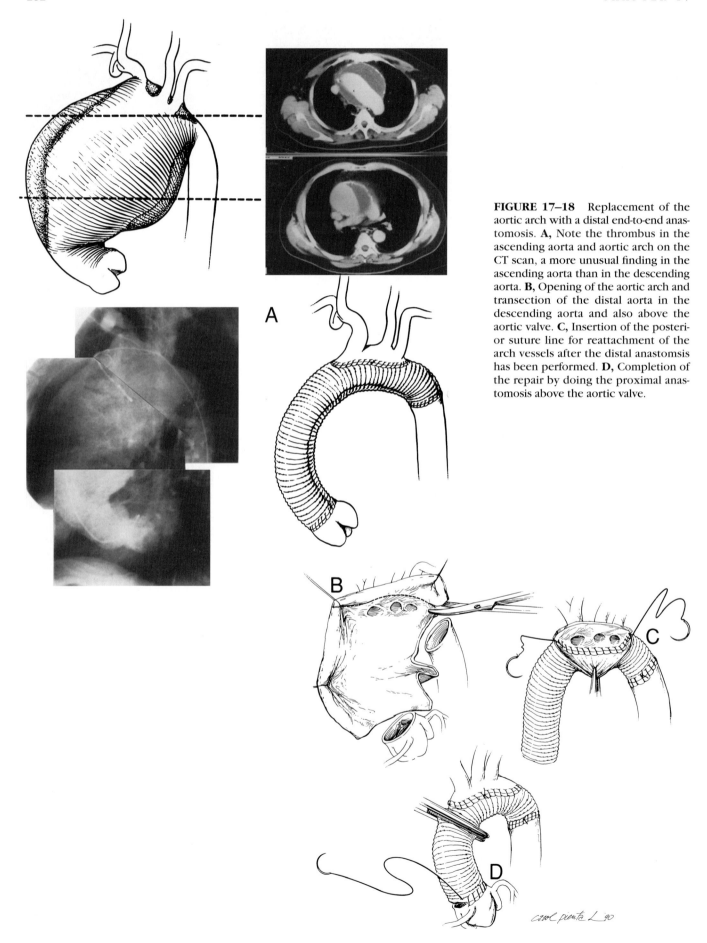

FIGURE 17–18 Replacement of the aortic arch with a distal end-to-end anastomosis. **A,** Note the thrombus in the ascending aorta and aortic arch on the CT scan, a more unusual finding in the ascending aorta than in the descending aorta. **B,** Opening of the aortic arch and transection of the distal aorta in the descending aorta and also above the aortic valve. **C,** Insertion of the posterior suture line for reattachment of the arch vessels after the distal anastomosis has been performed. **D,** Completion of the repair by doing the proximal anastomosis above the aortic valve.

vessels to a tubular graft with a distal descending aorta end-to-end anastomosis (Fig. 17–18), reattachment of the arch vessels to a graft as part of an elephant trunk procedure (Fig. 17–10), or reattachment of the arch vessels to a graft without a proximal descending aortic anastomosis as part of an operation to replace the entire aorta during one operation. The arch vessels can also be reattached individually, if aneurysmal, by short interposition grafts as illustrated in Figure 17–19. In addition, the aortic arch can be replaced from the left chest, usually as a beveled anastomosis.[1-3, 7, 54-58]

The use of deep hypothermic circulatory arrest with retrograde brain perfusion has allowed aortic arch replacements to be safely done with a low mortality and stroke rate. With this technique, the previously safe period of approximately 40 minutes of circulatory arrest in a study of 656 patients[8] can probably be extended to 50 or 60 minutes with retrograde perfusion of the brain (Fig. 17–20).[8, 25, 59] An aortic arch operation should be performed with a minimal period of circulatory arrest and yet all aneurysmal parts of the aortic arch should be resected. This should engender the least risk to both the patient's life and neurological function during both the early and late postoperative periods.

OPERATIVE PREPARATION AND ANESTHESIA

The femoral artery and vein are exposed in the groin, usually the right groin, and the vessels are looped with umbilical tape. The chest is opened through a standard midline incision and the pericardium is opened. In patients who have had multiple previous cardiac operations or who have extensive aneurysms eroding the sternum, femorofemoral bypass is instituted prior to sternal entry. The patient is then cooled until electroencephalographic (EEG) activity is absent, the circulation is arrested, and the sternum is opened.

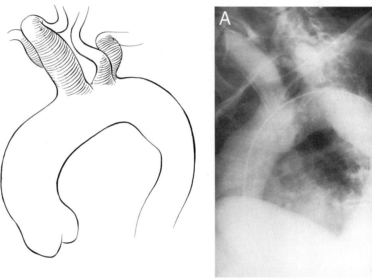

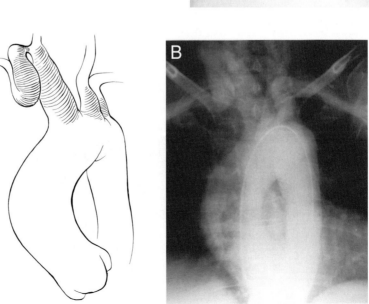

FIGURE 17–19 **A,** Diagram and preoperative arteriogram of a patient with an ascending aortic aneurysm and also dilatation of the arch arteries. **B,** The anteroposterior view.

Illustration continued on following page

Two "cardiotomy suckers" should be available in case the aneurysm should be inadvertently opened. The aortic arch is then exposed on its left anterior lateral surface, and the plane of surgical dissection is kept close to the aorta so that the phrenic nerve is not damaged and the left pleura is not entered. Furthermore, electrocautery is best avoided to reduce the risk of phrenic nerve damage. The vagus nerve and the recurrent laryngeal nerves are also preserved by dissection close to the aorta. The vessels of the head are not dissected out or mobilized because this causes unnecessary bleeding and they are well visualized from inside the aorta. Next, the patient is placed in a steep Trendelenburg position to prevent accumulation of air in the arch vessels.[1, 3, 4, 8, 25, 54, 58] A 23 to 30 mm woven Dacron tubular prosthesis is selected for insertion, depending on the size of the aorta, and a 10 mm woven tube side graft is used for perfusion of the arch. If a collagen-impregnated graft is not used, the graft should be painted with a 25% solution of albumin while being thoroughly stretched to ensure that the albumin penetrates the interstices of the graft, and then baked by flash sterilization for 5 minutes. This should result in a graft that is neither wet nor flaky, so that it will neither ooze nor result in embolization of albumin flakes to the brain. The 10 mm graft is anastomosed end-to-side to the larger aortic graft with a running 4-0 Prolene suture.[1, 3, 4, 8, 25, 54, 58, 60]

During cooling, the ascending aorta and arch should be gently palpated regularly to ensure that the measured radial arterial pressures correlate with the palpated pressures. In addition, we now use TEE routinely to evaluate blood flow when bypass is commenced, particularly in patients with aortic dissection. The reason for this is to detect, particularly in patients with aortic dissection, whether the aortic arch

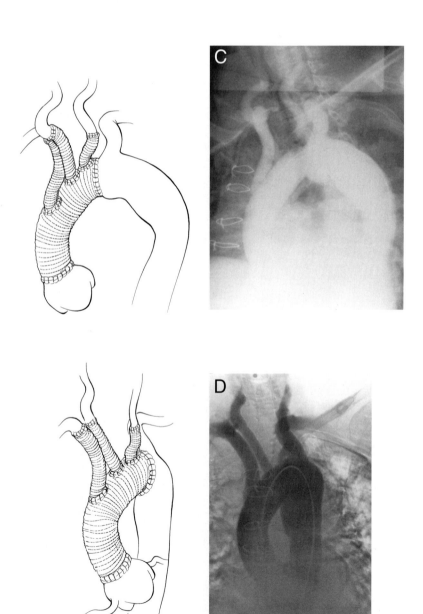

FIGURE 17–19 *Continued* **C** and **D,** Postoperative diagrams and arteriograms after placement of individual tube grafts to the right subclavian, right common carotid, and left common carotid arteries. Note that the distal aortic anastomosis was done proximal to the left subclavian artery.

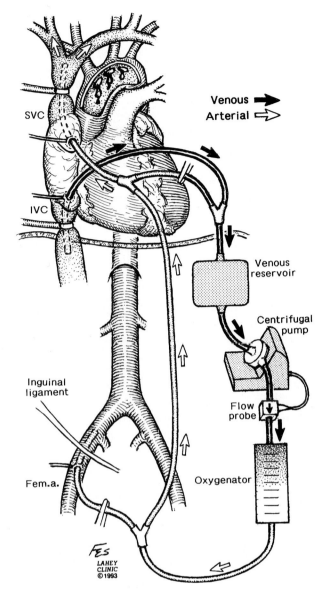

FIGURE 17–20   Cardiopulmonary bypass cannulae for retrograde perfusion of the brain. Note that the femoral arterial line has a Y for perfusion of the superior vena cava retrograde with a tape around the vena cava.

vessels and brain are being adequately perfused. Although regular monitoring of the right radial artery pressure will usually alert the surgeon to the potential problem of an inadequate aortic arch perfusion pressure, this is not always the case. For example, the innominate artery may be perfused by one lumen of the dissected aorta with no communication with the other lumen, or if the aortic dissection septum acts as a flutter valve, selective nonperfusion of the head vessels can occur. Furthermore, the EEG may be unreliable because it may show no brain activity suggesting that hypothermia is adequate when, in fact, there is brain ischemia. The nasopharyngeal and esophageal temperatures should usually decrease more rapidly than the rectal and bladder temperatures. Indeed, a failure of esophageal and nasopharyngeal temperatures to fall adequately and rapidly

should alert the surgeon to check for nonperfusion of the head vessels.[1, 3, 4, 8, 25, 54, 58]

Patients are cooled until the EEG shows no activity at 2 microvolt sensitivity for 5 minutes, and bladder, rectal, nasopharyngeal, and esophageal temperatures are all below 20° C.[61] The patient's head is also surrounded by ice packs. Cardiopulmonary bypass is stopped and the patient is placed in a steep Trendelenburg position with circulatory arrest. The aneurysm is opened between two stay sutures and all blood is evacuated, assisted by the left atrioventricular sump drainage.[1, 3, 4, 8, 25, 54, 58]

Hyperkalemic blood retrograde and antegrade cardioplegia aided by topical hypothermic saline solution without ice is used for arresting cardiac contractions. Topical hypothermic saline solution is removed from the pericardial well, both because it runs into the operative field and also because it increases the risk of phrenic nerve damage in association with deep hypothermia. The aorta is opened along the arch approximately 1 cm from the origin of the greater vessels, and a stay suture is placed through the aorta proximal to the innominate artery. Distally, the aortic incision is taken to an anterior lateral position to allow resection of all dilated segments; if a beveled anastomosis is to be performed, then the aorta is usually completely transected. As discussed in the next chapter, in those patients with chronic aortic dissection the septum is excised as far as possible in the descending thoracic aorta so that both true and false lumina are perfused distally.[1, 3, 4, 8, 25, 54, 58]

Once the arch greater vessel reattachment is completed as described below, the proximal ascending repair is performed. With the patient remaining in a steep Trendelenburg position, the cardiopulmonary bypass pump is slowly restarted through the femoral artery cannula. Potential embolic material in the initial blood return is suctioned from the arch, and the greater vessels are allowed to fill. Gentle compression of the vessels ensures that no air pockets are present. The blood is allowed to exit through both the proximal aortic graft and from the 10 mm side arm. When the return is free of air or any possible emboli, the other arterial arm of the cardiopulmonary bypass pump is connected to the 10 mm side arm. All air is carefully evacuated from the aortic graft and the 10 mm side arm. A plastic band should be applied to secure the cannula in position in the side arm, the proximal aortic tube graft is then clamped, cardiopulmonary bypass is restored to normal flow, and warming is commenced. The aortic graft, at the highest point above the innominate artery but proximal to the clamp, should be punctured with a needle a couple of times to allow any possible remaining air in the graft or descending aorta to escape from the graft. If no valve or coronary artery bypasses are needed, the blood in the cardiopulmonary bypass pump is warmed before the cardiopulmonary bypass is restarted unless retrograde brain perfusion is being used.

The ascending aorta is replaced by complete transection of the aorta just above the coronary artery sinuses and use of a running suture without Teflon felt. By abandoning the inclusion technique, especially the Bentall composite valve graft technique for proximal anastomosis, the incidence of false aneurysms is reduced, even in those patients with aortic dissection and Marfan syndrome. For composite valve graft replacements (the technique is described previously in this chapter), the preferred methods should be either reanastomosis of the coronary arteries as buttons containing the ostia or placement of a tube graft to the left main coronary artery with use of the button technique for the right coronary artery as previously described. Occasionally, in a patient with acute aortic dissection in whom the coronary arteries cannot be reattached, the ostia must be oversewn and distal coronary artery vein bypasses have to be performed to the coronary arteries as necessary.[1, 3, 4, 8, 25, 54, 58]

It is important to ensure that hemostasis is achieved at all the anastomoses before cardiopulmonary bypass is discontinued and this is conveniently done during rewarming of the patient. After administration of protamine, the plasmapheresis concentrate is reinfused, and every 20 to 30 minutes blood samples are sent for coagulation analysis to guide the administration of blood products until all clotting deficiencies are corrected. During the postoperative period, the patient is treated, if necessary, with inotropes, vasodilators, and blood products. The standard postoperative care is similar to that for any patient after a cardiopulmonary bypass or a coronary artery bypass operation. Blood products, however, must be used freely if there is any evidence of excess bleeding, and thus any deficiencies in the coagulation profile are corrected to normal. Since these patients are usually overloaded with fluid by the end of the procedure, dopamine is used liberally, as is Lasix, to encourage diuresis.[1, 3, 4, 8, 25, 54, 58]

ARCH REPAIRS

The beveled anastomosis is the easiest and safest and usually will require a circulatory arrest period of 10 to 15 minutes. Before insertion, the tube graft is beveled so that all the aneurysmal parts of the proximal aortic arch are replaced. This will usually mean that the distal end of the graft is sutured into position, starting at the lesser curve of the aortic arch with a forehand suture run up the posterior wall followed by an anterior suture along the anterior part of the incision immediately below the greater vessels. If more than this section of the aortic arch, but not the descending aorta, is involved, then either replacement with an aortic tongue or reattachment of the arch vessels to a tube graft is required.

For replacement of the aortic arch with a tongue of graft, the graft is opened along the length that will be attached around the arch vessels, with excision of approximately 2 cm along the slit. The distal end is then beveled to match the distal aorta, usually the proximal descending aorta, to which it will be sutured. The graft is sutured into position by a method similar to that used for a beveled anastomosis, but care must be taken not to damage the phrenic and recurrent laryngeal nerves. We have used this technique

since the late 1980s and have found it to be useful in selected patients when the aorta beyond the left subclavian artery is not heavily diseased or aneurysmal. We have found, however, that it is difficult to clamp the distal aortic arch if a subsequent descending or thoracoabdominal aortic repair is required, even if a good proximal neck for clamping appears to be present. Under these circumstances, it is usually better to perform an elephant trunk repair with a later staged operation.

If the proximal descending aorta is dilated but not beyond the proximal third of the descending aorta, then the arch vessels should be reattached as a separate aortic island with a distal end-to-end anastomosis. This is best done by selecting a graft that matches the distal uninvolved aorta and suturing it into position with a running suture. If the aorta is one that holds sutures well, transecting it is useful but the recurrent nerve must be protected. The anastomosis is best achieved by starting on the outer curve of the descending aorta with a forehand suture on the posterior superior aorta, followed by a forehand suture on the inferior anterior wall. Thereafter a hole to match the greater vessels is excised, and the greater vessels are reattached with suturing of first the posterior wall and then the anterior wall immediately below the greater vessels.

Our modification of the elephant trunk technique[1, 3, 54] is used as described previously for patients who have aneurysmal disease distal to the left subclavian artery that needs repair at a subsequent staged procedure.

ELEPHANT TRUNK PROCEDURE

Rationale

A problem that we noted with the standard elephant trunk technique was that some patients undergoing the procedure suffered torn aortas at the distal suture line with rupture just beyond the left subclavian artery. The reason for this was that suturing within the confines of the aorta sometimes resulted in tearing of the aortic wall because of the great torsion exerted on the needle during suturing at a difficult angle. Having noted this technical difficulty and the rupture of the descending thoracic aorta in the postoperative period in two patients when the above procedure was used, we devised a new technique, as described previously,[1, 3, 4, 8, 25, 54, 58] of inverting the proximal part of the graft into the distal graft. This modification has resulted in easier suturing of the graft into position at the subclavian artery with a concomitant improvement in results,[1, 3, 4, 8, 25, 54, 58] particularly in patients with aortic dissection[1, 3, 4, 8, 25, 54, 58] in whom the operative mortality rate for the modified elephant trunk technique has been reduced to only 5%. In addition to simplifying insertion of the prostheses, the technique makes possible a greater surface contact area between the graft and the aortic wall when the inverted tube graft is withdrawn for the aortic arch replacement and the distal suture line is automatically tightened during withdrawal. This results in a reduced risk of bleeding at the distal anastomosis because there is no need for torsion on the needle to suture through the graft and the aortic wall. Furthermore, sites of possible weakness can easily be strengthened. Thus the risk of tearing of the aorta is also considerably lessened. In summary, the modification of the elephant trunk procedure, as described below, is the preferred method whereby the aortic arch can be replaced within a circulatory arrest period of approximately 30 to 40 minutes with a reduced risk of bleeding both at the distal anastomosis and at the aortic arch anastomotic sites.[1, 3, 4, 8, 25, 54, 58]

To simplify anastomosis of the tube graft to the aorta distal to the left subclavian artery, a stay suture is placed on the proximal end of the tube graft (Fig. 17–21). The anastomosis of the 10 mm graft to the proximal tubular graft is performed and then inverted into the distal graft prior to circulatory arrest to save time during the circulatory arrest period. Then the suture and the proximal end are inverted so that the proximal part with the adherent 10 mm side graft is invaginated into the more distal tubular graft. A hemostat is kept on the stay suture for later withdrawal of the inverted part of the tube graft. The end-to-side anastomosed 10 mm

FIGURE 17–21 Replacement of the entire aorta by our modification of the elephant trunk technique. **A,** A midline incision is made, and the patient is placed on cardiopulmonary bypass with two venous cannulae and cooled until the circulation can be arrested and retrograde brain perfusion and cardioplegia achieved. The aorta is then opened along the stippled line. **B,** According to the size of the distal aortic arch, prior to circulatory arrest, a 10 mm side graft is anastomosed end-to-side to the larger tube graft. A collagen-impregnated graft works best for this, because it is softer and easier to sew to. The proximal tube graft with the side graft is then inverted into the distal tube graft. **C,** After the aorta is incised between stay sutures, the proximal aorta is transected. **D,** The distal aorta can also be transected to improve exposure distally if bleeding should occur at the arch anastomosis.

Illustration continued on following page

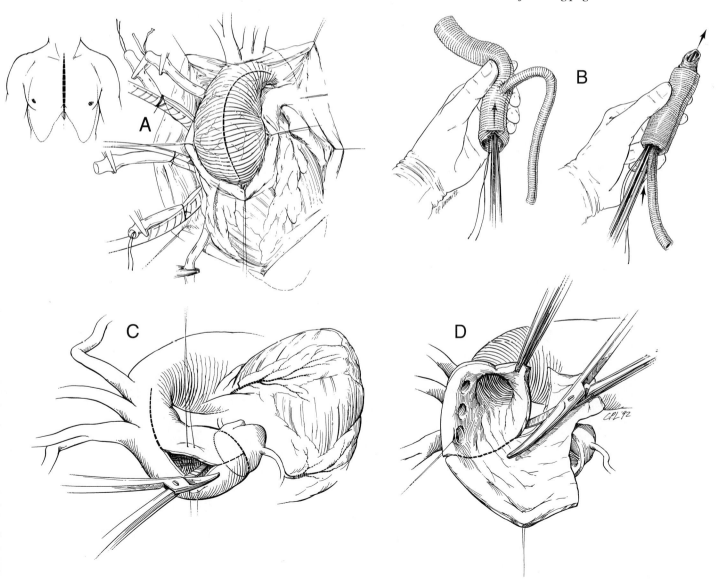

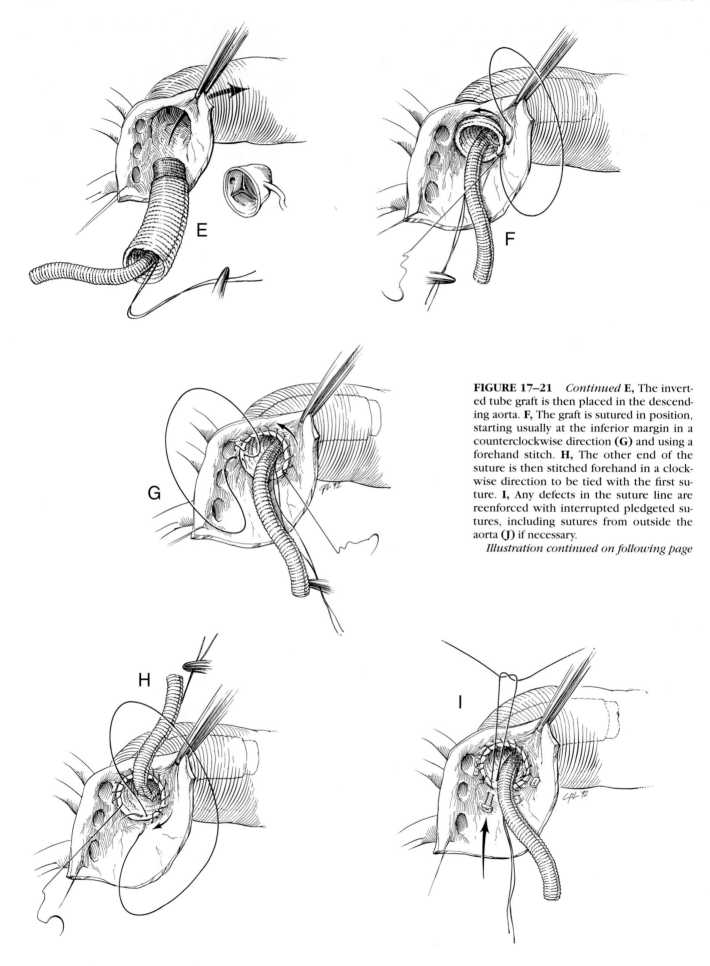

FIGURE 17–21 *Continued* **E,** The inverted tube graft is then placed in the descending aorta. **F,** The graft is sutured in position, starting usually at the inferior margin in a counterclockwise direction **(G)** and using a forehand stitch. **H,** The other end of the suture is then stitched forehand in a clockwise direction to be tied with the first suture. **I,** Any defects in the suture line are reenforced with interrupted pledgeted sutures, including sutures from outside the aorta **(J)** if necessary.

Illustration continued on following page

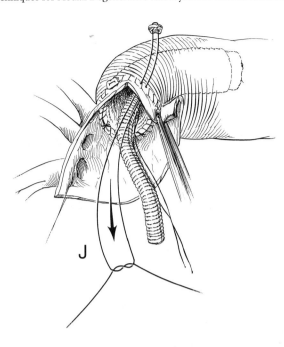

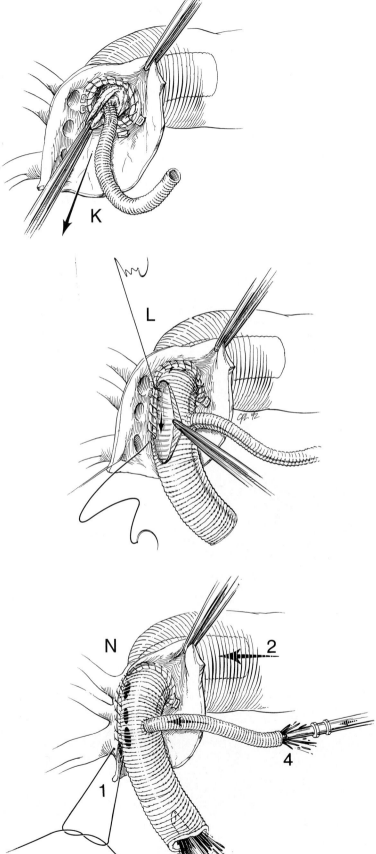

FIGURE 17–21 *Continued* **K,** The tube graft is then withdrawn from the distal aorta. **L,** Next a hole is cut in the tube graft for the arch vessels, which are then reattached to the tube graft by first performing the posterior suture line. **M,** The anterior suture line is then performed, initially with a backhand stitch followed by a forehand stitch along the anterior anastomosis. **N,** The knot is tied down **(1)** and slow perfusion through the femoral artery is commenced to evacuate any debris or air **(2).** The ascending graft is aspirated to remove embolic material **(3),** and then the side graft is perfused with the arterial cannula **(4)** and secured in position with a plastic banding gun.

Illustration continued on following page

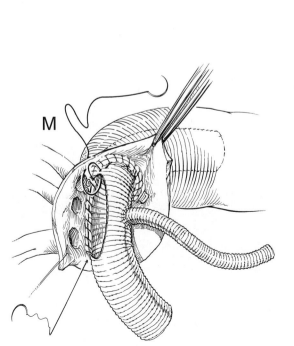

tube graft is also inverted for a distance of approximately 5 cm leaving the outer graft approximately 15 cm long. The 10 mm graft can easily be moved around during suturing without obscuring the field. Furthermore, during removal of the proximal inverted end, the 10 mm graft can also be gently tugged upon. Since the 10 mm tube graft is already anastomosed to the aortic arch graft, the period of circulatory arrest is shortened.[1, 3, 4, 8, 25, 54, 58]

The invaginated graft is placed in the descending aorta, and a secure suture is placed just beyond the subclavian artery between the aorta and the doubled-over edge of the tube graft (Fig. 17–21), usually starting at the inferior margin. Whenever possible, along the left inferior lateral, left lateral, and superior margins of the aorta, the suture is placed

forehand from outside the aorta through the doubled-over graft and then backhand over the top of the graft edge out through the aortic wall to the outer side. The advantage of this procedure is that a hemostatic atraumatic suture is inserted without torsion on the aortic wall. Furthermore, when the inner tube graft is pulled out, the suture line is automatically tightened by unfolding at the suture line and the contact surface areas at the anastomosis are increased (Fig. 17–21). The suture line is further strengthened at areas of weakness or gaps by a few pledgeted 2-0 Ticron valve sutures, which are placed from outside the aorta through the graft and then tied. This is particularly important at the inferior margin. One or two may have to be placed in the subclavian artery through the aortic wall and then through the graft,

FIGURE 17–21 *Continued* **O,** The proximal anastomosis is thereafter completed, with the distal ascending tube graft clamped. **P,** A few weeks or months later the patient returns for repair of the descending thoracic (**1**) or thoracoabdominal aorta (**2**). **Q,** The elephant trunk is grasped through the clot and clamped after the aorta is opened. **R,** If needed, an interposition graft is attached to the elephant trunk and the rest of the repair is performed, including reattachment of the intercostal patch and the visceral arteries. (From Svensson LG. J Cardiac Surg 1992;7:301–12.)

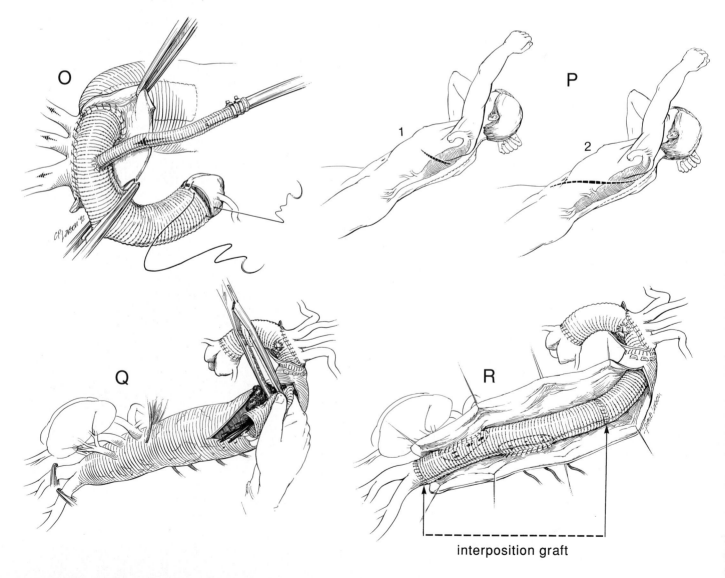

interposition graft

since these are the two areas where it has been noted that leaks are present during the second-stage procedure of the aortic repair. In patients with acute dissection or a flimsy aorta, it is sometimes useful to transect the aorta beyond the left subclavian artery and then perform the distal anastomosis with an over-and-over continuous suture. With transection, the distal aorta anastomosis can be strengthened by placement of a strip of Teflon felt outside the aorta so that the aortic wall is sandwiched between the outer Teflon strip layer and the inner inverted tube graft.

After completion of the anastomosis, the stay suture and side arm are gently tugged upon to remove the inverted proximal graft from the distal elephant trunk and the arch vessels are then ready to be reanastomosed. No more than approximately 15 cm should have been placed in the descending aorta, because this increases the risk of postoperative paraplegia and paresis (see Chapter 27 on Statistical Analysis of Operative Results). An oval hole is cut in the graft opposite the arch vessels. Reattachment of the arch vessels is then performed by placing the first suture through the opening in the graft through the graft wall and the aorta, exiting at the origin of the subclavian artery, and tying a secure knot. Next, the suture is run continuously by a forehand over-and-over technique along the lower margin of the graft edge and then up the posterior margin of the greater vessels. The suturing is performed from inside the aorta approximately 0.5 cm from the origin of the greater vessels and ending at the innominate artery. From inside the aorta, the other suture is sutured backhand near the origin of the subclavian artery through to the outside of the aorta and then back through the graft into the graft lumen (Fig. 17–21). Once the corner has been rounded, the anastomosis is rapidly completed by a forehand over-and-over suture on the outside of the aorta. This suture line is accessible for later insertion of pledgeted interrupted horizontal sutures, should any bleeding occur. Furthermore, because the sutures are spaced farther apart, the period of ischemia to the brain is reduced. Next, the two sutures are tied together at the origin of the innominate artery. The proximal aortic or graft-to-graft end-to-end anastomosis is then completed.[1, 3, 4, 8, 25, 54, 58]

Some 6 weeks to 3 months later, the patient is readmitted for the second stage of the elephant trunk procedure. The use of the elephant trunk technique has simplified the second-stage operation, as a proximal indurated aorta does not have to be mobilized or cross-clamped and often, especially with descending thoracic aortic aneurysms, only one distal anastomosis is necessary. Whenever possible, we reattach segmental intercostal and lumbar arteries from vertebral levels T7 to L2 to enable reestablishment of blood flow to the spinal cord by both the artery of Adamkiewicz and higher thoracic spinal radicular arteries (Fig. 17–21). The operative technique for the second-stage procedure is essentially the same as that for the standard descending thoracic or thoracoabdominal aortic aneurysm repair, as described in later chapters.[1, 3, 4, 8, 25, 54, 58]

The patient is placed in a left thoracotomy position, with the pelvis tilted approximately 60 degrees to the table,

depending on how far down on the aorta the distal anastomosis is going to be performed. Both groins are prepared so that they are in the sterile operative field in the event that the femoral arteries have to be cannulated for pump bypass. The chest is opened through a standard thoracotomy incision unless the abdominal part of the aorta also has to be replaced. For replacement of the abdominal section of the aorta, the incision is directed toward the umbilicus. This is in contrast to the usual thoracic incision along the ribs because, at the angle formed by the junction of the abdominal midline incision and the thoracotomy incision, the lower skin flap tends to necrose resulting in a large defect. The sixth rib is resected, and if more exposure of the aorta is needed at the subclavian artery, the fifth rib can be divided posteriorly. This is rarely necessary for second-stage elephant trunk procedures. The subcostal margin can be divided and the diaphragm preserved for repairs above the celiac artery, although for aneurysms extending below the superior mesenteric artery division of the diaphragm is usually needed. Either an extraperitoneal or an intraperitoneal approach to the abdominal aorta can be used, since there appear to be no differences in the incidence of respiratory complications, according to a prospective study of respiratory failure.[1, 3, 4, 8, 25, 54, 58]

The aorta at the site of the distal anastomosis is mobilized and encircled, but no umbilical tapes are passed around it. If feasible, an atriofemoral bypass centrifugal pump is inserted. The site of the previous distal elephant trunk anastomosis is identified immediately beyond the left subclavian artery, and then the anterior lateral aorta is opened longitudinally with a knife (Fig. 17–21). The thrombus surrounding the distal elephant trunk will usually allow the surgeon to identify the graft without the loss of blood, after which the graft is encircled and clamped. If bleeding should occur on opening of the aorta, the graft is quickly clamped by what is sometimes called the "slash and grab" procedure. Since there is a possibility that the patient may exsanguinate during this maneuver, it is advisable to have two autotransfusion devices available for aspirating blood and venous access sufficient for rapid reinfusion of blood. Of particular note, blood loss may be as much as stroke volume times the number of heart beats it takes to obtain control of the graft. To reduce blood loss, the systemic pressure and heart rate can be lowered by a short-acting beta-blocker or the patient can be partially exsanguinated into the atriofemoral bypass pump prior to opening of the aorta, especially since this latter technique allows for rapid reinfusion of blood. The blood lost in the chest does not need to be washed as long as protamine is administered at a later stage to reverse effects of the heparin mixed with the blood during suctioning. The distal anastomosis is performed either to the circumferentially transected aorta in a standard manner or to an interposition graft if the elephant trunk is not long enough to bridge the gap to the distal aortic anastomosis site.[1, 3, 4, 8, 25, 54, 58]

Results

We used the elephant trunk operative technique in 84 patients with a 30-day survival rate of 92%, as previously reported by us.[1, 3, 4, 8, 25, 54, 58] Of the patients who survived the surgery, 56 patients had undergone a second-stage operative procedure with a 30-day survival rate of 96%. The median interval between procedures was 62 days, with a range of 0 (second stage done immediately after the first-stage procedure) to 358 days. Two of the initial deaths from the first procedure were due to rupture at the distal suture line, but this has not been a problem since the elephant trunk technique was modified in 1988. The net result is that nine patients have had replacement of the entire (total) aorta, 27 have had replacement of the ascending aorta, aortic arch, descending thoracic aorta, and upper abdominal aorta, and 22 patients have had the entire thoracic aorta replaced. Seven of the 84 patients died within 30 days of the elephant trunk procedure. Four deaths were the result of ruptures in the distal aneurysmal aorta (two at the distal elephant trunk anastomosis at the subclavian artery, as noted above), one death was due to multiple organ failure,

one to stroke, and one to respiratory failure. One patient developed permanent paraplegia after the elephant trunk procedure, and two developed paraparesis. This was probably due to the distal elephant trunk in the descending aorta being too long, with formation of thrombus around the graft and occlusion of critical intercostal arteries supplying the spinal cord.[1, 3, 4, 8, 25, 54, 58]

Although patients with aortic aneurysmal disease requiring replacement of the ascending aorta, aortic arch, and distal aorta have to undergo very extensive and high-risk surgery, with our modified elephant trunk technique a survival rate of 90% to 95% can be expected. This includes similar survival rates for the second-stage procedure, resulting in a good quality of life after this type of surgery and a reduced risk of death due to rupture. This type of salvage surgery is recommended in those patients who are good-risk candidates for extensive aortic surgery. The technique of replacing the entire aorta from, or including, the aortic

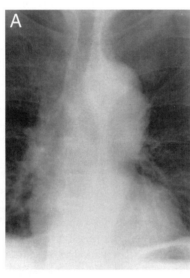

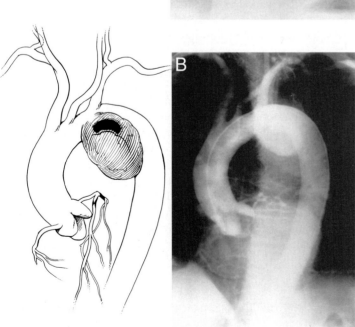

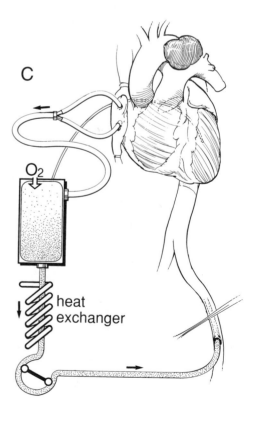

FIGURE 17–22 Patient with distal aortic arch aneurysm seen on the chest radiograph (**A**) and arteriogram (**B**) along with coronary artery disease. **C,** The patient was placed on cardiopulmonary bypass with femoral artery cannulation, and venous drainage was from both cavae with a right superior pulmonary vein cannula decompressing the left ventricle. (From Svensson LG, Crawford ES. Curr Probl Surg 1993;30:1–172.)

valve to the aortic bifurcation during a single operation through both a mediastinal and a left thoracoabdominal incision will be discussed in a subsequent chapter.

REPLACEMENT OF THE DISTAL AORTIC ARCH

Repair of the distal aortic arch in patients with degenerative aneurysms and superimposed atherosclerosis can be a particularly hazardous procedure because in these usually elderly patients there is frequently loose atheroma in the aortic lumen, and thus the risk of stroke is increased with cross-clamping. The options for repairing these aneurysms are (1) left lateral thoracotomy and clamping of the aorta, if possible, between the innominate artery and the left carotid artery and insertion of the graft with reattachment of the left carotid artery and left subclavian artery (see Chapter 18); (2) left lateral thoracotomy, cardiopulmonary bypass, deep hypothermia with circulatory arrest, and then repair of the distal arch; (3) median sternotomy, cardiopulmonary bypass, deep hypothermia with circulatory arrest, and repair of the arch and proximal descending aorta (Figs. 17–22 and 17–23). We have used all these methods successfully, provided that careful assessment is made with regard to the approach that will give the best access for the repair. For example, the anterior approach can prove difficult if a

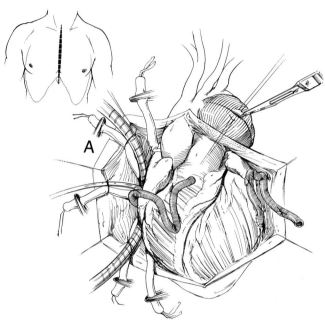

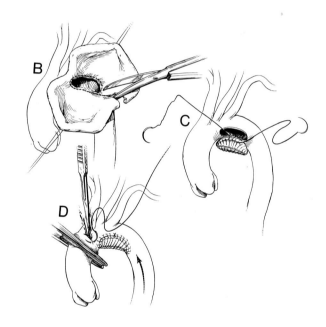

FIGURE 17–23 During cooling, vein bypasses were performed to the coronary arteries, and when brain electrical silence had been established by EEG, the distal aortic arch aneurysm was opened **(A)**, the aneurysm wall was excised **(B)**, a Dacron patch was sutured into position **(C)**, and the proximal aorta was de-aired **(D)** after reestablishment of blood flow. The proximal graft anastomoses were performed during rewarming **(E)** completing the operation. **F** shows a diagram and the arteriogram of the completed repair

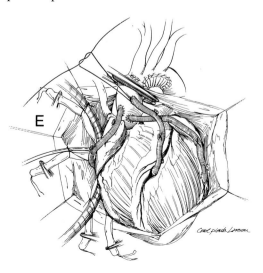

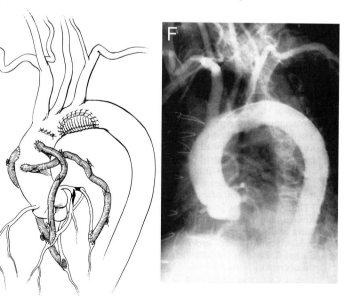

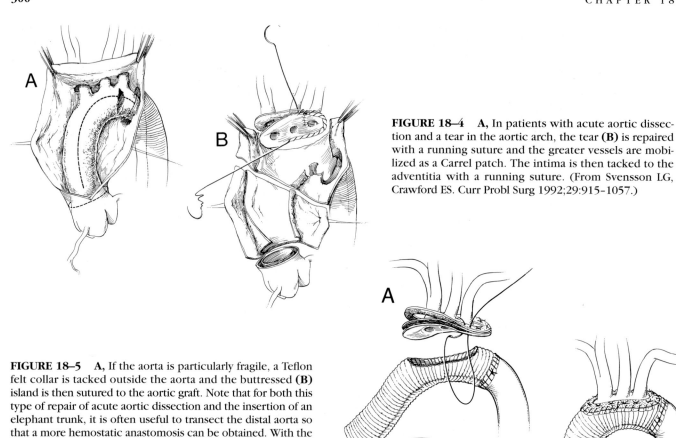

FIGURE 18–4 **A,** In patients with acute aortic dissection and a tear in the aortic arch, the tear **(B)** is repaired with a running suture and the greater vessels are mobilized as a Carrel patch. The intima is then tacked to the adventitia with a running suture. (From Svensson LG, Crawford ES. Curr Probl Surg 1992;29:915–1057.)

FIGURE 18–5 **A,** If the aorta is particularly fragile, a Teflon felt collar is tacked outside the aorta and the buttressed **(B)** island is then sutured to the aortic graft. Note that for both this type of repair of acute aortic dissection and the insertion of an elephant trunk, it is often useful to transect the distal aorta so that a more hemostatic anastomosis can be obtained. With the elephant trunk technique, the aorta can also be sandwiched between an outer Teflon felt strip or interrupted pledgeted sutures and the inner inverted tube graft. (From Svensson LG, Crawford ES. Curr Probl Surg 1992;29:915–1057.)

FIGURE 18–6 Patient with acute dissection associated with a saccular aneurysm of the aortic arch. **A** and **B,** Preoperative CT scan and angiogram showing acute dissection and associated clot-lined saccular aneurysm. A year before the patient had initially presented with a saccular aneurysm and an associated infrarenal aneurysm. The infrarenal aneurysm was repaired, but the patient did not wish to have his arch repaired.

Illustration continued on following page

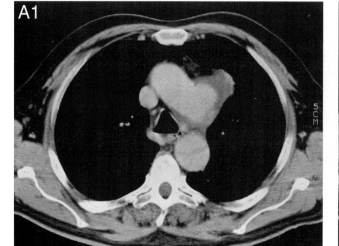

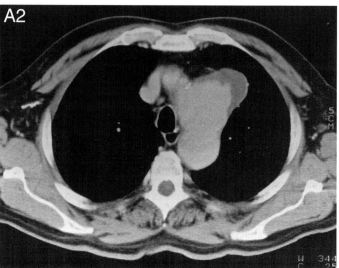

valve to the aortic bifurcation during a single operation through both a mediastinal and a left thoracoabdominal incision will be discussed in a subsequent chapter.

REPLACEMENT OF THE DISTAL AORTIC ARCH

Repair of the distal aortic arch in patients with degenerative aneurysms and superimposed atherosclerosis can be a particularly hazardous procedure because in these usually elderly patients there is frequently loose atheroma in the aortic lumen, and thus the risk of stroke is increased with cross-clamping. The options for repairing these aneurysms are (1) left lateral thoracotomy and clamping of the aorta, if possible, between the innominate artery and the left carotid artery and insertion of the graft with reattachment of the left carotid artery and left subclavian artery (see Chapter 18); (2) left lateral thoracotomy, cardiopulmonary bypass, deep hypothermia with circulatory arrest, and then repair of the distal arch; (3) median sternotomy, cardiopulmonary bypass, deep hypothermia with circulatory arrest, and repair of the arch and proximal descending aorta (Figs. 17–22 and 17–23). We have used all these methods successfully, provided that careful assessment is made with regard to the approach that will give the best access for the repair. For example, the anterior approach can prove difficult if a

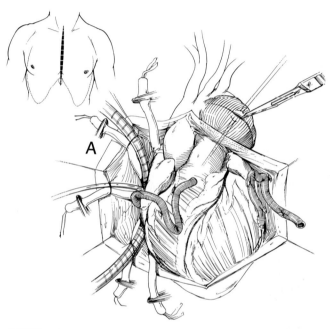

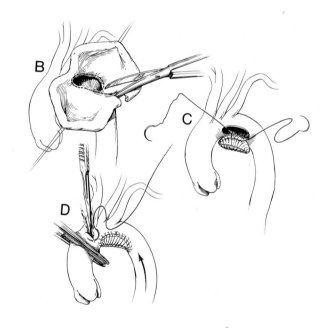

FIGURE 17–23 During cooling, vein bypasses were performed to the coronary arteries, and when brain electrical silence had been established by EEG, the distal aortic arch aneurysm was opened **(A),** the aneurysm wall was excised **(B),** a Dacron patch was sutured into position **(C),** and the proximal aorta was deaired **(D)** after reestablishment of blood flow. The proximal graft anastomoses were performed during rewarming **(E)** completing the operation. **F** shows a diagram and the arteriogram of the completed repair

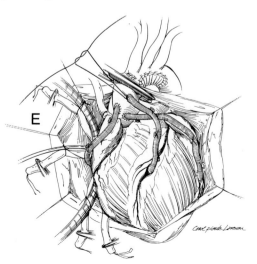

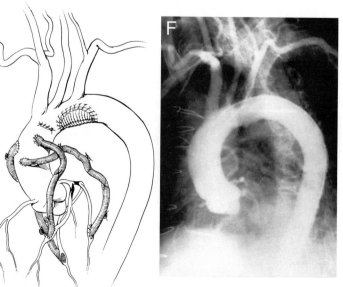

substantial part of the descending thoracic aorta needs repair. Furthermore, oversewing of the intercostal arteries is often awkward. Regardless of which procedure is used, however, the mortality rate is approximately 15% for all the approaches and the stroke rate is also about 15%.[6,8] On the whole, our preference tends toward repair of these lesions from an anterior approach because there is better control of the patient's hemodynamics.[1,3,4,8,25,54,58]

REFERENCES

1. Svensson LG, Crawford ES, Hess KR, et al. Dissection of the aorta and dissecting aortic aneurysms: improving early and long-term surgical results. Circulation 1990;82(5 Supp):IV 24-38.
2. Svensson LG, Crawford ES. Aortic dissection and aortic aneurysm surgery: clinical observations, experimental investigations and statistical analyses. Part I. Curr Probl Surg 1992;29:819-912.
3. Svensson LG, Crawford ES. Aortic dissection and aortic aneurysm surgery: clinical observations, experimental investigations, and statistical analyses. Part II. Curr Probl Surg 1992;29:915-1057.
4. Svensson LG, Crawford ES. Aortic dissection and aortic aneurysm surgery: clinical observations, experimental investigations, and statistical analyses. Part III. Curr Probl Surg 1993;30:1-172.
5. Crawford ES, Crawford JL. Diseases of the Aorta Including an Atlas of Angiographic Pathology and Surgical Technique. Baltimore: Williams & Wilkins, 1984.
6. Crawford ES, Svensson LG, Coselli JS, et al. Surgical treatment of aneurysm and/or dissection of the ascending aorta, transverse aortic arch, and ascending aorta and transverse aortic arch: factors influencing survival in 717 patients. J Thorac Cardiovasc Surg 1989; 98:659-73.
7. Crawford ES, Coselli JS, Svensson LG, et al. Diffuse aneurysmal disease (chronic aortic dissection, Marfan, and mega aorta syndromes) and multiple aneurysm: treatment by subtotal and total aortic replacement emphasizing the elephant trunk operation. Ann Surg 1990;211:521-37.
8. Svensson LG, Crawford ES, Hess KR, et al. Deep hypothermia with circulatory arrest: determinants of stroke and early mortality in 656 patients. J Thorac Cardiovasc Surg 1992;106:19-31.
9. Wheat MN Jr, Wilson JR, Bartley TD. Successful replacement of the entire ascending aorta and aortic valve. JAMA 1964;188:717-9.
10. David TE, Feindel CM. An aortic valve-sparing operation for patients with aortic incompetence and aneurysm of the ascending aorta. J Thorac Cardiovasc Surg 1992;103:617-21.
11. Robicsek F, Thubrikar MJ. Conservative operation in the management of annular dilatation and ascending aortic aneurysm. Ann Thorac Surg 1994;57:1672-4.
12. Barnett MG, Fiore AC, Vacca KJ, et al. Tailoring aortoplasty for repair of fusiform ascending aortic aneurysm. Ann Thorac Surg 1995; 59:497-501.
13. Gott VL, Pyeritz RE, Cameron DE, et al. Composite graft repair of Marfan aneurysm of the ascending aorta: results in 100 patients. Ann Thorac Surg 1991;52:38-44.
14. Svensson LG, Crawford ES, Coselli JS, et al. Impact of cardiovascular operation on survival in the Marfan patient. Circulation 1989;80(3 Pt 1):i233-42.
15. Svensson LG, Crawford ES, Hess KR, et al. Composite valve graft replacement of the proximal aorta: comparison of techniques in 348 patients. Ann Thorac Surg 1992;54:427-39.
16. Kouchoukos NT, Marshall WG Jr, Wedige STA. Eleven-year experience with composite graft replacement of the ascending aorta and aortic valve. J Thorac Cardiovasc Surg 1986;92:691-705.
17. Kouchoukos NT. Inclusion (aneurysm wrap) technique for composite graft replacement of the ascending aorta and aortic valve 'letter.' J Thorac Cardiovasc Surg 1988;96:967.
18. Kouchoukos NT. Composite graft replacement of the ascending aorta and aortic valve with the inclusion-wrap and open techniques. Semin Thorac Cardiovasc Surg 1991;3:171-6.
19. Cabrol C, Pavie A, Gandjbakhch I, et al. Complete replacement of the ascending aorta with reimplantation of the coronary arteries. J Thorac Cardiovasc Surg 1980;79:388-401.
20. Cabrol C, Pavie A, Mesnildrey P, et al. Long-term results with total

replacement of the ascending aorta and reimplantation of the coronary arteries. J Thorac Cardiovasc Surg 1986;91:17-25.
21. Coselli JS, Crawford ES. Composite valve-graft replacement of aortic root using separate Dacron tube for coronary artery reattachment. Ann Thorac Surg 1989;47:558-65.
22. Svensson LG. Approach to the insertion of composite valve graft. Ann Thorac Surg 1992;54:376-8.
23. Svensson LG. Aortic surgery, coarctation of the aorta, and aortic dissection. Curr Opin Cardiol 1993;8:254-61.
24. Svensson LG, Patel V, Coselli JS, et al. Preliminary report of localization of spinal cord blood supply by hydrogen during aortic operations. Ann Thorac Surg 1990;49:528-36.
25. Svensson LG, Sun J, Nadolny E, Kimmel WA. Prospective evaluation of minimal blood use for ascending aorta and aortic arch operations. Ann Thorac Surg 1995;59:1501-8.
26. McKowen RL, Campbell DN, Woelfel GF, et al. Extended aortic root replacement with aortic allografts. J Thorac Cardiovasc Surg 1987; 93:366-74.
27. Livi U, Abdulla AK, Parker R, et al. Viability and morphology of aortic and pulmonary homografts: a comparative study. J Thorac Cardiovasc Surg 1987;93:755-60.
28. Angell WW, Angell JD, Oury JH, et al. Long-term follow-up of viable frozen aortic homografts. A viable homograft valve bank. J Thorac Cardiovasc Surg 1987;93:815-22.
29. Gunning AJ. Ross' first homograft replacement of the aortic valve. Ann Thorac Surg 1992;54:809-10.
30. Belcher P, Ross D. Aortic root replacement—20 years experience of the use of homografts. Thorac Cardiovasc Surg 1991;39:117-22.
31. Kirklin JK, Smith D, Novick W, et al. Long-term function of cryopreserved aortic homografts: a ten year study. J Thorac Cardiovasc Surg 1993;106:154-66.
32. O'Brien MF, McGiffin DC, Stafford EG, et al. Allograft aortic valve replacement: long-term comparative clinical analysis of the viable cryopreserved and antibiotic 4 degrees C stored valves. J Cardiac Surg 1991;6:534-43.
33. Jones EL, Shah VB, Shanewise JS, et al. Should the freehand allograft be abandoned as a reliable alternative for aortic valve replacement? Ann Thorac Surg 1995;59:1397-404.
34. Daicoff GR, Botero LM, Quintessenza J. Allograft replacement of the aortic valve versus the miniroot and valve. Ann Thorac Surg 1993; 55:855-9.
35. Gross RE, Hurwitt ES, Bill AH Jr, Peirce E. Preliminary observations on the use of human arterial grafts in the treatment of certain cardiovascular defects. N Engl J Med 1948;239:578-9.
36. Swan H, Maaske C, Johnson M, et al. Arterial homografts. II. Resection of thoracic aortic aneurysm using a stored human arterial transplant. Arch Surg 1950;61:732-7.
37. Oudot J, Beaconfield P. Thrombosis of the aortic bifurcation treated by resection and homograft replacement: report of five cases. Arch Surg 1959;66:365.
38. Dubost C. The first successful resection of an aneurysm of the abdominal aorta followed by re-establishment of continuity using a preserved human arterial graft. Ann Vasc Surg 1986;1:147-9.
39. Dubost C, Allanz M, Oeconomos N. Resection of an aneurysm of thoracoabdominal aorta: reestablishment of the continuity by a preserved human arterial graft, with results after five months. Arch Surg 1952;64:405-8.
40. DeBakey ME, Cooley DA. Surgical treatment of aneurysm of abdominal aorta by resection and restoration of continuity with homograft. Surg Gynecol Obstet 1953;97:257-66.
41. DeBakey ME, Cooley DA. Successful resection of aneurysm of thoracic aorta and replacement by graft. JAMA 1953;152:673-6.
42. DeBakey ME, Creech OJ, Cooley DA. Occlusive disease of the aorta and its treatment by resection and homograft replacement. Ann Surg 1954;140:290-310.
43. Cornelissen PHJ, Hamerlijnck RP, Vermeulen FE. Aneurysmatic dilatation of an aortic homograft more than 30 years after implantation into the thoracic aorta. Eur J Cardiothorac Surg 1994;8:447-8.
44. Robles A, Vaughan M, Lau JK, et al. Long-term assessment of aortic valve replacement with autologous pulmonary valve. Ann Thorac Surg 1985;39:238-42.
45. Ross D, Jackson M, Davies J. Pulmonary autograft aortic valve replacement: long-term results. J Cardiac Surg 1991;6:529-33.
46. Santangelo K, Elkins RC, Stelzer P, et al. Normal left ventricular function following pulmonary autograft. J Cardiac Surg 1991;6: 633-7.

47. Lamberti JJ, Mainwaring RD, Billman GF, et al. The cryopreserved homograft valve in the pulmonary position: mid-term results and technical considerations. J Cardiac Surg 1991;6:627-32.

48. Kouchoukos NT, Davila-Roman VG, Spray TL, et al. Replacement of the aortic root with a pulmonary autograft in children and young adults with aortic-valve disease. N Engl J Med 1994;330:1-6.

49. DeBakey ME, Cooley DA, Crawford ES, et al. Successful resection of fusiform aneurysm of aortic arch replacement by homograft. Surg Gynecol Obstet 1957;105:656-64.

50. Barnard CN, Schire V. The surgical treatment of acquired aneurysms of the thoracic aorta. Thorax 1963;18:101-5.

51. Griepp RB, Stinson EB, Hollingsworth JF, et al. Prosthetic replacement of the aortic arch. J Thorac Cardiovasc Surg 1975;70:1051-63.

52. Borst HG, Walterbusch G, Schaps D. Extensive aortic replacement using "elephant trunk" prosthesis. Thorac Cardiovasc Surg 1983;31:37-40.

53. Borst HG, Frank G, Schaps D. Treatment of extensive aortic aneurysms by a new multiple-stage approach. J Thorac Cardiovasc Surg 1988;95:11-3.

54. Svensson LG. Rationale and technique for replacement of the ascending aorta, arch, and distal aorta using a modified elephant trunk procedure. J Cardiac Surg 1992;7:301-12.

55. Crawford ES, Saleh SA. Transverse aortic arch aneurysm: improved results of treatment employing new modifications of aortic reconstruction and hypothermic cerebral circulatory arrest. Ann Surg 1981;194:180-8.

56. Crawford ES, Snyder DM. Treatment of aneurysms of the aortic arch: a progress report. J Thorac Cardiovasc Surg 1983;85:237-46.

57. Crawford ES, Stowe CL, Crawford JL, et al. Aortic arch aneurysm: a sentinel of extensive aortic disease requiring subtotal and total aortic replacement. Ann Surg 1984;199:742-52.

58. Svensson LG, Shahian DM, Davis FG, et al. Replacement of entire aorta from aortic valve to bifurcation during one operation. Ann Thorac Surg 1994;58:1164-6.

59. Lytle BW, McCarthy PM, Meaney KM, et al. Systemic hypothermia and circulatory arrest combined with arterial perfusion of the superior vena cava: effective intraoperative cerebral protection. J Thorac Cardiovasc Surg 1995;109:738-43.

60. Kouchoukos NT. Adjuncts to reduce the incidence of embolic brain injury during operations to the aortic arch. Ann Thorac Surg 1994;57:243-5.

61. Coselli JS, Crawford ES, Beall ACJ, et al. Determination of brain temperatures for safe circulatory arrest during cardiovascular operation. Ann Thorac Surg 1988;45:638-42.

18

Techniques for Dissection Involving the Proximal Aorta

The management of the aorta in patients with aortic dissection depends on whether the dissection is an acute or a chronic process. Thus, the operative techniques will be described separately. The diagnosis, preoperative management, hypothermic circulatory arrest with retrograde brain perfusion, and anesthesia techniques are described in different chapters. To check that the arterial inflow does not preferentially perfuse only one lumen, an intraoperative transesophageal echo is useful to show that both lumina are perfused. Examples of aortic dissection and false-positives that may result in operation are shown in Figure 18-1.

ACUTE PROXIMAL DISSECTION

Proximal Aortic Arch Anastomosis

In patients with acute proximal dissection, the distal anastomosis is performed initially in the proximal arch by the open technique with the use of deep hypothermia and circulatory arrest and a beveled anastomosis along the principles described in Chapter 17.[1-8] The patient is placed in a head-down (Trendelenburg) position. The virtue of the deep hypothermic circulatory arrest technique is that the inner aortic lumen can be visualized, including the origins of the aortic arch vessels, and thus more accurate suturing can be performed without traumatizing the delicate aorta with a clamp (Figs. 18-2 and 18-3). This method also facilitates the distal transection of the aorta and tacking of the true lumen to the outer aortic wall as described previously. The distal anastomosis is angled so that the anastomosis is just proximal to the innominate artery and ends in the lesser curve of the arch. The anastomosis is performed with a running suture of 4-0 or 5-0 Prolene without the use of pledgets or Teflon to buttress it (Fig. 18-3).[8, 9]

Aortic Arch Management

On occasion an intimal tear may be present in the aortic arch and, provided that the aorta is not aneurysmal and the tear is small, the tear can be oversewn with Prolene or inter-

rupted pledgeted sutures, and a proximal anastomosis is performed as described previously. More often, however, rupture has occurred in the arch or the arch is aneurysmal, and in this situation the aortic arch must be replaced. Replacement of the aortic arch is a hazardous procedure in the presence of acute aortic dissection, particularly if the arch has been destroyed by rupture of the aorta and the tissues are fragile.[8, 9]

If the aortic arch has to be replaced, the distal end-to-end anastomosis between the tubular graft and the aorta is fashioned just beyond the left subclavian artery, with the transected aorta tacked as described previously (Figs. 18-4 and 18-5). The brachiocephalic vessels are excised as a Carrel patch with a 1 cm rim of aorta (Figs. 18-4 and 18-5) and attached to the graft by a technique that we have previously described.[8] A Teflon patch that has been tailored with a buttonhole for the brachiocephalic arteries is threaded over the Carrel patch so that it sits on the adventitia.[8, 9] The inner septum is tacked to the outer wall and a Teflon patch is inserted as described previously (Figs. 18-4 and 18-5). This buttressed free island is then sutured to an opening in the aortic tubular graft with a running suture.[8, 9] Occasionally, when acute dissection is associated with a classic saccular aneurysm of the aortic arch, the distal aorta does not have to be transected circumferentially but can be fixed with a large patch by means of a running suture line followed by supporting horizontal mattress sutures (Fig. 18-6).

In patients with acute dissection, replacement of the entire aortic arch by the elephant trunk technique is usually avoided (Figs. 18-7 and 18-8). In the exceptional cases in which we have used the technique either the descending aorta is very aneurysmal or there is a danger that the descending thoracic aorta may rupture and result in the patient's death. If the aortic arch has to be replaced, then a Carrel patch with a 1 cm margin around the greater vessels is mobilized as described previously. A matching piece of Teflon doughnut patch is cut with an inner hole to fit the greater vessels. The Carrel patch is then threaded through the Teflon doughnut opening and secured with a few interrupted sutures to sandwich the layers.[8, 9] The distal elephant

Text continued on page 303

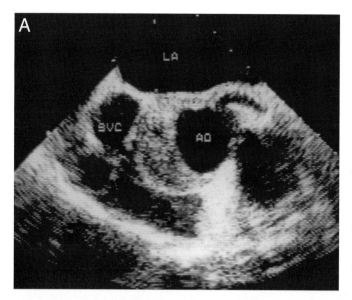

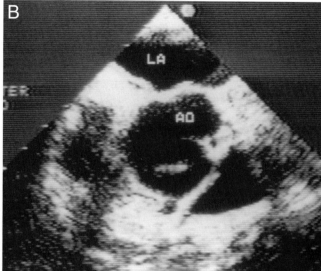

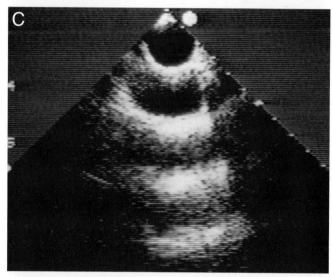

FIGURE 18–1 TEE and aortic dissection. **A,** Findings on TEE in a patient with aortic dissection. Note the true aortic lumen *(AO),* with the left main coronary artery arising at the 2 o'clock position. On the left-hand part of the aorta, there is an extensive clot involving half the aortic lumen as a result of aortic dissection. **B,** Example of the anterior left atrial wall *(LA)* causing an echo in the aorta *(AO)* that has the appearance of an aortic septum, suggesting aortic dissection. This false-positive finding can be differentiated by the equal distance between the probe and the atrial wall and between the atrial wall and the false septum. Furthermore, the false septum does not extend across the entire aortic lumen. **C,** The appearance of multiple echoes from the descending thoracic aorta that are clearly not due to an aortic dissection septum. **D,** The line transversely across the echo image in this example is due to a Swan–Ganz catheter and does not have the appearance of a septum. **E,** TEE of the descending aorta with extensive calcification. As seen at the 4 o'clock position on the scan, an intramural aortic hematoma, possibly related to a penetrating ulcer, needs to be excluded. The calcification causes radial echo shadows. (From Svensson LG, Labib S. Curr Opinion Cardiol 1994;9:191–9.)

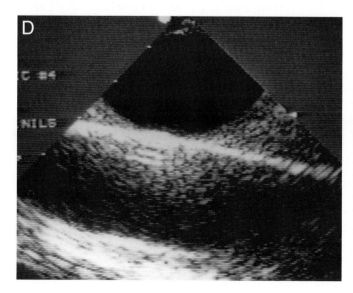

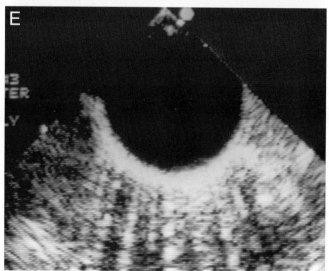

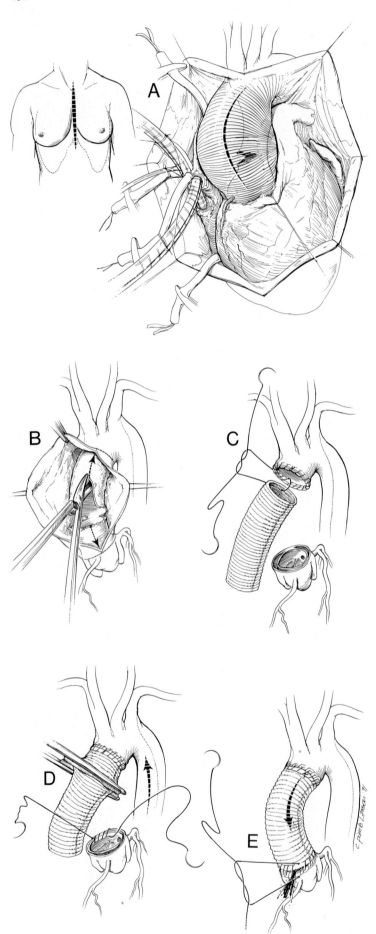

FIGURE 18–2 **A,** Steps in the repair of acute aortic dissection. First the patient is cooled until the EEG is flat, and then retrograde brain perfusion is commenced and the aorta is incised. **B,** The inner intimal septum is incised, and the aorta is transected both proximally and distally. **C,** The intimal layers are reapproximated to the adventitia if needed, either with a continuous over-and-over suture or with interrupted mattress sutures, and then the distal anastomosis is performed with a 4-0 or 5-0 suture and as atraumatic an over-and-over stitch as possible. No Teflon strips are used because of the risk of a gradient resulting from stenosis at the anastomosis site or because of hemolysis from the intraaortic Teflon. This also shortens the time of circulatory arrest that is required for the repair to about 10 to 15 minutes. **D,** The brain is then reperfused and the patient is rewarmed. In most patients we place a side graft or an arterial cannula directly into the ascending aorta graft to reperfuse the aorta antegrade, although this is not shown here. Antegrade perfusion reduces the risk of disruption of the distal anastomosis, malperfusion of the aortic arch, the risk of a residual false channel remaining in the rest of the dissected aorta, and also the risk of embolism to the brain. **E,** The proximal repair is then performed and air is evacuated from the graft. (From Svensson LG, Crawford ES. Curr Probl Surg 1992;29:915–1057.)

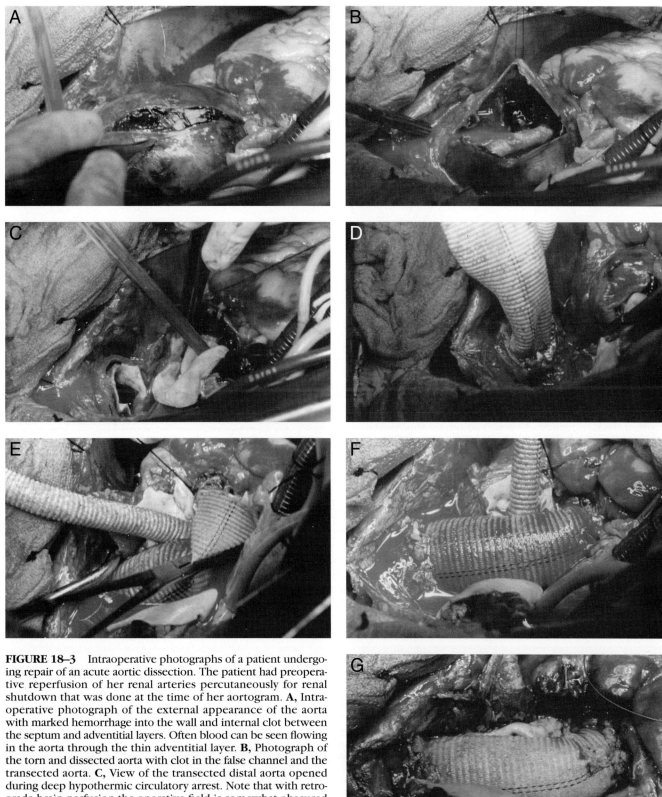

FIGURE 18–3 Intraoperative photographs of a patient undergoing repair of an acute aortic dissection. The patient had preoperative reperfusion of her renal arteries percutaneously for renal shutdown that was done at the time of her aortogram. **A,** Intraoperative photograph of the external appearance of the aorta with marked hemorrhage into the wall and internal clot between the septum and adventitial layers. Often blood can be seen flowing in the aorta through the thin adventitial layer. **B,** Photograph of the torn and dissected aorta with clot in the false channel and the transected aorta. **C,** View of the transected distal aorta opened during deep hypothermic circulatory arrest. Note that with retrograde brain perfusion the operative field is somewhat obscured by blood. **D,** Photograph of the distal anastomosis at the end of circulatory arrest without the use of Teflon strips although Teflon pledgeted horizontal mattress sutures have been used to strengthen the anastomosis. **E,** Construction of the proximal anastomosis to the transected aorta. Note that an arterial line has been placed to a tube graft attached end-to-side to the aorta to reperfuse the dissected aorta antegrade. **F,** Photograph of the completed repair with the side graft in place. **G,** Photograph of the repair after bypass was discontinued and hemostasis was obtained.

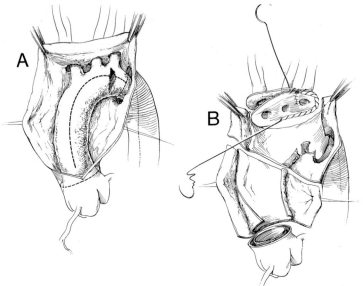

FIGURE 18–4 **A,** In patients with acute aortic dissection and a tear in the aortic arch, the tear **(B)** is repaired with a running suture and the greater vessels are mobilized as a Carrel patch. The intima is then tacked to the adventitia with a running suture. (From Svensson LG, Crawford ES. Curr Probl Surg 1992;29:915–1057.)

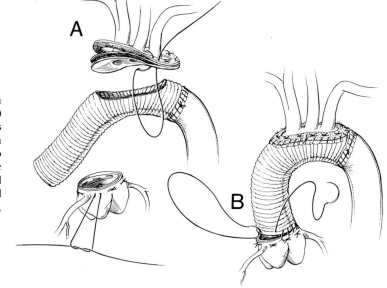

FIGURE 18–5 **A,** If the aorta is particularly fragile, a Teflon felt collar is tacked outside the aorta and the buttressed **(B)** island is then sutured to the aortic graft. Note that for both this type of repair of acute aortic dissection and the insertion of an elephant trunk, it is often useful to transect the distal aorta so that a more hemostatic anastomosis can be obtained. With the elephant trunk technique, the aorta can also be sandwiched between an outer Teflon felt strip or interrupted pledgeted sutures and the inner inverted tube graft. (From Svensson LG, Crawford ES. Curr Probl Surg 1992;29:915–1057.)

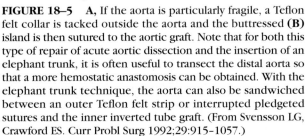

FIGURE 18–6 Patient with acute dissection associated with a saccular aneurysm of the aortic arch. **A** and **B,** Preoperative CT scan and angiogram showing acute dissection and associated clot-lined saccular aneurysm. A year before the patient had initially presented with a saccular aneurysm and an associated infrarenal aneurysm. The infrarenal aneurysm was repaired, but the patient did not wish to have his arch repaired.

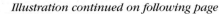

Illustration continued on following page

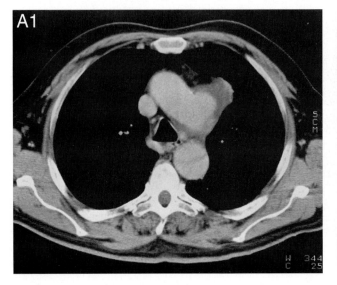

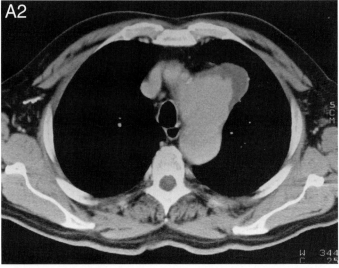

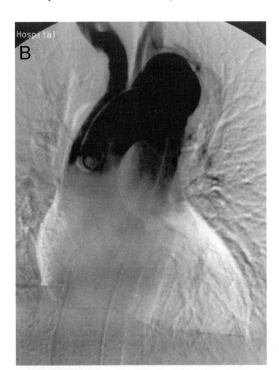

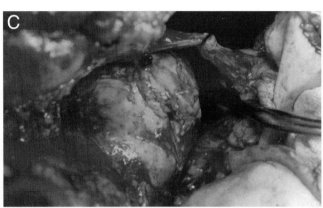

FIGURE 18–6 *Continued* **A** and **B**, Preoperative CT scan and angiogram showing acute dissection and associated clot-lined saccular aneurysm. A year before the patient had initially presented with a saccular aneurysm and an associated infrarenal aneurysm. The infrarenal aneurysm was repaired, but the patient did not wish to have his arch repaired. **C**, Intraoperative photograph of the aneurysm. Note that the phrenic nerve has been retracted to improve exposure. **D** and **E**, Photograph of the specimen. **F** and **G**, Postoperative CT after patch repair of the ascending aorta, the aortic arch, and the descending aorta as far as the hilum of the lung with also a coronary artery bypass to the left anterior descending coronary artery. Note that the descending aortic dissection is still visible **(G)**.

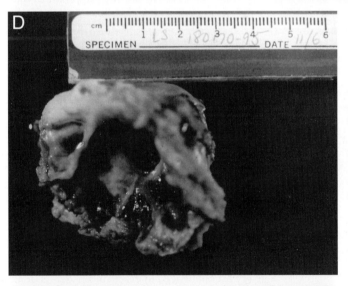

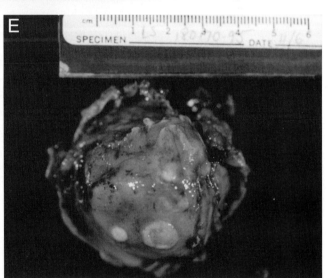

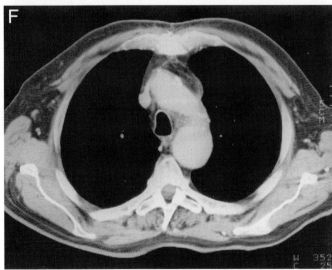

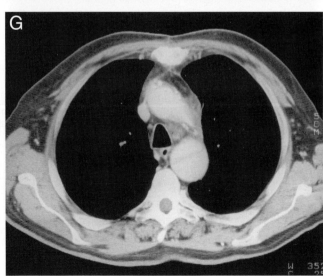

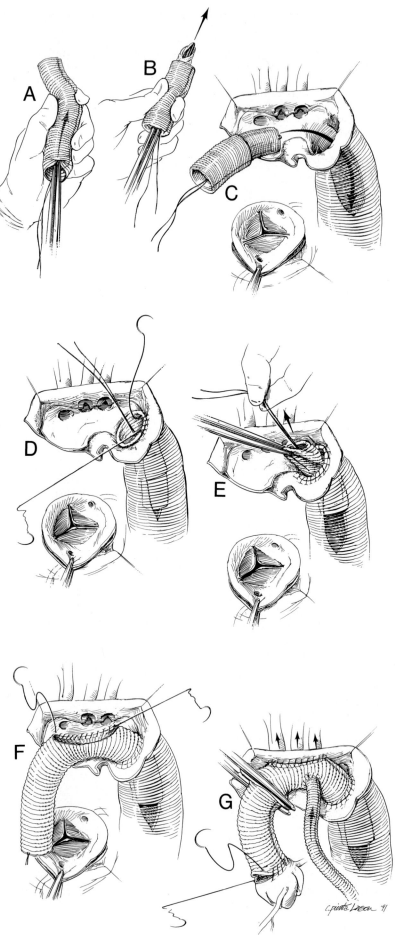

FIGURE 18–7 Replacement of the entire aorta with our modification of the elephant trunk technique. After a midline incision is made, the patient is placed on cardiopulmonary bypass with two venous cannulae and cooled until the circulation can be arrested and retrograde brain and cardioplegia can be perfused. **A,** According to the size of the distal aortic arch, prior to circulatory arrest a side 10 mm graft is anastomosed end-to-side to the larger tube graft. Alternatively, a graft can either be reattached later or be cannulated with an arterial cannula. A collagen-impregnated graft works best for this because it is softer and easier to sew. **B,** The proximal tube graft with the side graft is then inverted into the distal tube graft **(C). D,** After the aorta has been incised between stay sutures, the proximal aorta is transected. The distal aorta can also be transected to improve exposure distally if bleeding should occur at the arch anastomosis. **E,** The graft is sutured in position, starting usually at the inferior margin in a counterclockwise direction using a forehand stitch. The other end of the suture is then sutured forehand in a clockwise direction to be tied with the first suture. Any defects in the suture line are reenforced with interrupted pledgeted sutures, even from outside the aorta if necessary. **E,** The tube graft is then withdrawn from the distal aorta. **F,** Next a hole is cut in the tube graft for the arch vessels, which are then reattached to the tube graft by the posterior suture line. **G,** The anterior suture line is then created, initially with a backhand stitch followed by a forehand stitch along the anterior anastomosis. The knot is tied down, and slow perfusion through the femoral artery is commenced to evacuate any debris or air. The ascending graft is aspirated to remove embolic material and then the side graft is perfused with the arterial cannula **(G)** and secured in position with a plastic banding gun. The proximal anastomosis is thereafter completed with the distal ascending tube graft clamped. (Svensson LG[20]) (From Svensson LG, Crawford ES. Curr Probl Surg 1992;9:191–9.)

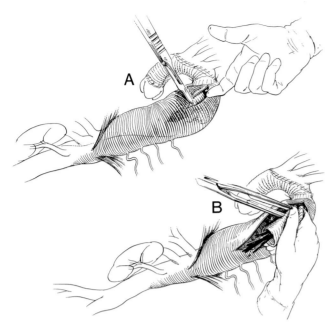

FIGURE 18–8 A, The descending thoracic or thoracoabdominal aortic repair. The elephant trunk is grasped through the clot after the aorta is opened and clamped. **B,** If necessary, an interposition graft is attached to the elephant trunk and the rest of the repair is performed, including reattachment of the intercostal patch and the visceral arteries (Svensson LG[20]). (From Svensson LG, Crawford ES. Curr Probl Surg 1992;29:915–1057.)

trunk procedure is then performed. This is often done optimally by transection of the descending aorta and placement of a strip of Teflon on the outside of the aorta, and then the aorta is sutured so that it is sandwiched between the outer Teflon and the inner doubled-over tube graft. The Carrel patch is thereafter reattached. After completion of this first stage, the patient is then redraped for a left thoracotomy and the descending aorta is repaired (Fig. 18–8). The other option under these circumstances is to perform both procedures during a single operation with a circulatory arrest period as described in Chapter 24.[8, 9]

Once the aortic arch anastomoses have been completed, the cardiopulmonary pump is restarted with the patient still in a head-down position. Any debris is carefully sucked away as it is flushed out of the distal aorta. A side arm is placed to the aortic arch part of the graft for perfusion of the head vessels. Once flow has been reestablished, the proximal graft is cross-clamped immediately proximal to the innominate artery (Fig. 18–2) so that blood flow can be fully established.[8, 9]

Aortic Valve Management

Several options are available, although experience usually dictates which technique is best applied to the individual patient. Several guidelines may be of value. If a minimal amount of clot is present either in the proximal extent or in the crevice of the dissection below the apex of the aortic commissures, then it is recommended that the aorta be mobilized circumferentially, freed from the right atrium,

and transected approximately 1 cm above the commissural attachments, including above the right coronary ostium (Fig. 18–2). The clot in the wall can then be teased out with a pair of forceps. The edge of the transected aorta may be handled in one of two ways. Either a running over-and-over tacking suture of 4-0 Prolene is used in the transected edge of the aorta to obliterate the dissected aortic wall or several interrupted sutures are placed with double-ended needles from the inside of the true lumen, through the area of dissection, out onto the adventitia (Fig. 18–2). These sutures are then gently tied without pledgets to avoid tearing the fragile inner intima. The latter method of using interrupted sutures without pledgets is preferable if the intima is particularly thin and fragile or if dissection has been present for a few days, resulting in inflammation, and if the aortic root is small. With the over-and-over suturing technique, the aorta tends to become narrowed, and thus this method is useful if some minimal annuloaortic ectasia or aneurysmal formation is present. If both the outer adventitial layer and the inner intimal layers (the septum) are fairly firm, then these tacking sutures may not be necessary. Once the transected aorta has been managed by the most appropriate method, a collagen-impregnated or baked woven Dacron graft is then anastomosed with a running suture of 4-0 Prolene to the transected edge of the aorta. Discrepancies in size are compensated for by taking closer-spaced, although equidistant, bites on the graft because the aorta is usually the larger of the two. Particular care should be taken when suturing in the vicinity of the right coronary artery, the position of which can be checked by gentle probing with a right-angled forceps or a probe, so that its origin is not oversewn.[8, 9]

If the commissures have been lifted away from the aortic outer wall by the dissection, then they can be resuspended with placement of a few valve sutures with pledgets from the apex of the commissure to approximately 1 cm above the point where they are situated in the abnormal dissected aorta (Fig. 18–9). The two needles with the suture can then be passed through the outer aortic wall and tied with a pledget on the outside. Next the valve is carefully inspected and tested. The proximal anastomosis may then be performed as described above.[8, 9]

Sometimes the aortic valve is destroyed as a result of the dissection process, particularly if the dissection extends deeply into the aortic root or ventricular septum or if a perforation occurs at the proximal extent of the dissection. Similarly, if either a bicuspid aortic valve or an otherwise diseased valve is present, or if the patient has Marfan syndrome, then the aortic valve should be replaced with a prosthetic valve to reduce the risk of later reoperation (Fig. 18–10). In patients without significant annuloaortic ectasia, the valve and reconstruction can be performed by the Wheat technique as described in Chapter 17[10] (Fig. 18–11). By this approach, the aortic wall is excised down to approximately 1 cm above both coronary arteries and the aortic annulus. The edge of the transected aorta is managed by tacking sutures as described above. Next the aortic valve is excised and interrupted, pledgeted valve sutures are placed

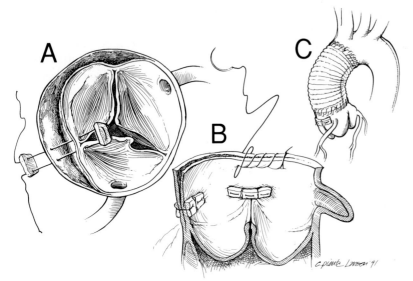

FIGURE 18–9 **A,** In patients with aortic regurgitation due to aortic dissection because the commissures have been dissected away from the aortic wall, the commissures are resuspended with interrupted sutures pledgeted with either Teflon or pericardial pledgets. **B,** The proximal aorta is reapproximated if needed and the repair completed **(C).** (From Svensson LG, Crawford ES. Curr Probl Surg 1992;29:915–1057.)

FIGURE 18–10 **A,** Type I aortic dissection and rupture of the aorta in the abdomen as seen by the abdominal CT scan in a patient who had undergone previous aortic valve replacement with a biological valve. **B,** The ruptured abdominal aorta was first repaired with a bifurcated tube graft, and then a composite valve graft was inserted with a tube graft to the left main coronary artery and the right coronary artery was reattached as an aortic button with also a distal vein bypass for coronary artery disease. In addition, the aortic arch was replaced with our modification of the elephant trunk technique. The patient required no operative homologous blood transfusion, although he did require cryoprecipitate for a low fibrinogen level. Subsequently, the rest of the thoracic aorta was replaced with the use of intraoperative hydrogen mapping of the intercostal arteries supplying the spinal cord and intrathecal papaverine with CSF drainage to protect the spinal cord. The postoperative angiogram is shown. (Reprinted with permission from the Society of Thoracic Surgeons. From Svensson LG, Sun J, Nalodny E, Kimmel WA. Ann Thorac Surg 1995;59:1501–8.)

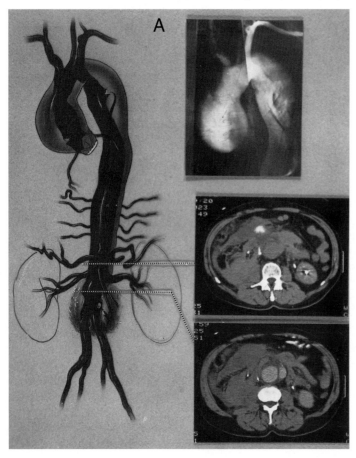

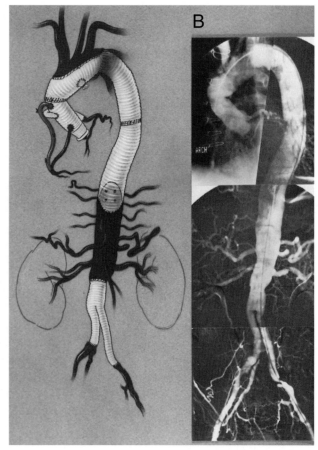

with the pledget seated on the annulus and the suture exiting on the ventricular side. The prosthetic valve is appropriately sized, seated, and tied down. The proximal end of the tubular graft is then trimmed to follow the contour of the scalloped aorta and secured in position with a running 4-0 Prolene suture. Particular care should be taken around the coronary ostia, and the graft should be sutured directly to the valve suturing ring and noncoronary sinus to avoid tearing these fragile areas. Indeed, this is our preferred technique for elderly patients in whom the occurrence of annuloaortic ectasia is less common and the longer clamp time required for a composite graft is likely to be more deleterious.[8, 9]

If the entire aortic root is diseased, either destroyed by dissection or by marked annuloaortic ectasia, or if the dissection process extends into the ventricular septum, then a composite graft should be inserted. The native valve is excised, and then it becomes necessary to decide how the coronary ostia will be managed. If the coronary arteries appear to be well attached to the aortic wall and not narrowed at the ostia, then in the acute situation placing a graft to the left main coronary ostium and mobilizing the right coronary artery as a button as described in detail in Chapter 17 is the preferred technique (Figs. 18–12 to 18–14). The reason for this is that excising the left ostium as an aortic button and attempting to reattach it to the aortic graft can be hazardous because the inflamed buttons often tear and

any tension on it will result in bleeding. First an 8 mm or 10 mm baked woven Dacron tube graft is attached around the left coronary ostium with 4-0 Prolene sutures, and then valve sutures are placed as described above. The left main coronary artery ostium should be carefully inspected and, if the dissection extends into it, should be repaired with pledgeted sutures. Distal bypasses may also be needed. Next the previously sized composite baked tube graft is seated and tied in position. The tube graft is then brought around behind the composite graft, and the distal aortic anastomosis is performed, usually to a previously placed tube graft (see below). Thereafter, a generous length of 8 mm or 10 mm tube graft is loosely coiled around the composite graft and the distal end is transected at an angle so that flow is directed down the course of the graft. The right coronary artery button is reattached and checked for patency, and then the tube graft is attached to the composite graft. If the marking line on the tube graft is anastomosed at the toe of the left coronary anastomosis at approximately the 12 o'clock position from the surgeon's viewpoint, then the heel should be at approximately the 6 o'clock position. However, some allowance must be made for variations in the individual patient's anatomy, particularly if the coronary ostia are well displaced out of the coronary sinuses. Before the aortic clamps are removed, it is advisable to place a soft vascular clamp on the right coronary artery anastomosis so that air will not embolize down the right coronary

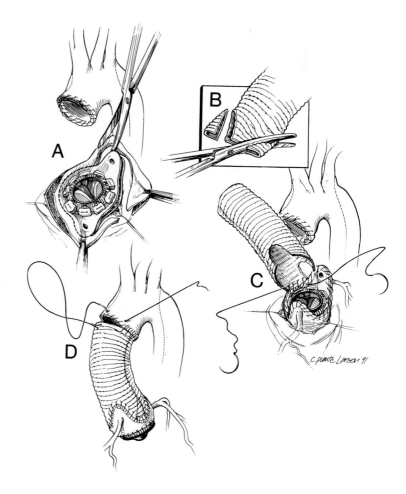

FIGURE 18–11 Proximal repair using the Wheat method. **A,** First the aortic valve is seated and then the aorta is transected circumferentially, with the aortic ostia being carefully preserved and the aortic layers being carefully reapproximated with a running suture. **B,** Scallops are excised from the graft to match the coronary artery ostia. **C,** The graft is then sutured into position, and the distal anastomosis **(D)** is completed. (From Svensson LG, Crawford ES. Curr Probl Surg 1992;29:915–1057.)

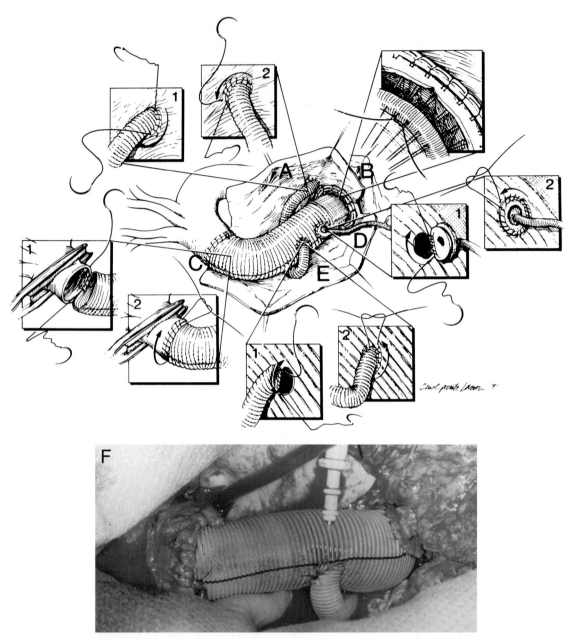

FIGURE 18–12 Insertion of a composite graft consisting of an interposition graft to the left main coronary artery ostium and an aortic button for the right coronary artery. **A. 1,** First the 10 mm tube graft is sutured to the left main coronary artery ostium with 4-0 Prolene material while the composite graft is being prepared for insertion after the annulus has been sized. A convenient point to start is at the 1 or 2 o'clock position with the right side run forehand to the heel. Next **(A.2)** the left side is run forehand. **B,** The composite valve graft is then seated, with the midcusp section tied down so that the valve is well seated in the annulus. **C,** The distal anastomosis is then performed with either 3-0 or 4-0 Prolene suture; the posterior layer is first done forehand from the inside followed by the anterior layer forehand from the outside. **D,** Next the mobilized right coronary artery ostial button is threaded through the center of a Teflon doughnut and fastened to the graft with a running 4-0 Prolene suture forehand from the inside for the inferior margin *(1)*. The suture is continued forehand from the outside to the superior margin. **D.2,** The suture is tightened and then run forehand up to the other end and tied down. Through a hole in the ascending graft where the left main graft will be anastomosed, the right coronary artery is probed to check for patency. The left main graft is then stretched so that there is approximately 1 to 1.5 cm of extra length to allow for when the graft is distended with blood and the ostia retract. The beveled graft is then sutured to the ascending aortic graft; the left side is done first **(E.1)** followed by forehand suturing of the inferior margin with 4-0 Prolene. For illustrative purposes, the 10 mm graft is shown as being longer than it actually is. An intraoperative photograph is shown in **F.** (Reprinted with permission from the Society of Thoracic Surgeons. From Svensson LG. Ann Thorac Surg 1992;54:376–8.)

FIGURE 18–13 Intraoperative photograph of a 38-year-old patient with Marfan syndrome who presented with an inferior myocardial infarction. The photograph shows the intimal aortic tear without undermining of the intima; this is not an uncommon finding in patients with Marfan syndrome and may precede classic aortic dissection. An embolus of either intima or clot may have embolized down the right coronary artery, since no coronary artery disease was found on cardiac catheterization. TEE had missed the diagnosis because no aortic wall hematoma or septum ("flap") was found. The aortogram done with the catheterization, however, revealed bulging of the aorta in the vicinity of the tear. The aorta was repaired with insertion of a composite valve graft by the technique we have described, with a tube graft to the left main coronary artery as seen in the photograph, and the right coronary artery was reattached as a button buttressed with a Teflon felt doughnut.[21]

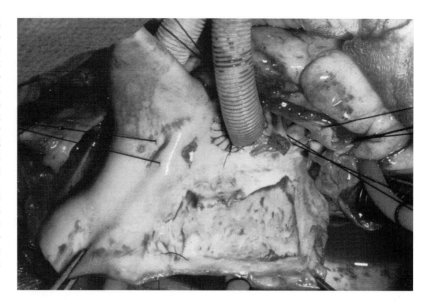

artery.[8, 9] The Bentall method is particularly prone to late false aneurysm formation if used in the acute situation for patients with Marfan syndrome (Fig. 18–15).

If the coronary arteries are dissected or tears are seen through the ostia inside the coronary lumina, then the ostia can be oversewn with generous figure-of-eight 3-0 Prolene sutures. Conventional coronary anastomoses are then performed to the distal coronary arteries. Since induction of cardioplegia can be a problem under these circumstances when the ostia cannot be cannulated or cannulation must be avoided because of the fragile ostia, retrograde cardioplegia has proved to be very effective. The composite valve graft is seated as described previously.[8, 9]

CHRONIC PROXIMAL DISSECTION

The important difference between acute and chronic dissection is that in acute dissection the inner lumen is still pliable and elastic and can be stretched to reconstruct the aorta, whereas the tissue is very friable. With chronic dissection, reconstruction of the aorta by tacking the intima to the adventitial layer is generally more difficult because scar tissue has usually formed in the aortic wall and does not allow stretching of the intimal flap, although the adventitia holds sutures better and with less risk of bleeding.[8, 9]

Ascending Aorta Reconstruction

Ascending aorta reconstruction is usually performed in those patients who either have type II aortic dissection or occasionally type I dissection when the remaining aorta is not aneurysmal or when the patient is elderly. The patient is placed on bicaval and femoral artery cardiopulmonary bypass as described previously. The aorta is then cross-clamped immediately proximal to the innominate artery, opened, and inspected, and cardioplegia is given in the coronary ostia provided that retrograde cardioplegia has not already been achieved. The aorta is then completely transected as described by Kouchoukos and associates,[11] so that the anastomosis can be inspected circumferentially for better hemostasis and less risk of later false aneurysm fo mation. Thus in the last 10 years the inclusion technique for repairs of the ascending aorta has virtually been abandoned in favor of the above procedure. During the repair, the septum is excised so that approximately a 1 mm ridge remains on the inner surface of the false lumen. The proximal aorta should also be similarly transected. Next an appropriate tubular graft is anastomosed both distally and proximally with 3-0 Prolene sutures; neither Teflon patches nor pledgets are used for the anastomoses. With the patient in a Trendelenburg position, air is meticulously evacuated from the heart and graft, and then the aorta is unclamped.[8, 9]

Ascending and Aortic Arch Repair

Frequently the aortic arch needs to be repaired in patients with chronic dissection of the proximal aorta, often after previous repairs to the ascending aorta. For this, the patient is placed on cardiopulmonary bypass as described, deep hypothermia is established, and the circulation is arrested with the patient in a head-down (Trendelenburg) position. The aorta is then opened and the inner septum is excised, leaving a 1 mm edge (Fig. 18-16). The aorta is transected proximal to the innominate artery, and the incision is extended down to the level of the subclavian artery. In the segment of the aorta beyond the left subclavian artery, a generous wedge of the septum is excised so that blood flow will perfuse both lumina (Fig. 18-16). Similarly, if the arch

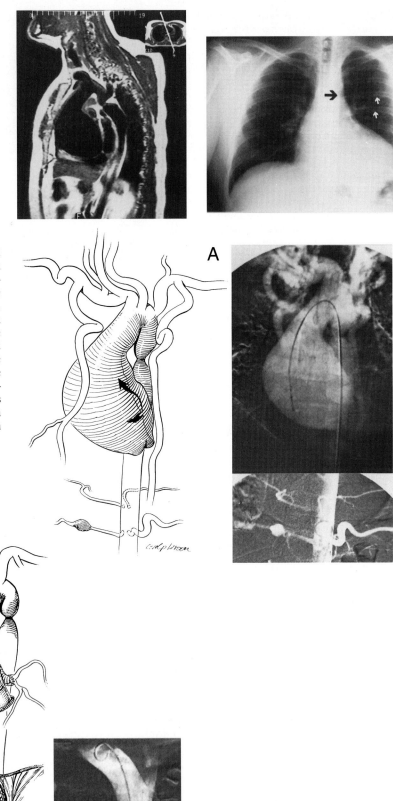

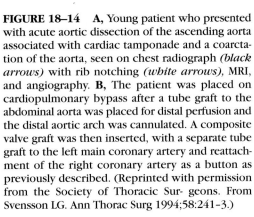

FIGURE 18–14 **A,** Young patient who presented with acute aortic dissection of the ascending aorta associated with cardiac tamponade and a coarctation of the aorta, seen on chest radiograph *(black arrows)* with rib notching *(white arrows)*, MRI, and angiography. **B,** The patient was placed on cardiopulmonary bypass after a tube graft to the abdominal aorta was placed for distal perfusion and the distal aortic arch was cannulated. A composite valve graft was then inserted, with a separate tube graft to the left main coronary artery and reattachment of the right coronary artery as a button as previously described. (Reprinted with permission from the Society of Thoracic Surgeons. From Svensson LG. Ann Thorac Surg 1994;58:241–3.)

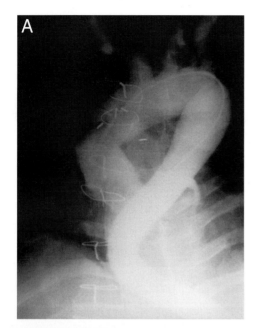

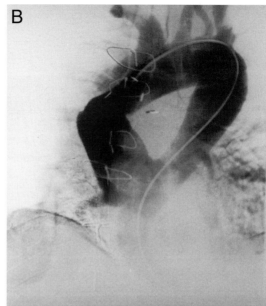

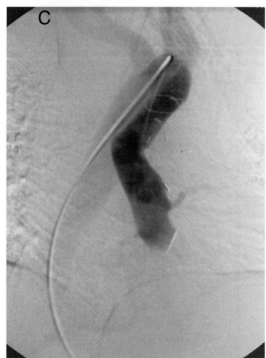

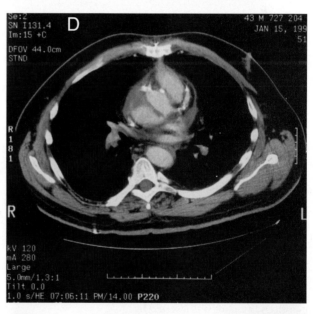

FIGURE 18–15 **A,** Aortogram of a patient with Marfan syndrome who underwent emergency surgery for repair of acute aortic dissection with insertion of a composite valve by the Bentall technique. The patient subsequently was referred because of pain associated with a false aneurysm arising from the left main coronary artery anastomosis (**A, B,** and **C**), also seen on CT scan with contrast (**D**). **E,** A lateral radiograph of the chest shows the positioning of the heart and aorta in relation to the sternum. The patient underwent reoperation, with the right subclavian artery used for arterial blood inflow during cardiopulmonary bypass.

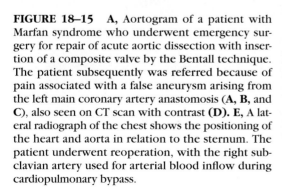

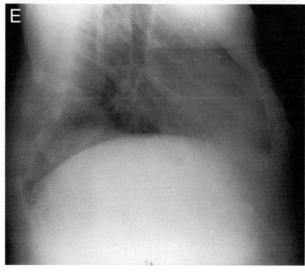

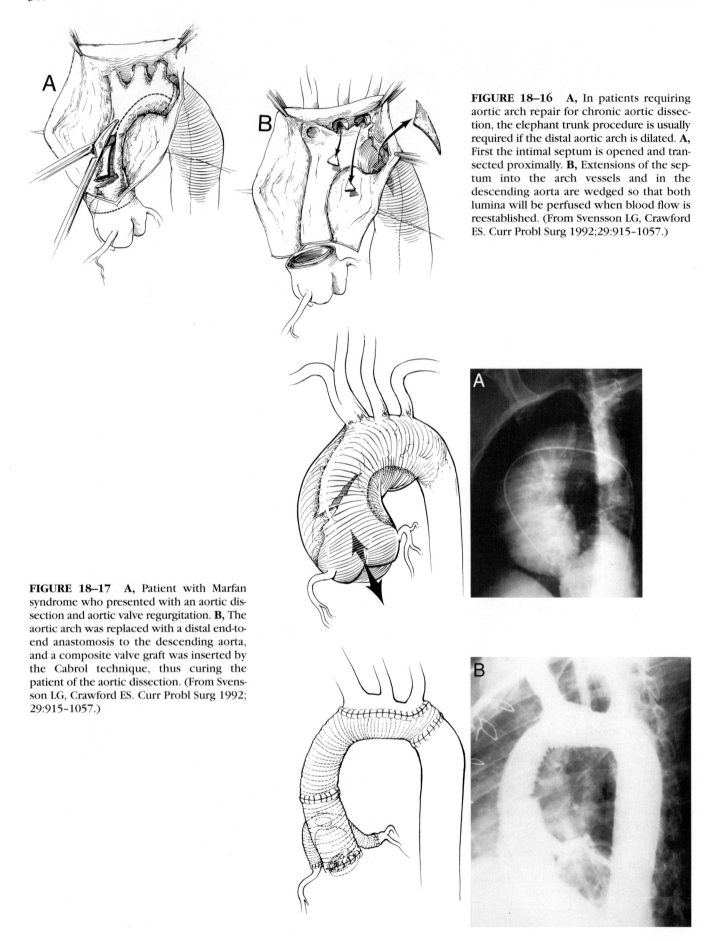

FIGURE 18–16 **A,** In patients requiring aortic arch repair for chronic aortic dissection, the elephant trunk procedure is usually required if the distal aortic arch is dilated. **A,** First the intimal septum is opened and transected proximally. **B,** Extensions of the septum into the arch vessels and in the descending aorta are wedged so that both lumina will be perfused when blood flow is reestablished. (From Svensson LG, Crawford ES. Curr Probl Surg 1992;29:915–1057.)

FIGURE 18–17 **A,** Patient with Marfan syndrome who presented with an aortic dissection and aortic valve regurgitation. **B,** The aortic arch was replaced with a distal end-to-end anastomosis to the descending aorta, and a composite valve graft was inserted by the Cabrol technique, thus curing the patient of the aortic dissection. (From Svensson LG, Crawford ES. Curr Probl Surg 1992; 29:915–1057.)

vessels are dissected at their origins, a wedge can be excised (Fig. 18-16). The distal anastomosis is performed with a running 3-0 Prolene suture without Teflon felt. Thereafter, a piece of the graft is excised to match the arch vessels, which are then anastomosed to the graft without excision of a Carrel patch island. A side arm is placed to the arch segment of the graft and flow is reestablished to the arch vessels, once air has been evacuated, and the graft is clamped proximal to the innominate artery. If indicated, the entire aortic arch can also be replaced (Fig. 18-17) (see Chapter 17 for a more detailed discussion of arch repairs). The proximal repair can then be performed.[8, 9]

Aortic Valve Management

In patients with chronic dissection, many of whom will have had previous surgery, we have found the supporting tissues around the aortic valve to be less pliable. Therefore, we do not advise valve repairs or resuspension in most patients because of the markedly increased risks of death and of serious complications associated with a second or third reoperation. Therefore the aortic valve should be replaced with a durable prosthetic valve, either separately or as a composite valve graft. In the elderly, a Wheat type of repair is the preferred approach. Tacking sutures are usually not necessary at the proximal transected aorta, although often a coronary artery bypass with autogenous vein to the distal right coronary artery is required because the right coronary artery ostium has been destroyed. In younger patients who have either extensive destruction, Marfan syndrome, or large aneurysms, the insertion of a composite graft is the procedure of choice. One of two methods of reattaching coronary artery ostia is usually used. Either a tube graft to the left main coronary ostium is placed and a right coronary button is modified as described above (Fig. 18-3) or excised coronary artery buttons are mobilized and attached to the graft (Fig. 18-18). In patients who are undergoing reoperation or those in whom the ostia are close to the annulus or tension on the anastomoses may occur, the first technique is preferred. In our experience, the long-term results with both of these methods have been favorable; in fact, no patients with either type of anastomosis have required reoperation. The previously popular Bentall technique of repair is hardly ever used now because of the high risk of reoperation (approximately 10% at 5 years) (Fig. 18-19).[8, 12] This is probably because leaks and false

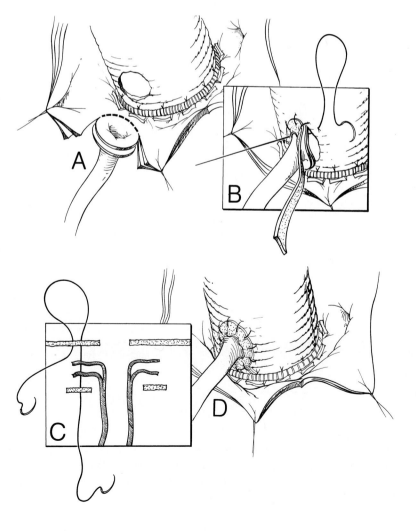

FIGURE 18–18 Details of the coronary ostia during reattachment by the button technique. **A,** The ostia are mobilized as buttons, and a hole is cut in the graft opposite the ostia. **B,** The ostium, supported by Teflon felt strip or a Teflon doughnut, is then sutured to the graft, in this case compressing the dissected aortic wall. **C,** The dissected aortic wall is sandwiched between the graft and the Teflon to give greater strength to the anastomosis and reduce the risk of bleeding. **D,** The completed repair. (From Svensson LG, Crawford ES. Curr Probl Surg 1992;29:915–1057.)

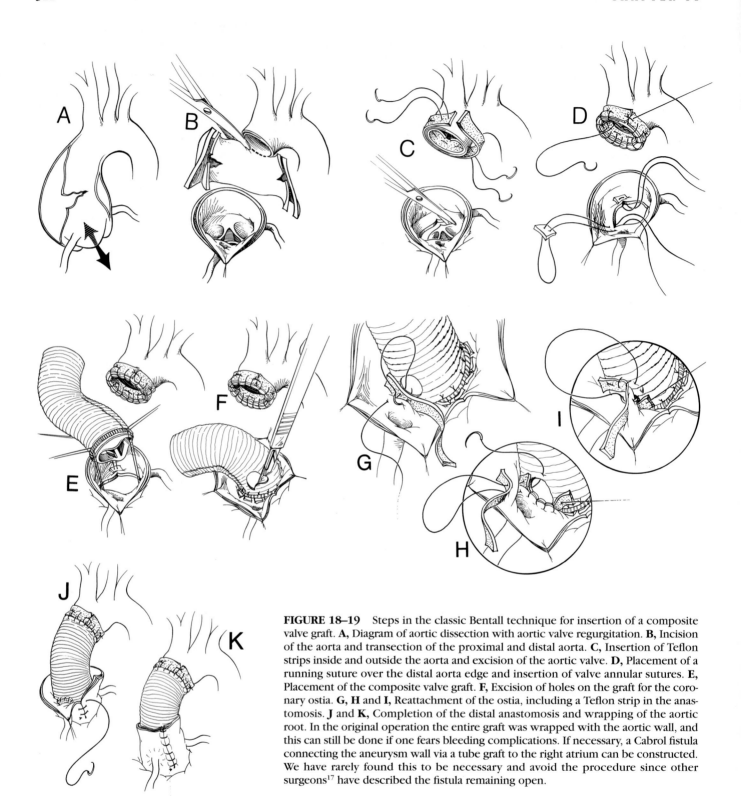

FIGURE 18–19 Steps in the classic Bentall technique for insertion of a composite valve graft. **A,** Diagram of aortic dissection with aortic valve regurgitation. **B,** Incision of the aorta and transection of the proximal and distal aorta. **C,** Insertion of Teflon strips inside and outside the aorta and excision of the aortic valve. **D,** Placement of a running suture over the distal aorta edge and insertion of valve annular sutures. **E,** Placement of the composite valve graft. **F,** Excision of holes on the graft for the coronary ostia. **G, H** and **I,** Reattachment of the ostia, including a Teflon strip in the anastomosis. **J** and **K,** Completion of the distal anastomosis and wrapping of the aortic root. In the original operation the entire graft was wrapped with the aortic wall, and this can still be done if one fears bleeding complications. If necessary, a Cabrol fistula connecting the aneurysm wall via a tube graft to the right atrium can be constructed. We have rarely found this to be necessary and avoid the procedure since other surgeons[17] have described the fistula remaining open.

aneurysms form at the direct coronary ostia to composite graft anastomoses, which are often under tension and thus pull free from the aortic wall, particularly in patients with Marfan syndrome.[8, 12] The Cabrol technique, although sometimes used when the right coronary artery ostium cannot be mobilized adequately, is usually not used now because of the risk of right coronary artery occlusion and resultant right heart ischemia (see Figs. 18-20 to 18-23). The preceding chapter discusses in greater detail the techniques for composite graft insertion.[8, 9]

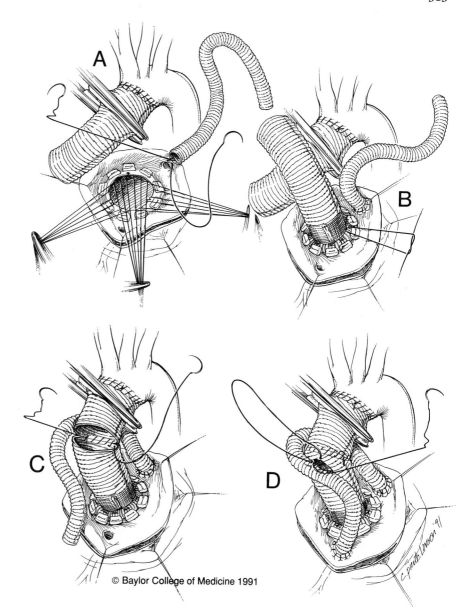

FIGURE 18–20 Steps in the insertion of a composite valve graft by the Cabrol method in patients with aortic dissection. **A,** The dissected wall of the aorta is retracted with stay sutures, and then the aortic arch is repaired with the use of deep hypothermia and circulatory arrest. Thereafter, the annular sutures are placed and the tube graft to the left main artery is sutured in position. If required, as when the ostium is dissected, pledgeted sutures are used to strengthen the suture line. **B,** Next the composite valve graft is seated and tied into position. **C,** The aortic arch graft is anastomosed to the composite valve graft. **D,** The tube graft is then anastomosed to the right coronary artery, followed by a side-to-side anastomosis of the interposition tube graft to the ascending composite valve graft. (From Svensson LG, Crawford ES. Curr Probl Surg 1992;29:915–1057.)

© Baylor College of Medicine 1991

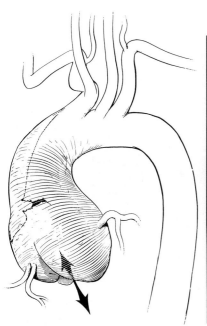

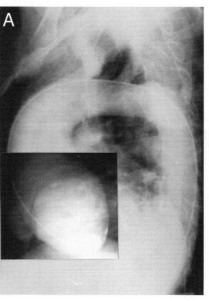

FIGURE 18–21 A, Patient with type II aortic dissection and aortic valve regurgitation.

Illustration continued on following page

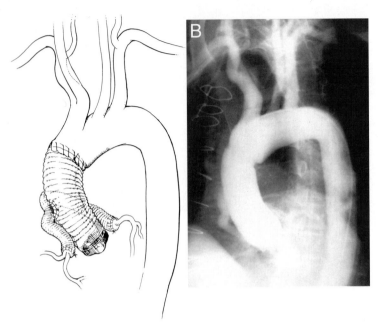

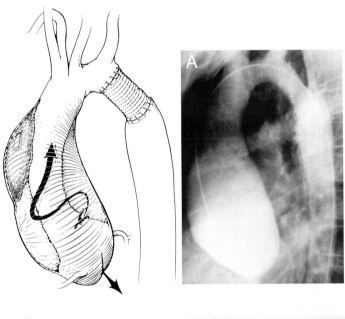

FIGURE 18–21 *Continued* **B,** Angiogram after insertion of composite valve graft. Note the sharp angle at the right coronary artery anastomosis.

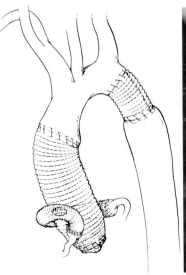

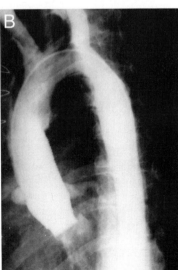

FIGURE 18–22 **A,** Patient with type II aortic dissection and previous descending aortic repair for coarctation, a not uncommon combination. **B,** Diagram and angiogram after repair by the Cabrol technique.

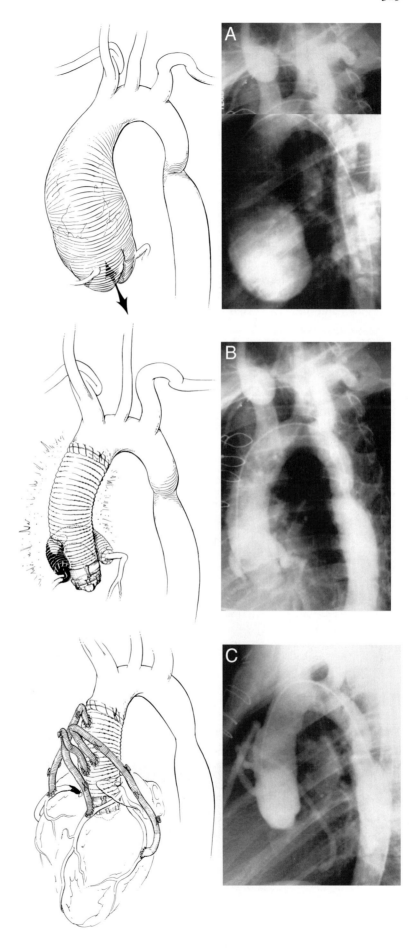

FIGURE 18–23 **A,** Young patient with ascending aortic aneurysm with aortic valve regurgitation and asymptomatic descending aortic pseudocoarctation. **B,** The patient underwent a Cabrol type of composite graft insertion but later returned with a graft infection; in addition, the graft to the right coronary artery had occluded. **C,** The old graft was excised, the surrounding tissues and aorta were debrided, and the coronary artery origins were oversewn. Next saphenous vein bypasses to the distal coronary arteries were done and omentum was "swung up" to fill the dead space. (Reprinted with permission from the Society of Thoracic Surgeons. From Svensson LG, Crawford ES, Hess KR, et al. Ann Thorac Surg 1992;54:427–39.)

Elephant Trunk Technique

The elephant trunk technique described previously by us[8, 9] has considerably improved both the ease and safety of performing extensive aortic arch replacements (Figs. 18-7, 18-8, 18-16 and 18-24; see also Chapter 17). We have noted, however, that with end-to-end anastomoses beyond the left subclavian artery or with the original elephant trunk technique,[7] tears of the aorta at the anastomosis have often occurred at the time of insertion. Such tears increase the serious risk of postoperative rupture of the distal aorta into the left chest.[8, 9]

To reduce the risk of tearing the aorta and also to simplify the technique of performing the anastomoses, a stay suture should be placed on the proximal end of the graft, which is then inverted into the distal part of the graft. Next the graft is placed in the descending aorta and a secure running suture is sewed to the aorta. The graft can then be withdrawn and the arch vessels reattached as described in the preceding chapter.[8, 9]

The arterial graft for perfusing the arch can be anastomosed to the arch before inversion into the distal graft in order that the circulatory arrest time may be shortened. The use of the 10 mm end-to-side graft for the arterial inflow instead of the femoral artery reduces the risk of embolization resulting from distal debris and air to the brain. Furthermore, the risk of the distal elephant trunk obstructing flow by functioning as a flutter valve is reduced. Sometimes one of the lumina is not perfused by the elephant trunk because not enough of a wedge has been excised or because the graft preferentially perfuses only one lumen. To avoid these complications, the lumina distal to the graft can be checked intraoperatively by transesophageal echocardiography (TEE), which will reveal the pattern of flow and show whether both lumina are being adequately perfused.[8, 9]

Reoperations

Reoperations on patients who have had previous cardiac or aortic surgery is becoming more frequent as the patient

FIGURE 18–24 **A,** Patient with Marfan syndrome and aortic dissection, including aneurysm formation of the aorta and innominate artery. **B,** As a first-stage operation, the aortic arch was replaced by the elephant trunk technique with insertion of a tube graft to the innominate artery and repair of the proximal aorta with a composite valve graft by the Cabrol method.

Illustration continued on following page

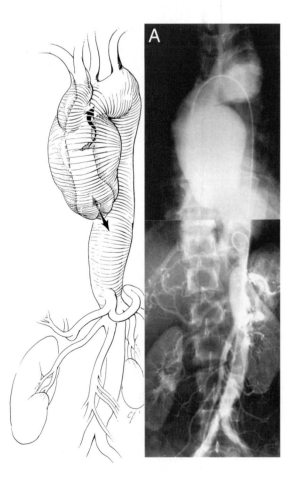

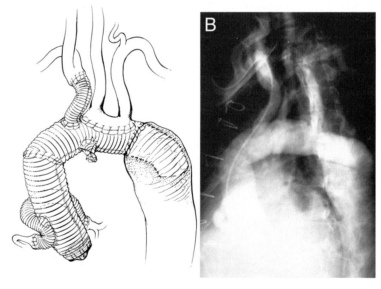

population ages and as more patients have undergone successful aortic surgery in the past. The most frequent reasons for the original operations are acute dissection, coronary artery disease, valve destruction, and Marfan syndrome. Patients later return requiring reoperation for chronic dissection associated with aneurysm formation distal to the previous repair (a frequent cause), biological valve failure, failed composite graft insertions and false aneurysms, failure to resect ascending aortic aneurysms at the time of aortic valve replacements, complications related to intraluminal grafts (the senior author [E.S.C.] has reported 17 cases causing partial luminal obstruction, kinking, chronic hemolysis, anemia, and persistence of aneurysms outside the graft[13]), prosthetic graft infections, progression of coronary artery disease, and unsuccessful lesser procedures such as separate valve graft replacements, valve repairs, aortoplasties, aortic valve resuspensions, and aortic valve remodeling or reimplantations.[8, 12, 14–18]

The operative technique for patients who have had previous cardiac or cardioaortic surgery is similar to that for a primary operation once the chest has been opened. However, for patients in whom a minor procedure is required, femorofemoral bypass with circulatory arrest is used and the heart and aorta are not fully dissected free.

Reoperations through the mediastinum for those patients who have had previous cardioaortic surgery require precautions similar to those for any cardiac reoperations. Some of these were dealt with in Chapter 16. The important principles can be summarized by the following points:

1. A detailed history and physical examination and the old operative reports are required.

2. Noninvasive studies, such as a lateral chest radiograph, carotid studies, pulmonary function tests, and an echocardiogram should be available if indicated.

3. A magnetic resonance imaging (MRI) or computer tomography (CT) study should be obtained.

4. Cardiac catheterization and an aortogram should have been done in most patients.

FIGURE 18–24 *Continued* **C,** and **D,** Aortogram after the second-stage repair of the thoracoabdominal aorta with reimplantation of intercostal arteries. (From Svensson LG, Crawford ES, Coselli JS, et al. Impact of cardiovascular operation on survival in the Marfan patient. Circulation 1989;80(3Pt1):I233–42. Reproduced with permission. Copyright 1989 American Heart Association.)

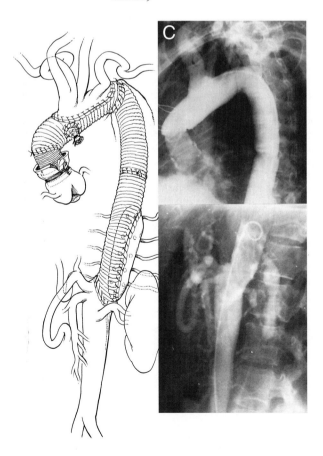

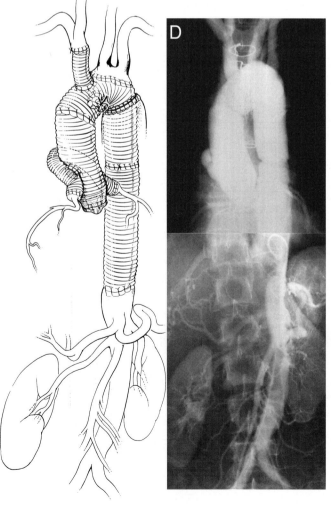

5. If the patient is undergoing reoperation for sepsis, bacterial cultures should be available to determine antibiotic sensitivities. Cultures may have to be obtained from fluid aspirated by CT or echocardiographic needle aspiration.

For the reoperation, femorofemoral cardiopulmonary bypass is useful if only the aorta and the aortic valve need to be replaced or if there is an increased danger of entering a false aneurysm during reentry (Fig. 18-25). The right subclavian artery may also be used in those patients in whom use of the femoral arteries is contraindicated (see illustrations). To check the positioning of the venous cannula in the right atrium after it has been threaded through the femoral vein, TEE can be performed to visualize the cannula in the left atrium. We also use a centrifugal pump on the venous line to improve venous drainage.

We have found that the best method of opening the sternum is to place the patient in a Trendelenburg position, use rake retractors to lift the sternum off the heart, and dissect with long scissors under the sternum before using the sternal saw (Fig. 18-26). With this approach, even in those patients with aneurysms abutting against the posterior table of the sternum, the sternum can be opened with low risk.

FIGURE 18–25 Cardiopulmonary bypass setup for femorofemoral bypass for sternal reentry. Note the venous line centrifugal pump to aid venous drainage, the tip of the venous line in the right atrium positioned with TEE, and the "Y" arterial line for antegrade perfusion into the aortic arch graft after repair of the arch.

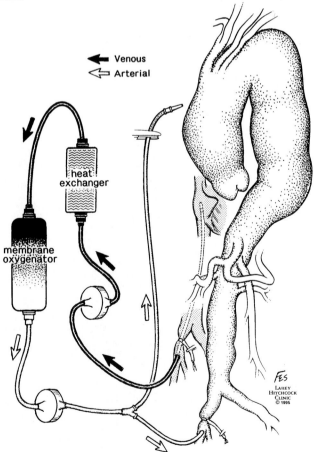

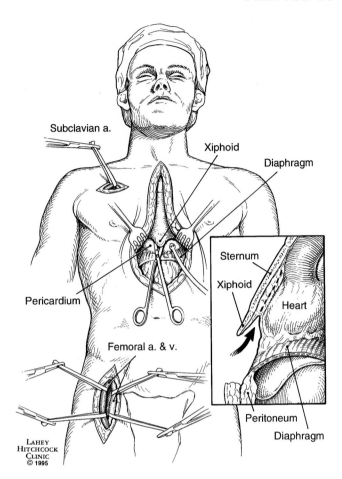

FIGURE 18–26 Incisions and our preferred method for mediastinal reentry after previous cardiac operations. If patients do not have iliac artery stenoses or occlusion, then the femoral artery and vein are routinely exposed and encircled with umbilical tape. If there is a possibility of problems with perfusion through the femoral artery, then the subclavian artery is also exposed. An alternative in some patients is to cannulate the aneurysm directly in the aortic arch and, after the repair, to reperfuse the aortic arch with a side graft. After removal of the old sternal wires, a tunnel is created under the breast bone by means of a pair of scissors, and cutting on the periosteum is done with the patient in a head-down position. At the same time, the subcostal margin and later the sternal edge are retracted with rake retractors. The xiphoid is often excised before the tunneling is commenced. Once a tunnel of a few inches has been produced, a sternal saw is used to open the sternum from below to the end of the tunnel. Further tunneling is then done under the sternum, and the saw is again used to open the sternum. This is continued in stages until the whole sternum has been divided. We have found this to be the safest method for patients who have aortic aneurysms impinging on the back of the sternum.

The operative principles, as in primary operations, can be summarized as follows:

1. All dilated segments of the aorta should be resected. If necessary, an elephant trunk type of procedure should be performed for later staged operations.

2. All proximal extents of dissection should be resected so that no false lumen can form and cause later problems

3. Blood flow should be rerouted distally in patients with chronic aortic dissection into both lumina except in the unusual patient who is having a reoperative repair for acute dissection (for example, after a previous aortic valve replacement).

4. The aortic valve should be replaced if it is leaking. Chronic dissected aortic valves are more difficult to repair successfully. Furthermore, a third operation to replace an aortic valve carries a higher risk of death.

5. If annuloaortic ectasia is present, then a composite aortic valve should be inserted.

6. If sepsis is present (for example, in an infected graft), all old graft material must be removed, the area thoroughly debrided, the new repair performed, and then all dead space and the new graft covered with omentum and, if necessary, also muscle flaps (see Chapter 8).

The methods of repair are illustrated in Figs. 18-10, 18-15, 18-23, and 18-27 to 18-40.

RESULTS

The results of ascending aorta and aortic arch surgery have continued to improve over time. In the recent experience of one of us (L.G.S.) in a series of 97 patients, there was one death (1%) and one stroke (1%) in a patient who did not have retrograde brain perfusion. In this group of patients, 68 had valve replacement (including 40 composite grafts), 43 had aortic dissection repairs, 19 had acute dissections, 41 had aortic arch repairs including the descending aorta in 19 and 2 had simultaneous thoracoabdominal repairs involving two incisions; see later chapter), 28 required coronary artery bypasses, 7 had elephant

Text continued on page 334

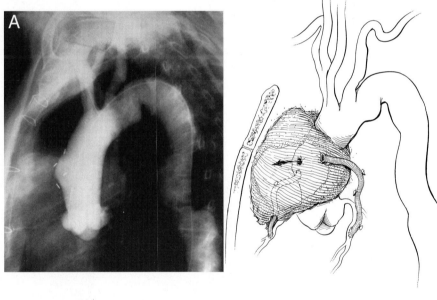

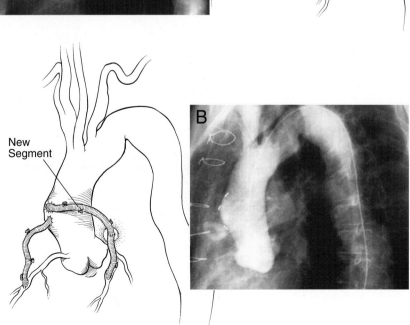

FIGURE 18–27 A, Preoperative angiogram and diagram of a patient who had previously undergone a coronary artery bypass operation and subsequently presented with a false aneurysm arising from the proximal anastomosis of the saphenous vein bypass to the left anterior descending coronary artery. **B,** Postoperative result after repair of the false aneurysm and insertion of an interposition segment of vein graft.

New Segment

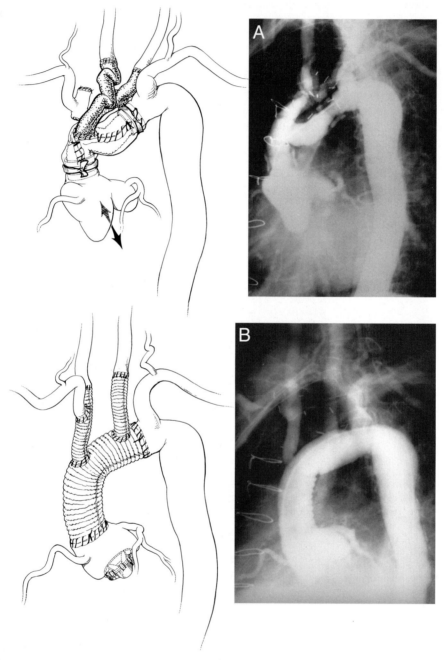

FIGURE 18–28 Patient requiring reoperation after previous repair of acute dissection with an intraluminal graft and vein bypasses to the right and left common carotid arteries **(A). B,** Diagram and arteriogram after aortic valve replacement, repair of ascending aorta and aortic arch, and insertion of tube grafts to the greater vessels.

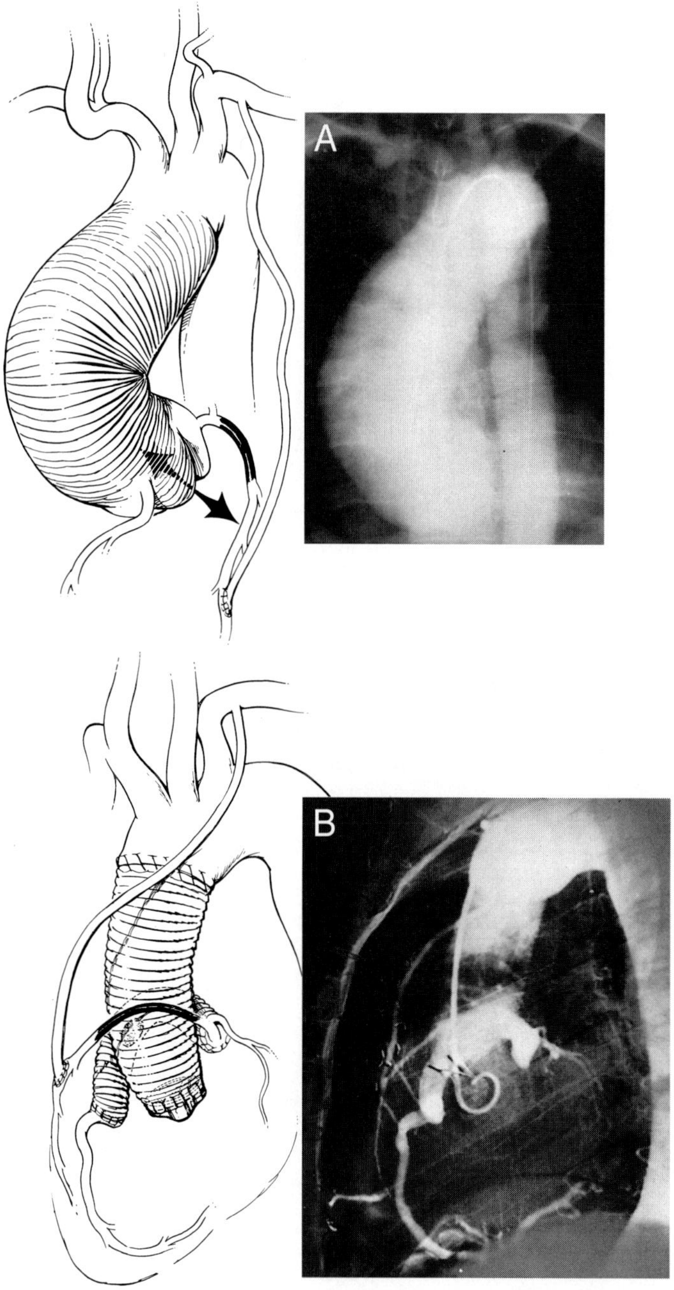

FIGURE 18–29 **A,** Aortic valve regurgitation and ascending aortic aneurysm in a patient with previous internal mammary bypass to the left anterior descending coronary artery. **B,** Postoperative diagram and angiogram after reoperation and insertion of a composite valve graft with preservation of the left mammary artery graft.

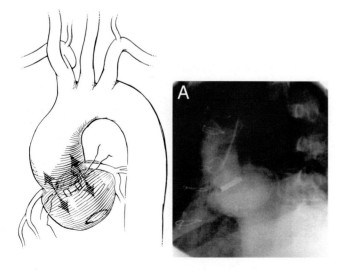

FIGURE 18–30 **A,** Patient with previous tilting disk aortic valve insertion who presented with perivalvular leaks and aortic aneurysm.

Illustration continued on following page

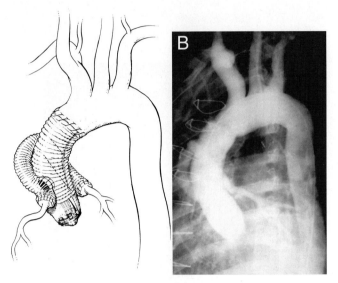

FIGURE 18–30 *Continued* **B,** Postoperative angiogram after insertion of a composite valve graft by the Cabrol method.

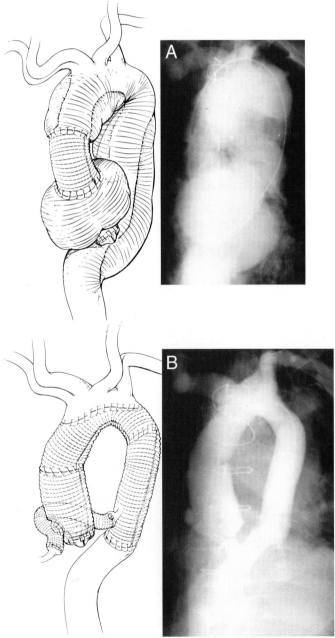

FIGURE 18–31 **A,** Middle-aged man with Marfan syndrome who had a separate valve and tube graft inserted elsewhere and was referred for aortic dissection beyond the repair. **B,** The aorta was repaired with a Cabrol type of composite valve graft insertion and the aortic arch was replaced by the elephant trunk method. Subsequently, the descending aorta was repaired.

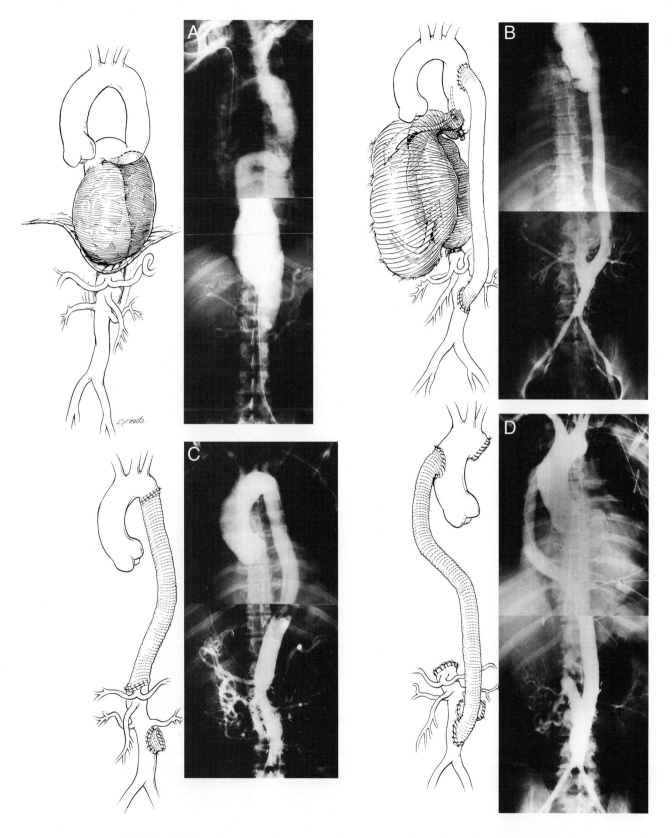

FIGURE 18–32   Diagram and aortogram of a patient with Marfan syndrome and a thoracoab-dominal aneurysm **(A).** A descending aorta-to-abdominal aorta bypass and attempted exclusion of the aneurysm was performed elsewhere in 1975 **(B). C,** The old graft was removed and the thoracoabdominal aorta was repaired, although 6 weeks later the patient had a *Staphylococcus epidermidis* infection of the graft that did not respond to intravenous antibiotics and irrigation of the aneurysm cavity with gentamicin. **D,** Subsequently, an ascending aorta-to-abdominal aorta graft was inserted, and 2 weeks later the old thoracoabdominal graft was removed.

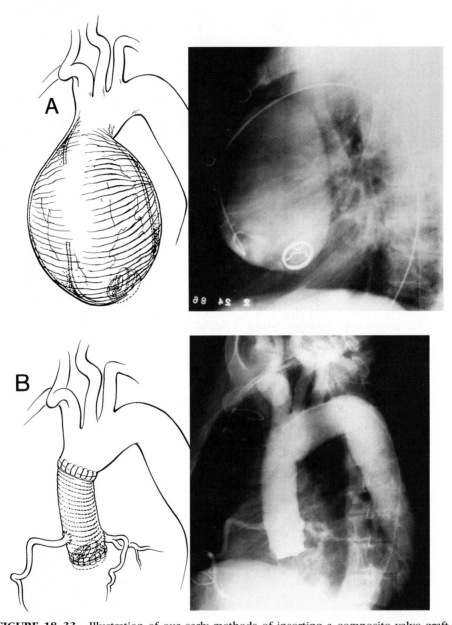

FIGURE 18–33 Illustration of our early methods of inserting a composite valve graft in patients with aortic dissection by the button technique. **A,** Patient with dissection of the ascending aorta after insertion of a tilting disk valve. **B,** Diagram and aortogram after insertion of a composite valve graft with a tilting disk and reattachment of the coronary artery ostia as buttons.

Illustration continued on following page

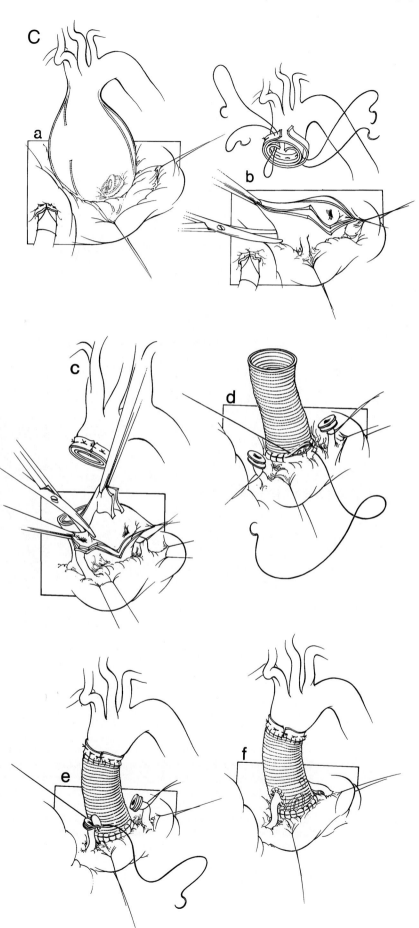

FIGURE 18–33 *Continued* **C,** First the patient is placed on bypass and the right ventricle and pulmonary outflow tract are retracted to expose the aorta *(a).* The aorta in this illustration is sandwiched between an inner and an outer layer of Teflon felt *(b).* This technique has since been abandoned because the Teflon can cause hemolysis or result in a pressure gradient across the anastomosis. We now use interrupted sutures without Teflon to tack up the intima if necessary. The coronary artery ostia are mobilized *(b* and *c)* and then the composite valve graft is seated. This is shown as being done with a continuous suture *(d).* We have found, however, that patients with a continuous suture line at the annulus in conjunction with classic Bentall repairs are more likely to develop paravalvular leaks. None of the patients, however, in whom the button technique with a continuous suture was used have since required reoperation; this may have been because the aorta was not reapproximated as a tight watertight wrap around the composite valve graft.[17] The coronary artery buttons are reattached to the composite graft after the distal anastomosis is performed *(e).* However, we would now recommend that Teflon felt be used to strengthen the anastomosis of the buttons to the graft. Appearance of the completed repair *(f).*

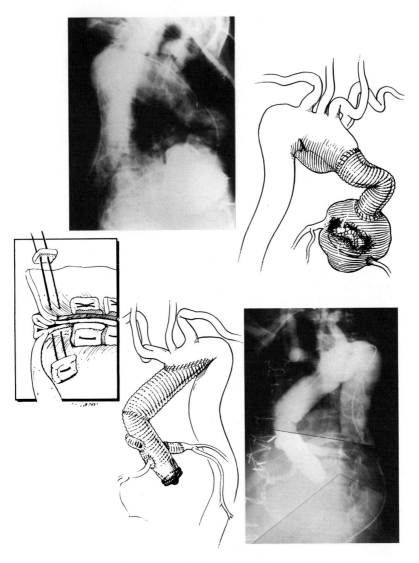

FIGURE 18–34   Patient in whom an initial valve replacement was followed by aortic dissection and then attempted repair with another biological valve and a separate ascending aorta tube graft. The repair became infected with *Staphylococcus aureus* with an annular abscess involving two thirds of the annulus and free pus around the graft. The patient, who was referred with septicemic shock and heart failure, underwent extensive debridement of all graft tissue and of surrounding tissue, including the aorta, with use of circulatory arrest. The aortic arch was then repaired and the aorta was built up by bringing down normal aortic tissue to the left ventricle outflow tract with pledgeted sutures. The composite valve graft was seated after placement of a tube graft to the left main coronary artery, as described previously.[22] The right coronary artery was reattached as a buttressed button. The repair was then wrapped with omentum, and irrigation catheters were placed around the graft for perfusion of the repair with antibiotics. On a regimen of permanent antibiotics for life, the patient has not had a recurrence of infection. (From Svensson LG, Labib S. Curr Opinion Cardiol 1994;9:191–9.)

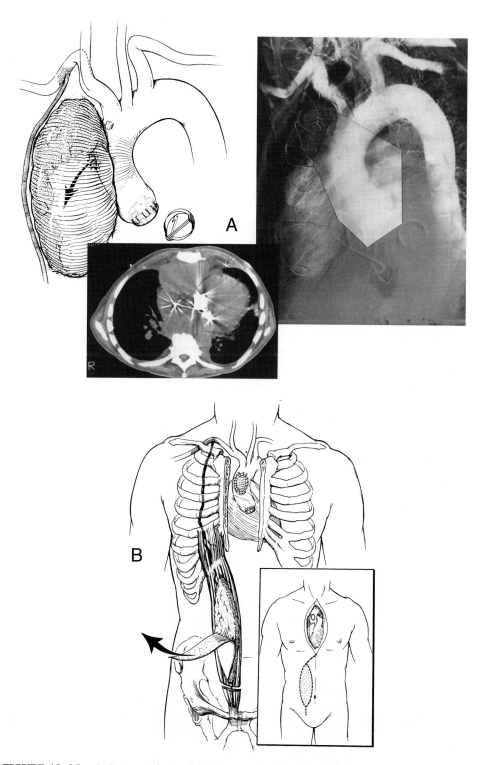

FIGURE 18–35 **A,** Patient who had double valve replacement followed by ascending aortic false aneurysm, with 13 attempts made to control sepsis associated with the false aneurysm and infected pledgets. The patient had also become HIV positive from blood transfusions. **B,** After induction of deep hypothermia with circulatory arrest, the false aneurysm was excised and, after debridement, the aorta was repaired with a patch. The right rectus muscle was then mobilized, and the overlying skin excised.

Illustration continued on following page

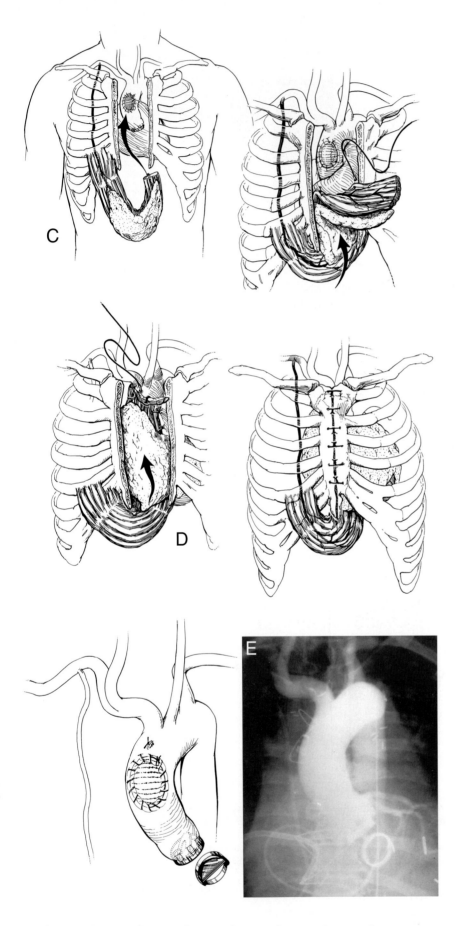

FIGURE 18–35 *Continued* **C,** The rectus was swung up to fill the dead space and sutured into position (**D**), and the sternum was closed. **E,** Postoperative angiogram after the repair.

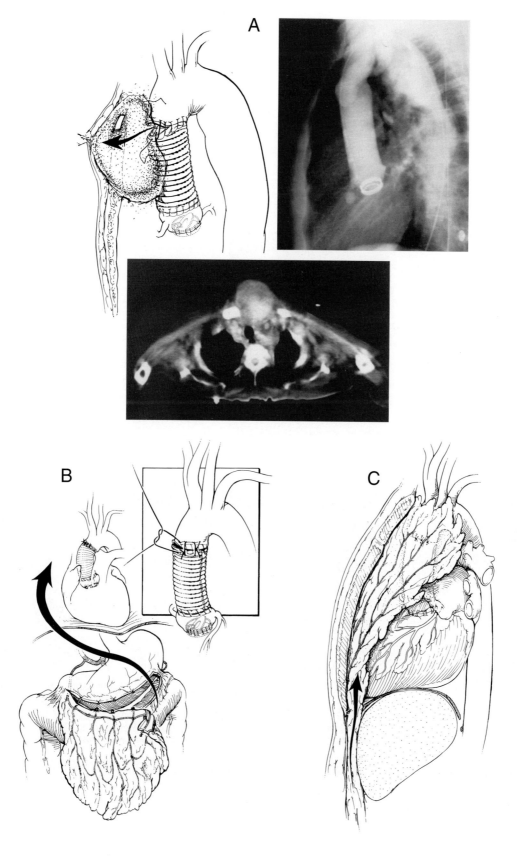

FIGURE 18–36 **A,** Patient with aortocutaneous fistula after previous valve and ascending aortic graft replacement. On the CT scan, note the false aneurysm outside the mediastinum. **B,** The false aneurysm neck at the distal anastomosis was oversewn, and the omentum was swung up to fill the dead space. **C,** The lateral diagram illustrates positioning of the omental flap.

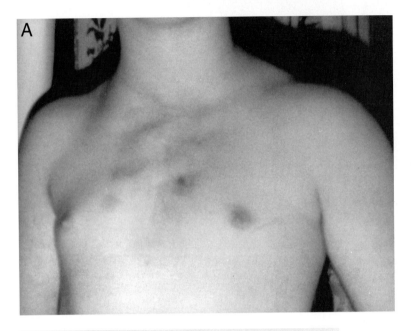

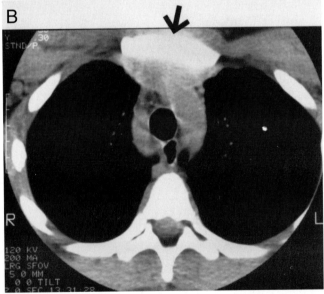

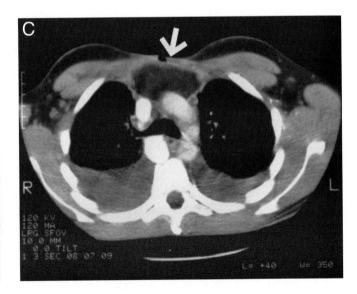

FIGURE 18–37   **A,** Teenager who had a methacrylate prosthesis placed to repair the manubrium after chest trauma and who later presented with a false aneurysm under the skin. **B,** On CT, the prosthesis *(arrow)* was seen impinging on the aorta and causing the false aneurysm **(C)**.

Illustration continued on following page

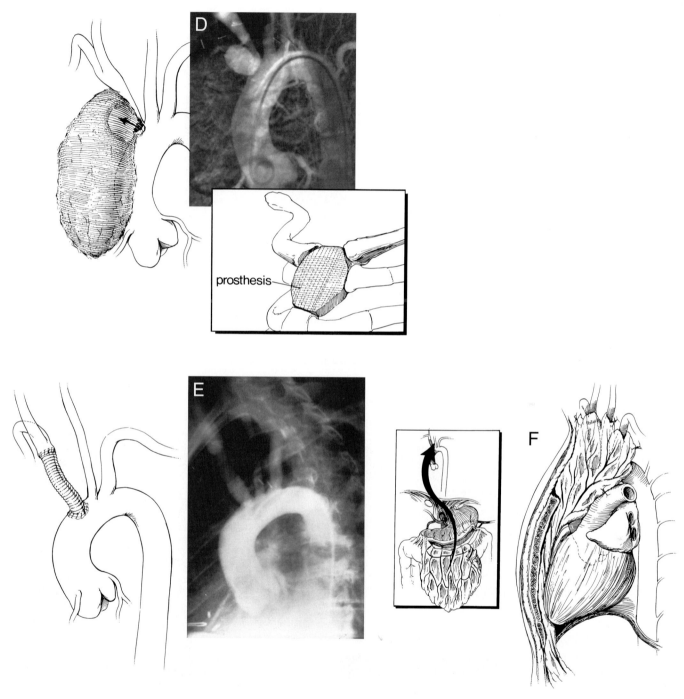

FIGURE 18–37 *Continued* **D,** Most of the false aneurysm is filled with clot but arises from the origin of the innominate artery. **E,** The innominate artery was replaced with a tube graft. **F,** the omentum was swung up to fill the dead space left after evacuation of clot from the false aneurysm.

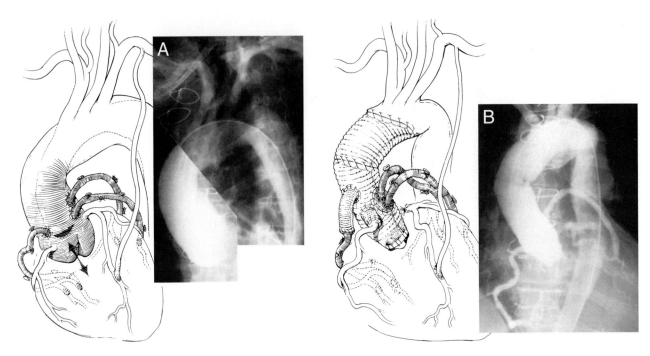

FIGURE 18–38 **A,** Patient with a previous coronary artery bypass, including with a left internal mammary artery, who presented with aortic dissection and aortic valve regurgitation. **B,** The aortic arch was repaired after induction of deep hypothermia with circulatory arrest, and a composite valve graft was inserted with interposition tube grafts to the right coronary artery ostium and to the vein bypass graft for the right coronary artery system. The vein bypasses to the obtuse marginal arteries were reimplanted as an aortic button, and the left main coronary artery ostium was oversewn.

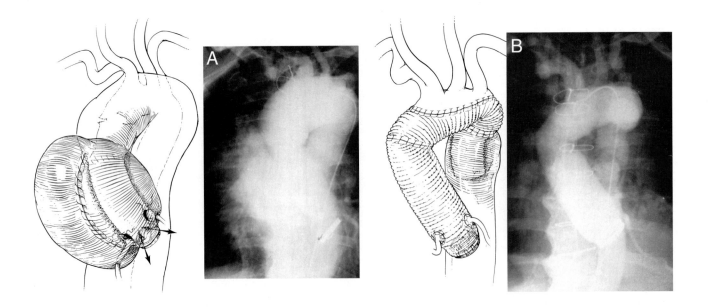

FIGURE 18–39 **A,** Patient who underwent classic Bentall repair for both the coronary artery anastomoses and wrapping of the ascending aorta and later presented with a false aneurysm, a paravalvular leak, disruption of the coronary anastomoses, and distal aortic dissection beyond the composite valve graft. **B,** The patient underwent reoperation in which the aortic arch was replaced by the elephant trunk technique, and the button technique used for the reanastomoses of the coronary artery ostia.

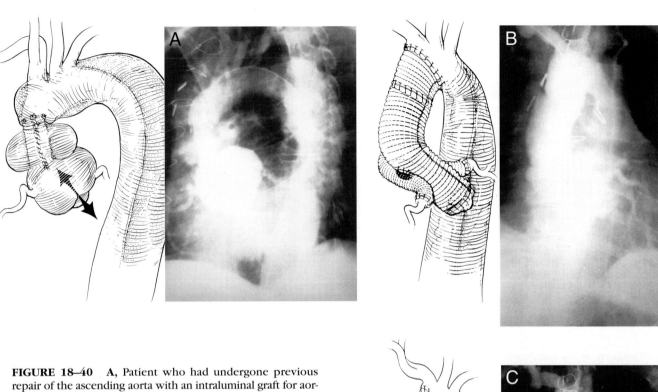

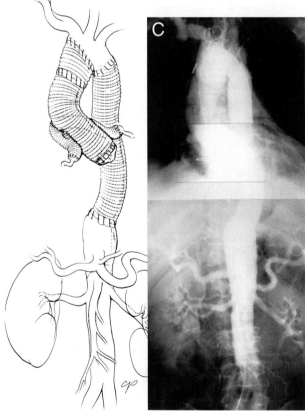

FIGURE 18–40   A, Patient who had undergone previous repair of the ascending aorta with an intraluminal graft for aortic dissection elsewhere and who later presented with aortic valve regurgitation and aneurysm formation. **B,** The aortic arch was repaired with a beveled tube graft after induction of hypothermic circulatory arrest and the proximal aorta was repaired with a composite valve graft by the Cabrol technique. **C,** Later the descending thoracic aorta was repaired, with resection of all aneurysmal parts of dissected aorta

trunk type repairs, and 6 had preoperative sepsis, because of either previous aortic surgery or mycotic aneurysms. Approximately two thirds of these patients who had elective operations did not require blood transfusions.[19]

REFERENCES

1. Barnard CN, Schire V. The surgical treatment of acquired aneurysms of the thoracic aorta. Thorax 1963;18:101-5.
2. Griepp RB, Stinson EB, Hollingsworth JF, et al. Prosthetic replacement of the aortic arch. J Thorac Cardiovasc Surg 1975;70:1051-63.
3. Cooley DA, Ott DA, Frazier OH, et al. Surgical treatment of aneurysms of the transverse aortic arch: experience with 25 patients using hypothermic techniques. Ann Thorac Surg 1981;32:260-72.
4. Cooley DA, Livesay JJ. Technique of "open" distal anastomosis for ascending and transverse arch resection. Cardiovasc Dis (Bull Tex Heart Inst) 1981;8:421.
5. Antunes MJ, Colsen PR, Kinsley RH. Hypothermia and circulatory arrest for surgical resection of aortic arch aneurysms. J Thorac Cardiovasc Surg 1983;86:576-81.
6. Crawford ES, Crawford JL. Diseases of the Aorta Including an Atlas of Angiographic Pathology and Surgical Technique. Baltimore, MD: Williams & Wilkins. 1984.
7. Borst HG, Frank G, Schaps D. Treatment of extensive aortic aneurysms by a new multiple-stage approach. J Thorac Cardiovasc Surg 1988;95:11-3.
8. Svensson LG, Crawford ES, Hess KR, et al. Dissection of the aorta and dissecting aortic aneurysms: improving early and long-term surgical results. Circulation 1990;82(5 Supp):IV 24-38.
9. Svensson LG, Crawford ES. Aortic dissection and aortic aneurysm surgery: clinical observations, experimental investigations, and statistical analyses. Part II. Curr Probl Surg 1992;29:915-1057.
10. Wheat MW Jr, Harris PD, Malm JR, et al. Acute dissecting aneurysms of the aorta: treatment and results in 64 patients. J Thorac Cardiovasc Surg 1969;58:344-51.
11. Kouchoukos NT, Marshall WG Jr, Wedige STA. Eleven-year experience with composite graft replacement of the ascending aorta and aortic valve. J Thorac Cardiovasc Surg 1986;92:691-705.
12. Svensson LG, Crawford ES, Coselli JS, et al. Impact of cardiovascular operation on survival in the Marfan patient. Circulation 1989;80(3 Pt 1):I233-42.
13. Crawford ES. Commentary on Oz MC, et al. Twelve-year experience with intraluminal sutureless ringed graft replacement of the descending thoracic and thoracoabdominal aorta. J Vasc Surg 1990;11:331-8.
14. Crawford ES, Svensson LG, Coselli JS, et al. Surgical treatment aneurysm and/or dissection of the ascending aorta, transverse aortic arch, and ascending aorta and transverse aortic arch: factors influencing survival in 717 patients. J Thorac Cardiovasc Surg 1989;98:659-74.
15. Crawford ES, Coselli JS, Svensson LG, et al. Diffuse aneurysmal disease (chronic aortic dissection, Marfan, and mega aorta syndromes) and multiple aneurysm: treatment by subtotal and total aortic replacement emphasizing the elephant trunk operation. Ann Surg 1990;211:521-37.
16. Svensson LG, Crawford ES, Hess KR, et al. Deep hypothermia with circulatory arrest: determinants of stroke and early mortality in 656 patients. J Thorac Cardiovasc Surg 1992;106:19-31.
17. Svensson LG, Crawford ES, Hess KR, et al. Composite valve graft replacement of the proximal aorta: comparison of techniques in 348 patients. Ann Thorac Surg 1992;54:427-39.
18. Coselli JS, LeMaire SA, Buket S. Marfan syndrome: the variability and outcome of operative managment. J Vasc Surg 1995;21:432-43.
19. Svensson LG, Sun J, Nadolny E, Kimmel WA. Prospective evaluation of minimal blood use for ascending aorta and aortic arch operations. Ann Thorac Surg 1995;59:1501-8.
20. Svensson LG. Rationale and technique for replacement of the ascending aorta, arch, and distal aorta using a modified elephant trunk procedure. J Cardiac Surg 1992;7:301-12.
21. Svensson LG. Approach to the insertion of composite valve graft. Ann Thorac Surg 1992;54:376-8.

Techniques for Degenerative Disease of the Distal Aorta

Distal repairs are defined as those involving repair of the aorta distal to the left subclavian artery. There is, however, an overlap between distal and proximal operations, because proximal operations through the mediastinum may extend down into the descending thoracic aorta, as discussed in Chapters 17 and 18. Similarly, some patients require extensive replacements of the distal ascending aorta or aortic arch and also the thoracoabdominal or descending thoracic aorta that are most easily done through the left side of the chest using hypothermic circulatory arrest, as illustrated (Figs. 19-1 to 19-3).

REPAIRS OF THE DISTAL AORTA COMBINED WITH REPAIRS OF THE PROXIMAL AORTA THROUGH THE LEFT CHEST

Most of these operations will require hypothermic circulatory arrest for repair of the aortic arch, although occasionally the distal aortic arch to immediately beyond the innominate artery can be repaired without bypass (Figs. 19-1 to 19-6).

For patients who require hypothermic circulatory arrest, the procedure is similar to that described in previous chapters. The patient is positioned so that the groins are accessible for femoro-femoral cannulation and bypass. We use a long venous cannula to reach into the right atrium and check positioning of the tip of the cannula in the right atrium with transesophageal echocardiography (TEE) monitoring. TEE is also useful for checking brain perfusion and the quality of the thoracic aorta during the operation. Sometimes we have placed a two-stage cannula into the right atrial auricle from the left side of the chest for venous drainage and have found this to be surprisingly easy to do. In some patients who had been cannulated for atriofemoral bypass, we have added cannulae to either the femoral vein, the pulmonary artery, or the right atrium to increase venous drainage. To further improve venous drainage, we also find it useful to have a centrifugal pump on the venous line to aid venous drainage by suction. A left ventricular apex cannula for drainage and prevention of left ventricular distention is not always necessary unless there is aortic valve regurgita-

tion. If the condition of the aortic valve is documented on preoperative studies to have moderate to severe regurgitation, then a different operative approach is needed. The patient's shoulders are positioned as for a descending thoracic or thoracoabdominal repair and the chest is opened (see below).

Once EEG monitoring shows that there is no electrical activity, the circulation is arrested and the patient is placed head-down in a Trendelenburg position. The aorta is incised and blood is drained without cross-clamping the aorta. Two options for performing the proximal anastomosis are available. The graft can be sutured end-to-end in the ascending aorta by the inclusion technique, or the graft can be beveled and sutured as a patch from the ascending aorta and then around the aortic arch vessels. The latter method is both easier and quicker because, after the end-to-end anastomosis is sutured, the aortic arch vessels have to be attached to the graft as a separate anastomosis. Once the proximal anastomosis is completed, air is removed from the aortic arch and blood flow to the brain is reestablished by means of an arterial cannula placed either into the aortic arch part of the graft directly or into a side branch attached to the aortic arch. The rest of the repair is then performed as described below for descending thoracic or thoracoabdominal operations.

DISTAL REPAIRS

Most operations involving the descending thoracic aorta do not require cardiopulmonary bypass but should, whenever possible, be done with atriofemoral bypass, as discussed in previous chapters, in addition to temperature control with a heat exchanger. The preoperative work-up has also been dealt with in previous chapters. By the time they come to surgery, most patients will have had an imaging study (computed tomography, magnetic resonance imaging, angiography) and cardiac evaluation (thallium stress test, dobutamine echocardiography, or cardiac catheterization). Also, patients undergoing descending thoracic or thoracoabdominal repairs, will usually have had routine angiography. For abdominal aneurysms, however, this is controversial, and it is likely that noninvasive imaging such

Text continued on page 343

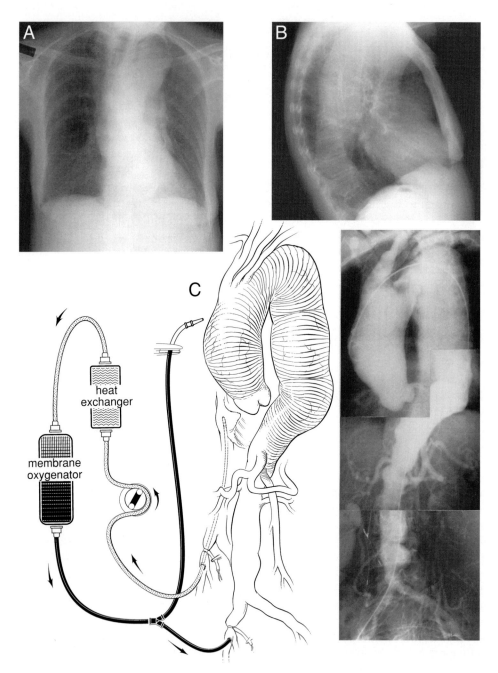

FIGURE 19–1 Patient with mega aorta requiring extensive repair. **A** and **B** show the preoperative chest radiographs and **C** shows a diagram of the cardiopulmonary bypass arrangement with a Y arterial graft for attachment to a side graft.

Illustration continued on following page

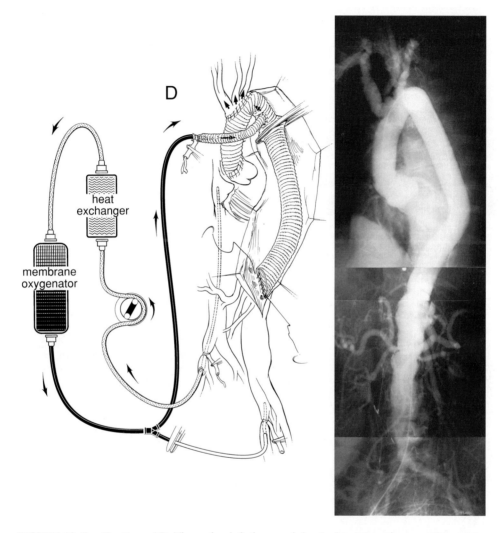

FIGURE 19–1   *Continued* **D,** Through a left thoracoabdominal incision, the ascending aorta, the aortic arch, and the rest of the aorta can be replaced, although the aortic valve is not accessible. A side graft is attached to the aortic arch or the proximal descending aorta to perfuse the brain while the rest of the repair is completed.

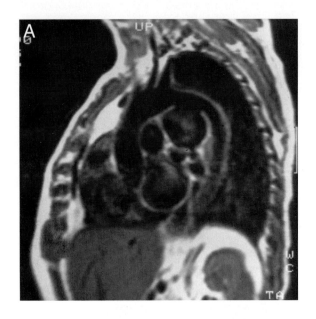

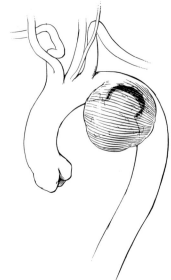

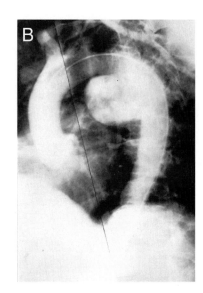

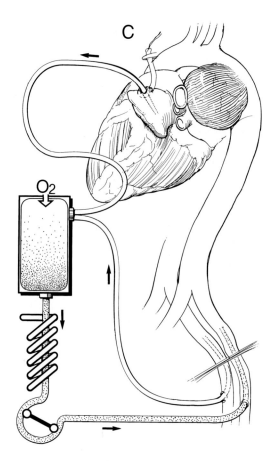

FIGURE 19–2 Repair of distal aortic arch aneurysm with use of hypothermic arrest. Patient with a distal aortic arch saccular aneurysm on MRI **(A)**, and on aortography **(B)**. **C,** The patient was placed on atriofemoral cardiopulmonary bypass with additional venous drainage from the femoral vein and cooled for hypothermic circulatory arrest.

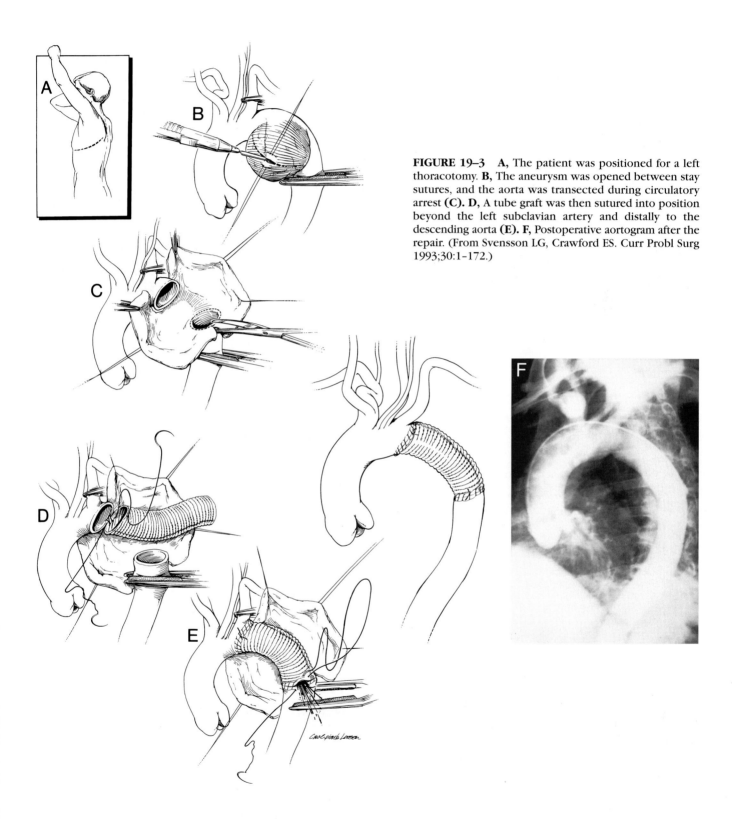

FIGURE 19–3 **A,** The patient was positioned for a left thoracotomy. **B,** The aneurysm was opened between stay sutures, and the aorta was transected during circulatory arrest **(C). D,** A tube graft was then sutured into position beyond the left subclavian artery and distally to the descending aorta **(E). F,** Postoperative aortogram after the repair. (From Svensson LG, Crawford ES. Curr Probl Surg 1993;30:1–172.)

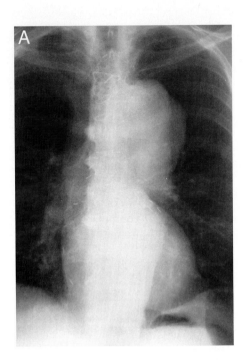

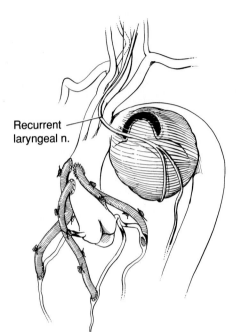

Recurrent
laryngeal n.

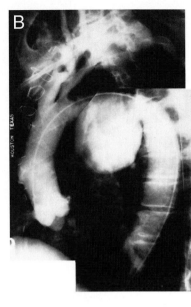

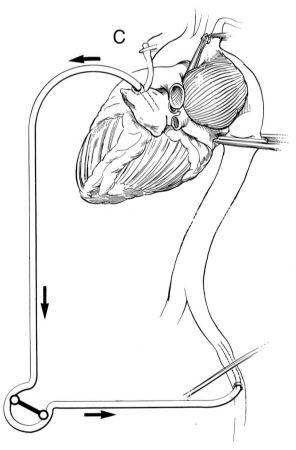

C

FIGURE 19–4 Repair of distal aortic arch aneurysm with atriofemoral bypass. **A,** Chest radiograph showing aortic arch aneurysm after previous coronary artery bypass surgery. **B,** Aortography showing a saccular aneurysm. The displacement and stretching of the recurrent laryngeal nerve by aortic arch aneurysms often result in left vocal cord paralysis and hoarseness. **C,** Insertion of atriofemoral bypass and clamping of the distal aortic arch, the left subclavian artery, and the descending aorta. (From Svensson LG, Crawford ES. Curr Probl Surg 1993;30:1–172.)

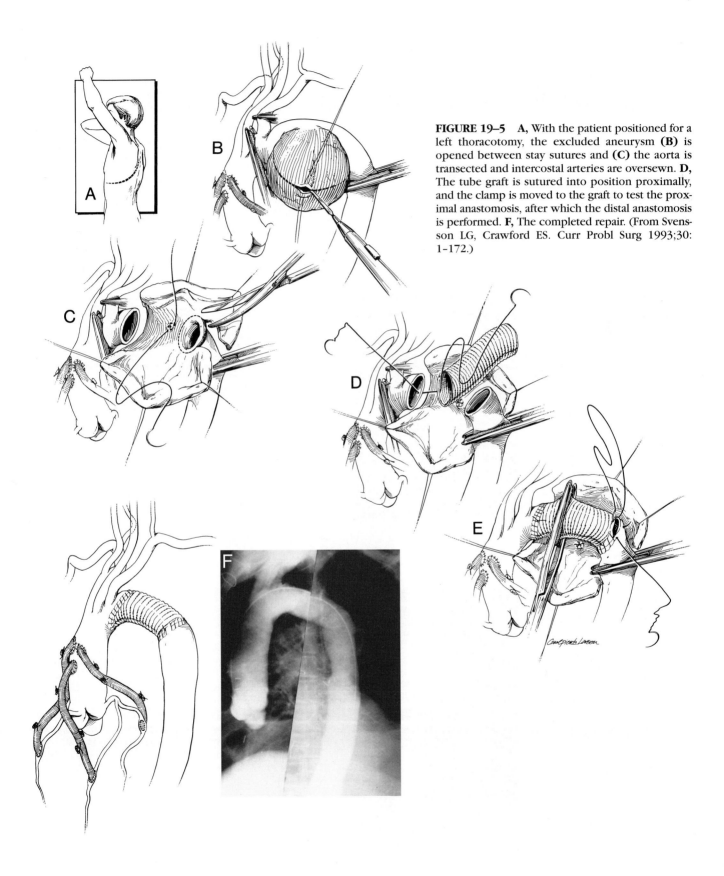

FIGURE 19–5 **A,** With the patient positioned for a left thoracotomy, the excluded aneurysm **(B)** is opened between stay sutures and **(C)** the aorta is transected and intercostal arteries are oversewn. **D,** The tube graft is sutured into position proximally, and the clamp is moved to the graft to test the proximal anastomosis, after which the distal anastomosis is performed. **F,** The completed repair. (From Svensson LG, Crawford ES. Curr Probl Surg 1993;30: 1–172.)

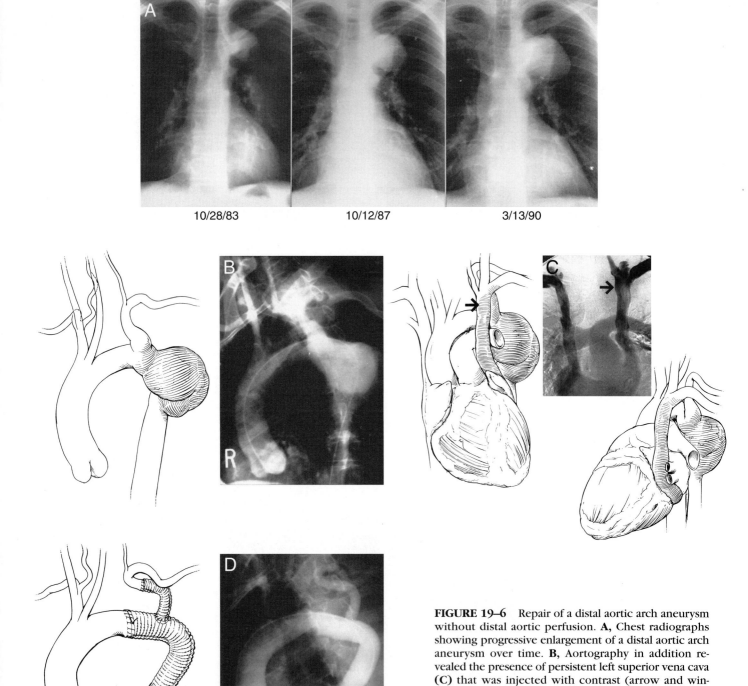

10/28/83   10/12/87   3/13/90

FIGURE 19–6 Repair of a distal aortic arch aneurysm without distal aortic perfusion. **A,** Chest radiographs showing progressive enlargement of a distal aortic arch aneurysm over time. **B,** Aortography in addition revealed the presence of persistent left superior vena cava (**C**) that was injected with contrast (arrow and window). **D,** Postoperative aortogram after insertion of a descending aortic graft and a separate tube graft to the left subclavian artery. (From Svensson LG, Crawford ES. Curr Probl Surg 1993;30:1–172.)

as spiral computed tomography (CT), magnetic resonance imaging (MRI), or magnetic resonance angiography (MRA) will replace dye-contrast angiography.

DESCENDING THORACIC AORTA REPLACEMENT

The operative technique for repair of degenerative aneurysms is similar to that for aortic dissection with the exception that for the latter the dissected septum does have to be excised (Figs. 19–7 and 19–8).

The patient is intubated with a double-lumen tube and then placed in a left thoracotomy position with the chest at about an 80- to 90-degree angle to the table, depending on how far distally the repair needs to be taken. The draping should include the left groin in the field so that a left atriofemoral bypass circuit can be established. The femoral artery is first dissected out and mobilized. Next the skin is incised from behind the scapula, around the inferior margin of the scapula, and then across the front of the chest. If a proximal descending aorta repair is planned, then the line is in the submammary fold. If the more distal descending aorta is also to be repaired, then the incision is best aimed more toward the umbilicus in the event that the diaphragm has to be divided. For proximal descending aortic repairs the fifth rib is resected, whereas if more distal parts have to be repaired then the sixth rib is resected. The aorta proximal to the site of the proximal anastomosis is then mobilized and encircled so that it can be cross-clamped when necessary. The lung is then retracted laterally to expose the phrenic nerve and the hilum of the lung. The pericardium is incised posterior to the phrenic nerve to expose the left auricle. A pursestring suture is then placed around the base of the auricle. The cannula for blood drainage is inserted into the auricle and secured in position, after which the arterial end is inserted into the previously mobilized femoral artery and secured in position. Alternatively, the left inferior pulmonary vein can be used for cannulation if adhesions are dense. However, care should be taken that the vein is not

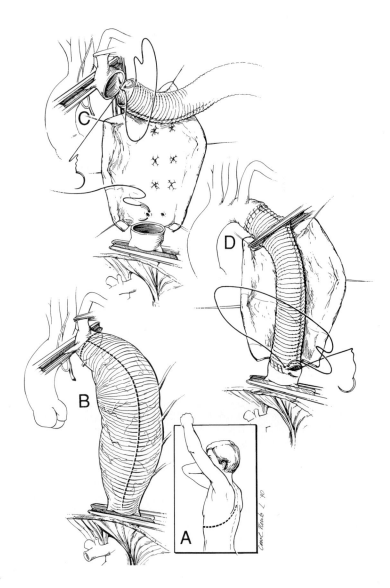

FIGURE 19–7 Steps in the repair of a descending thoracic aortic aneurysm. **A,** The incision for the left thoracotomy is aimed obliquely toward the umbilicus in case a full thoracoabdominal repair is necessary. The costal margin is also divided if additional exposure is required for the distal anastomosis. **B,** After distal aortic perfusion is established, usually with atriofemoral bypass, the aorta is cross-clamped proximally and distally and then transected. For segmental repairs, which we do whenever possible, the shortest proximal segment of aorta is cross-clamped so that most of the intercostal arteries are perfused while the proximal anastomosis is performed **(C).** The tube graft is then sutured into position proximally after the intercostal arteries are oversewn above T7. **D,** The clamp is moved to the tube graft and the distal anastomosis is completed. If an intercostal artery patch has been reattached, the clamp is moved to below the intercostal arteries so that a segmental repair can be made, with a shorter period of ischemia to the spinal cord. (From Svensson LG, Crawford ES. Curr Probl Surg 1993;30:1–172.)

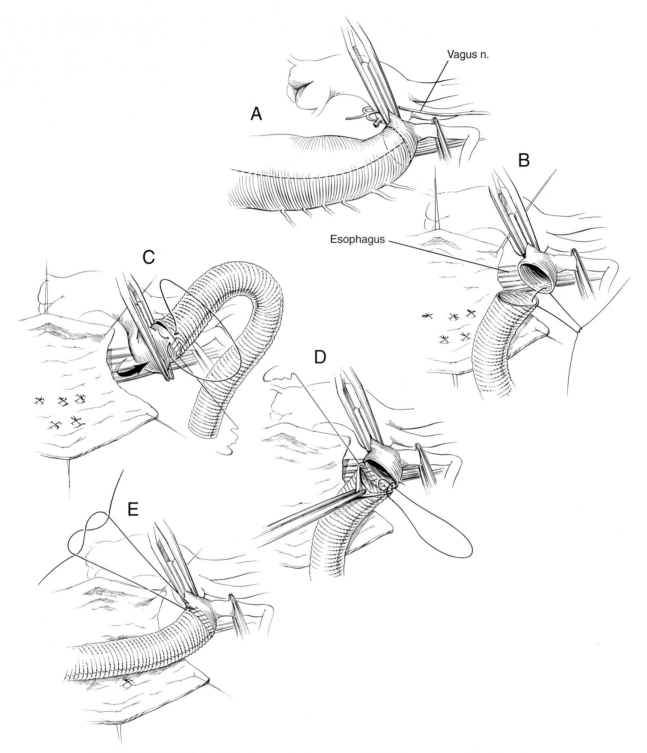

FIGURE 19–8 Technique for the proximal anastomosis of either a descending thoracic or thoracoabdominal repair at the left subclavian artery. **A,** The aorta is cross-clamped between the left common carotid and left subclavian arteries, and the left subclavian artery is also clamped. The vagus nerve is preserved by medial retraction. The recurrent nerve is also identified and preserved where it wraps around the lower margin of the atretic ductus arteriosis. The *dotted lines* mark the incisions. **B,** After transection of the proximal aorta, the esophagus lying posteromedially is noted. The upper intercostals are oversewn, and then the anastomosis is started on the posterior aspect of the outer curve of the aorta. **C,** The posteromedial suture line is first performed; in this illustration it is done by suturing forehand on the outside, but it can also be done by suturing forehand within the aorta. **D,** The anterolateral aspect of the anastomosis is then completed with a running forehand stitch. **E,** The knot is then tied on the medial aspect. (From Svensson LG, Crawford ES. Curr Probl Surg 1993;30: 1–172.)

constricted because of the danger that lung infarction could occur. More recently, one of us (L.G.S.) has recommended the use of a heat exchanger in the circuit to cool the patient with atriofemoral bypass and a heat exchanger to warm the patient after aortic unclamping.[1]

The aorta is cross-clamped at a convenient site. The aorta at the proximal suture line is then transected, and the chosen tube graft is held in position with a 3-0 Prolene suture. This is conveniently done by tying the suture at the posterior outer curve of the aorta for proximal descending anastomoses and then running it along the posterior anastomosis in a forehand manner. This can be done from inside the anastomosis or from the outside with the graft retracted over the patient's upper incision. The anterior suture line is then completed with a running forehand suture and tied to the other end at the medial margin of the aorta. When the proximal anastomosis is more distal, however, it is more convenient to start the suture line at the medial margin and run the posterior suture line to the outer lateral edge of the aorta. The distal aorta is then transected and the distal

suture line is constructed. This is usually best done by starting at the medial margin, with the posterior wall sutured first, followed by the anterior part of the anastomosis. Care should be taken when the anastomoses are sutured that the esophagus, bronchus, and recurrent laryngeal nerves are not damaged during the repair.

THORACOABDOMINAL AORTIC REPAIR

The operative technique for thoracoabdominal aneurysms was developed by one of us (E.S.C.) (Fig. 19–9)[2-7] to simplify the operative technique previously described by Etheredge and colleagues[8] and DeBakey and colleagues.[9] In our review of 1509 patients, the operative technique appears to be safe and durable.[1] More recently, the results have become even better with a 30-day mortality rate of 4% for type I and II aneurysms.[10, 11] In the experience of one of us (L.G.S.) during the last 2 years in a series of 26 patients with distal

FIGURE 19–9   **A,** Diagram and anteroposterior angiogram of the first patient in whom the senior author (E.S.C.) performed a thoracoabdominal repair by the inclusion technique. **B,** Left anterior oblique view. The left renal artery was reattached with a separate tube graft, and the ostia of the other visceral arteries were reattached as separate anastomoses. To save time, more often these are usually now done as a single Carrel patch with three or four of the visceral arteries arising from the patch.

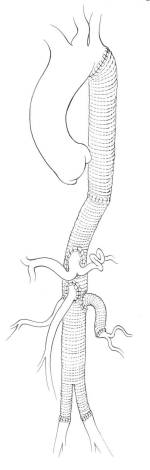
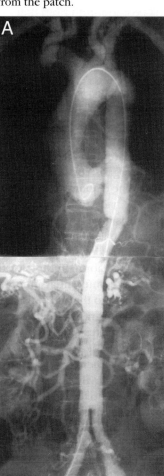
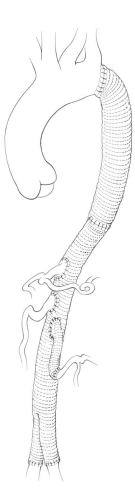
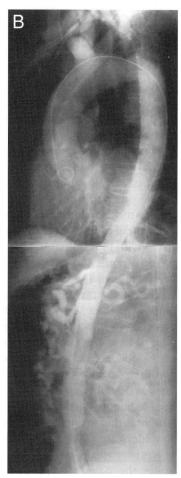

the end of it can be inserted over the fifth rib and the scapula and then pulled upward to hook over a sterile anesthetic screen. Next the lower rib margin is held outward by means of a vertical bar with a connected horizontal bar running the length of the lower rib. The second option is to use a flexible wishbone retractor to spread the chest incision. The third alternative is to use two retractor sets with two wishbones (one for the chest and one for the abdomen). A flexible retractor is used to keep the abdominal contents from falling back while the spleen is shielded with a large abdominal towel.[1, 17, 18]

The atrial inflow of the atriofemoral bypass is inserted as described, and flow is commenced as soon as the femoral artery is cannulated. For gentle mobilization of the proximal aorta, the remnant of the atretic ductus arteriosus is divided; this preserves the recurrent laryngeal nerve and frees up the vagus nerve. Care should be taken not to perforate the posterior distal arch while the aorta between the left carotid and left subclavian arteries is being mobilized. The aorta is also encircled at a point where it narrows more distally, usually at the diaphragm, so that a clamp can be temporarily placed there while the proximal aorta is repaired and atriofemoral bypass is used to perfuse the kidneys and lower abdominal aorta. The aorta is also encircled at the bifurcation, with care taken not to damage the inferior vena cava and iliac veins lying posterior to the aorta. No umbilical tapes are passed around the aorta, since they tend to get caught in the clamps and may be accidentally sutured into

FIGURE 19–11 Steps for repair of a type II thoracoabdominal aortic aneurysm. **A,** The line of incision for a thoracoabdominal aortic repair. **B,** If distal aortic perfusion is not being used, the aorta is cross-clamped proximally and distally or at the iliac arteries and the aorta is transected circumferentially. **C,** The intercostal arteries at levels T3 to T6 are oversewn and those below are preserved. Cannulae can be placed in the lower intercostal arteries, but care must be taken that the arteries are not damaged and that the catheters are not sewn in position. The visceral arteries are also cannulated and the renal arteries are injected with cold Ringer's solution to cool the kidneys. **D,** After completion of the proximal anastomosis, the clamp is moved onto the graft and the intercostal arteries are reattached. **E,** The visceral arteries are then reattached; often, as in this illustration, the superior mesenteric, celiac, and right renal arteries are attached as one Carrel patch and the left renal artery as a separate anastomosis. The distal anastomosis is then performed. When atriofemoral bypass is being used and a segmental repair can be performed, then a short segment of the proximal descending thoracic aorta is cross-clamped while the atriofemoral bypass perfuses the more distal intercostal arteries and the proximal anastomosis is performed. After the proximal anastomosis is completed, the intercostal arteries are reattached and then reperfused by clamping below the intercostal patch. While the intercostal arteries are being reattached, the visceral arteries are perfused by means of a clamp immediately above the celiac artery. After completion of the visceral artery repair, they are reperfused from proximally while the distal anastomosis is completed. Our studies with hydrogen and intrathecal platinum electrodes have clearly shown that intercostal blood flow to the spinal cord can be maintained for a large part of the repair if a segmental arterial repair is used. (From Svensson LG, Crawford ES. Curr Probl Surg 1993;30:1-172.)

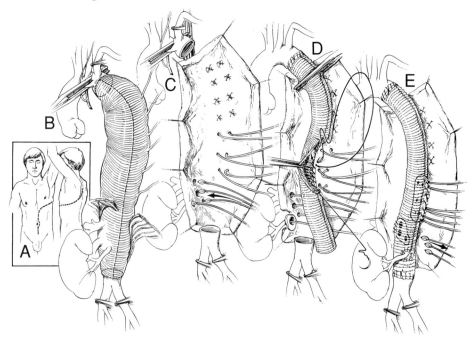

constricted because of the danger that lung infarction could occur. More recently, one of us (L.G.S.) has recommended the use of a heat exchanger in the circuit to cool the patient with atriofemoral bypass and a heat exchanger to warm the patient after aortic unclamping.[1]

The aorta is cross-clamped at a convenient site. The aorta at the proximal suture line is then transected, and the chosen tube graft is held in position with a 3-0 Prolene suture. This is conveniently done by tying the suture at the posterior outer curve of the aorta for proximal descending anastomoses and then running it along the posterior anastomosis in a forehand manner. This can be done from inside the anastomosis or from the outside with the graft retracted over the patient's upper incision. The anterior suture line is then completed with a running forehand suture and tied to the other end at the medial margin of the aorta. When the proximal anastomosis is more distal, however, it is more convenient to start the suture line at the medial margin and run the posterior suture line to the outer lateral edge of the aorta. The distal aorta is then transected and the distal

suture line is constructed. This is usually best done by starting at the medial margin, with the posterior wall sutured first, followed by the anterior part of the anastomosis. Care should be taken when the anastomoses are sutured that the esophagus, bronchus, and recurrent laryngeal nerves are not damaged during the repair.

THORACOABDOMINAL AORTIC REPAIR

The operative technique for thoracoabdominal aneurysms was developed by one of us (E.S.C.) (Fig. 19–9)[2-7] to simplify the operative technique previously described by Etheredge and colleagues[8] and DeBakey and colleagues.[9] In our review of 1509 patients, the operative technique appears to be safe and durable.[1] More recently, the results have become even better with a 30-day mortality rate of 4% for type I and II aneurysms.[10, 11] In the experience of one of us (L.G.S.) during the last 2 years in a series of 26 patients with distal

FIGURE 19–9   **A,** Diagram and anteroposterior angiogram of the first patient in whom the senior author (E.S.C.) performed a thoracoabdominal repair by the inclusion technique. **B,** Left anterior oblique view. The left renal artery was reattached with a separate tube graft, and the ostia of the other visceral arteries were reattached as separate anastomoses. To save time, more often these are usually now done as a single Carrel patch with three or four of the visceral arteries arising from the patch.

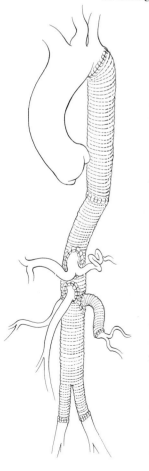
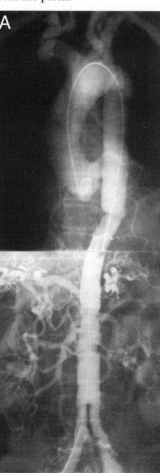
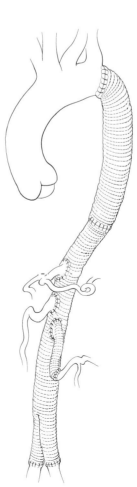
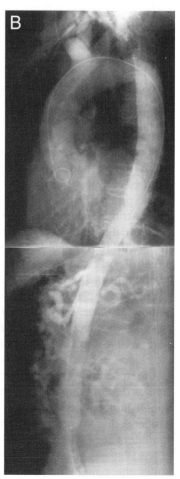

the end of it can be inserted over the fifth rib and the scapula and then pulled upward to hook over a sterile anesthetic screen. Next the lower rib margin is held outward by means of a vertical bar with a connected horizontal bar running the length of the lower rib. The second option is to use a flexible wishbone retractor to spread the chest incision. The third alternative is to use two retractor sets with two wishbones (one for the chest and one for the abdomen). A flexible retractor is used to keep the abdominal contents from falling back while the spleen is shielded with a large abdominal towel.[1, 17, 18]

The atrial inflow of the atriofemoral bypass is inserted as described, and flow is commenced as soon as the femoral artery is cannulated. For gentle mobilization of the proximal aorta, the remnant of the atretic ductus arteriosus is divided; this preserves the recurrent laryngeal nerve and frees up the vagus nerve. Care should be taken not to perforate the posterior distal arch while the aorta between the left carotid and left subclavian arteries is being mobilized. The aorta is also encircled at a point where it narrows more distally, usually at the diaphragm, so that a clamp can be temporarily placed there while the proximal aorta is repaired and atriofemoral bypass is used to perfuse the kidneys and lower abdominal aorta. The aorta is also encircled at the bifurcation, with care taken not to damage the inferior vena cava and iliac veins lying posterior to the aorta. No umbilical tapes are passed around the aorta, since they tend to get caught in the clamps and may be accidentally sutured into

FIGURE 19–11 Steps for repair of a type II thoracoabdominal aortic aneurysm. **A,** The line of incision for a thoracoabdominal aortic repair. **B,** If distal aortic perfusion is not being used, the aorta is cross-clamped proximally and distally or at the iliac arteries and the aorta is transected circumferentially. **C,** The intercostal arteries at levels T3 to T6 are oversewn and those below are preserved. Cannulae can be placed in the lower intercostal arteries, but care must be taken that the arteries are not damaged and that the catheters are not sewn in position. The visceral arteries are also cannulated and the renal arteries are injected with cold Ringer's solution to cool the kidneys. **D,** After completion of the proximal anastomosis, the clamp is moved onto the graft and the intercostal arteries are reattached. **E,** The visceral arteries are then reattached; often, as in this illustration, the superior mesenteric, celiac, and right renal arteries are attached as one Carrel patch and the left renal artery as a separate anastomosis. The distal anastomosis is then performed. When atriofemoral bypass is being used and a segmental repair can be performed, then a short segment of the proximal descending thoracic aorta is cross-clamped while the atriofemoral bypass perfuses the more distal intercostal arteries and the proximal anastomosis is performed. After the proximal anastomosis is completed, the intercostal arteries are reattached and then reperfused by clamping below the intercostal patch. While the intercostal arteries are being reattached, the visceral arteries are perfused by means of a clamp immediately above the celiac artery. After completion of the visceral artery repair, they are reperfused from proximally while the distal anastomosis is completed. Our studies with hydrogen and intrathecal platinum electrodes have clearly shown that intercostal blood flow to the spinal cord can be maintained for a large part of the repair if a segmental arterial repair is used. (From Svensson LG, Crawford ES. Curr Probl Surg 1993;30:1–172.)

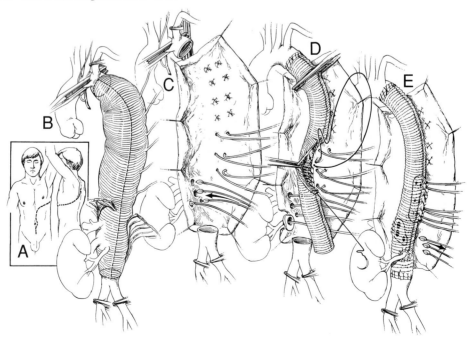

constricted because of the danger that lung infarction could occur. More recently, one of us (L.G.S.) has recommended the use of a heat exchanger in the circuit to cool the patient with atriofemoral bypass and a heat exchanger to warm the patient after aortic unclamping.[1]

The aorta is cross-clamped at a convenient site. The aorta at the proximal suture line is then transected, and the chosen tube graft is held in position with a 3-0 Prolene suture. This is conveniently done by tying the suture at the posterior outer curve of the aorta for proximal descending anastomoses and then running it along the posterior anastomosis in a forehand manner. This can be done from inside the anastomosis or from the outside with the graft retracted over the patient's upper incision. The anterior suture line is then completed with a running forehand suture and tied to the other end at the medial margin of the aorta. When the proximal anastomosis is more distal, however, it is more convenient to start the suture line at the medial margin and run the posterior suture line to the outer lateral edge of the aorta. The distal aorta is then transected and the distal

suture line is constructed. This is usually best done by starting at the medial margin, with the posterior wall sutured first, followed by the anterior part of the anastomosis. Care should be taken when the anastomoses are sutured that the esophagus, bronchus, and recurrent laryngeal nerves are not damaged during the repair.

THORACOABDOMINAL AORTIC REPAIR

The operative technique for thoracoabdominal aneurysms was developed by one of us (E.S.C.) (Fig. 19–9)[2-7] to simplify the operative technique previously described by Etheredge and colleagues[8] and DeBakey and colleagues.[9] In our review of 1509 patients, the operative technique appears to be safe and durable.[1] More recently, the results have become even better with a 30-day mortality rate of 4% for type I and II aneurysms.[10, 11] In the experience of one of us (L.G.S.) during the last 2 years in a series of 26 patients with distal

FIGURE 19–9   **A,** Diagram and anteroposterior angiogram of the first patient in whom the senior author (E.S.C.) performed a thoracoabdominal repair by the inclusion technique. **B,** Left anterior oblique view. The left renal artery was reattached with a separate tube graft, and the ostia of the other visceral arteries were reattached as separate anastomoses. To save time, more often these are usually now done as a single Carrel patch with three or four of the visceral arteries arising from the patch.

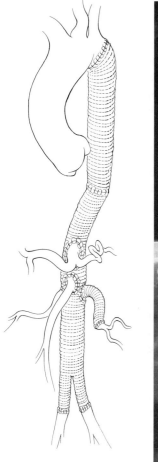
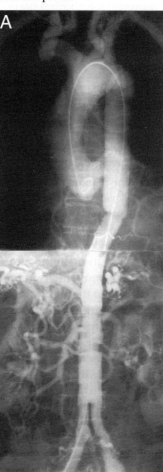
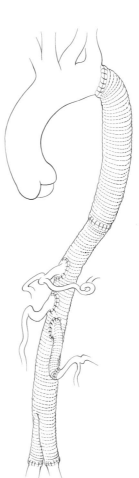
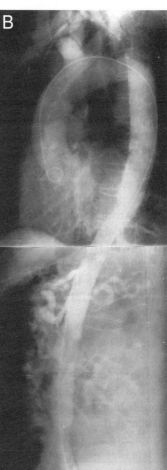

the end of it can be inserted over the fifth rib and the scapula and then pulled upward to hook over a sterile anesthetic screen. Next the lower rib margin is held outward by means of a vertical bar with a connected horizontal bar running the length of the lower rib. The second option is to use a flexible wishbone retractor to spread the chest incision. The third alternative is to use two retractor sets with two wishbones (one for the chest and one for the abdomen). A flexible retractor is used to keep the abdominal contents from falling back while the spleen is shielded with a large abdominal towel.[1, 17, 18]

The atrial inflow of the atriofemoral bypass is inserted as described, and flow is commenced as soon as the femoral artery is cannulated. For gentle mobilization of the proximal aorta, the remnant of the atretic ductus arteriosus is divided; this preserves the recurrent laryngeal nerve and frees up the vagus nerve. Care should be taken not to perforate the posterior distal arch while the aorta between the left carotid and left subclavian arteries is being mobilized. The aorta is also encircled at a point where it narrows more distally, usually at the diaphragm, so that a clamp can be temporarily placed there while the proximal aorta is repaired and atriofemoral bypass is used to perfuse the kidneys and lower abdominal aorta. The aorta is also encircled at the bifurcation, with care taken not to damage the inferior vena cava and iliac veins lying posterior to the aorta. No umbilical tapes are passed around the aorta, since they tend to get caught in the clamps and may be accidentally sutured into

FIGURE 19–11 Steps for repair of a type II thoracoabdominal aortic aneurysm. **A,** The line of incision for a thoracoabdominal aortic repair. **B,** If distal aortic perfusion is not being used, the aorta is cross-clamped proximally and distally or at the iliac arteries and the aorta is transected circumferentially. **C,** The intercostal arteries at levels T3 to T6 are oversewn and those below are preserved. Cannulae can be placed in the lower intercostal arteries, but care must be taken that the arteries are not damaged and that the catheters are not sewn in position. The visceral arteries are also cannulated and the renal arteries are injected with cold Ringer's solution to cool the kidneys. **D,** After completion of the proximal anastomosis, the clamp is moved onto the graft and the intercostal arteries are reattached. **E,** The visceral arteries are then reattached; often, as in this illustration, the superior mesenteric, celiac, and right renal arteries are attached as one Carrel patch and the left renal artery as a separate anastomosis. The distal anastomosis is then performed. When atriofemoral bypass is being used and a segmental repair can be performed, then a short segment of the proximal descending thoracic aorta is cross-clamped while the atriofemoral bypass perfuses the more distal intercostal arteries and the proximal anastomosis is performed. After the proximal anastomosis is completed, the intercostal arteries are reattached and then reperfused by clamping below the intercostal patch. While the intercostal arteries are being reattached, the visceral arteries are perfused by means of a clamp immediately above the celiac artery. After completion of the visceral artery repair, they are reperfused from proximally while the distal anastomosis is completed. Our studies with hydrogen and intrathecal platinum electrodes have clearly shown that intercostal blood flow to the spinal cord can be maintained for a large part of the repair if a segmental arterial repair is used. (From Svensson LG, Crawford ES. Curr Probl Surg 1993;30:1–172.)

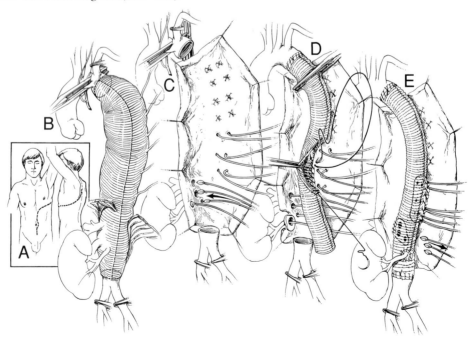

FIGURE 19–12 Steps in the insertion of a graft for a type IV thoracoabdominal aortic aneurysm. The distal descending aorta is cross-clamped above the diaphragm, and the proximal anastomosis is performed. The visceral arteries are then implanted, in this case with a separate hole for the celiac and superior mesenteric arteries, and separate holes for each of the left and right renal arteries. The distal anastomosis is then performed.

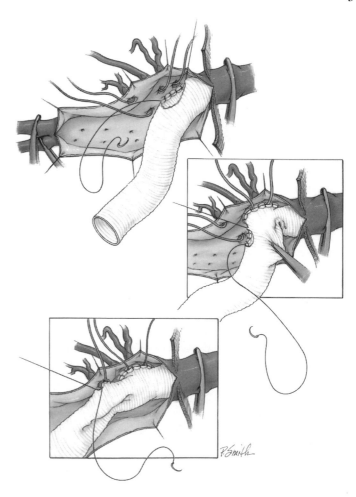

the anastomosis, particularly if the tapes are proximally placed around the aorta. The anesthesiologist should be informed when the aorta is ready to be cross-clamped. After appropriate preparations by the anesthesiologist (see previous discussion in Chapter 16) the aorta is gently cross-clamped between the left carotid and subclavian arteries (Figs. 19–9 to 19–11), with close attention paid to the proximal pressures. The anesthesiologist should palpate the left carotid artery in the neck to check for continued perfusion of the brain. The aorta is then cross-clamped distally at the most convenient site. Next electrocautery is used to open the lumen. The proximal aorta is then transected just distal to the left subclavian artery. The aorta should be completely transected so that no lumina are missed on the medial side of the aorta, particularly with aortic dissection. This exposes the esophagus, which is protected. More posteriorly, lower, and deeper is the left main bronchus. If bleeding is excessive from the segmental intercostal arteries, particularly if atriofemoral bypass is being used, then the intercostal arteries from the level of the aortic transection to the level of T7 (first intercostal space below the incision) should be oversewn. The handling of segmental arteries under a novel experimental protocol that we are conducting with the use of hydrogen[19] has been discussed.

The insertion of the atriofemoral bypass pump and the construction of the proximal anastomosis are described above. The repair is performed in a sequential manner with the aorta up to the proximal anastomosis being perfused, whenever possible, while this anastomosis is constructed. The clamp is then moved more distally, usually above the celiac artery, the aorta is opened, and the intercostal arteries are exposed. Although we have found the use of hydrogen to identify which arteries supply the spinal cord both accurate and useful, this is an experimental technique that is used at this stage if planned.[19, 22] For most patients, the intercostal arteries up to and including T6 are oversewn and those below are reattached to the new graft.[10, 19, 20, 22] This should result in reattachment of the lower thoracic radicular arteries and the arteria radicularis magna to reperfuse the spinal cord (see Chapter 15). In patients with degenerative type aneurysms, the number of patent segmental intercostal or lumbar arteries are, however, less than those of patients with aortic dissection and thus reattachment of aortic patches with segmental arteries is usually not as extensive.[1, 17, 18]

The part of the graft with reattached segmental arteries is then reperfused, and the visceral repair is performed. The four major arteries are identified, inspected, and checked for emboli since there is often extensive thrombus formation around the arteries. A perfusion catheter is placed in each renal artery, and then cold Ringer's lactate solution is injected to cool the kidney. We have also used cooling pads from outside the kidney to protect it and temperature probes in the kidney to check for the renal temperature. In our initial study[23] of renal function after descending thoracic or thoracoabdominal aneurysm repairs, we were unable to show that either cooling or bypass protected the kidneys. However, in later studies[1, 16, 24] with more statistical power, we have found that both atriofemoral bypass and cooling of the kidneys are protective.[1, 17, 18]

Greater care should be taken in the reanastomosis of the visceral arteries, particularly since occlusive disease at the ostia or atherosclerotic material increases the risk of end-organ embolization or dysfunction. When occlusive disease of the visceral arteries (either total occlusion or stenosis) is present, repair is usually required.[16] Stenoses at the origin of the visceral arteries should be treated with endarterectomy, even if the stenosis is causing no apparent symptoms,[16] because an early intervention is prudent and the procedure is easy to perform. Total occlusion or distal stenoses of the renal arteries with preserved renal size or with renal dysfunction is best treated by suturing Dacron 8 mm bypass grafts to the distal uninvolved arteries.[16] Similarly, symptomatic distal stenoses of the superior mesenteric artery should be treated with the use of Dacron tube grafts. If only the celiac artery is totally occluded or distally stenotic and the patient has no symptoms then usually no bypasses are performed for the celiac artery.[16] The reason for this is that it is most uncommon for a single occluded celiac artery to cause symptoms or postoperative problems. When a bypass is needed for the left renal artery, this can simply be performed from the aortic prosthesis to the renal artery. For the right renal artery, 8 mm bypass grafts are anastomosed end-to-side to the iliac artery and then end-to-end to the right renal artery, which is exposed by a Kocher maneuver.[16]

Once the visceral repair has been performed, the clamp is moved to below the visceral arteries to reperfuse them and the distal aortic anastomosis is done either at the aortic bifurcation or, if necessary, at the external iliac or femoral arteries with a bifurcated graft. After hemostasis is obtained, the aorta is loosely wrapped over the graft and the incisions are closed.

INFRARENAL AORTIC AND JUXTARENAL AORTIC REPAIR OF ANEURYSMS

For both infrarenal and juxtarenal aortic repairs of aneurysms, the aorta is exposed through a midline incision. For complex repairs, a left thoracoabdominal incision or even a right retroperitoneal exposure can be used.[25] An exploratory laparotomy is performed, particularly to check for undiagnosed malignant lesions, gallstones, and patency of the superior mesenteric artery. Manipulation of the aneurysm is kept to a minimal amount until the aneurysm is clamped off. To expose the aneurysm the transverse colon is reflected over the chest wall and the small intestine

is reflected over to the right of the patient. The duodenum is mobilized to the right, the aorta is exposed anteriorly and laterally below the renal arteries, and the proximal iliac arteries are identified below the aneurysm. No attempt is made to encircle either the aorta proximally or the iliac arteries. Sometimes the inferior mesenteric vein may have to be ligated to improve exposure. The iliac arteries are clamped with vascular clamps, and then the aorta is clamped below the renal arteries with a vertically placed Crafoord clamp. The aorta is next opened with the use of electrocautery. If the iliac arteries are calcified, no attempt should be made to clamp them, and they must be allowed to back-bleed freely. The back-bleeding will fall to a minimal rate within a few minutes. No heparin is usually administered. The aorta is transected around two thirds of the circumference, for both the proximal and distal anastomoses, and a tube graft is selected for insertion. Bleeding lumbar arteries are oversewn, as is the origin of the inferior mesenteric artery in most patients. In patients with no middle colic artery, a history of transverse colectomy (Figs. 19-13 and 19-14), an occluded superior mesenteric artery, or intraoperative damage to the middle colic artery,[26] the inferior mesenteric artery is usually anastomosed to the graft as a Carrel patch.[27] The tube graft is then inserted with a running 3-0 Prolene suture, starting usually posterolaterally for both the proximal and distal anastomoses. Before the suture is tied down distally, the graft is flushed by alternate release of the angled vascular clamps and then the aortic clamp. Next the suture is tied down and all the clamps are released. The aneurysm wall and fatty material in the vicinity are used to reperitonealize the aorta, and the abdomen is closed in a routine manner. With this technique, the procedure can be carried out within 40 minutes skin-to-skin.[18]

For patients with juxtarenal or suprarenal aneurysms, the infradiaphragmatic aorta is exposed by separation of the crura of the diaphragm just to the right of the midline of the aorta (Figs. 19-15 and 19-16). The aorta is then clamped at this position until the proximal aortic anastomosis has been performed, and then the graft is clamped below the proximal anastomosis. Any tube grafts that have to be placed to other visceral arteries can be taken off the infrarenal aorta as illustrated (Fig. 19-17).[18]

Patients with ruptured aneurysms of the infrarenal aorta are taken at once to the operating room, where the abdomen is rapidly opened immediately after the induction of anesthesia (Fig. 19-18).[28] The abdominal aorta must be quickly clamped at the diaphragm, and thereafter, resuscitation of the patient commences with the insertion of venous access catheters.[28] There should be no delay in getting hemodynamically unstable patients to surgery, and there should be no attempt at resuscitation until the aorta has been clamped. Once the proximal anastomosis is completed, the clamp is moved to below the anastomosis on the aortic graft.[28] The remaining procedure is performed as described above. We do not favor clamping the thoracic aorta through a left thoracotomy because bleeding from the collateral

Text continued on page 358

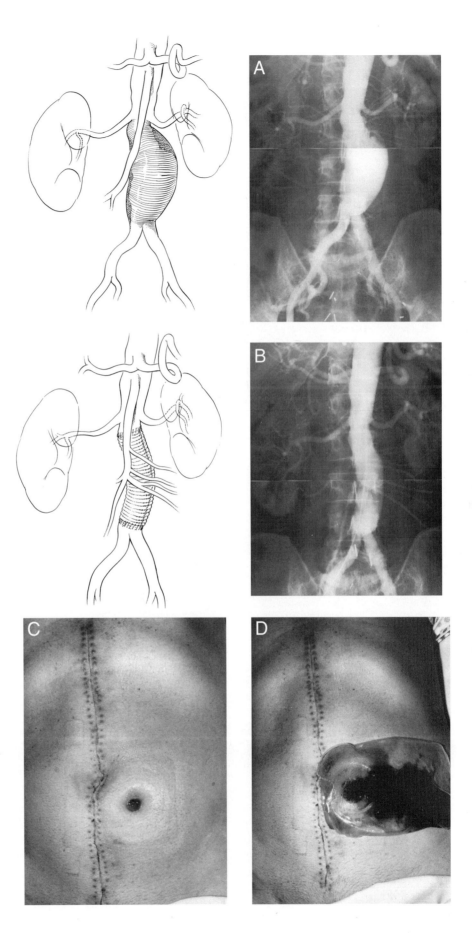

FIGURE 19–13 Preoperative diagram and arteriogram (**A**) and postoperative illustrations (**B**) after infrarenal abdominal aneurysm repair in a patient who had previously undergone a colectomy. **C,** The patient had no wound complications and (**D**) the colostomy bag was clear of the incision.

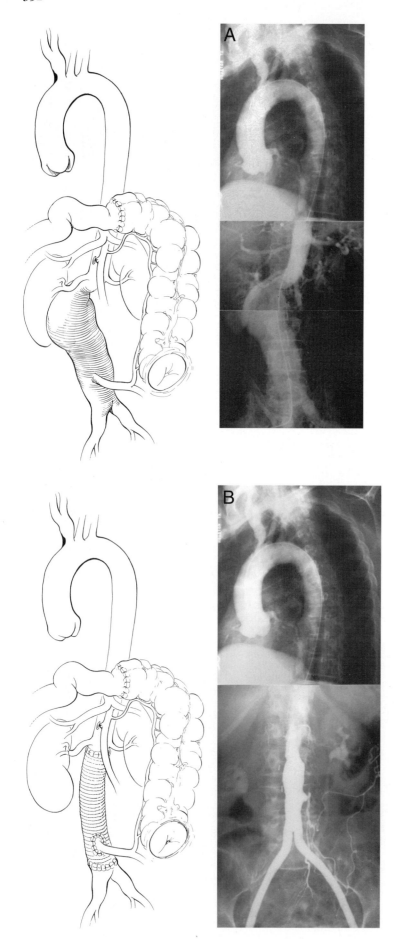

FIGURE 19–14 **A,** Diagram and arteriogram of a patient who had previously undergone a colectomy and who now presented with an infrarenal abdominal aortic aneurysm. **B,** Postoperative diagram and arteriogram after reimplantation of the inferior mesenteric artery into the infrarenal graft.

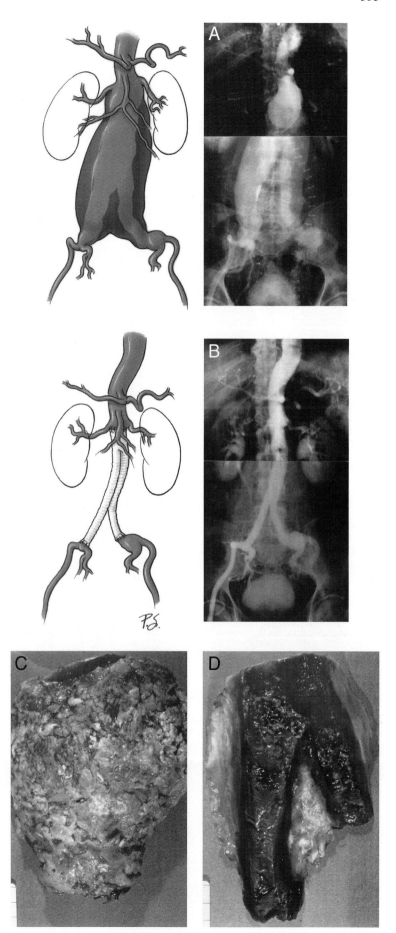

FIGURE 19–15 Steps in the repair of a juxtarenal abdominal aortic aneurysm. **A,** Preoperative aortogram of a patient who had been explored elsewhere (note skin clips) for a juxtarenal abdominal aortic aneurysm. **B,** Postoperative arteriogram after insertion of a bifurcated graft. **C,** Photograph shows the clot removed from the aorta and **(D)** the aortic bifurcation.

Illustration continued on following page

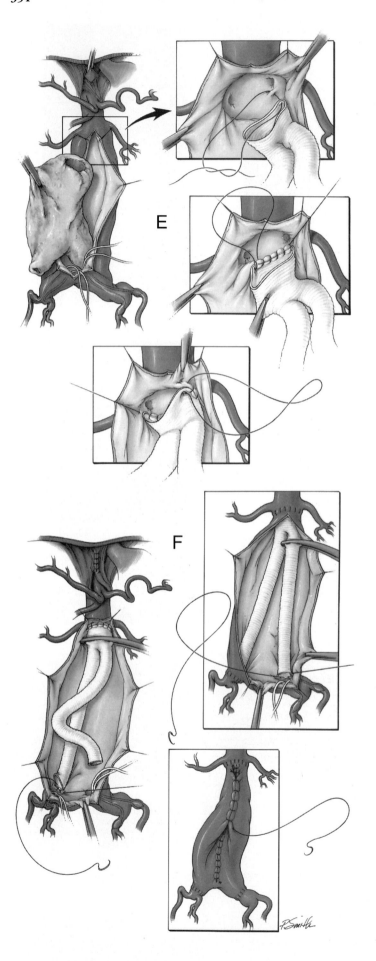

E

F

FIGURE 19–15 *Continued* **E,** The aorta is first cross-clamped at the diaphragm and opened, and the clot lining the aneurysm is removed. The graft is then sutured into position below the renal arteries, with care taken to preserve the renal ostia. A right-angled clamp is useful for checking patency of the arteries. The posterior and anterior suture lines are then completed. **F,** The graft is then clamped below the renal arteries, reestablishing blood flow to the kidneys, and the distal anastomoses are performed with the graft finally being wrapped with the old aneurysm wall.

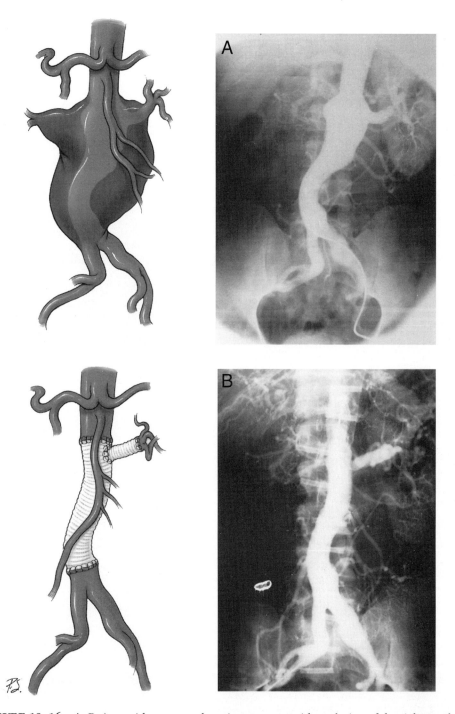

FIGURE 19–16   A, Patient with suprarenal aortic aneurysm with occlusion of the right renal artery. **B,** The aneurysm was repaired with supraceliac aortic cross-clamping and placement of an aortic tube graft with a separate graft to the left renal artery.

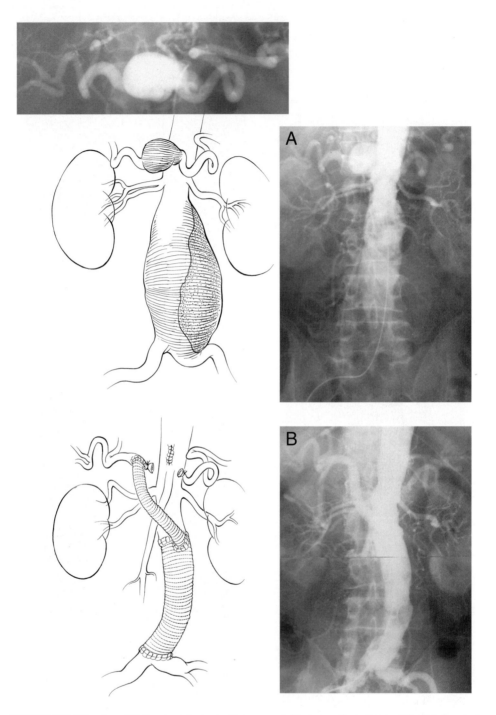

FIGURE 19–17   **A** and **B,** Preoperative arteriogram and diagrams of a patient with an infrarenal aneurysm and celiac artery aneurysm treated with infrarenal aortic repair and insertion of a tube graft to the artery with ligation of the splenic artery.

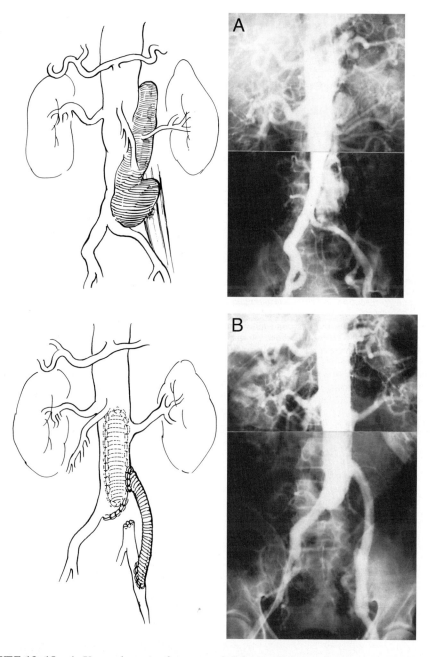

FIGURE 19–18 **A,** Unusual repair of a ruptured abdominal aortic aneurysm as seen on aortography with extension of the tear above the left renal artery. **B,** The tear was repaired with a patch, and a separate tube graft was placed to the left iliac artery

blood supply to the distal aorta will frequently continue to occur at the site of the ruptured aorta.[17, 18]

REFERENCES

1. Svensson LG, Crawford ES, Hess KR, et al. Experience with 1509 patients undergoing thoracoabdominal aortic operations. J Vasc Surg 1993;17:357-70.
2. Crawford ES. Thoracoabdominal and abdominal aortic aneurysm involving renal, superior mesenteric, and celiac arteries. Ann Surg 1974;179:763-72.
3. Crawford ES, Morris GC, Myhre HO, Roehm JO Jr. Celiac axis, superior mesenteric artery occlusion: surgical considerations. Surgery 1977;82:856-66.
4. Crawford ES, Snyder DM, Cho GC, et al. Progress in treatment of thoraco-abdominal and abdominal aortic aneurysms involving celiac, superior mesenteric, and renal arteries. Ann Surg 1978;188:404-22.
5. Crawford ES, Crawford JL. Diseases of the Aorta: Including an Atlas of Angiographic Pathology and Surgical Technique. Baltimore: Williams & Wilkins, 1984.
6. Crawford ES, Crawford JL, Safi HJ, et al. Thoracoabdominal aortic aneurysms: preoperative and intraoperative factors determining immediate and long-term results of operation in 605 patients. J Vasc Surg 1986;3:389-404.
7. Crawford ES, DeNatale RW. Thoracoabdominal aortic aneurysm: observations regarding the natural course of the disease. J Vasc Surg 1986;3:578-82.
8. Etheredge SN, Yee J, Smith JV, et al. Successful resection of a large aneurysm of the upper abdominal aorta and replacement with homograft. Surgery 1955;38:1071-81.
9. DeBakey ME, Creech O, Morris GC. Aneurysm of thoracoabdominal aorta involving the celiac, superior mesenteric, and renal arteries: report of four cases treated by resection and homograft replacement. Ann Surg 1956;144:549-73.
10. Svensson LG, Hess KR, Coselli JS, Safi HR. Influence of segmental arteries, extent, and atriofemoral bypass on postoperative paraplegia after thoracoabdominal aortic aneurysm repairs. J Vasc Surg 1994;20:255-62.
11. Crawford ES, Svensson LG, Hess KR, et al. A prospective randomized study of cerebrospinal fluid drainage to prevent paraplegia after high-risk surgery on the thoracoabdominal aorta. J Vasc Surg 1991;13:36-45.
12. Svensson LG, Shahian DM, Davis FG, et al. Replacement of entire aorta from aortic valve to bifurcation during one operation. Ann Thorac Surg 1994;58:1164-6.
13. Crawford ES, Coselli JS, Safi HJ. Partial cardiopulmonary bypass, hypothermic circulatory arrest, and posterolateral exposure for thoracic aortic aneurysm operation. J Thorac Cardiovasc Surg 1987;94: 824-7.
14. Crawford ES, Coselli JS. Thoracoabdominal aneurysm surgery. Semin Thorac Cardiovasc Surg 1991;3:300-22.
15. Crawford ES, Hess KR, Cohen ES, et al. Ruptured aneurysm of the descending thoracic and thoracoabdominal aorta: analysis according to size and treatment. Ann Surg 1991;213:417-25.
16. Svensson LG, Crawford ES, Hess KR, et al. Thoracoabdominal aortic aneurysms associated with celiac, superior mesenteric and renal artery occlusive disease: methods and analysis of results in 271 patients. J Vasc Surg 1992;16:378-90.
17. Svensson LG, Crawford ES. Aortic dissection and aortic aneurysm surgery: clinical observations, experimental investigations, and statistical analyses. Part II. Curr Probl Surg 1992;29:915-1057.
18. Svensson LG, Crawford ES. Aortic dissection and aortic aneurysm surgery: clinical observations, experimental investigations, and statistical analyses. Part III. Curr Probl Surg 1993;30:1-172.
19. Svensson LG, Patel V, Robinson MF, et al. Influence of preservation or perfusion of intraoperatively identified spinal cord blood supply on spinal motor evoked potentials and paraplegia after aortic surgery. J Vasc Surg 1991;13:355-65.
20. Svensson LG, Crawford ES. Aneurysms involving the descending and upper abdominal aorta. Chest Clin North Am 1992;2:311-28.
21. Svensson LG, Hess KR, Coselli JS, et al. A prospective study of respiratory failure after high-risk surgery on the thoracoabdominal aorta. J Vasc Surg 1991;14:271-82.
22. Svensson LG, Patel V, Coselli JS, Crawford ES. Preliminary report of localization of spinal cord blood supply by hydrogen during aortic operations. Ann Thorac Surg 1990;49:528-35.
23. Svensson LG, Coselli JS, Safi HJ, et al. Appraisal of adjuncts to prevent acute renal failure after surgery on the thoracic or thoracoabdominal aorta. J Vasc Surg 1989;10:230-9.
24. Svensson LG, Crawford ES, Hess KR, et al. Variables predictive of outcome in 832 patients undergoing repairs of the descending thoracic aorta. Chest 1993;104:1248-53.
25. Davidson BR, Gardham R. Selective use of a right retroperitoneal approach to abdominal aortic aneurysm. Br J Surg 1992; 79:639-40.
26. Crawford ES. Symposium: prevention of complications of abdominal aortic reconstruction (Introduction). Surgery 1983;93:91-6.
27. Carrel A. Technique and remote results of vascular anastomoses. Surg Gynecol Obstet 1912;14:246.
28. Crawford ES. Ruptured abdominal aortic aneurysm [Editorial]. J Vasc Surg 1991;13:348-50.

Techniques for Dissection Involving the Distal Aorta

ACUTE DISTAL AORTIC DISSECTION

For acute distal aortic dissection, should medical therapy fail or other indications arise as discussed in Chapter 4, then it is advisable to repair the descending aorta from the proximal extent of the dissection (usually at the left subclavian artery) to where the aortic diameter is less than 4 cm. The proximal aorta should be completely transected at the left subclavian artery, with exposure of the esophagus (Fig. 20-1). This reduces the risk of a later aortoesophageal fistula developing. This also ensures that all dissected lumina are divided if extending proximal to the left subclavian artery and are not missed as illustrated previously. Similarly, it is advisable to transect the distal aorta circumferentially because this ensures that all lumina, which in the distal aorta may number more than two, will be included in the anastomosis. As with the proximal aorta, the inner elastic lumen is tacked to the outer aortic wall as described previously (Fig. 20-1) so that the blood is rerouted into the true lumen. In the acute situation, intercostal arteries are usually oversewn and not reattached because the aortic wall is very fragile and tends to tear. A soft collagen-impregnated graft or a baked woven Dacron tube graft is then inserted. A graft that is slightly smaller than the aorta (22 or 20 mm) may be preferable, because it reduces the distal pulse wave (dP/dt) and thus decreases the risk of subsequent distal aneurysm formation in the dissected aorta.[1, 2]

Atriofemoral bypass is used to reduce high proximal aortic pressures, thus lowering the risk that the aortic clamp will tear the acute dissected aorta. The distal anastomosis, however, is easier to do without clamping of the distal aorta. This also reduces the risk of the distal clamp damaging the fragile dissected aorta during manipulation. Usually the distal anastomosis is performed in the chest. However, if the aorta is aneurysmal into the abdomen, then the distal anastomosis is made to the abdominal aorta.[1, 2]

In our experience, the intraluminal ring prosthesis for the repair of either proximal or distal aortic dissection has little advantage and may, in fact, be hazardous. On one occasion the fragile aorta at the left subclavian artery was torn twice and the distal aorta was torn once when the intraluminal ring was tied into position. The prosthesis had to be removed and the patient placed on deep hypothermia with circulatory arrest so that the aorta could be replaced with a conventional tubular graft. A further problem is that, to remove all of the proximal dissected aorta at the subclavian artery, the proximal graft anastomosis has to be angled (Fig. 20-1), but this cannot be done with an intraluminal ring prosthesis. Similarly, the distal anastomosis for repair of the ascending and proximal aortic arch has to be angled (beveled), and this also cannot be done with an intraluminal graft. Nor can a proximal ring be used satisfactorily to resuspend or obliterate a proximal dissection at the commissures. In fact, the prosthesis may interfere with valve functions. On late follow-up, we[1, 3, 4] have observed many patients in whom gradients have developed across the stenotic ring prostheses; when particularly severe, this has resulted in hemolysis, heart failure, and poststenotic aneurysm formation. A carefully and meticulously inserted tube graft is far better than a ringed prosthesis, and seldom can a satisfactory ringed prosthesis be inserted in less time than a tubular graft. On late follow-up, erosion of the ring through the aortic wall is also a problem.[1, 2]

CHRONIC DISTAL AORTIC DISSECTION

Descending Thoracic Aorta

For patients who have aneurysmal involvement of only the descending thoracic aorta, the same technique is used as for acute dissection, with the exception that the distal anastomosis has to be fashioned so that both true and false lumina are perfused (Fig. 20-2). For this, a wedge is excised and fixed in position with sutures (Fig. 20-2). For dissection involvement of the left subclavian artery, an interposition graft can be inserted (Fig. 20-3). If there is concern as to whether both lumina are perfused, intraoperative transesophageal echocardiography can be performed to check for blood flow to both lumina.[1, 2]

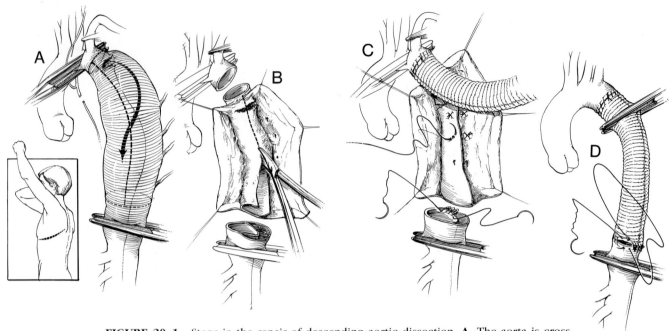

FIGURE 20–1 Steps in the repair of descending aortic dissection. **A,** The aorta is cross-clamped between the left common carotid and subclavian arteries proximally, the left subclavian artery is also clamped, and the aorta is transected. **B,** The aorta is then opened, with care taken to make sure that the true lumen is opened. This is ensured by complete transection of the aorta. **C,** In patients with acute dissection the true lumen is reapproximated to the outer adventitial layer at the distal anastomotic site. **D,** The aorta is then sutured to the aortic graft to complete the repair. (From Svensson LG, Crawford ES. Curr Probl Surg 1992;29:915–1057.)

Thoracoabdominal Aortic Repair

If the patient has had both imaging studies (computed tomography or magnetic resonance imaging) and aortography, the surgeon is well prepared for many of the potential hazards of thoracoabdominal aortic aneurysm surgery, as stated in Chapter 19. The surgeon should have a reasonable idea of whether the proximal aorta can be cross-clamped at the left carotid artery (Fig. 20–4). If not, preparation should be made for deep hypothermia and circulatory arrest, as

described previously. Similarly, if the aneurysm extends out to the chest wall or if extensive scarring is present from previous pleural effusions and leakage, then deep hypothermia and circulatory arrest may be needed before the chest can be entered. For those patients in whom the aorta is expected to be friable and prone to tear from the proximal clamp, consideration should be given to the use of circulatory arrest, since this may reduce the risk of the aorta tearing as a result of the proximal hypertension during clamping. Should tearing occur, then cardiopulmonary bypass and deep

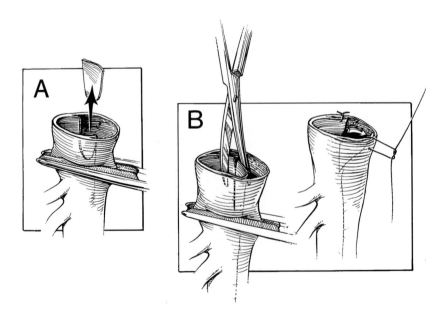

FIGURE 20–2 Management of the distal aorta in patients with chronic dissection. **A,** A wedge of the septum is excised to ensure that both the true lumen and the false lumen are perfused. Most often the false lumen perfuses the left kidney and the true lumen perfuses the other visceral organs. **B,** If, after the lumen is excised, there is concern as to whether both lumina will be perfused, the septum is tacked down to ensure that the septum does not act as a flutter valve. If the aorta is fragile, pledgeted sutures are useful for tacking the septum to the adventitia. (From Svensson LG, Crawford ES. Curr Probl Surg 1992;29:915–1057.)

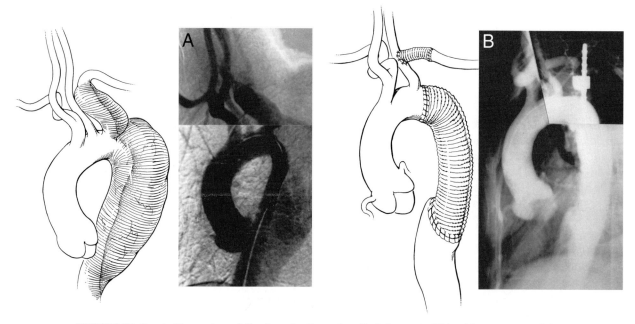

FIGURE 20–3   A, Illustration of distal aortic dissection (DeBakey type IIIa) with extension of the dissection into the left subclavian artery as far as the internal mammary artery in a patient with Marfan syndrome. In most patients with distal aortic dissection, the dissection may involve the inferior lateral aspect of the left subclavian artery, but extension for a considerable distance into the left subclavian artery is unusual. **B,** The aorta was repaired by insertion of a tube graft to repair the distal aortic arch beyond the left common carotid artery and extending into the descending aorta. The left subclavian artery was reimplanted into the left common carotid artery with an interposition graft. Note that the upper extent of a Harrington rod for correction of scoliosis is present.

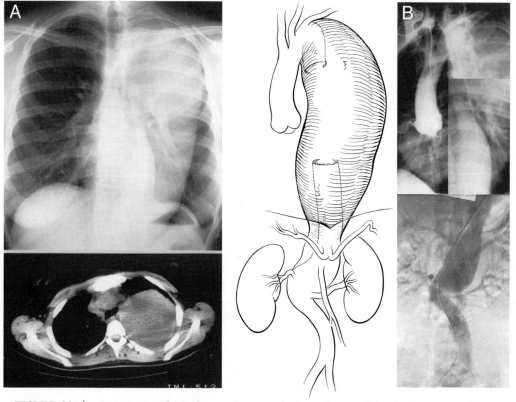

FIGURE 20–4   A, Patient with Marfan syndrome and a large thoracoabdominal aneurysm due to aortic dissection seen on the chest radiograph and CT scan. **B,** The aortogram revealed that the aorta could be cross-clamped between the left subclavian artery and the left common carotid artery and, therefore, deep hypothermia with circulatory arrest was not necessary before thoracotomy or aortic cross-clamping. (From Svensson LG, Crawford ES. Curr Probl Surg 1992;29:915–1057.)

hypothermia can be established by cannulation of the ascending aorta for arterial inflow to the upper body (the aorta would be cross-clamped and possibly open at this stage); thus blood cannot be pumped from below via the femoral artery to the brain. In those patients who have had previous proximal aortic repairs, atriofemoral bypass is usually used because of the risk of further retrograde dissection of the arch with distal repairs and because the outer adventitial aortic wall is often thin and prone to tear. The atrial cannula should be carefully inserted through an atrial pursestring with tourniquet because the pericardium will often be densely adherent to the left auricle from previous proximal aortic repairs. Alternatively, the inferior pulmonary vein can be used for outflow drainage. If atriofemoral bypass is used and the planned thoracoabdominal aortic repair is extensive, then it is wise to have two cell savers available to adequately handle the blood loss from the patent segmental arteries.[1, 2]

The repair of a thoracoabdominal aortic dissection is similar to that described in Chapter 19. However, there are usually more intercostal and lumbar arteries that are patent and that need to be reattached. The skin incision for thoracoabdominal aneurysms is aimed from the inferior margin of the left scapula toward the umbilicus with a gentle curve upward as it crosses the costal margin (Figs. 20-5 and 20-6). The sixth rib and the diaphragm are resected. The peritoneum can be reflected off the diaphragm and the rectus muscle to allow for a complete extraperitoneal and retroperitoneal repair, which is useful in patients who have undergone multiple previous intraabdominal procedure. Alternatively, the peritoneal cavity can be entered anteriorly and the bowel reflected to the right side of the patient.[5] Protection and inspection of the spleen at the end of the operation are easier with this method.[1, 2]

The atrial inflow of the atriofemoral bypass is inserted as described, and flow is commenced as soon as the femoral artery is cannulated. After the anesthesiologist has been notified (see discussion in Chapter 19), the aorta is gently cross-clamped between the left carotid and subclavian arteries (Figs. 20-5 and 20-6). Next, electrocautery is used to open the outer false lumen and the inner true lumen is opened with a pair of scissors (Figs. 20-5 and 20-6). The proximal aorta is then transected just distal to the left subclavian artery. The aorta should be completely transected so that no lumina are missed on the medial side of the aorta. This exposes the esophagus, which should be protected. More posteriorly, lower, and deeper is the left main bronchus. A baked or collagen-impregnated graft is then selected for insertion. If an extensive repair is required, then a 60 cm graft is used. The proximal end is beveled at an angle so that the toe is anastomosed at the base of the subclavian artery (Figs. 20-5 and 20-6). This allows for a wider orifice with less risk of stenosis and easier suturing of the anastomosis inside the chest. No pledgets or felt are used. After completion of the anastomosis, the graft is tested for hemostasis. The graft is placed under gentle tension and a hole that will accommodate the intercostal arteries from T6 to

T12 is excised. The reason for anastomosing these arteries is that, as discussed previously, this will ensure the likelihood that 90% of the time the arteria radicularis magna (ARM), also known as the artery of Adamkievicz, is adequately reperfused after unclamping.[1, 2] After this anastomosis has been performed, the distal aorta should be clamped either at a lower level or at the aortic bifurcation. The remaining aorta that needs repair is then opened, with care taken that all lumina are located and opened. The visceral vessels are cannulated with No. 9 balloon catheters to prevent bleeding, for the injection of cold Ringer's solution, and to aid with the exposure. Caution should be taken that the balloon catheters are not overinflated, since this can result in rupture of the vessels with retroperitoneal hemorrhage that may not be detected in time to prevent exsanguination. The visceral artery ostia are anastomosed as a patch, including the renal arteries, after excision of the dissection septum separating the ostia (Figs. 20-5 and 20-6). Occasionally, the distance between the renal arteries is excessive and the left renal artery has to be reanastomosed as a separate Carrel patch. After completion of this anastomosis, a clamp is placed on the graft below the renal arteries after air and clot have been carefully removed from the graft. The proximal clamp, which usually is below the intercostal patch, is removed so that the viscera, kidneys, and part of the spinal cord are reperfused. The remaining anastomosis is performed to the aortic bifurcation and, as described previously, adequate blood flow to both lumina must be ensured. Sometimes a bifurcated graft has to be attached and the anastomosis performed to the distal common iliac, external iliac, or femoral arteries. The external iliac artery on the right can be reached either behind the mesentery of the colon and ureters or via a counterincision to the right iliac fossa. The latter procedure is more cumbersome, however. After completion of the remaining anastomoses, all clamps are removed after timely warning to the anesthesiologist. The wound is then closed layer by layer once hemostasis has been achieved.[1, 2]

Second-Stage Elephant Trunk Procedure

This technique is different in that the proximal aorta is not cross-clamped because of the previous distal arch surgery and the distal elephant trunk lying in the descending aorta can be cross-clamped after the aorta is opened with a knife just distal to the previous suture line and the graft is identified (see previous chapters for a detailed description). Frequently clot has accumulated around the graft and thus the graft can be exposed without much bleeding. Failing that, the graft must be quickly cross-clamped. The remainder of the procedure is performed as described earlier except that there is no need to transect the proximal aorta.[1, 2]

Peripheral Vascular Procedures

We[1] are in agreement with others[6, 7] that there is little role for peripheral vascular procedures in the management of aortic dissection prior to thoracic repairs of either the proximal ascending aorta or distal dissections starting at the left subclavian artery. Rarely, as illustrated (Fig. 20-7), a patient may have a ruptured abdominal aorta from the dissection, and this must be repaired before the definitive proximal aortic repair is performed. Repair of the aortic dissection as described above will reestablish blood flow to most organs or arteries that are obstructed and thus will reverse ischemia. Therefore strokes, spinal ischemia, renal failure, and leg ischemia are best treated by repairing the aortic

lesion that has the greatest chance of resulting in recovery. This approach has the long-term advantage of reducing the risk of rupture of the dilated aneurysmal segments of the aorta. Occasionally there is the exceptional case in which percutaneous techniques are of value in a patient who is about to undergo surgery or who has had surgery and organ perfusion is still not reestablished. For example, in a patient of ours (L.G.S.) who was about to have repair of a type I acute aortic dissection and who had renal shutdown as a result of renal artery dissection, our invasive angiographers

Text continued on page 370

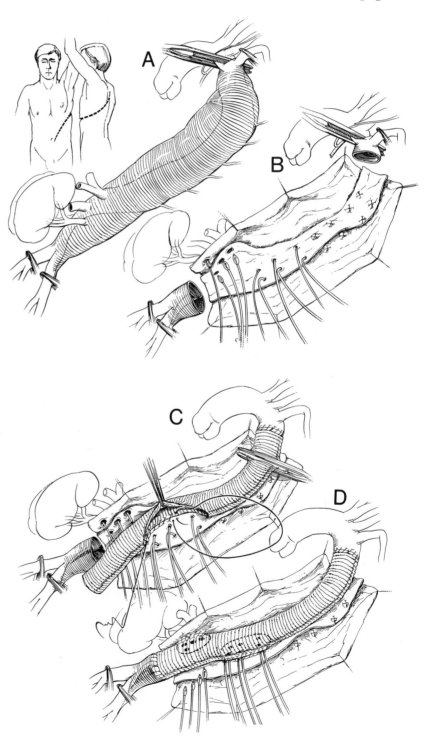

FIGURE 20–5 Steps in repair of the thoracoabdominal aorta for aortic dissection. **A,** The line of incision is indicated, with the incision aimed toward the umbilicus. The aorta is then cross-clamped as for descending aortic dissections. **B,** The upper intercostal arteries are oversewn and the intercostal arteries below T7 are preserved. **C,** The intercostal arteries are reimplanted, followed by the visceral arteries **(D),** and then the distal aortic anastomosis is performed. Whenever possible, atriofemoral bypass is used and a segmental repair is performed as described for thoracoabdominal aneurysms without aortic dissection. (From Svensson LG, Crawford ES. Curr Probl Surg 1992;29:915–1057.)

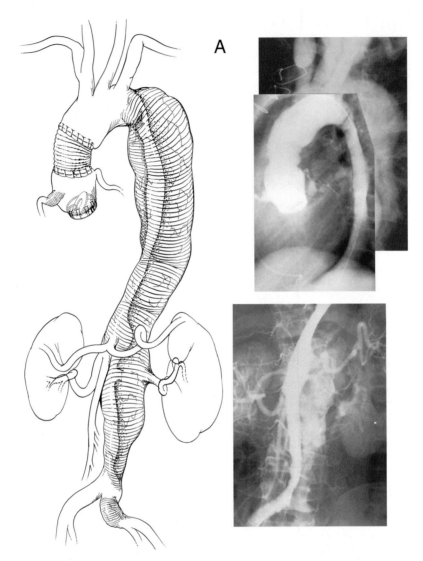

FIGURE 20–6 Illustration of a type II thoracoabdominal aneurysm repair for a distal aortic dissection. **A,** Diagram and preoperative angiogram of a patient who had previously had an ascending aorta and aortic valve replacement.

Illustration continued on following page

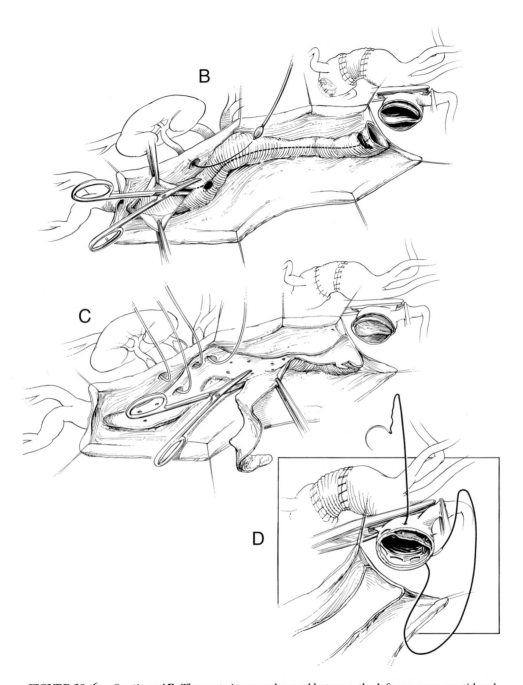

FIGURE 20–6 *Continued* **B,** The aorta is cross-clamped between the left common carotid and left subclavian arteries and then transected proximally. The false lumen is opened, and balloon catheters are placed in the visceral arteries. **C,** The septum is excised to expose all patent intercostal and lumbar arteries. **D,** If necessary (for example, in patients with type I aortic dissection), the intimal layer is tacked to the outer advential layer.

Illustration continued on following page

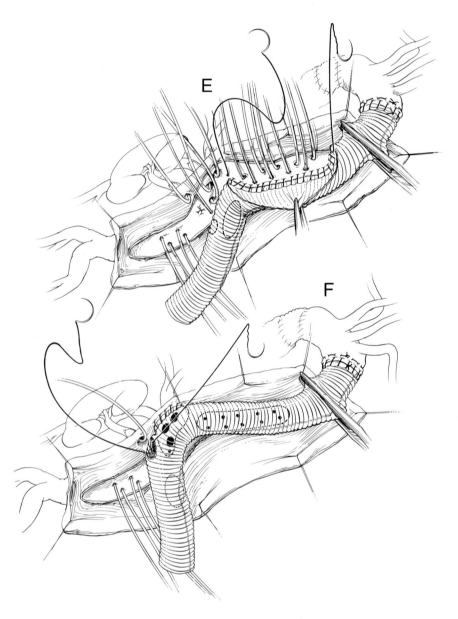

FIGURE 20–6 *Continued* **E,** After completion of the proximal anastomosis, the intercostal arteries are reattached to the graft as a patch. Catheters can be placed in the intercostal arteries to control back-bleeding, but they may damage the arteries. **F,** The visceral arteries are thereafter attached as a Carrel patch, as are any major lumbar arteries.

Illustration continued on following page

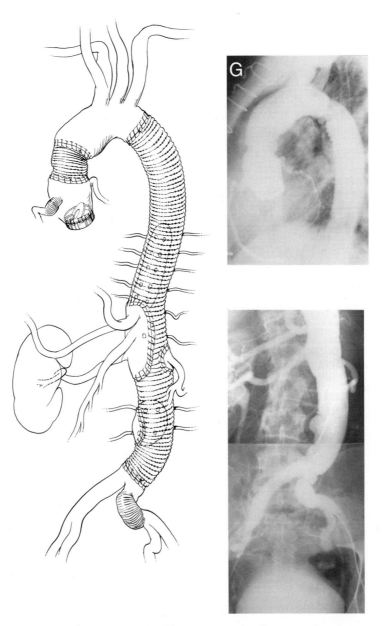

FIGURE 20–6 *Continued* **G,** The postoperative diagram and angiogram.

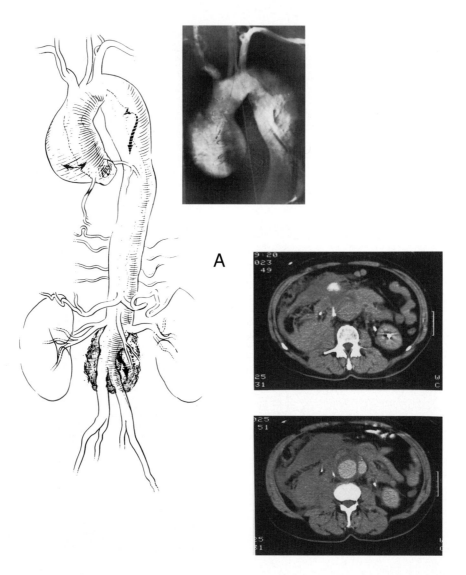

A

FIGURE 20–7   A, Patient with type I aortic dissection and rupture of the aorta in the abdomen as seen by the abdominal CT scan; this patient had undergone a previous aortic valve replacement with a biological valve.

Illustration continued on following page

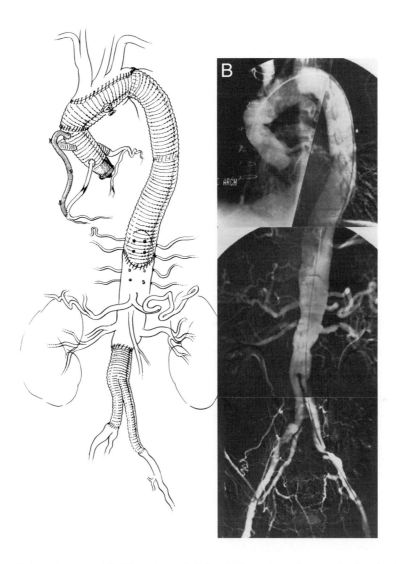

FIGURE 20–7 *Continued* **B,** The ruptured abdominal aorta was first repaired with a bifurcated tube graft. Then a composite valve graft was inserted with a tube graft to the left main coronary artery, and the right coronary artery was reattached as an aortic button. A distal vein bypass was also performed because of coronary artery disease. In addition, the aortic arch was replaced by our modification of the elephant trunk technique. The patient required no operative homologous blood transfusion, although he did require cryoprecipitate for a low fibrinogen level. Subsequently, the rest of the thoracic aorta was replaced with the use of intraoperative hydrogen mapping of the intercostal arteries supplying the spinal cord and intrathecal papaverine with drainage of cerebrospinal fluid to protect the spinal cord. The postoperative angiogram is shown. (Reprinted with permission of the Society of Thoracic Surgeons. From Svensson LG, Sun J, Nadolny E, Kimmel WA. Ann Thorac Surg 1995;59:1501–8.)

established blood flow to the kidneys during aortography prior to surgery. In other patients with type III dissections, organ perfusion has been established by such techniques as fenestration of the septum, so that an open operative procedure could be avoided or postponed. The availability of stents and percutaneous methods of establishing organ perfusion or of stenting the dissection septum in the aorta, even if not clad with a tube graft, should result in safer medical management of acute distal dissections in the early period after dissection and allow for elective repair of the aorta when the aorta will hold sutures better.[1, 2]

Very rarely, after performing a central aortic repair where there have been technical problems, we have had to perform either a descending aortic graft-to-left renal artery bypass, a right iliac-to-right renal artery bypass, or an axillofemoral bypass to an ischemic limb. Occasionally, in patients with type I dissection, a clot may be found in the greater vessels with occlusion of the artery, most often the innominate artery. In this situation, the clot should be removed and a distal bypass performed to less involved segments of the arteries. It is remarkable that these patients, who often appear to have had a severe stroke, awake after surgery with no or minimal neurological deficits. The probable reason for this is that the comatose state arises from the low-flow collateral flow to the brain from unoccluded arteries and may also be due to the hypotension or shock that is often present. Thus, since unconsciousness may not be the result of an irreversible embolic stroke, the low-flow state of the brain is reversed by surgery with recovery of the patient.[1, 2]

We stress, however, that correction of the central aortic lesion should precede correction of any peripheral vascular problems. As discussed above, however, the availability of percutaneous techniques will often allow for the correction of organ malperfusion. We[1] do not consider that there is a role for aortic bypasses with the exclusion of the dissected segment by means of clamps or staplers during the initial operative procedure. Aortic bypass will not reduce the risk of rupture or prevent the complications of paraplegia or renal failure, as has also been shown by others.[1, 2, 8, 9]

REFERENCES

1. Svensson LG, Crawford ES, Hess KR, et al. Dissection of the aorta and dissecting aortic aneurysms: improving early and long-term surgical results. Circulation 1990;82(5 Supp):IV 24–38.
2. Svensson LG, Crawford ES. Aortic dissection and aortic aneurysm surgery: clinical observations, experimental investigations, and statistical analyses. Part II. Curr Probl Surg 1992;29:915–1057.
3. Crawford ES, Svensson LG, Coselli JS, et al. Aortic dissection and dissecting aortic aneurysms. Ann Surg 1988;208:254–73.
4. Crawford ES, Svensson LG, Coselli JS, et al. Surgical treatment of aneurysm and/or dissection of the ascending aorta, transverse aortic arch, and ascending aorta and transverse aortic arch: factors influencing survival in 717 patients. J Thorac Cardiovasc Surg 1989;98:659–73.
5. Svensson LG, Hess KR, Coselli JS, et al. A prospective study of respiratory failure after high-risk surgery on the thoracoabdominal aorta. J Vasc Surg 1991;14:271–82.
6. Lawrie GM. In discussion of vascular complications associated with spontaneous aortic dissection. J Vasc Surg 1988;7:207–8.
7. Sarris GE, Miller DC. Peripheral vascular manifestations of acute aortic dissection. In: Rutherford RB, ed. Vascular Surgery. ed 3. Philadelphia: WB Saunders, 1989:942–951.
8. Patra P, Petiot JM, Mainguene C, et al. Retrograde dissections of the aortic arch after exclusion-bypass of the descending thoracic aorta: a report of three cases. Ann Vasc Surg 1989;3:341–4.
9. Carpentier A, Fabiani JN. La thrombo-exclusion dans les dissections et les anevrysmes de l'aorte thoracique descendante. In: Kieffer E, ed. Chirugie de l'aorte throracique descendante et thoraco-abdominale. Expansion Scientifique Francaise, Paris 1986:245–251.

Procedures for Occlusive Disease of the Aorta

PROXIMAL AORTA

Occlusive disease of the ascending aorta as a result of atherosclerosis does not occur. Nonetheless, with the aging of Western populations, the occurrence of atherothrombotic material or calcification in the ascending aorta or aortic arch is of importance. Increasingly, we are seeing patients with embolic strokes who, on transesophageal echocardiography (TEE), are found to have atherothrombotic material in their aortas. Our approach in these patients, who have no other indications for surgery, is to recommend anticoagulation with Coumadin. It is of interest that, on follow-up TEE a few months later, the material is no longer visible or is considerably reduced and persistent free-floating fronds of material are unusual. For those patients with other indications for surgery, including endarterectomy or graft replacement of the aorta, this problem is addressed at the same time. In a subgroup of patients with severe calcification resulting in a porcelain aorta, we have performed endarterectomies of the aortic calcification at the same time that we have inserted an aortic valve for predominantly aortic valve stenosis. It is interesting that many of these patients have a history of various types of advanced arthritis or of chest radiotherapy. Coronary artery disease is also often associated with this calcification.

In our experience with eight patients who had this calcification problem, including two in whom circulatory arrest was used for dealing with the aortic arch, one patient had a new episode of mild confusion after surgery. That patient had had a previous hemiplegic stroke and, on a computed tomography (CT) scan, was found to have a new frontal infarct. All the patients survived without significant complications. Kouchoukos and colleagues[1] reported the use of intraoperative ultrasound, deep hypothermic circulatory arrest, and graft replacement of the ascending aorta in 47 patients who required coronary artery bypass grafting in association with severe atherosclerotic disease of the ascending aorta. The 30-day mortality rate was 4.3%, and none of the surviving patients suffered a stroke, in spite of the severity of the disease. The treatment of these cases and of occlusive disease of the aortic arch (Fig. 21–1) and descending thoracic or thoracoabdominal aorta is also discussed in Chapter 9.[2]

The management of occlusive disease of the greater vessels is discussed in Chapter 9. For most patients, we perform bypass grafts from the ascending aorta if a donor artery is not available, but, when available and feasible, subclavian carotid artery transposition gives the best long-term results.[3-5]

VISCERAL OCCLUSIVE DISEASE

Sudden total occlusion of the visceral arteries can result in disastrous complications, such as gangrene of the intestines or renal failure. Stenoses of the visceral arteries, with the concomitant risk of sudden total occlusion, is seldom detected before they become symptomatic, except as an incidental finding during arteriography of the abdominal aorta. Clearly, for those patients who have symptoms and who can undergo operation, surgical repair of the occlusive segment is usually warranted.[6]

Crawford and colleagues[7] have previously reported that if occlusive disease (either total occlusion or stenosis) of the arteries was bypassed with tube grafts in patients with symptomatic disease and operation was limited to an abdominal procedure, the risks of operation were low and a 5-year survival rate of 63% could be achieved. Excellent results with surgical repair of symptomatic disease of the superior mesenteric and celiac arteries have also been published by several other authors.[8-21] Nevertheless, opinions differ as to whether asymptomatic superior mesenteric plus celiac artery disease or renal artery occlusive disease should be repaired at the time of abdominal aortic operation. For patients undergoing infrarenal abdominal aortic operation, Connolly and Kwaan[22] have strongly argued in favor of prophylactic bypass or endarterectomy of the superior mesenteric artery and celiac artery if occlusive disease is present because, in their experience, the occurrence of early and late postoperative intestinal gangrene or symptoms was frequent if the disease was not treated. The opinion that asymptomatic occlusive disease should be repaired during infrarenal aortic operation has also been endorsed by other surgeons.[6, 7, 15, 18, 19, 23]

Endarterectomy or bypass for renal artery occlusive disease in most patients is performed via a midline abdominal approach with the patient in the supine position.

Endarterectomy is preferable in patients in whom the occlusive disease involves the proximal third of the renal artery. Bypass is used for more distal disease or when endarterectomy fails.[6, 24]

Extensive occlusive disease of the visceral arteries, including the celiac and superior mesenteric arteries, is best treated by means of a thoracoabdominal incision, incision of the posterior lateral aorta, endarterectomy of the visceral arteries, closure of the aortic incision with a running suture, and then repair of the infrarenal aorta with an aortic prosthesis. However, if this visceral artery segment is aneurysmal, then the entire aorta should be replaced with a prosthetic graft.

Usually, 8 mm tube grafts are used for the bypasses from the aorta to the visceral arteries in an antegrade direction. If both the celiac and superior mesenteric arteries are occluded or stenosed, then it is wise to bypass both since, on long-term follow-up, there is a high incidence of reocclusion with the need for reoperation, and the degree of symptoms is lessened if two grafts have been inserted.[25] Bypasses to the right renal artery, however, are usually performed from the right iliac artery or the right limb of a bifurcated aortic graft during thoracoabdominal repairs. Figures 21-2 to 21-9 illustrate the operative technique in patients who underwent such repairs.[6, 24]

Text continued on page 380

FIGURE 21–1   Patient with stenosis of the right subclavian artery and the innominate artery (**A** to **C**). The repair involved placement of a tube graft from the ascending aorta to the distal innominate artery and a PTFE graft from the right common carotid artery to the distal subclavian artery (**D** and **E**).

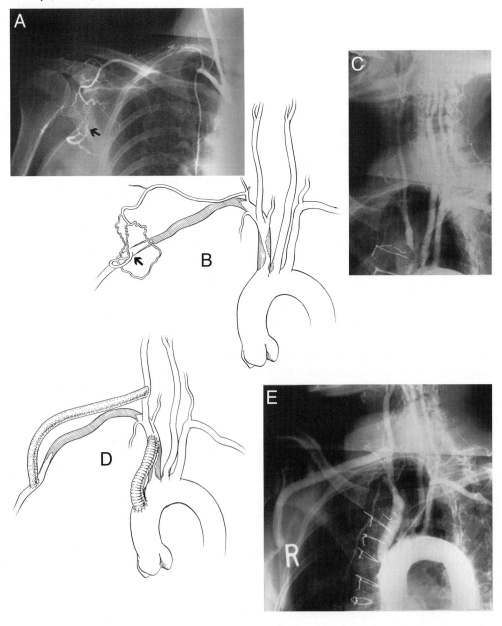

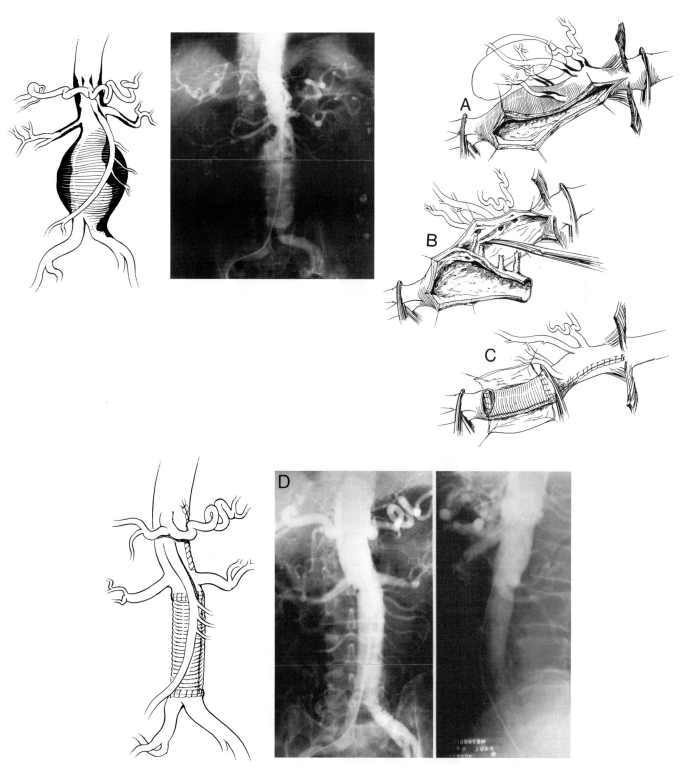

FIGURE 21–2   Patient with extensive atherosclerosis of the abdominal aorta and stenoses of the celiac, superior mesenteric, and renal arteries. **A,** With the aorta cross-clamped, the aorta was opened and stay sutures were placed. **B,** An endarterectomy of the aorta and visceral arteries was then performed. **C,** The upper suprarenal aorta was closed with a running suture and blood flow was established to the visceral arteries, after which the infrarenal aorta was repaired with a tube graft. **D,** Postoperative appearance of the aorta.

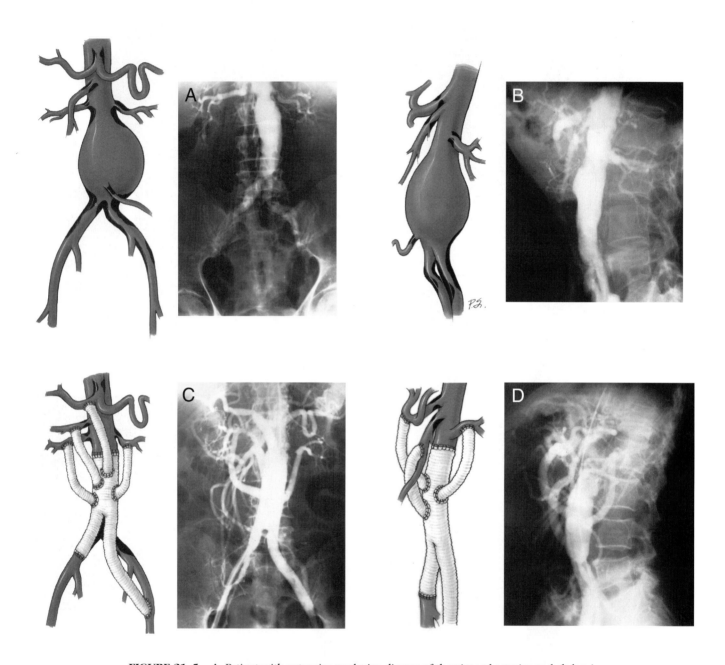

FIGURE 21–5   **A,** Patient with extensive occlusive disease of the visceral arteries and abdominal aortic aneurysm. **B,** Lateral abdominal view showing tight stenoses of the superior mesentera and celiac arteries. **C** and **D,** Postoperative anterior and lateral views after placement of an infrarenal graft and bypasses to the visceral arteries.

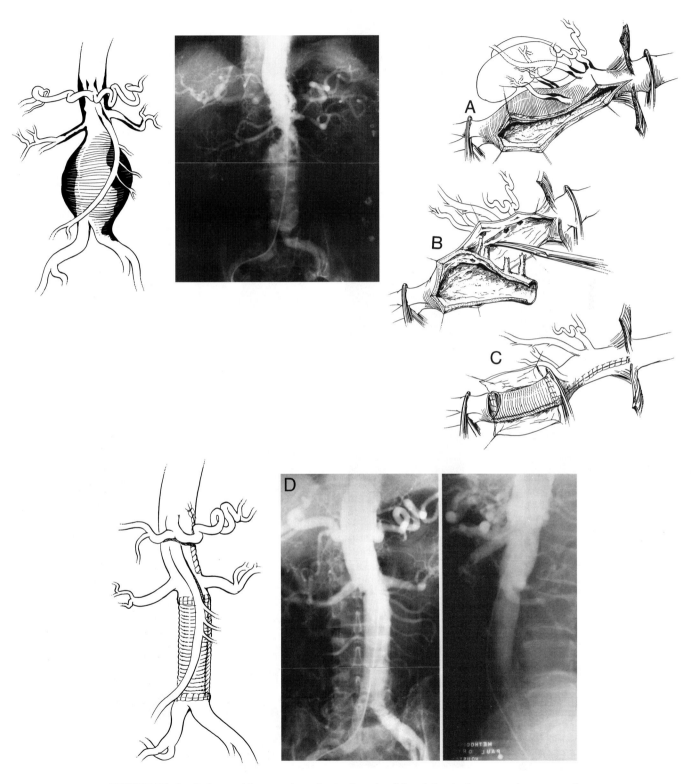

FIGURE 21–2 Patient with extensive atherosclerosis of the abdominal aorta and stenoses of the celiac, superior mesenteric, and renal arteries. **A,** With the aorta cross-clamped, the aorta was opened and stay sutures were placed. **B,** An endarterectomy of the aorta and visceral arteries was then performed. **C,** The upper suprarenal aorta was closed with a running suture and blood flow was established to the visceral arteries, after which the infrarenal aorta was repaired with a tube graft. **D,** Postoperative appearance of the aorta.

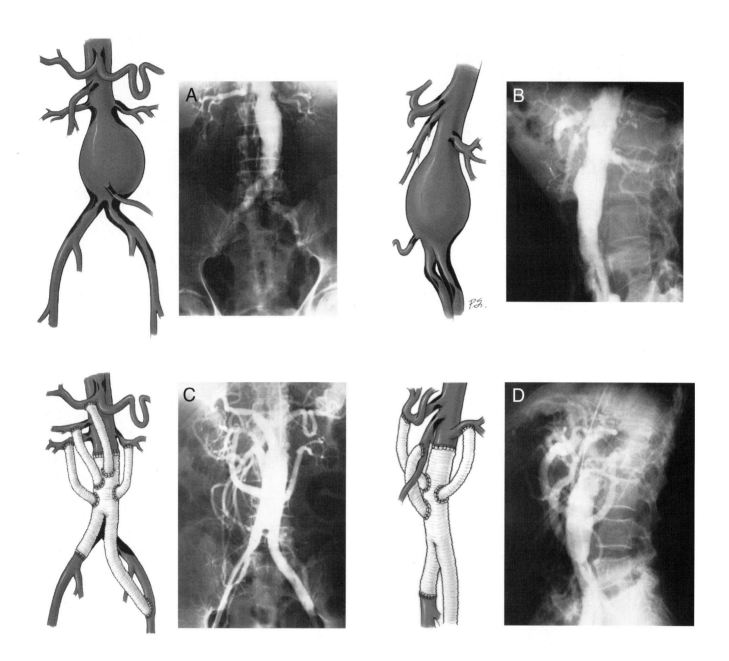

FIGURE 21–5   A, Patient with extensive occlusive disease of the visceral arteries and abdominal aortic aneurysm. **B,** Lateral abdominal view showing tight stenoses of the superior mesentera and celiac arteries. **C** and **D,** Postoperative anterior and lateral views after placement of an infrarenal graft and bypasses to the visceral arteries.

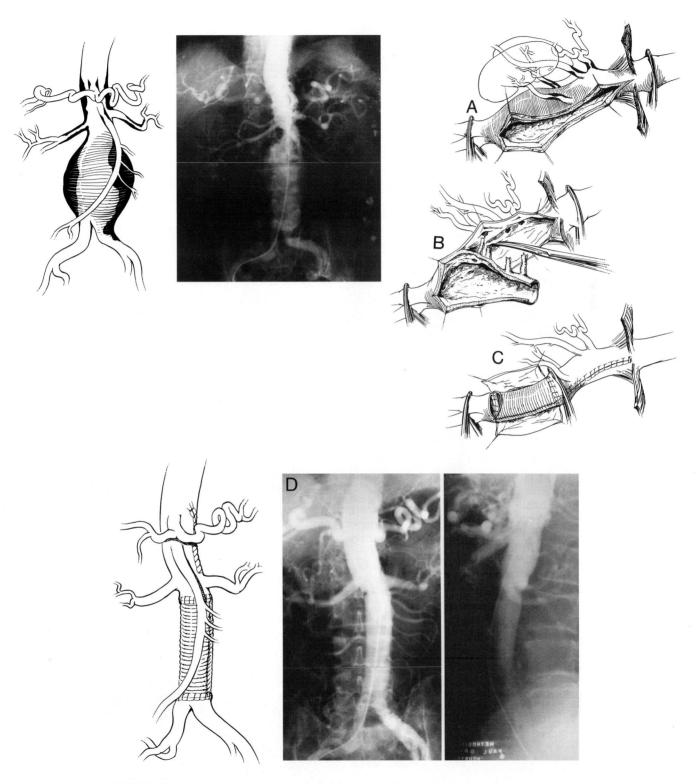

FIGURE 21–2 Patient with extensive atherosclerosis of the abdominal aorta and stenoses of the celiac, superior mesenteric, and renal arteries. **A,** With the aorta cross-clamped, the aorta was opened and stay sutures were placed. **B,** An endarterectomy of the aorta and visceral arteries was then performed. **C,** The upper suprarenal aorta was closed with a running suture and blood flow was established to the visceral arteries, after which the infrarenal aorta was repaired with a tube graft. **D,** Postoperative appearance of the aorta.

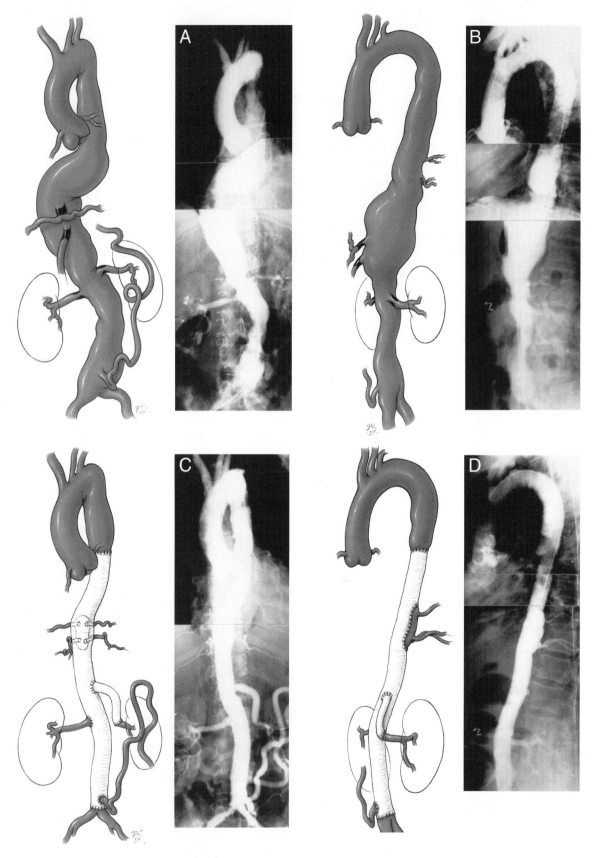

FIGURE 21–3 **A** and **B,** Patient with thoracoabdominal aortic aneurysm with visceral artery stenoses, including occlusion of the superior mesenteric and celiac arteries, with a large inferior mesenteric artery providing collateral blood flow. **C** and **D,** Postoperative aortogram after reimplantation of the intercostal arteries, reimplantation of the right renal artery, bypass to the left renal artery, and reimplantation of the inferior mesenteric artery.

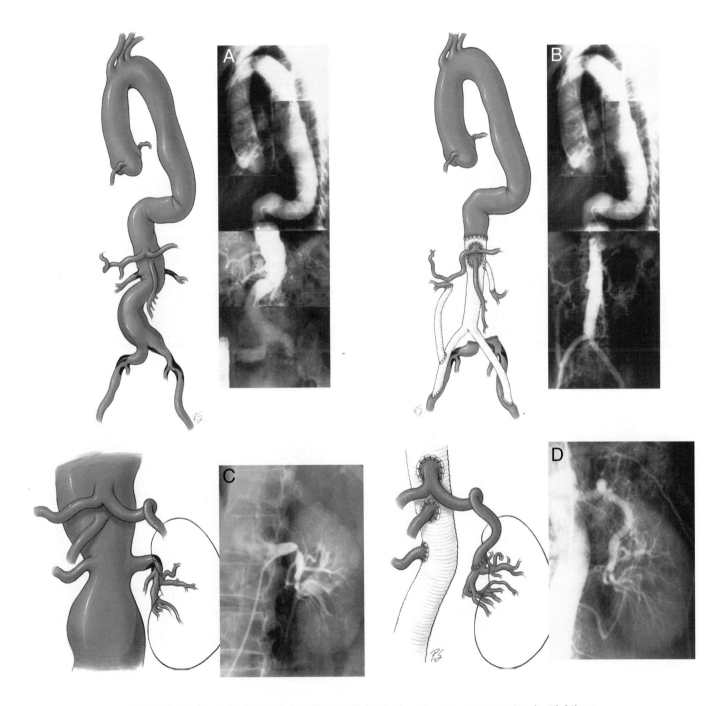

FIGURE 21–4 **A,** Patient with low thoracoabdominal aortic aneurysm associated with bilateral renal artery stenoses and stenoses of the iliac arteries. **B,** Aortogram after repair with a bifurcated graft, reimplantation of the superior mesenteric and celiac arteries, and bypasses to the renal arteries. Note that with a thoracoabdominal incision, the easiest way to perform a distal bypass to the right renal artery is to take the bypass off the right iliac artery and to perform a Kocher maneuver to expose the renal artery. **C,** The other option for patients with renal artery stenoses is to perform distal bypasses with either the splenic or hepatic arteries. In the patient shown, who had a left renal artery stenosis, a splenorenal artery bypass was done during a thoracoabdominal aortic aneurysm repair. **(D)**

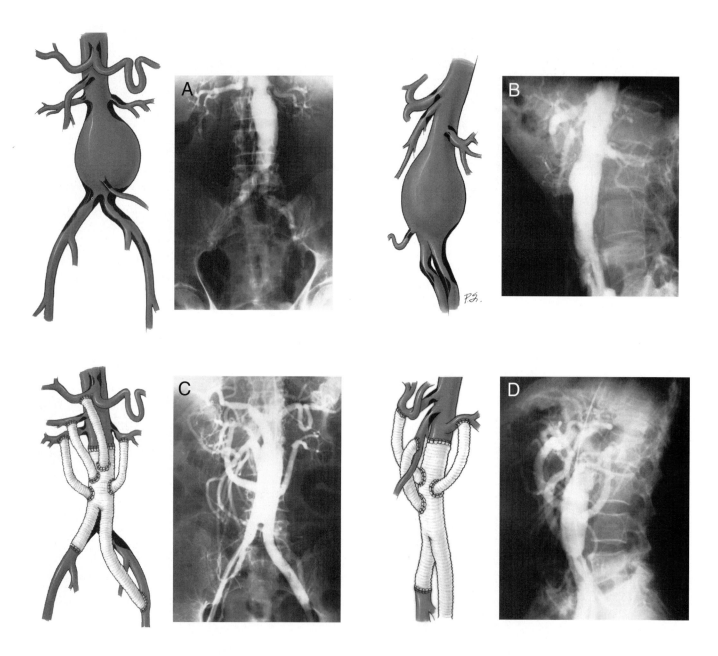

FIGURE 21–5   **A,** Patient with extensive occlusive disease of the visceral arteries and abdominal aortic aneurysm. **B,** Lateral abdominal view showing tight stenoses of the superior mesentera and celiac arteries. **C** and **D,** Postoperative anterior and lateral views after placement of an infrarenal graft and bypasses to the visceral arteries.

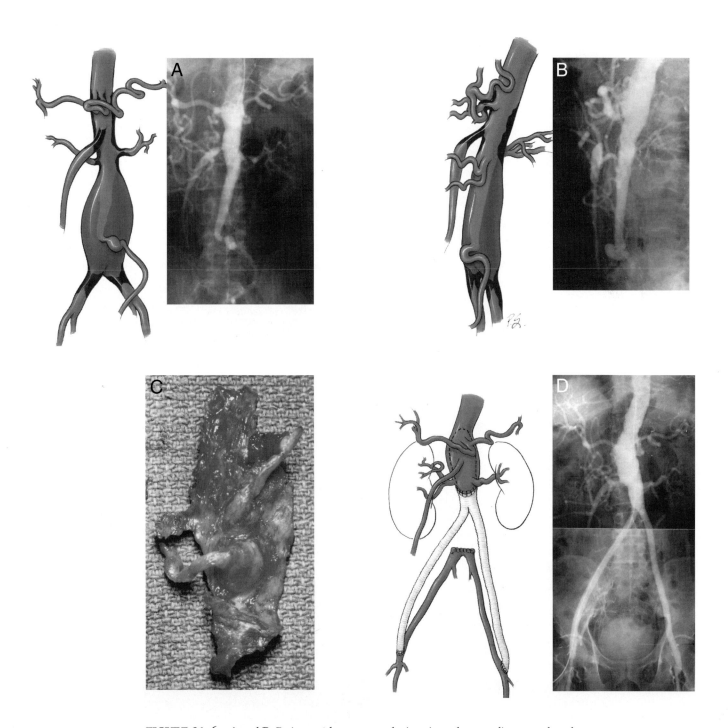

FIGURE 21–6 **A** and **B,** Patient with severe occlusive visceral artery disease and occlusion of the infrarenal aorta. **C,** Endarterectomy specimen. **D,** Aortogram and diagram after reimplantation of the visceral arteries and distal bypass to the femoral arteries.

Illustration continued on following page

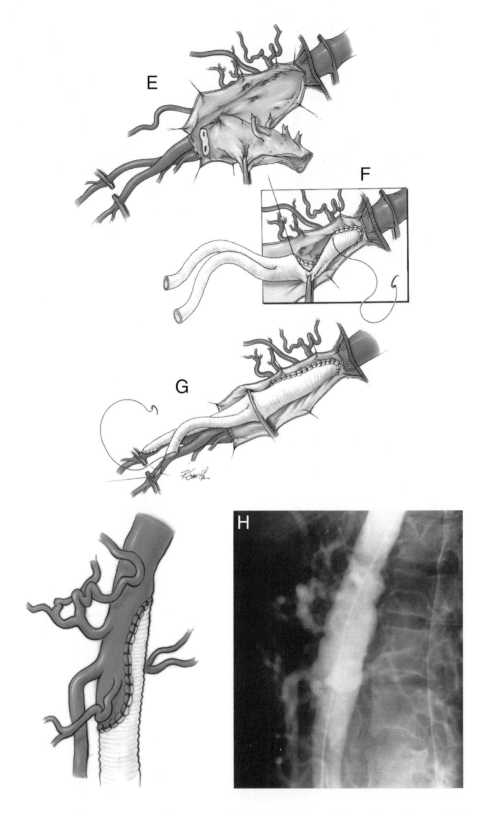

FIGURE 21–6 *Continued* **E,** Illustration of the endarterectomy, **F,** Insertion of the graph that has been beveled behind the visceral arteries. **G,** Construction of the distal anastomoses with perfusion of the abdominal viscera. **H,** Lateral view of the repair.

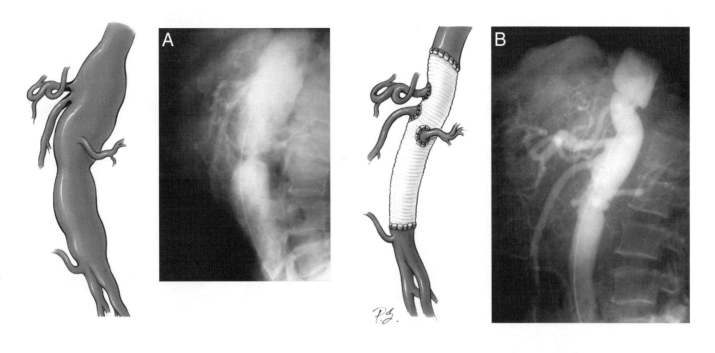

FIGURE 21–7   A, Patient with aortic aneurysm and superior mesenteric and celiac artery stenoses. B, Postoperative lateral view after endarterectomy of the proximal arteries and separate reimplantation into the graft. C, First the proximal anastomosis was inserted and then (D) the ostia were subjected to endarterectomy and (E) sutured to the graft, and the aorta was finally wrapped (F).

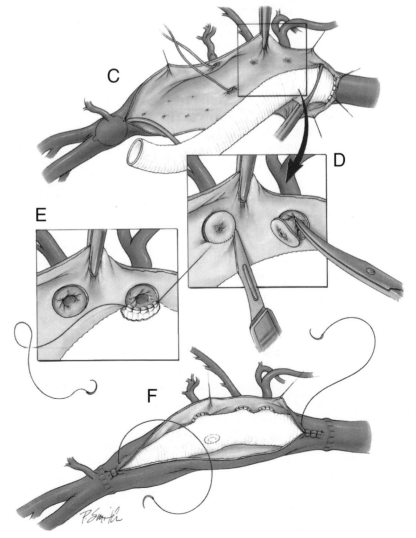

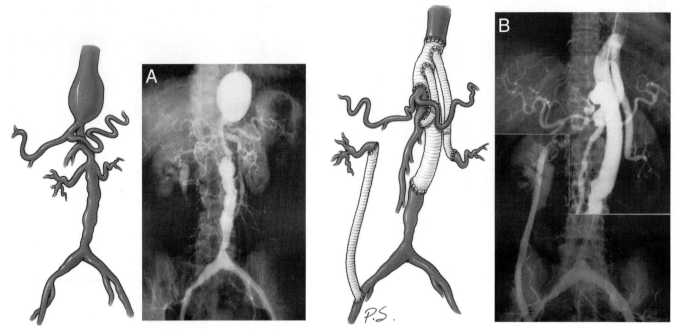

FIGURE 21–8   A, Preoperative aortogram of a patient with severe occlusive disease of the aorta. **B,** Postoperative aortogram after insertion of bypasses to the distal visceral arteries, including a bypass from the right iliac artery to the right renal artery. (From Svensson LG, Crawford ES, Hess KR, et al. J Vasc Surg 1992;16:378–90.)

THORACOABDOMINAL AORTIC ANEURYSMS ASSOCIATED WITH CELIAC, SUPERIOR MESENTERIC, AND RENAL ARTERY OCCLUSIVE DISEASE

Of 1509 patients in our experience who underwent thoracoabdominal aortic repairs, 271 had either celiac, superior mesenteric, or renal artery occlusive disease. After 1987, the 30-day survival rate was 93% (79/85) compared with 90% (245/271) before 1988. Multivariate predictors of death were age, postoperative reoperation for bleeding, and cardiac complications ($p < 0.05$). Renal complications (13% dialysis, 35/271) were associated with preoperative renal dysfunction, an elevated preoperative serum creatinine level, a prolonged urine clearance time of dye (particularly if more than 30 minutes), extent of the aorta replaced, coagulopathy, and paraplegia or paraparesis ($p < 0.05$). The incidence of postoperative renal dysfunction was reduced by renal artery endarterectomy ($p < 0.05$). On univariate analysis ($p < 0.05$), the risk of renal failure was reduced by renal artery perfusion with cold Ringer's lactate solution. Gastrointestinal complications (9%, 25/271) were associated with a history of peptic ulcer disease on multivariate

FIGURE 21–9 Of 271 patients that we reviewed who had stenoses of the visceral arteries, 86 had stenotic disease of the superior mesenteric or celiac arteries and 43 had both arteries repaired. The results are discussed in the texts. (From Svensson LG, Crawford ES, Hess KR, et al. J Vasc Surg 1992;16:378–90.)

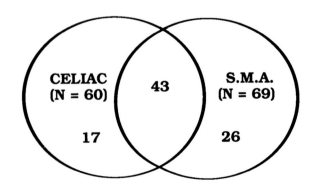

analysis ($p < 0.05$). The Kaplan-Meier 5-year survival rates for patients with and without occlusive disease were 53% and 60% and, at 10 years, 37% and 30%, respectively ($p = 0.08$). From this study, we concluded that endarterectomy or bypass of occlusive visceral disease reduces the risk of renal failure after thoracoabdominal aortic aneurysm repairs, does not decrease early or late survival, and does not increase the risk of gastrointestinal complications.[6, 24]

In this study the 30-day survival rate over the entire time period was 90%, which compares favorably with the survival rate of 92% in those patients without visceral occlusive disease operated on during the same time interval (Table 21-1). These data should, however, be interpreted with some reservation since this was not a prospective study. More recently, in our experience, the 30-day survival rate has improved to 97% in patients undergoing thoracoabdominal aortic operations.[22, 26] We did not find that the risk of gastrointestinal complications was significantly increased in the present study as a result of the repair of the superior mesenteric or celiac arteries (Table 21-1). The incidence of renal complications, however, was increased (29% versus 15%, $p < 0.0001$) in these patients compared with those who did not undergo repair of the visceral arteries because of occlusive disease. Nevertheless, in those patients with occlusive visceral disease, if renal artery endarterectomies were performed ($p = 0.0045$) or if a renal artery was repaired ($p = 0.05$), the incidence of renal complications was reduced. Furthermore, on stepwise logistic regression analysis with adjustment for the influence of the other variables, renal artery endarterectomy was also significantly associated with a lower risk of renal failure. Thus, in our opinion, this justifies the performance of either a renal artery endarterectomy or bypass of occlusive disease of the renal arteries at the time of a thoracoabdominal aortic operation, even if there were no symptoms of occlusal visceral disease. This study does not, however, address the question of whether asymptomatic occlusive disease of the renal, celiac, or superior mesenteric artery should be treated in

patients who are not undergoing thoracoabdominal aortic repairs, namely, infrarenal abdominal aortic operation.[6]

Our approach to occlusive disease of the superior mesenteric, the celiac artery, or both has been to perform endarterectomies for ostial stenoses at the time of the thoracoabdominal aortic repair. Thus while 60 patients had celiac artery repairs, this was usually combined with superior mesenteric artery repair ($N = 43$) or the patient had a stenosis of the celiac artery ostium that could easily be treated by endarterectomy ($N = 17$). Now, as in the past, if only one vessel is totally occluded, particularly if the celiac artery is occluded, and the patient has no symptom, no attempt is usually made to bypass the occlusion of the artery. If, however, both arteries are occluded, then by preference a bypass is done to the distally patent superior mesenteric artery and, often, to the celiac artery, especially in patients with symptoms. If the aortic graft has to be extended to below the origin of the inferior mesenteric artery, an attempt is always made to reimplant it, because it is often the source of collateral blood flow to a proximally obstructed superior mesenteric or celiac artery. The superior mesenteric and celiac arteries are also bypassed or subjected to endarterectomy since the long-term results appear to be better with complete revascularization.[7, 15, 21] On the basis of our results, this approach appears to have been satisfactory. Nevertheless, even with repair of both major arteries and reimplantation of the inferior mesenteric artery, postoperative bowel ischemia may occur. Indeed, this occurred in one patient with symptoms who was surviving on her inferior mesenteric artery and then postoperatively developed bowel ischemia, liver failure, and the unusual postoperative complication of pancreatitis after thoracoabdominal aortic operation, which ultimately resulted in her death. Nevertheless, despite the high incidence of stress ulceration in experimental animals after aortic cross-clamping,[27] gastrointestinal complications after similar thoracoabdominal aortic operations in humans are surprisingly uncommon.[28] A similar difference in the sensitivity of the bowel to ischemic injury between animals and humans has been noted by Bergan and colleagues.[10] The reason for this is unclear but may be related to species differences in the tolerance of reperfusion injuries and the generation of oxygen derived free radicals, as has been documented in both the gastrointestinal tract,[20, 27] and the heart[6, 29] (see Chapter 12).

In our patients we did not perform studies to determine patency of vessels after operation. However, McMillan and associates[30] reported that in 25 patients with angiography or duplex scans, there was no difference in patency at 72 months (89%) according to antegrade or retrograde perfusion, vein versus polytetrafluoroethylene (PTFE) graft, and acute or chronic ischemia.

In a previous study we reported the variables influencing the development of renal complications after 1525 descending thoracic aortic or thoracoabdominal aortic repairs.[31] The significant variables were similar to those in the present study, including the protective effect of renal

TABLE 21–1 COMPARISON OF OUTCOMES AFTER THORACOABDOMINAL AORTA REPAIRS IN PATIENTS WITH AND WITHOUT OCCLUSIVE DISEASE OF THE VISCERAL ARTERIES[6]

Outcome	Occlusive disease $N = 271$	No occlusive disease $N = 1238$	p value
30-day survival	245 (90%)	1139 (92%)	NS
Renal complications	78 (29%)	191 (15%)	< 0.0001
GI complications	25 (9%)	76 (6%)	0.07
Postoperative dialysis	35 (13%)	101 (8%)	0.013
In-hospital survival	235 (87%)	1119 (90%)	NS

GI, gastrointestinal complications.

TABLE 21–2   INCIDENCE OF POSTOPERATIVE COMPLICATIONS AND ASSOCIATION OF THE VARIABLES WITH EARLY DEATH, RENAL COMPLICATIONS, AND GASTROINTESTINAL COMPLICATIONS ON UNIVARIATE ANALYSIS IN THE 271 PATIENTS[6]

Compli-cation	Incidence N (%)	Death (*p* value)	Renal (*p* value)	Gastro-intestinal (*p* value)
Pulmonary	99 (37)	0.05	0.008	0.21
Cardiac	36 (13)	< 0.0001	0.0087	0.67
Reoperation	32 (12)	0.0016	0.25	0.54
Sepsis	25 (9)	0.01	0.0071	0.23
Coagulopathy	14 (5)	0.0007	0.072	0.5
Paraplegia/P	41 (15)	0.23	0.02	0.19
GI	25 (9)	0.78	0.026	—
Renal	78 (29)	0.0001	—	—

GI, gastrointestinal complications; *Paraplegia/P,* paraplegia/paraparesis.

artery endarterectomy for occlusive disease. In the previous older study, despite a larger sample size, we were unable to show that the routine use of cold Ringer's lactate solution to perfuse the kidneys reduced the risk of postoperative renal complications.[31] In the latter report, however, we showed that in patients with occlusive disease the additional use of cold perfusion of the renal arteries with cold (4° C) Ringer's solution appears to protect the kidneys from ischemia during operations. We usually do this by injecting 120 ml of solution into each renal artery and then keep the left kidney cold by placing it in a cooling jacket. Alternatively, 1.5 L of cold solution can be administered and the temperature monitored by a thermistor needle in the left kidney as previously described.[6, 31]

In conclusion, our data support the principle that occlusive disease of the renal arteries should be treated by endarterectomy or bypass at the time of thoracoabdominal aortic operation and that superior mesenteric or celiac artery repairs can be performed without an increased risk of death or postoperative gastrointestinal complications. (See Tables 21–1 to 21–3.)

AORTOILIAC DISEASE

Endarterectomy of the aortoiliac segment is achievable but has fallen increasingly into disfavor because of the progression of disease and the good results achieved with aortoiliac or aortobifemoral bypass grafts.[32, 33] Nevertheless, endarterectomy is feasible when disease is localized to the distal abdominal aorta and to the iliac arteries without extension beyond the iliac bifurcations. If endarterectomy is performed, it is important that a clean distal end point be achieved, and if a flap is present it must be tacked down

with sutures. Endarterectomy is inadvisable when either the aorta is totally occluded or the aorta or iliac arteries are aneurysmal.[6]

Van den Akker and colleagues[34] reviewed their series of 747 patients who had undergone aortoiliac operations for occlusive disease, of whom 229 had undergone endarterectomies and 518 had undergone prosthetic repairs, including aorto-bi-iliac repairs in 339. The respective mortality rates were 1.6%, 3%, and 3.1%. Critical ischemia because of heart disease was the most common cause of both early and late death. Twenty-one percent required later reoperative procedures. Van den Akker and colleagues concluded that the results of using endarterectomy extensively were comparable with other published results but, unfortunately, they did not compare their patients who had endarterectomy with those who had prosthetic bypasses.

The usual operative technique for aortoiliac disease is to perform an aorto-bi-femoral bypass graft.[32, 33] Aorto-bi-iliac grafts are generally not recommended because of the risk of progression of distal disease in the iliac or femoral arteries.[32, 33] The method of performing the proximal anastomosis to the aorta should be decided on an individual basis to match the patient's problems. Either an end-to-side or an end-to-end anastomosis can be performed.[6]

End-to-side anastomoses allow continued perfusion of the lumbar arteries, the middle sacral arteries, and often the internal iliac (hypogastric) arteries. The advantage of this is that sacral and buttock ischemia and spinal cord ischemia are less likely to occur, particularly if the external iliac arteries are occluded and there is no retrograde flow from the femoral arteries. Since the end-to-side anastomosis can be placed with minimal disruption of either the hypogastric nerves or the native internal iliac artery blood flow, the incidence of postoperative sexual dysfunction is also reduced.

TABLE 21–3   CAUSES OF EARLY (N = 26) AND LATE DEATHS (N = 63)[6]

	Early	Late	Total
Cardiac	19	24	43
Pulmonary	11	11	22
Renal	9	7	16
Sepsis	5	6	11
Hemorrhage	4		4
Stroke	1	3	4
Pulmonary embolus	1	2	3
Rupture	1	8	9
Other	3	9	12
Aortointestinal fistula		4	4
Unknown		3	3
Cancer		2	2
GI hemorrhage		2	2

GI, gastrointestinal.

If patent major arteries arise from the infrarenal aorta, such as a large accessory renal artery or inferior mesenteric artery, particularly if the celiac or superior mesenteric arteries are occluded, then an end-to-side anastomosis will help maintain antegrade blood flow down such patent arteries. Thus the preoperative aortogram should be carefully examined for important arteries, including collateral arteries to the bowel or internal iliac arteries, indicating that the blood supply of the distal aorta or proximal iliac arteries has to be maintained. This technique is also preferable when there is concern about the later development of graft infection, because the graft can be removed and the aorta repaired while the infection is cleared. Furthermore, in some patients an ancillary axillobifemoral bypass may not be necessary to maintain limb viability. This is also important if the bypass graft should later occlude and reoperation is not feasible. In such patients, an amputation stump is more likely to heal if severe limb ischemia should occur. The disadvantages are that the graft is more difficult to retroperitonealize with surrounding tissue, and thus aortointestinal or graft intestinal fistulae are more likely to occur. Hemodynamically, more turbulence is likely in the graft and may predispose it to earlier occlusion, although this has not been proven in any prospective randomized studies.[6, 32, 33]

End-to-end anastomosis to the aorta immediately below the renal arteries is indicated when the distal aorta is occluded at the renal arteries, the aorta or iliac arteries are aneurysmal, or the patient is thin. This is the preferred technique in most patients because the hemodynamic results are better and long-term patency may be improved.[6] It should be noted, however, that in patients with a small or hypoplastic infrarenal aorta, whether male or female, occlusions of their grafts are more likely to develop after repair,[35] and the addition of a profundoplasty may ameliorate patency.

A standard midline incision is used for the repair. The aorta immediately below the renal arteries is clamped after exposure of the anterior and lateral circumference. A curved clamp is then placed obliquely below the first clamp with sufficient space to perform an end-to-end or end-to-side anastomosis. The oblique clamp is placed so that it will occlude the distal aorta and also prevent blood flow from the lumbar arteries. The proximal aorta is then divided anteriorly and laterally for approximately two thirds of the circumference if an end-to-end anastomosis is going to be performed. The distal aortic stump is oversewn with 3-0 Prolene sutures in two layers in patients in whom an end-to-end anastomosis is going to be constructed. The selected bifurcation graft is then sutured to the aortic stump with a running 3-0 Prolene suture. The anastomosis is tested and the graft is flushed of any blood, after which it is tunneled behind the ureters and peritoneum down to the previously exposed femoral arteries. After the common femoral artery and the superficial femoral and profunda arteries have been clamped, the common femoral artery is opened and, if necessary, the incision is extended on to the profunda for prox-imal profunda occlusive disease. Each of the graft limbs is then anastomosed to the femoral artery in an end-to-side fashion with 4-0 or 5-0 Prolene sutures. The distal end of the graft should be beveled with a gentle S curve to give a wide-open anastomosis. If a later femoropopliteal or distal bypass is envisioned, the distal graft anastomosis can be performed side-to-side and the end ligated. The ligated stump is then later used for the distal bypass. In patients in whom an end-to-side anastomosis is to be performed, the anterior aorta is opened a sufficient distance for the beveled aortic graft to be anastomosed. Either the toe or the heel can be first anastomosed, depending on whichever is easiest in the individual patient.[6]

In some patients either the infrarenal aorta is completely occluded or atheroma extends up to the orifices or involves the renal arteries. In these patients the aorta should be cross-clamped at the diaphragm while the aorta and the renal arteries are cleared of atheroma. If a renal artery procedure is required, the left renal vein is skeletonized, including ligation of the gonadal veins, and then encircled with a vessel loop for traction. An endarterectomy of the renal arteries can conveniently be performed by extension of a T incision up to the base of the superior mesenteric artery to gain exposure of the renal arteries. After the endarterectomy the longitudinal incision is then closed with Prolene sutures down to the circumferential incision in the aorta. The end-to-end anastomosis is then performed and the aortic cross-clamp is moved to the infrarenal aorta with reperfusion of the kidneys.[6]

Clair and colleagues[36] reported their experience with transaortic renal endarterectomy in 43 patients with aortic aneurysm repair in 30 and treatment of occlusive disease in nine. Two endarterectomies (2.6%) required bypass because of poor flow, and in 3.9% reimplantation or bypasses were performed because of fragile ostia. The 30-day mortality rate was 4.7%, hypertension was cured or improved in 83%, and renal function was improved in 19% but worsened in 23%. In patients with juxtarenal occlusion, Tapper and colleagues[37] reported that in a series of 103 patients, 26 presented with acute occlusion, 66 with chronic occlusion, and 21 with occlusion of old grafts and the respective mortality rates were 31%, 9%, and 4.7%. Those authors speculated that the better results in the latter two groups were due to the availablity of more collateral arteries that protected against distal ischemia during aortic occlusion. For chronic occlusions of the aortic bifurcation, thrombolytic treatment with balloon angioplasty has been reported in 25 patients, with complete lysis in 20% (5/25), partial lysis in 40%, of whom 8 of 10 had mechanical reopening of the aorta with an overall 52% success rate. TPA tended to work quicker than streptokinase or urokinase. Ten patients (40%) underwent surgery.

Figures 21–10 to 21–15 illustrate various techniques used to treat some unusual problems associated with occlusive disease involving the infrarenal aorta.

Text continued on page 389

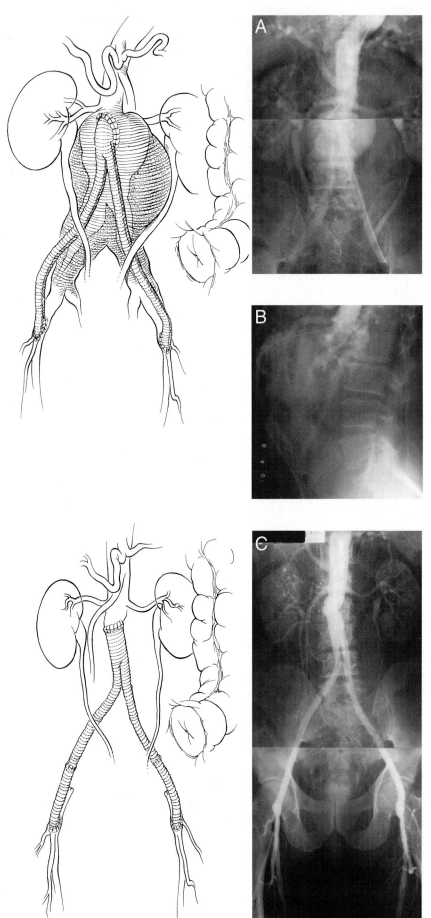

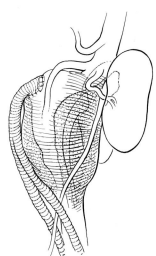

FIGURE 21–10 Patient with iliac occlusive disease, an abdominal aneurysm, and colostomy who was treated elsewhere with an end-to-side tube graft because of the fear of graft infection. **A,** Anteroposterior view. **B**, Lateral view. The patient was operated on again by us because of pain and early ureteric obstruction, and an infrarenal bifurcated graft was inserted **(C).**

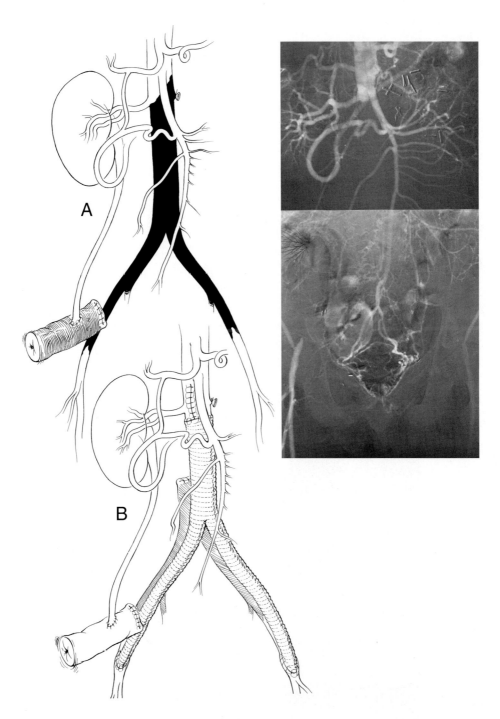

FIGURE 21–11 A, Patient with occluded distal aorta, left nephrectomy, and right ureter anastomosed to an ileal conduit. **B,** Postoperative result after endarterectomy of the aorta and insertion of bifurcated tube graft.

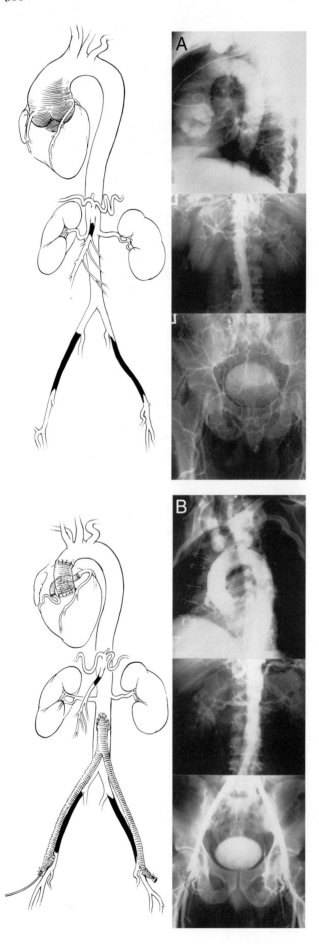

FIGURE 21–12 **A,** Patient with an ascending aortic aneurysm requiring a composite valve graft repair and associated bilateral iliac artery stenoses. **B,** To establish arterial bypass inflow, an aortofemoral bypass was first performed with the right arterial limb cannulated for cardiopulmonary bypass. Next the ascending aorta was repaired by the Cabrol method of coronary artery ostial reattachment. (Reprinted with permission from the Society of Thoracic Surgeons. From Coselli JS, Crawford ES. Ann Thoracic Surg 1987;43:437-9.)

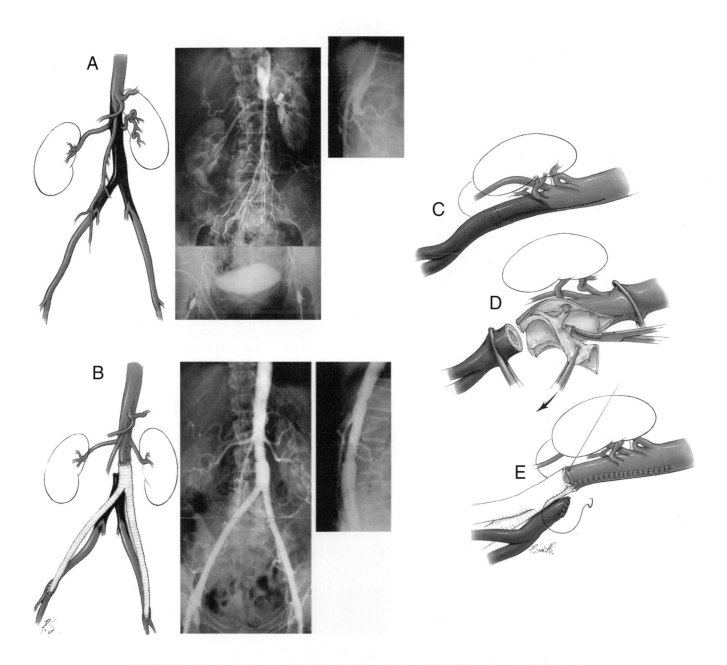

FIGURE 21–13 **A,** Aortogram of a patient with occlusion of the infrarenal aorta. **B,** Illustration of the postoperative result after endarterectomy and distal bifurcation graft bypass to the femoral arteries. **C,** Line of the posterior incision for the endarterectomy. **D,** Performance of the endarterectomy. **E,** Repair of the visceral segment of the aorta and insertion of an infrarenal aortic graft.

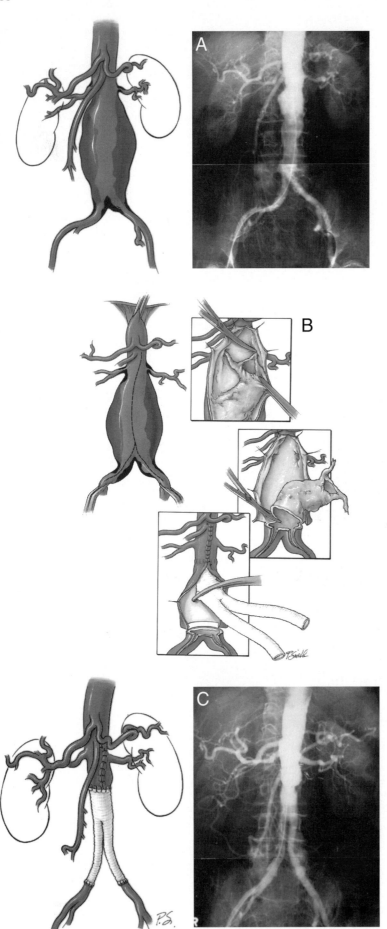

FIGURE 21–14 **A,** Patient with infrarenal aortic aneurysm and renal artery stenoses. **B,** Stages of repair with supraceliac artery clamping and then endarterectomy of the renal arteries with an incision extended up alongside the left aspect of the superior mesenteric artery. The left renal vein can be mobilized and encircled with a sling to aid exposure. A bifurcated graft is sutured into position after repair of the suprarenal aorta. **C,** Postoperative aortography showing the result.

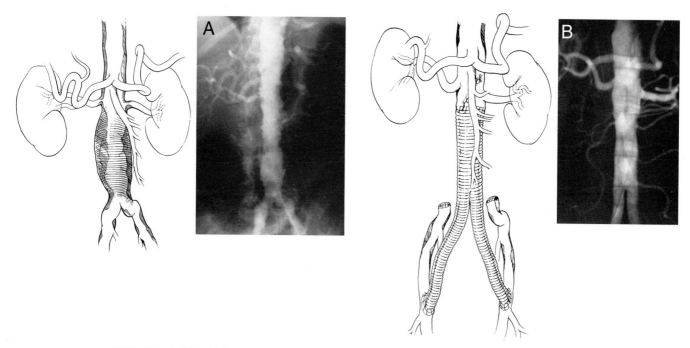

FIGURE 21–15 **A,** Patient with a clot-lined infrarenal aortic aneurysm and renal artery stenoses. **B,** The aorta was repaired by means of an incision extending up as a flap door above the renal arteries so that an endarterectomy of the renal arteries could be performed, and then a distal bifurcated graft was inserted

REFERENCES

1. Kouchoukos NT, Wareing TH, Daily BB, Murphy SF. Management of the severely atherosclerotic aorta during cardiac operations. J Cardiac Surg 1994;9:490-4.
2. Svensson LG, Sun J, Cruz H, Shahian DM. Endarectomy for aortic valve stenosis and calcified porcelain aorta. Ann Thorac Surg 1996; 61:149-52.
3. Crawford ES, Stowe CL, Powers RWJ. Occlusion of the innominate, common carotid, and subclavian arteries: long-term results of surgical treatment. Surgery 1983;94:781-91.
4. Edwards WH Jr, Tapper SS, Edwards WH Sr, et al. Subclavian revascularization: a quarter century experience. Ann Surg 1994;219: 673-8.
5. Law MM, Colburn MD, Moore WS, et al. Carotid-subclavian bypass for brachiocephalic occlusive disease: choice of conduit and long-term follow-up. Stroke 1995;26:1565-71.
6. Svensson LG, Crawford ES, Hess KR, et al. Thoracoabdominal aortic aneurysms associated with celiac, superior mesenteric and renal artery occlusive disease. Methods and analysis of results in 271 patients. J Vasc Surg 1992;16:378-90.
7. Crawford ES, Morris GC, Myhre HO, Roehm JO Jr. Celiac axis, superior mesenteric artery occlusion: surgical considerations. Surgery 1977;82:856-66.
8. Shaw RS, Maynard EP. Acute and chronic thrombosis of mesenteric arteries associated with malabsorption: report of two cases successfully treated by thromboendarterectomy. N Engl J Med 1958; 258:874-8.
9. Morris GC, DeBakey ME. Abdominal angina, diagnosis and surgical treatment. JAMA 1961;176:88-92.
10. Bergan JJ, Dean RH, Conn JJ, Yao ST. Revascularization in treatment of mesenteric infarction. Ann Surg 1975;182:430-8.
11. McCollum CH, Graham JM, DeBakey ME. Chronic mesenteric arterial insufficiency: results of revascularization in 33 cases. South Med J 1976;69:1266-8.
12. Boley SJ, Sprayregan S, Siegelmann SS, et al. Initial results from an aggressive roentgenological and surgical approach to acute mesenteric ischemia. Surgery 1977;82:848-55.
13. Stoney RJ, Ehrenfeld WK, Wylie EJ. Revascularization methods in chronic visceral ischemia caused by atherosclerosis. Ann Surg 1977; 186:468-76.
14. Hertzer NA, Beven EG, Humphries AW. Chronic intestinal ischemia. Surg Gynecol Obstet 1977;145:321-8.
15. Hollier LH, Bernatz PE, Pairolero PC, et al. Surgical management of chronic intestinal ischemia: a reappraisal. Surgery 1981;90:940-3.
16. Rogers DM, Thompson JE, Garret WV, et al. Mesenteric vascular problems. Ann Surg 1982;195:554-65.
17. Stanton PE, Hollier PA, Seidel TW, et al. Chronic intestinal ischemia: diagnosis and therapy. J Vasc Surg 1986;4:338-44.
18. Rapp JH, Reilly LM, Qvarfordt PG, et al. Durability of endarterectomy and antegrade grafts in the treatment of chronic visceral ischemia. J Vasc Surg 1986;3:799-806.
19. Van Dongen JM. Renal and intestinal artery occlusive disease. World J Surg 1988;12:777-87.
20. Bourchier RG, Gloviczki P, Larson MV, et al. The mechanisms and prevention of intravascular fluid loss after occlusion of the supraceliac aorta in dogs. J Vasc Surg 1991;13:637-45.
21. Geelkerken RH, Van Bocket JH, De Roos WK, et al. Chronic mesenteric vascular syndrome: results of reconstructive surgery. Arch Surg 1991;126:1101-6.
22. Conolly JE, Kwaan HM. Prophylactic revascularization of the gut. Ann Surg 1979;190:514-22.
23. Rheudasil JM, Stewart MT, Schellack JV, et al. Surgical treatment of chronic mesenteric arterial insufficiency. J Vasc Surg 1988;8:495-500.
24. Svensson LG, Crawford ES. Aortic dissection and aortic aneurysm surgery: clinical observations, experimental investigations, and statistical analyses. Part III. Curr Probl Surg 1993;30:1-172.
25. Morris GC Jr, Crawford ES, Cooley DA, et al. Revascularization of the celiac and superior mesenteric arteries. Arch Surg 1962;84:95.
26. Crawford ES, Crawford JL. Diseases of the Aorta Including an Atlas of Angiographic Pathology and Surgical Technique. Baltimore: Williams & Wilkins, 1984.
27. Svensson LG, Ritter CV, Oosthuizen MMJ, et al. Prevention of gastric mucosal lesions following aortic cross-clamping. Br J Surg 1987; 74:282-5.

28. Svensson LG, Hess KR, Coselli JS, et al. A prospective study of respiratory failure after high-risk surgery on the thoracoabdominal aorta. J Vasc Surg 1991;14:271-82.

29. McCord JM. Oxygen-derived free radicals in post-ischemic tissue injury. N Engl J Med 1985;312:159-63.

30. McMillan WD, McCarthy WJ, Bresticker MR, et al. Mesenteric artery bypass: objective patency determination. J Vasc Surg 1995;21:729-41.

31. Svensson LG, Grum DF, Bednarski M, et al. Appraisal of cerebrospinal fluid alterations during aortic surgery with intrathecal papaverine administration and cerebrospinal fluid drainage. J Vasc Surg 1990;11:423-9.

32. Crawford ES, Manning LG, Kelly TF. "Redo" surgery after operations for aneurysm and occlusion of the abdominal aorta. Surgery 1977;81:41.

33. Crawford ES, Bomberger RA, Glaeser DH, et al. Aortoiliac occlusive disease: factors influencing survival and function following reconstructive operation over a twenty-five year period. Surgery 1981;90:1555-67.

34. van den Akker PJ, von Schilfgaarde R, Brand R, et al. Long term success of aortoiliac operation for arteriosclerotic obstructive disease. Surg Gynecol Obstet 1992;174:485-96.

35. Valentine RJ, Hansen ME, Myers SI, et al. The influence of sex and aortic size on late patency after aortofemoral revascularization in young adults. J Vasc Surg 1995;21:296-306.

36. Clair DG, Belkin M, Whittemore AD, et al. Safety and efficacy of transaortic renal endarterectomy as an adjunct to aortic surgery. J Vasc Surg 1995;21:926-34.

37. Tapper SS, Jenkins JM, Edwards WH, et al. Juxtarenal aortic occlusion. Ann Surg 1992;215:443-50.

38. Coselli JS, Crawford ES. Femoral artery perfusion for cardiopulmonary bypass in patients with aortoiliac artery obstruction. Ann Thorac Surg 1987;43:437-9.

Repair of Aortic Fistulae

Fistulae can develop at any site where the aorta is in close proximity to an adjacent hollow epithelial or endothelium-lined structure. Thus sites include the cardiac chambers, the pulmonary artery, the trachea, the superior or inferior vena cava, innominate, renal, or iliac veins, esophagus, bronchus, gastrointestinal tract, and ureters.

The cause of the fistulae is previous trauma, either penetrating or blunt injury, previous surgery in the vicinity, pressure necrosis of surrounding structures, rupture of the aorta into the adjacent structure, or (rarely) a congenital malformation. The more commonly seen lesions include rupture of a dissected aorta or a sinus of Valsalva aneurysm into one of the adjacent cardiac chambers (usually the right ventricle); an aortoesophageal fistula from previous descending or thoracoabdominal repairs by the inclusion technique and not transection of the aorta[1, 2]; aortointestinal fistulae after infrarenal repairs; and aortocaval fistulae from rupture of abdominal aortic aneurysms into the inferior vena cava.

Aorta–to–cardiac chamber fistulae can usually be repaired with relative ease, at the time of repair of the ascending aorta, by closing off the communication with pledgeted sutures. Treatment of aortoesophageal fistulae is a more complex problem, and, because the patients usually present in shock or die immediately from upper intestinal exsanguination, survival is rare. Occasionally, primary aortoesophageal fistulae have been treated successfully.[3, 4] The descending thoracic or thoracoabdominal aortic repair is done in a standard fashion after the esophagus has been repaired, and then an omental flap is placed between the graft and the esophagus.

AORTOCAVAL FISTULAE

Aortocaval fistulae are rare complications of aortic aneurysms (Figs. 22-1 and 22-2). The entity was first documented by Syme[5] in a 22-year-old patient. In 1972 Reckless[6] had managed to collect 71 cases in the world literature. Subsequently, Baker and colleagues[7] and Brewster and colleagues[8] have reported large series of patients. The diagnosis is important because of the high mortality rate associated with the condition, which may approach 50%.[9] Most cases are due to atherosclerotic aneurysms eroding into the inferior vena cava or, more infrequently, into adjacent veins or are the result of trauma.[10] For example, lumbar disc surgery is

particularly associated with the complication. Rarely, malignant tumors may be the cause of aortocaval fistulae.[11] Fifty percent of the patients who have aortocaval fistulae present with associated high-output heart failure, characterized by a hyperdynamic circulation and a low diastolic pressure. Venous hypertension of the lower torso below the fistula may occur, resulting in the distinctive feature of blue, bloated, and edematous lower limbs coupled with cool, clammy, and pale upper limbs. Renal vein hypertension may be associated with hematuria and proteinuria. Occasionally patients present with pulmonary emboli related to aneurysmal thrombus breaking off and embolizing to the lungs. In addition, a continuous murmur may sometimes be heard over the abdomen.[12] Computer tomography (CT) scans, as we have documented (Fig. 22-2),[9] or aortography will often demonstrate the fistula with filling of the inferior vena cava. A Swan-Ganz catheter is essential for surgical repair since the large fluxes in fluid load to the heart during surgery must be carefully monitored. While the fistula is being closed, the increased cardiac afterload from aortic clamping and the reduced preload caused by venous occlusion of the inferior vena cava must be carefully managed. Furthermore, once the aortic clamps are removed, the situation is reversed and requires diligent attention by the anesthesiologist. The operative technique involves the use of at least one autotransfusion device and digital control of the fistula because excessive blood loss, air embolism, and thrombus embolism are great risks in these patients, especially those who have larger fistulae. An attempt should be made to control bleeding from the inferior vena cava by exerting pressure on it, although the aortic aneurysm is often large and obscures the vena cava, making control difficult. A technique (Fig. 22-1) that we have found useful is to place stay sutures on either side of the fistula while it is digitally controlled, carefully pull up on the stay sutures, and then oversewing the approximated fistula with either a running suture or interrupted sutures.[9, 13]

AORTOINTESTINAL FISTULAE

Most aortointestinal fistulae seen currently are the result of previous infrarenal aortic aneurysm repairs. They typically appear months to years after surgery. The incidence has been reported to be between 0.4% and 4%.[14-16] Patients present with either gastrointestinal bleeding or with evidence

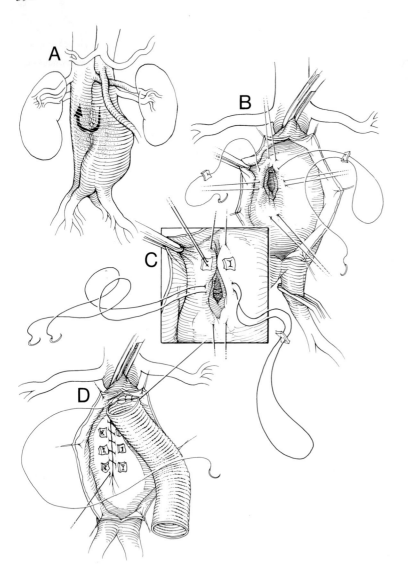

FIGURE 22–1 Steps in the repair of an aortovena caval or iliac vein fistula. Cell savers for reinfusion of lost blood are essential. **A,** After cross-clamping of the supraceliac or infrarenal aorta, the aneurysm is exposed. **B,** The fistula is exposed and the fistula is gently controlled digitally while two sutures are placed superior and inferior to the fistula and strong upward traction is exerted by an assistant. It is critically important that clot or air does not embolize while the fistula is digitally controlled and the stay sutures are being placed. **C,** Pledgeted sutures on a large needle, such as a MH needle, are then used to close the fistula while traction is maintained on the stay sutures to reduce bleeding and the risk of air embolism. **D,** The fistula repair is further strengthened by a continuous over-and-over suture, and then the aortic tube graft is sutured into position in the usual manner. (From Svensson LG, Crawford ES. Curr Probl Surg 1993;30:1–172.)

FIGURE 22–2 Patient who presented with high-output cardiac failure, hematuria, bilateral leg swelling, and abdominal mass and later had an abdominal continuous bruit. CT scan with contrast revealed erosion of the aneurysm calcification into the inferior vena cava; furthermore, contrast was noted in both the aorta and the inferior vena cava at the same time, a sign that we documented in this patient in a previous publication. (From Svensson LG, Gaylis H, Barlow JB. S Afr Med J 1987;72:876-7.)

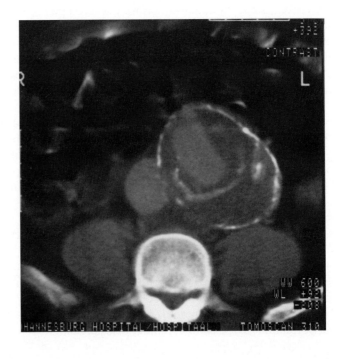

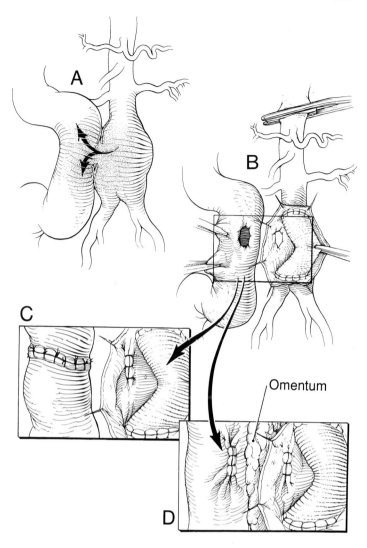

FIGURE 22–3 Steps in the repair of an aortoduodenal or intestinal fistula. **A,** The fistula is exposed through a standard laparotomy and **(B)** the supraceliac aorta is cross-clamped. The fistula is exposed through the aneurysm wall and the fistula to the intestine is divided and dissected free off the aorta. A tube graft is sutured into position after extensive debridement of the area. **C,** The section of intestine with the fistula is excised and then reanastomosed end-to-end. In addition, the hole in the aneurysm wall is closed. **D,** Omentum is placed between the aortic wall and the intestine to prevent further fistula formation. If there is evidence of extensive bacterial contamination and infection, then tubes placed alongside the repair can be left for irrigation with antibiotics in the postoperative period. The patient is then maintained on a lifetime regimen of antibiotics.

of graft infection, including systemic signs of sepsis. The diagnosis of the fistula can be difficult. Upper endoscopy may reveal the graft in the lumen of the bowel, but since the third and fourth parts of the duodenum are difficult to visualize, as is the proximal jejunum, the graft erosion may not be detected. Nevertheless, other causes of bleeding in the upper gastrointestinal tract can be excluded. Magnetic resonance imaging (MRI) or CT scanning may reveal a false aneurysm at the proximal anastomosis or the presence of gas or fluid surrounding the graft. Aortography rarely shows the bleeding site but may identify a false aneurysm. Radioisotope scans are useful in some patients. Carefully performed technetium-labeled red cell scans should identify a source of bleeding in the midline of the patient adjacent to the aorta. Also, indium III scans may identify inflammatory tissue surrounding the aorta in the late postoperative period, suggesting graft infection. Definitive diagnosis is made by urgent repair of the aorta and intestine.[17]

Repair involves clamping the aorta at the diaphragm and then exposing the fistula (Fig. 22–3). The bowel is repaired in a standard manner unless destruction is extensive, in which case a bowel resection may be necessary. The old aortic graft is removed and the surrounding tissues are extensively debrided. A new graft is inserted and managed as in patients with infected graft prostheses (see Chapter 7 on graft infections). The new graft is wrapped with the omentum to protect it from surrounding tissues and the bowel. If the original repair was an end-to-side bypass for aortoiliac disease, the old graft can be removed and the aorta repaired. Any ischemia that then develops in the lower limbs is treated, if necessary, with axillofemoral grafts. This method of repair was advocated by surgeons during the early experience with the problem,[18] and we have continued to use it.

The management of aortointestinal fistulae in the abdomen, however, is controversial. Others[15, 16, 19] have reported a high complication rate with in situ repairs and advocate removal of the old graft, closure of the aortic stump, and axillofemoral bypass. Of paramount importance with either approach is the debridement of all infected aortic tissue, because false aneurysms may form with the first approach or stump "blow-out" may occur with the latter if this is not done.[17]

REFERENCES

1. Svensson LG, Crawford ES, Hess KR, et al. Experience with 1509 patients undergoing thoracoabdominal aortic operations. J Vasc Surg 1993;17:357-70.

2. Svensson LG, Crawford ES, Hess KR, et al. Thoracoabdominal aortic aneurysms associated with celiac, superior mesenteric and renal artery occlusive disease: methods and analysis of results in 271 patients. J Vasc Surg 1992;16:378-90.

3. Coselli JS, Crawford ES. Primary aortoesophageal fistula from aortic aneurysm: successful surgical treatment by use of omental pedicle graft. J Vasc Surg 1990;12:269-77.

4. Crawford ES, Crawford JL. Diseases of the Aorta Including an Atlas of Angiographic Pathology and Surgical Technique. Baltimore: Williams & Wilkins, 1984.

5. Syme J. Case of spontaneous varicose aneurysm. Edinb Med Surg J 1831;36:104-5.

6. Reckless JPD. Aorto-caval fistulae: an uncommon complication of abdominal aortic aneurysm. Br J Surg 1972;59:461-2.

7. Baker EJ, Ayton V, Smith MA, et al. Magnetic resonance imaging of coarctation of the aorta in infants: use of a high field strength. Br Heart J 1989;62:97-101.

8. Brewster DC, Cambria RP, Moncure AC, et al. Aortocaval and iliac arteriovenous fistulas: recognition and treatment. J Vasc Surg 1991;13:253-64.

9. Svensson LG, Gaylis H, Barlow JB. Presentation and management of aortocaval fistula. A report of 6 cases. S Afr Med J 1987;72:876-7.

10. Calligaro KD, Savarese RP, DeLaurentis DA. Unusual aspects of aor-tovenous fistulas associated with ruptured abdominal aortic aneurysms. J Vasc Surg 1990;12:586-90.

11. Crawford ES, Turrel DJ, Alexander JK. Aorto-inferior vena caval fistula of neoplastic origin. Circulation 1963;27:414.

12. Svensson LG, Persson LA, Cohen PM, Gaylis H. Successful management of ruptured septic aortic aneurysm and horseshoe kidney with multiple renal arteries: a case report. S Afr J Surg 1987;25:161-3.

13. Svensson LG, Crawford ES. Aortic dissection and aortic aneurysm surgery: clinical observations, experimental investigations, and statistical analyses. Part III. Curr Probl Surg 1993;30:1-172.

14. Elliott JP Jr, Smith RF, Szilagyi DE. Proceedings: aortoenteric and para-prosthetic-enteric fistulas: problems of diagnosis and management. Arch Surg 1974;108:479-90.

15. Kleinman LH, Towne JB, Bernhard VM. A diagnostic and therapeutic approach to aortoenteric fistulas: clinical experience with twenty patients. Surgery 1979;86:868-80.

16. O'Mara CS, Williams GM, Ernst CB. Secondary aortoenteric fistula: a twenty year experience. Am J Surg 1981;142:203-9.

17. Svensson LG. Thoracoabdominal graft infections. In: Calligaro KD, Veith FJ, eds. Management of Infected Arterial Grafts. St. Louis: Quality Medical Publishing, 1994:65-81.

18. Garrett HE, Beall AC Jr, Jordan GL Jr, et al. Surgical considerations of massive gastrointestinal tract hemorrhage caused by aortoduodenal fistula. Am J Surg 1963;105:6.

19. Bunt TJ. Synthetic vascular graft infections. II. Graft-enteric erosions and graft-enteric fistulas. Surgery 1983;94:1-9.

23

Aortic Aneurysms Associated with a Horseshoe Kidney

The main difficulties in repairing an aneurysm associated with a horseshoe kidney, which occurs in approximately one in 710 patients,[1] involve exposure of the aorta for repair and the preservation of renal arteries (Figs. 23-1 to 23-5). The reasons for these problems are that both the position and the shape of the fused kidney are variable and the neck of the aneurysm is frequently at a higher level than a normal infrarenal aortic aneurysm. The

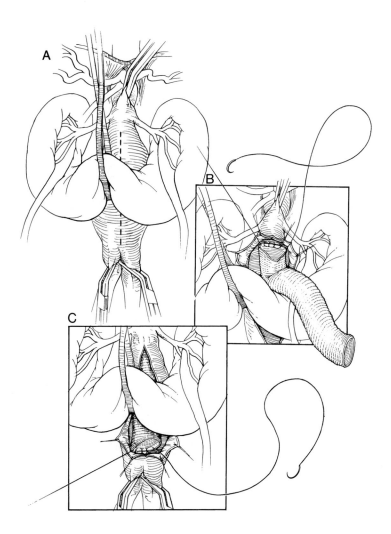

FIGURE 23–1   Steps in the repair of an uncomplicated abdominal aortic aneurysm associated with a horseshoe kidney. **A,** The aorta is cross-clamped in a suprarenal position, the horseshoe kidney is retracted with a umbilical tape sling, and the aorta is incised. **B,** The kidney is retracted downward for the proximal anastomosis and upward **(C)** for the distal anastomosis. (From Svensson LG, Crawford ES. Curr Probl Surg 1993;30:1-172.)

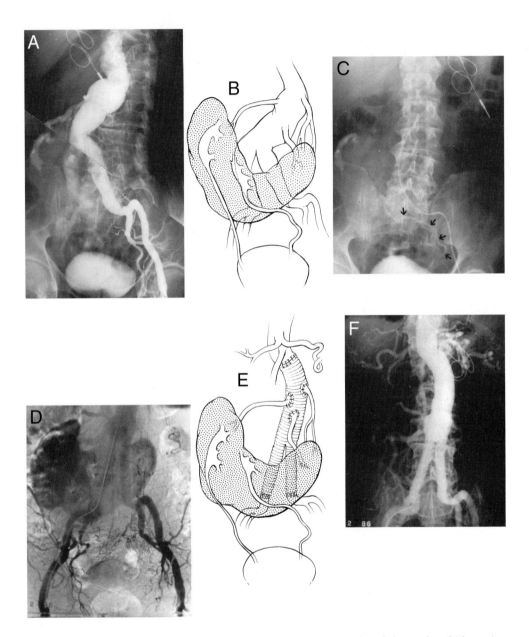

FIGURE 23–2   Repair of abdominal aortic aneurysm associated with horseshoe kidney. **A,** Preoperative angiogram, diagram **(B),** and ureterogram (ureter indicated by *arrows*) in a patient with a horseshoe kidney. The repair was done by cross-clamping of the supraceliac aorta and insertion of a bifurcated graft with reimplantation of the renal arteries as shown in figures **D, E,** and **F.**

FIGURE 23–3 A, Patient with horseshoe kidney and attempted repair of infrarenal aneurysm with a tube graft who presented to us with a rupture of the suprarenal component, a *Staphylococcus aureus* infection with frank pus, and shock. B, Diagram after repair with beveling of a graft behind the celiac artery and reimplantation of the renal arteries as a Carrel patch after division of the horseshoe kidney. The patient was irrigated with antibiotics retroperitoneally and recovered without any problems. He has remained on a life-time regimen of antibiotics. (From Svensson LG, Persson LA, Cohen PM, Gaylis H. S Afr J Surg 1987; 25:161–3.)

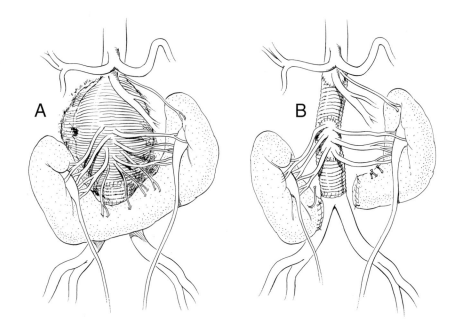

FIGURE 23–4 A, Patient with thoracoabdominal aneurysm and horseshoe kidney. B, Postoperative results after thoracoabdominal aneurysm extent type I repair through a retroperitoneal thoracoabdominal incision without disturbing the kidney.

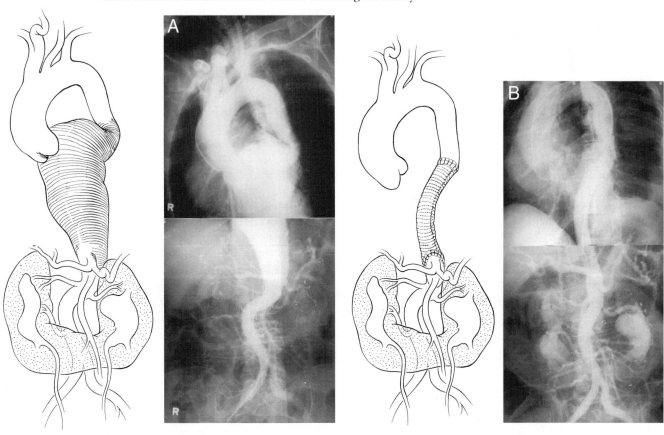

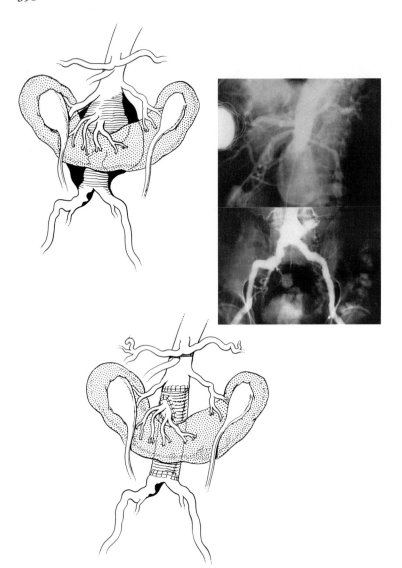

FIGURE 23–5 Preoperative angiogram and diagram of a patient with a horseshoe kidney and abdominal aortic aneurysm. The aneurysm was repaired by insertion of a tube graft and reimplantation of the renal arteries to the middle of the kidney as a Carrel patch.

risk of renal failure is also increased. In addition, the aberrant renal arteries and the abnormally located ureters can be damaged during surgery.

Typically, the lower poles of the kidney are fused and the calyces with ureters cross anteriorly over the isthmus of the horseshoe kidney. The blood supply of horseshoe kidneys occurs with five basic patterns,[1] of approximately equal incidence:

1. One renal artery for each side of the horseshoe kidney.

2. One renal artery for each side w3ith an aortic branch to the isthmus (the slightly more common pattern).

3. Two arteries for each side and one renal isthmus artery.

4. Two arteries for each side with one or more arising from the iliac arteries, including the isthmus branch.

5. Multiple renal arteries, sometimes too numerous to count accurately, originating from the aorta and the mesenteric and iliac arteries.[2] Venous abnormalities are less extensive and usually do not impede exposure of the aorta.

Preoperatively, the abnormal kidney is usually identified by ultrasound, computed tomography, magnetic resonance imaging, duplex scanning, or aortography. Where there is evidence of multiple arteries, selective cannulation of aortic branch arteries by angiography may be useful for both the intraoperative localization of arteries and the identification of safe planes through which to operate.

The repair is usually performed by one of two approaches, namely a thoracoabdominal approach,[3] particularly when most of the abdominal aorta is involved, or a transabdominal approach. With the abdominal approach through the midline, to aid exposure for better visualization, the supraceliac aorta can be cross-clamped and[4] either the horseshoe kidney can be reflected upward with a loop around the isthmus or the isthmus can be divided.[2] Urine leakage from the transected edges of the renal isthmus is rare if the raw surface is covered and sealed with the tough renal capsule.

Rarely, when a complex repair is required, cooling of the horseshoe kidney with cold Ringer's solution, as we have described previously,[2] is recommended. For a pelvic kidney, Schneider and Cronenwett[5] have described the use of double clamping to exclude the area of aortic repair and a temporary shunt for perfusion of the renal artery. Critical renal arteries usually need to be implanted as individual arteries if they arise from the aneurysmal aorta.[3] We have successfully reimplanted multiple renal arteries with a long Carrel patch.[2, 4]

REFERENCES

1. Eisendrath DN, Phifer FM, Culver HB. Horseshoe kidney. Ann Surg 1925;82:735-64.
2. Svensson LG, Persson LA, Cohen PM, Gaylis H. Successful management of ruptured septic aortic aneurysm and horseshoe kidney with multiple renal arteries: a case report. S Afr J Surg 1987;25:161-3.
3. Crawford ES, Coselli JS, Safi HJ, et al. The impact of renal fusion and ectopia on aortic surgery. J Vasc Surg 1988;8:375-83.
4. Svensson LG, Crawford ES. Aortic dissection and aortic aneurysm surgery: clinical observations, experimental investigations, and statistical analyses. Part III. Curr Probl Surg 1993;30:1-172.
5. Schneider JR, Cronenwett JL. Temporary perfusion of a congenital pelvic kidney during abdominal aortic aneurysm repair. J Vasc Surg 1993;17:613-7.

24

Replacement of the
Entire Aorta

Those patients who require replacement of the entire aorta either have had neglected type I aortic dissections or they present with a mega-aorta, most often due to chronic aortitis such as giant cell aortitis. Occasionally, patients who have Marfan syndrome without dissection require replacement of the entire aorta, although this is usually performed in stages.[1-3]

In this chapter, we refer to replacement of the *entire* aorta because the term *total replacement* has been used in the literature to describe replacement of segments of the aorta that have not included the entire aorta from the aortic valve commissures to the aortic bifurcation.[4, 5] Past descriptions of *total* aortic replacement through the left side of the chest have not included the proximal ascending aorta,[6] and others have described *total* aortic replacement when the infrarenal aorta has not been replaced with a tube graft to the aortic bifurcation.[1, 7]

The decision to replace the entire aorta is predicated on both the extent of aneurysm formation at the time of presentation and the severity of associated symptoms or complications of the aneurysm. There are three principal approaches to replacing the entire aorta.

First, the aorta can be replaced in stages as indicated by new aneurysm formation (Fig. 24-1).[6] Such repairs cannot be electively planned but quite often follow a general pattern. For example, a patient may first undergo replacement of the infrarenal abdominal aorta; then, with time, the ascending aorta and aortic arch are replaced and, even later, the thoracoabominal aorta is replaced. This is a common sequence of events for those patients with degenerative types of aneurysms that tend to evolve over several years.[1-3]

The second approach is the planned staged replacement of the entire aorta by our modification of the elephant trunk technique (Fig. 24-2).[6, 8] For the two-stage operations, two requirements usually have to be met. First, the aorta at the distal aortic arch must have a sufficient "neck" so that the graft can be sutured into position without the aorta tearing when the enlarged aorta at the distal aortic anastomosis is tailored down to the size of the aortic graft. Some careful judgment is required, depending on the quality of the aorta, anatomy, and acuity of the disease process, although the distal aortic arch usually should not be much larger than 7 or 8 cm in diameter to be tailored down to a 30 mm graft. The second criterion is that the distal aorta should not be at risk

of rupturing during the recovery period before the second-stage operation is performed. Thus patients who have severe back pain associated with the aneurysm are at risk and would not qualify as candidates for this procedure. Furthermore, those patients who have severe dysphagia or respiratory failure due to tracheal or bronchial compression (see below) require relief of pressure to prevent significant deterioration or death in the interval before a second-stage operation. The elephant trunk operative technique for either degenerative aneurysms or aortic dissection is discussed in detail in Chapters 17, 18, and 20.[1-3]

In a review of extensive aortic replacements, we reported replacement of the entire aorta in stages in 53 patients.[6] In the group of 82 patients who had subtotal replacements or entire aorta replacements, the 5-year survival rate was 65%, including the operative deaths. One patient had an attempted replacement of the entire aorta, excluding the segment immediately above the aortic valve, through a left thoracoabdominal incision but later died of multiple organ failure.

The third approach, which we (L.G.S.) pioneered and first performed on May 4, 1993 (Figs. 24-3 to 24-6) involves replacement of the entire aorta through a mediastinal and thoracoabdominal incision during a single operation.[1] The operation is extensive and exposes the patient to a procedure that requires a prolonged recovery period of several weeks. Clearly, it is indicated only for at-risk patients as outlined above. A patient undergoing an elephant trunk procedure can expect to be discharged from the hospital 6 to 10 days after the first operation if no complications occur and 4 to 10 days after an uncomplicated second-stage operation. For patients in whom the entire aorta is replaced during a single operation, however, a lengthy postoperative ventilation period is often required because of preoperative respiratory compromise in many patients and because of both a mediastinal and thoracoabdominal incision with division of the diaphragm is used for exposure. We have also noted that the sudden impedance to the heart caused by ejection of blood into a fairly noncompliant and nonelastic long graft does impose a strain on the heart. In patients undergoing staged repairs of the entire aorta, strain on the heart is mitigated by the time the heart has to hypertrophy to deal with the increased outflow impedance and because of the shorter graft. This lack of elasticity of the new graft replacing the

FIGURE 24–1 For extensive aortic replacements, reoperations because of previous cardiac procedures are frequent. The illustration shows the methods we use for reoperations. If patients do not have iliac artery stenoses or occlusion, the femoral artery and vein are routinely exposed and encircled with umbilical tape. If there is a possibility of problems with perfusion through the femoral artery, then the subclavian artery should also be exposed. An alternative in some patients is to cannulate the aneurysm directly in the aortic arch and then, after the repair, to reperfuse the aortic arch with a side graft. After removal of the old sternal wires, a tunnel is created under the breastbone with a pair of scissors and the periosteum is cut with the patient in a head down position. At the same time, the subcostal margin and later the sternal edge are retracted with rake retractors. The xiphoid is often excised before the tunneling is commenced. Once a tunnel of a few inches has been produced, the sternum is opened from below with an sternal saw to the end of the tunnel. Further tunneling is then done under the sternum, and the saw is used to open the sternum. This is continued in stages until the whole sternum has been divided. We have found that this is the safest method for patients who have aortic aneurysms impinging on the back of the sternum.

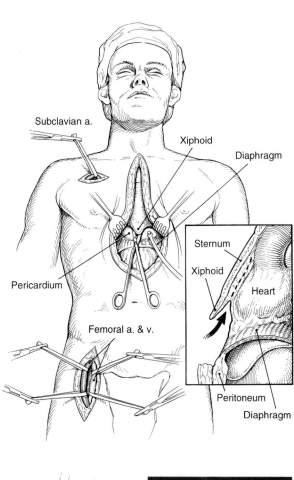

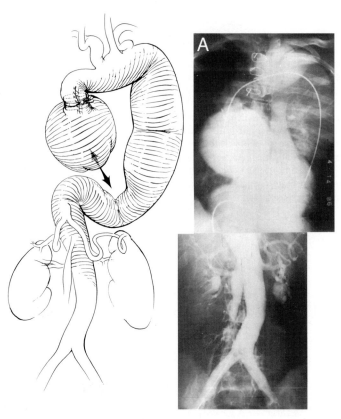

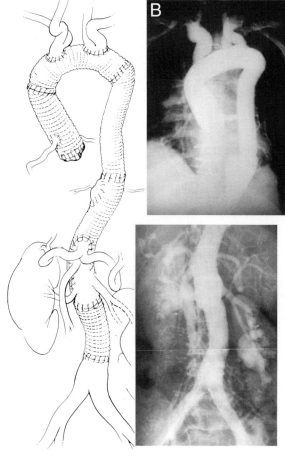

FIGURE 24–2 Replacement of the entire aorta in stages in a patient with Marfan syndrome. **A,** Initially an intraluminal prothesis was inserted for aortic dissection elsewhere and the patient was referred for aortic valve regurgitation with aneurysmal formation. **B,** First the aortic arch was replaced and a composite valve graft was inserted. The descending aorta was then replaced. A recurrent arch aneurysm developed and separate implantation of the greater vessels was required. Later the remaining thoracoabdominal aorta had to be replaced to complete the repair. The aortogram shows the completed repair. (From Svensson LG, Crawford ES, Coselli JS, et al. Impact of cardiovascular operation on survival in the Marfan patient. Circulation 1989;80(3Pt1):I233–42. Reprinted with permission. Copyright 1989 American Heart Association.)

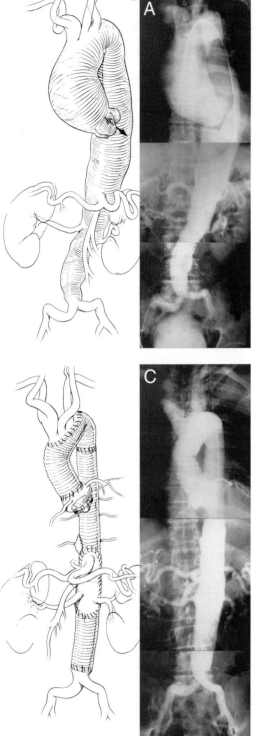

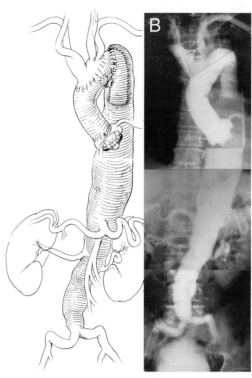

FIGURE 24–3 Replacement of the entire aorta by the elephant trunk technique. **A,** The middle-aged patient was seen in the emergency room with increasing dyspnea and chest discomfort and a history of temporal arteritis, a not infrequent presentation for patients with a mega-aorta. Aortography revealed aortic valve regurgitation and an extensive aneurysm. **B,** The first-stage elephant trunk procedure was performed, as described in previous chapters and, in addition, an aortic valve was inserted. The aortogram shows the elephant trunk in the descending aorta. **C,** Through a thoracoabdominal incision, the remaining aorta was repaired with reimplantation of the intercostal and visceral arteries.

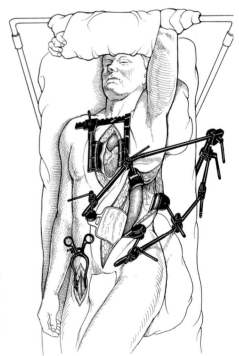

FIGURE 24–4 Positioning of the patient for replacement of the entire aorta during a single operation. Note that the left arm is elevated and the shoulder is padded with a pillow to position the patient at approximately a 30-degree angle. Both a mediastinal and a thoracoabdominal incision are made to give access to the aorta. The femoral artery and vein are exposed for cannulation

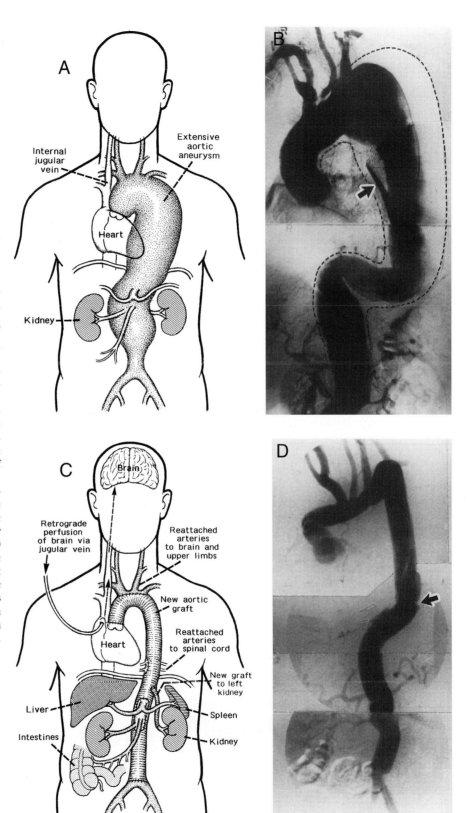

FIGURE 24–5 **A,** Illustrations of a patient who presented with a mega-aorta related to temporal and giant cell arteritis measuring 17 cm in diameter at the proximal descending thoracic aorta and 6 cm in the ascending and infrarenal aorta. The patient had dysphagia, weight loss, and severe pain that was unrelieved with narcotics. **B,** Aortography revealed an extensive aneurysm with contrast dye tracking under the clot in the descending aorta *(arrow)*. The *stippled line* indicates the outline of the aneurysm as seen on the original aortogram pictures. **C,** With the use of deep hypothermia, circulatory arrest, and retrograde brain perfusion, the arch vessels were first reattached. The brain was reperfused and then the proximal anastomosis above the aortic valve was performed. Through the left thoracoabdominal incision, the rest of the aorta was replaced, with reattachment of the intercostal arteries, visceral arteries, and finally the aortic bifurcation. In addition, a tube graft was used to reattach the left renal artery. **D,** The postoperative aortogram shows the completed repair with the *arrow* indicating where two 60 cm long grafts were joined to make the graft long enough. The graft in the chest appears to be redundant because of the size of the aneurysm cavity that was replaced. (Reprinted with permission from the Society of Thoracic Surgeons. From Svensson LG, Shahian DM, Davis FG, et al. Ann Thorac Surg 1994;58:1164-6.)

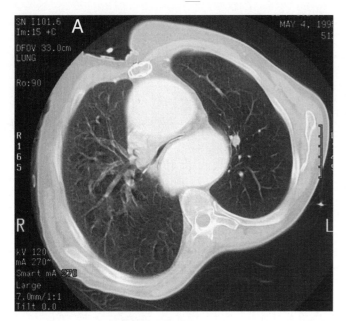 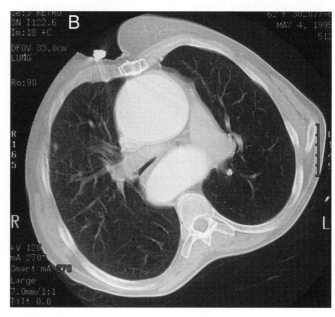

FIGURE 24–6 Preoperative CT scan of the chest showing compression of the trachea and bronchi by an aneurysm that had some displacement into the right chest. The patient had to be intubated for the CT scan and aortogram because of severe respiratory distress and the inability to lie flat. She had previously undergone cardiac surgery, was taking Coumadin for chronic atrial fibrillation, had 4+ aortic valve regurgitation, coronary artery disease, and also had dysphagia and weight loss. The ascending aorta, the aortic arch, and the thoracoabdominal aorta were replaced in a single operation and, in addition, a composite valve graft and coronary artery bypass were performed.

aorta results in a pressure wave, recorded in the femoral arteries, that is somewhat analogous to that observed with advanced aortic valve stenosis. The altered pulse wave has a slower upstroke, a slight plateau, and a slower fall in pressure resulting in a reduced (both positive and negative) *dP/dt.* Intraoperative measurements of blood pressure in the ascending aorta and the radial or femoral arteries usually reveals a 10 to 20 mm Hg gradient, whereas in a patient with a normal aorta undergoing, for example, a coronary artery bypass operation, femoral pressure will often be higher than the ascending aorta pressure. Despite the potential problems, the entire aorta replacement operation

has an important role for those selected patients who have previously been considered poor risks for extensive aortic repairs and, thus, often died during surgery or shortly afterwards because of operations that were inadequate to deal with the problem.[1, 8] The procedure of replacing the entire aorta in a single operation can be considered to be a combination of an elephant trunk type of operation without a distal arch anastomosis and a thoracoabdominal aortic repair, albeit with limited proximal exposure for the thoracoabdominal repair.[8]

As illustrated (Figs. 24–4 to 24–8), the patient is placed on the operating room table with a pillow positioned

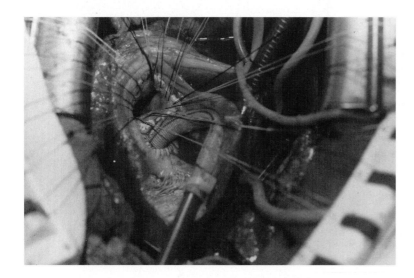

FIGURE 24–7 Intraoperative photograph of a patient having a composite valve graft and a coronary artery bypass done at the same time as replacement of the ascending aorta, aortic arch, and thoracoabdominal aorta through two incisions.

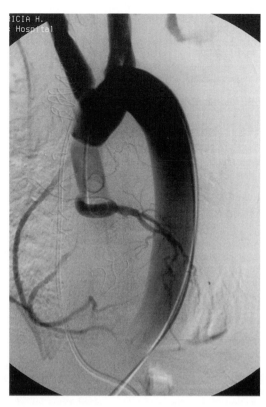

FIGURE 24–8   Postoperative aortogram of thoracic aorta showing composite valve graft with tube graft to left main, vein graft to right coronary, and replacement of the entire thoracic aorta. The abdominal aorta repair is not shown.

behind the left shoulder so that the shoulder is elevated for the thoracoabdominal incision, and the left arm is suspended on an anesthesia screen bar to keep the arm out of the sterile field. A conventional mediastinal incision and a thoracoabdominal incision are then made. The patient is placed on cardiopulmonary bypass and cooled until electroencephalographic electrical silence is achieved and the circulation is arrested. First the tube graft is placed in the descending aorta, and then a hole is excised for the greater vessels, which are reattached during circulatory arrest. Next the brain is reperfused, and the proximal ascending aortic anastomosis is performed either to the aorta or to a composite valve graft. Thereafter, through the thoracoabdominal incision, the tube graft is retrieved, the intercostal arteries are reimplanted, the visceral arteries are reimplanted, and the distal anastomosis is completed. After hemostasis is obtained, the incisions are closed. Postoperative care is the same as for any other thoracic aortic repair, with the exception that the period of postoperative ventilation tends to be lengthy, partly because of preoperative respiratory dysfunction. Nevertheless, in our limited experience, thus far our patients have survived and live a normal life with no or minimal medication, namely, Coumadin for valve anticoagulation.[1]

Credit should be given to the contributions of many surgeons who developed the operations on the ascending aorta, the aortic arch, and the thoracoabdominal aorta[4, 9-35] and to those under whom one of us (L.G.S.) trained and learned invaluable technical skills and lessons, particularly Drs. Floyd Loop, Delos Cosgrove, Bruce Lytle, Stanley Crawford, Michael DeBakey, Gerald Lawrie, James Jones, Gene Guinn, David Clarke, David Campbell, and colleagues Joseph Coselli and Hazim Safi, whose combined techniques resulted in the replacement of the entire aorta during a single operation.

REFERENCES

1. Svensson LG, Shahian DM, Davis FG, et al. Replacement of entire aorta from aortic valve to bifurcation during one operation. Ann Thorac Surg 1994;58:1164-6.
2. Crawford ES, Coselli JS, Svensson LG, et al. Diffuse aneurysmal disease (chronic aortic dissection, Marfan, and mega aorta syndromes) and multiple aneurysm: treatment by subtotal and total aortic replacement emphasizing the elephant trunk technique. Ann Surg 1990;211:521-37.
3. Svensson LG, Crawford ES, Coselli JS, et al. Impact of cardiovascular operation on survival in the Marfan patient. Circulation 1989;80(3 Pt 1):I233-42.
4. Massimo CG, Poma AG, Viligiardi RR, et al. Simultaneous total aortic replacement from arch to bifurcation: experience with six cases. Texas Heart Inst J 1986;13:147-51.
5. Massimo CE, Presenti LE, Favi PP, et al. Excision of the aortic wall in the surgical treatment of acute type-A aortic dissection. Ann Thorac Surg 1990;50:274-6.
6. Crawford ES, Coselli JS, Svensson LG, et al. Diffuse aneurysmal disease (chronic aortic dissection, Marfan, and mega aorta syndromes) and multiple aneurysm: treatment by subtotal and total aortic replacement emphasizing the elephant trunk operation. Ann Surg 1990;211:521-37.
7. Massimo CG, Presenti LF, Favi PP, et al. Simultaneous total replacement from valve to bifurcation: experience with 21 cases. Ann Thorac Surg 1993;56:1110-6.
8. Svensson LG. Rationale and technique for replacement of the

ascending aorta, arch, and distal aorta using a modified elephant trunk procedure. J Cardiac Surg 1992;7:301-12.

9. Barnard CN, Schire V. The surgical treatment of acquired aneurysms of the thoracic aorta. Thorax 1963;18:101-5.

10. Borst HG, Schaudig A, Rudolph W. Arteriovenous fistula of the aortic arch: repair during deep hypothermia and circulatory arrest. J Thorac Cardiovasc Surg 1964;48:443-7.

11. Borst HG, Walterbusch G, Schaps D. Extensive aortic replacement using "elephant trunk" prosthesis. Thorac Cardiovasc Surg 1983;31:37-40.

12. Cooley DA, DeBakey ME. Resection of the entire ascending aorta in fusiform aneurysm using cardiac bypass. JAMA 1956;162:1158-9.

13. Cooley DA, Ott DA, Frazier OH, et al. Surgical treatment of aneurysms of the transverse aortic arch: experience with 25 patients using hypothermic techniques. Ann Thorac Surg 1981;32:260-72.

14. Coselli JS, Crawford ES, Beall ACJ, et al. Determination of brain temperatures for safe circulatory arrest during cardiovascular operation. Ann Thorac Surg 1988;45:638-42.

15. Crafoord C, Nylin F. Congenital coarctation of aorta and its surgical treatment. J Thorac Surg 1945;14:347-61.

16. Crawford ES. Thoracoabdominal and abdominal aortic aneurysm involving renal, superior mesenteric, and celiac arteries. Ann Surg 1974;179:763-72.

17. Crawford ES, Palamara AE, Saleh SA, Roehm JOF. Aortic aneurysm: current status of surgical treatment. Surg Clin North Am 1979;59:597-636.

18. Crawford ES, Crawford JL, Safi HJ, et al. Thoracoabdominal aortic aneurysms: preoperative and intraoperative factors determining immediate and long-term results of operation in 605 patients. J Vasc Surg 1986;3:389-404.

19. DeBakey ME, Cooley DA. Successful resection of aneurysm of thoracic aorta and replacement by graft. JAMA 1953;152:673-6.

20. DeBakey ME, Cooley DA. Successful resection of aneurysms of distal aortic arch and replacement of graft. JAMA 1954;155:1398-403.

21. DeBakey ME, Cooley DA, Creech O Jr. Surgical considerations of dissecting aneurysms of the aorta. Ann Surg 1955;142:586-92.

22. DeBakey ME, Creech O, Morris GC. Aneurysm of thoracoabdominal aorta involving the celiac, superior mesenteric, and renal arteries: report of four cases treated by resection and homograft replacement. Ann Surg 1956;144:549-73.

23. DeBakey ME, Cooley DA, Crawford ES, et al. Successful resection of fusiform aneurysm of aortic arch replacement by homograft. Surg Gynecol Obstet 1957;105:656-64.

24. DeBakey ME, Cooley DA, Crawford ES, et al. The clinical application of a new flexible knitted Dacron arterial substitute. Arch Surg 1958;77:713-24.

25. Dubost C. The first successful resection of an aneurysm of the abdominal aorta followed by re-establishment of continuity using a preserved human arterial graft. Ann Vasc Surg 1986;1:147-9.

26. Etheredge SN, Yee J, Smith JV, et al. Successful resection of a large aneurysm of the upper abdominal aorta and replacement with homograft. Surgery 1955;38:1071-81.

27. Gibbon JH Jr. Application of a mechanical heart and lung apparatus to cardiac surgery. Minn Med 1954;37:171-80.

28. Griepp RB, Stinson EB, Hollingsworth JF, et al. Prosthetic replacement of the aortic arch. J Thorac Cardiovasc Surg 1975;70:1051-63.

29. Julian OC, Deterling RA Jr, Dye WS, et al. Dacron tube and bifurcation arterial prostheses produced to specification: II. Continued clinical use and the addition of microcrimping. Arch Surg 1952;78:260.

30. Kouchoukos NT, Karp RB, Blackstone EH, et al. Replacement of the ascending aorta and aortic valve with a composite graft: results in 86 patients. Ann Surg 1980;192:403-12.

31. Bentall H, DeBono A. A technique for complete replacement of the ascending aorta. Thorax 1968;23:338-9.

32. Lemole G, Strong M, Spagna P, Karmilowicz NP. Improved results for dissecting aneurysms: intraluminal sutureless prosthesis. J Thorac Cardiovasc Surg 1982;83:249-55.

33. Miller DC. Surgical management of aortic dissections: indications, perioperative management, and long-term results. In: Doroghazi RM, Slater EE, editors. Aortic Dissection. New York: McGraw-Hill, 1983:193-243.

34. Morris GC Jr, Henly WS, DeBakey ME. Correction of acute dissecting aneurysm of aorta with valvular insufficiency. JAMA 1963;184:63-4.

35. Swan H, Maaske C, Johnson M, et al. Arterial homografts. II. Resection of thoracic aortic aneurysm using a stored human arterial transplant. Arch Surg 1950;61:732-7.

Complications of Proximal Aorta Operations

The major complications and problems after proximal aortic surgery on the ascending aorta or aortic arch include hemorrhage (coagulopathy or for technical reasons); cardiac events (low cardiac output, infarction, ischemia, heart block, and arrhythmias); neurological problems (stroke, transient ischemic events, seizures, and neurocognitive dysfunction); respiratory problems (either complications or failure); renal failure, sometimes requiring dialysis; gastrointestinal complications, including hyperamylasemia; sepsis; and multiple organ failure. These complications are associated with an increased risk of death. We have reported[1] that hyperamylasemia is common after cardiopulmonary bypass and occurs in up to one third of patients, even if there is no evidence of pancreatitis, which is rare. Late complications related to the aorta are the development of aneurysms at a site distant from the original operation with the risk of rupture, false aneurysms, infection of aortic prostheses, occlusion of side branches, and organ-specific complications such as myocardial infarction and stroke.[2-22]

Postoperative bleeding complications have been dealt with previously in our discussion of blood conservation and autotransfusion in Chapter 16.[23] Control of postoperative bleeding, including that after proximal aortic surgery and other types of distal aortic surgery, can be summarized as follows. Approximately every 20 minutes, blood samples should be sent for testing of the prothrombin index (PT), partial thromboplastin time (PTT), platelet count, and fibrinogen level. If the PT is elevated, fresh frozen plasma is given. If both the PT and the PTT are elevated, fresh frozen plasma is initially given, and if heparin may have been given or is still circulating, then 50 mg of protamine is administered. If the PTT is still elevated and the fibrinogen level is decreased, especially if less than 150 mg/dl, then 10 units of cryoprecipitate are given. If active bleeding is occurring and the platelet count is less than 150,000 /mm³, or if the patient has received antiplatelet agents such as aspirin recently, 6 to 10 units of platelets are given. Amicar is used liberally, both as a bolus and subsequently as a continuous intravenous drip. Blood products continue to be prescribed as required. The use of aprotinin was discussed in Chapter 16. The drug clearly is effective,[24] but there are concerns regarding its safety.[25, 26] We have reported that, with meticulous surgical technique and blood-conservation methods, 87% of patients undergoing proximal operations do not require an intraoperative transfusion of homologous blood or blood product and, by the time of discharge from hospital, 69% will not have required a transfusion.[27]

CARDIAC COMPLICATIONS

Intraoperative low-output cardiac failure is mostly due to either inadequate myocardial preservation,[23] or myocardial infarction or technical problems. The latter include failure to perform coronary artery bypasses for coronary artery stenoses; poorly performed anastomoses; unsuccessful coronary endarterectomies; embolization to the coronary arteries; dissection of coronary arteries; and technical problems with reattachment of the coronary ostia during composite valve grafts or insertion of human valved conduits (homografts and autografts). In 348 composite valve grafts that we inserted,[21] technical problems resulting in myocardial ischemia were noted predominantly with the Cabrol technique. The problem arose when the interposition graft to the right coronary ostium either kinked or occluded with resultant thrombosis of the graft. In five patients, a reversed saphenous vein had to be inserted intraoperatively to the distal right coronary artery because of right ventricular dysfunction.[21] In our earlier experience with the use of high doses of thiopental (20 mg/kg) for neurological protection during deep hypothermia with circulatory arrest, we noted that some patients had low-output cardiac failure. Some of these patients were treated with left ventricular assist devices in the postoperative period and recovered. However, we now only use 5 mg/kg of thiopental.[19, 20] Furthermore, there is some evidence that thiopental may even be harmful when used in combination with deep hypothermia and circulatory arrest,[28] although for brain ischemia it appears to be protective.[29]

For reasons that are not entirely clear, patients in whom composite valve grafts are inserted appear to be particularly prone to postoperative ventricular arrhythmias.[6, 11, 14-16] In our own experience, 50 of 717 patients who underwent ascending or aortic arch surgery had either postoperative ventricular tachycardia or fibrillation.[6] Similarly, Kouchoukos[14] has noted a 22% incidence of ventricular arrhythmias. More recently, however, with our technique of placing a tube graft to the left main ostium and reattaching the right coronary ostium as a button in 34 patients, only two (6%) have had ventricular arrhythmias, one of them associated with Wolff-Parkinson-White (WPW) syndrome and supraventricular tachycardia.

There are several factors that cause or are associated with ventricular arrhythmias: myocardial ischemia, the propensity for arrhythmias in patients with Marfan syndrome, chronic aortic valve regurgitation with ventricular dilatation and fibrosis, undiagnosed myocardial infarctions, electrolyte abnormalities, long clamp-times, and pacemaker (R on T spikes)- induced arrhythmias. In addition, some patients exhibit an abnormal QT interval on electrocardiogram (ECG), an abnormal QTc by Bazett's formula, or even an abnormal correlation between the QT interval and the R-R interval that induces ventricular repolarization abnormalities and may lead to sudden death.[30] Undoubtedly, because these patients receive numerous blood products to increase coagulation, occlusion of vein grafts or the native coronary arteries may also play a role.

The use of signal-averaged ECGs after coronary artery bypass surgery has been reported to be 100% sensitive and 70% specific for predicting the occurrence of ventricular tachyarrhythmias.[31] The P-wave signal-averaged ECG has also been found to be 77% sensitive and 55% specific for predicting postoperative atrial fibrillation after cardiac surgery,[32] although its use after cardiac surgery has been questioned because of the high cost and low specificity.[33]

Sotalol, an agent newly introduced to the United States for the control of supraventricular tachycardia, is particularly effective in controlling postoperative atrial arrhythmias after open cardiac surgery.[34] The other alternative agents are digoxin, adenosine, beta-blockers, and verapamil.

NEUROLOGICAL COMPLICATIONS

Increasingly, studies document that cerebral embolization from aortic atheromatous plaques in the ascending aorta and aortic arch, observed on intraoperative echocardiography, is resulting in postoperative strokes.[35, 36] This complication is particularly likely to occur in elderly patients and in patients with peripheral vascular disease or diabetes. We have noted that the incidence of postoperative stroke after proximal aortic surgery was increased in our patients who, on the basis of aortic histology, were found to have evidence of atherosclerosis.[19] To reduce the incidence of postoperative stroke, deep hypothermia with circulatory arrest is an invaluable and relatively safe adjunct for proximal aortic operations. Aside from repair of the aortic arch and acute aortic dissection being indications for the application of deep hypothermia and circulatory arrest,[4, 6, 18, 23] patients with atheromatous disease of the ascending aorta should also be operated on by this technique. This procedure has

been advocated for the same problem associated with coronary artery bypass surgery.[35, 36] The pathophysiology and methods involved for establishing deep hypothermia with circulatory arrest were discussed in Chapter 13.

Factors that in our experience influence the results of deep hypothermia with circulatory arrest are discussed below. Of the 656 patients operated on between July 7, 1979, and January 30, 1991, with deep hypothermia and circulatory arrest, 13% had a history of cerebrovascular disease.[19] The median circulatory arrest time was 31 minutes (range, 7 to 120 minutes). The univariate predictors of transient or permanent stroke, either global or hemiparetic, which occurred in 44 patients (7%), were ($p < 0.05$) increasing age; a history of cerebrovascular disease; circulatory arrest time (7 to 29 minutes = 12/298, 4%; 30 to 44 minutes = 15/201, 7.5%; 45 to 59 minutes = 9/84, 10.7%; 60 to 120 minutes = 7/48, 14.6%); cardiopulmonary bypass time; and concurrent descending thoracic aorta repair. The independent determinants for stroke were ($p < 0.05$) a history of cerebrovascular disease; previous aortic surgery distal to the left subclavian artery; and cardiopulmonary bypass time. A history of aortic valve incompetence, however, was associated with a lower risk of stroke (adjusted odds ratio 0.42, $p = 0.015$). The incidence of stroke was observed to increase after 40 minutes of circulatory arrest and, furthermore, the mortality rate increased markedly after 65 minutes of circulatory arrest. Thus the "safe" period for strokes not developing appeared to be limited to approximately 40 minutes. The influences of selected continuous variables on the stroke incidence and mortality rate are shown (Fig. 25–1). Evident from the nonparametric curves were the marked increase in mortality after 65 minutes of circulatory arrest and the increase in stroke rate after 40 minutes of circulatory arrest.[19] The stroke rate beyond 65 minutes of circulatory arrest should be interpreted with caution, however, because the early mortality rate was high in this group of patients and thus the incidence of stroke could not be accurately determined.[19]

The major issues with deep hypothermia plus circulatory arrest and the prevention of complications are[19] (1) management of cardiopulmonary bypass and blood pH (acid-base balance) (discussed previously in Chapter 13); (2) the influence of time on the safety of circulatory arrest; (3) adjuncts that may extend the period of safety of circulatory arrest; and (4) the more subtle signs of deleterious neurological events in the form of neuropsychiatric and cognitive dysfunction.[19]

The second issue mentioned above is the period of safety of circulatory arrest. Contrary to expectation, the length of circulatory arrest was not an independent determinant of death or of postoperative stroke.[19] This was also noted in the study by Cameron and colleagues.[37] Clearly, this does not mean that the length of circulatory arrest is not important; rather, it is not one of the best independent predictors of the risk of stroke.[19] It may, however, be a better predictor of postoperative neurocognitive problems. Nevertheless, the univariate analysis, logistic regression

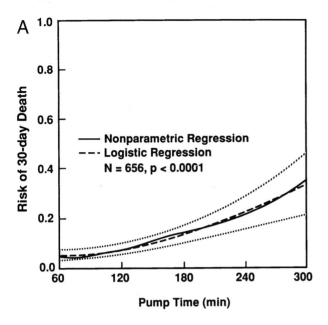

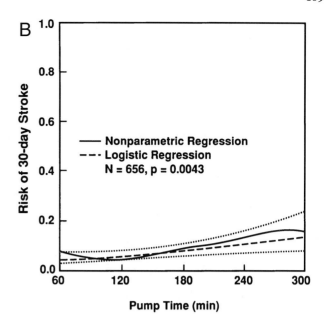

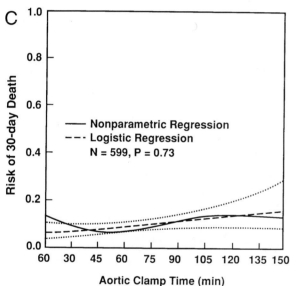

FIGURE 25–1 Influence of variables on the risk of death or stroke after deep hypothermic arrest. *Stippled lines* indicate logistic regression curves and *continuous lines* indicate the nonparametric curves. The 95% confidence limits are shown. Note that on univariate analysis pump time and circulatory arrest time were significant predictors of both death and stroke and that rewarming time and age were predictors of death. Also shown is the interaction between age and circulatory arrest time on the risk of stroke. (From Svensson LG, Crawford ES, Hess KR, et al. J Thorac Cardiovasc Surg 1992;106:19-31.)

Illustration continued on following two pages

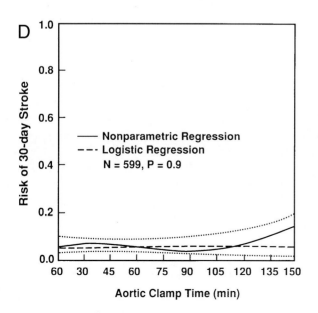

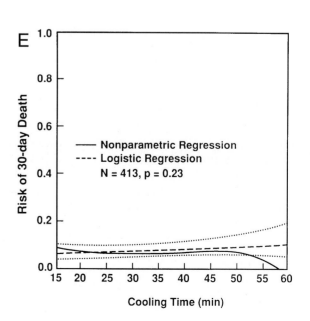

FIGURE 25–1 *Continued*

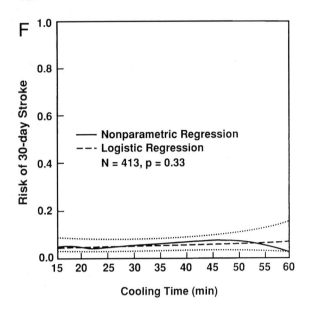

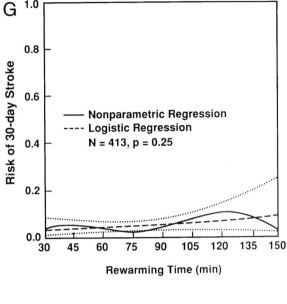

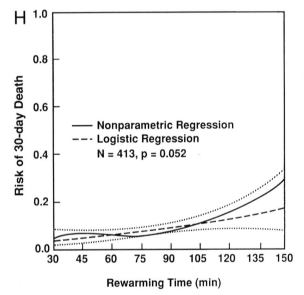

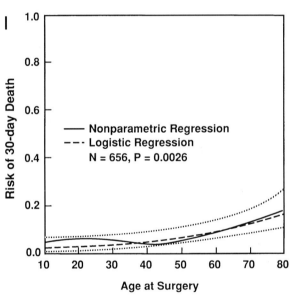

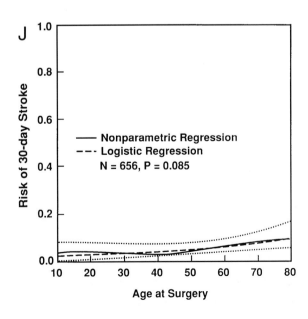

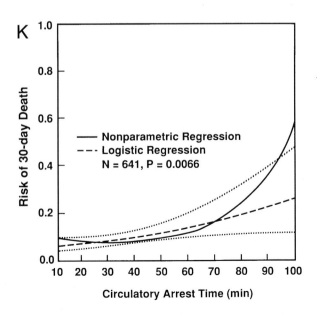

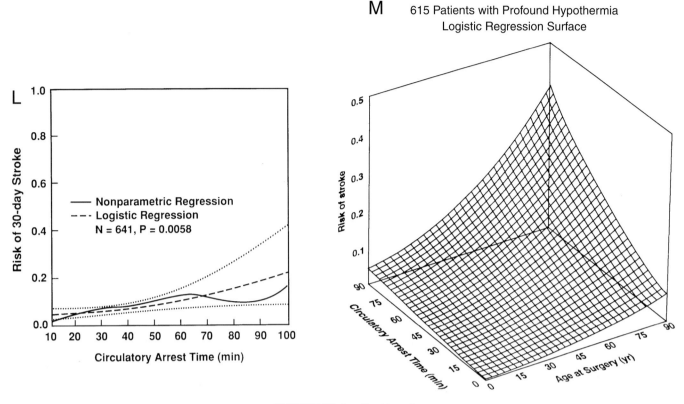

FIGURE 25–1 *Continued*

analysis of circulatory arrest time versus stroke, and both clinical and experimental research findings indicate that the time interval is important.[38, 39] The study by Treasure and colleagues[39] in gerbils showed that the risk of neurological dysfunction increased markedly after 45 minutes of circulatory arrest. Our data would suggest that after 40 minutes of circulatory arrest the risk of stroke increases and is particularly evident in older patients.

The use of deep hypothermia with circulatory arrest is not without potential complications. To minimize the risk, we recommend the following: air and debris should be meticulously aspirated from the aorta[6, 19, 20]; temperature gradients between the water bath and the blood should be kept below 10° C to reduce the incidence of gaseous microemboli[6, 19, 20]; 25 g of mannitol should be added to the pump on recommencement of flow for the possible scavenging of free radicals[6, 19, 20]; and 50 mEq of sodium bicarbonate should be added to the pump to correct for any acidosis that might have arisen due to the production of lactic acid during circulatory arrest.[6, 19, 20] The role of retrograde brain perfusion was discussed in Chapter 13.

The interesting finding that cardiopulmonary bypass time is a predictor of postoperative stroke raises the question of whether microembolization during prolonged cardiopulmonary bypass is a greater factor in the cause of strokes than the cerebrovascular ischemia time.[19] This is supported by research that has shown microembolization to be a problem with cardiopulmonary bypass[40] and that prolonged rewarming increases the risk of microembolism and is associated with cerebral hyperperfusion.[41] Some of the possible benefits arising from retrograde perfusion of the brain via veins during circulatory arrest may be the result of flushing out of microemboli in the brain capillary network and arterial system.[19] Thus the original report by Mills and Oschner[42] of retrograde perfusion to evacuate air from the arterial system may have great relevance to the use of retrograde brain perfusion, apart from the other possible but controversial benefits of either oxygenating the brain, providing metabolic substrates, removing metabolic pathway effluent, or keeping the brain cold. Since 1991, one of us (L.G.S.) has used retrograde perfusion of the superior vena cava as described by Mills and Oschner[42] and has been impressed with how mentally alert the patients were the day after surgery. Furthermore, when they were asked to do simple arithmetic calculations or memory tests, no gross deficit appeared to be present.

The third issue is the use of adjuncts to prolong or minimize the effects of circulatory arrest.[19] Animal research may yield clinically applicable adjuncts, including cerebroplegia,[43] blood substitutes, and retrograde perfusion of the brain.[19]

The fourth issue involves the subtle signs of neurological dysfunction that occur after deep hypothermia with circulatory arrest.[19] A high incidence of subtle neurocognitive deficits has been noted in previous studies of patients undergoing cardiopulmonary bypass[44, 45] and, of concern, the dysfunction in patients with pump times greater than 2 hours appears to be permanent.[46] In patients undergoing cardiopulmonary bypass, Engelman and colleagues[47] were unable to show, in their early data, that perfusate temperature (37° C, 32° C, 20° C) influenced the postoperative incidence of neurological dysfunction measured on the Mathew neurological scale, although all patients showed a decrease after surgery but returned to normal on late follow-up. Guyton and colleagues,[48] in a prospective randomized trial of warm cardioplegia versus cold crystalloid cardioplegia, found that neurological events were significantly ($p < 0.005$) higher with warm cardioplegia (4.5%) than with cold cardioplegia (1.4%). The reasons for this are unclear but may have been related to higher systemic glucose levels in the warm cardioplegia group. This aspect requires further research. As discussed in Chapter 12, there has been an explosion of research and information on the biochemistry involved in neurological deficits. It is clear that both the early causes, such as embolism, flow, and metabolism, and the secondary later events, such as mitochondrial DNA expression of disturbance, are important factors that should be considered.[49, 50]

The importance of carotid artery stenosis in the postoperative development of stroke and the question of whether concomitant carotid endarterectomy should be performed with cardiac surgery continue to be controversial. Gerraty and colleagues[51] studied 145 patients who had vascular and 213 who had coronary artery bypass operations and concluded that those with symptomatic carotid stenoses should undergo operation whereas those with asymptomatic stenoses do not need such intervention. We would agree with this policy for symptomatic stenoses, but we have found that the severity of carotid artery stenoses was an independent predictor of postoperative stroke in patients without symptoms. This finding is based on a series of more than 1300 patients we have recently evaluated with noninvasive Duplex carotid artery studies before coronary artery bypass operations.[52] The 30-day mortality rate was 2.2%, and the stroke rate was 2.5%. The independent predictors of postoperative stroke were severity of carotid stenoses according to Duplex studies, postoperative atrial fibrillation, unstable angina after myocardial infarction, history of stroke or transient ischemia attack, cardiopulmonary bypass time, peripheral vascular disease, and ascending aortic atherosclerosis. Thus we recommend that a more aggressive approach should be taken in operations on carotid stenoses, even when asymptomatic, particularly if the stricture is more than 80% or if bilateral carotid disease is present.

REFERENCES

1. Svensson LG, Decker G, Kinsley R. A prospective study of hyperamylasemia and pancreatitis after cardiopulmonary bypass. Ann Thorac Surg 1985;39:409-11.
2. Crawford ES, Crawford JL. Diseases of the Aorta Including an Atlas of Angiographic Pathology and Surgical Technique. Baltimore: Williams & Wilkins, 1984.
3. Crawford ES, Coselli JS, Safi HJ. Partial cardiopulmonary bypass, hypothermic circulatory arrest, and posterolateral exposure for thoracic aortic aneurysm operation. J Thorac Cardiovasc Surg 1987;94: 824-7.
4. Crawford ES, Svensson LG, Coselli JS, et al. Aortic dissection and dissecting aortic aneurysms. Ann Surg 1988;208:254-73.
5. Crawford ES, Coselli JS. Marfan's syndrome: combined composite valve graft replacement of the aortic root and transaortic mitral valve replacement. Ann Thorac Surg 1988;45:296-302.
6. Crawford ES, Svensson LG, Coselli JS, et al. Surgical treatment of aneurysm and/or dissection of the ascending aorta, transverse aortic arch, and ascending aorta and transverse aortic arch: factors influencing survival in 717 patients. J Thorac Cardiovasc Surg 1989; 98:659-73.
7. Crawford ES, Coselli JS, Svensson LG, et al. Diffuse aneurysmal disease (chronic aortic dissection, Marfan, and mega aorta syndromes) and multiple aneurysm: treatment by subtotal and total aortic replacement emphasizing the elephant trunk operation. Ann Surg 1990;211:521-37.
8. Coselli JS, Crawford ES, Beall ACJ, et al. Determination of brain temperatures for safe circulatory arrest during cardiovascular operation. Ann Thorac Surg 1988;45:638-42.
9. Coselli JS, Crawford ES. Composite valve-graft replacement of aortic root using separate Dacron tube for coronary artery reattachment. Ann Thorac Surg 1989;47:558-65.
10. Coselli JS, Crawford ES, Williams TWJ, et al. Treatment of postoperative infection of ascending aorta and transverse aortic arch, including use of viable omentum and muscle flaps. Ann Thorac Surg 1990;50:868-81.
11. Gott VL, Pyeritz RE, Cameron DE, et al. Composite graft repair of Marfan aneurysm of the ascending aorta: results in 100 patients. Ann Thorac Surg 1991;52:38-44.
12. Kouchoukos NT, Marshall WG Jr. Treatment of ascending aortic dissection in the Marfan syndrome. J Card Surg 1986;1:333-46.
13. Kouchoukos NT, Marshall WG Jr., Wedige STA. Eleven-year experience with composite graft replacement of the ascending aorta and aortic valve. J Thorac Cardiovasc Surg 1986;92:691-705.
14. Kouchoukos NT. Aortic graft-valve (composite) replacement at 20 years: wrap or no wrap? shunt or no shunt? Ann Thorac Surg 1989; 48:615-6.
15. Kouchoukos NT. Composite graft replacement of the ascending aorta and aortic valve with the inclusion-wrap and open techniques. Semin Thorac Cardiovasc Surg 1991;3:171-6.
16. Lytle BW, Mahfood SS, Cosgrove DM, Loop FD. Replacement of the ascending aorta: early and late results. J Thorac Cardiovasc Surg 1990;99:651-7.
17. Svensson LG, Crawford ES, Coselli JS, et al. Impact of cardiovascular operation on survival in the Marfan patient. Circulation 1989;80(3 Pt 1):i233-42.
18. Svensson LG, Crawford ES, Hess KR, et al. Dissection of the aorta and dissecting aortic aneurysms: improving early and long-term surgical results. Circulation 1990;82(5 Suppl):IV 24-38.
19. Svensson LG, Crawford ES, Hess KR, et al. Deep hypothermia with circulatory arrest: determinants of stroke and early mortality in 656 patients. J Thorac Cardiovasc Surg 1992;106:19-31.
20. Svensson LG. Rationale and technique for replacement of the ascending aorta, arch, and distal aorta using a modified elephant trunk procedure. J Cardiac Surg 1992;7:301-12.
21. Svensson LG, Crawford ES, Hess KR, et al. Composite valve graft replacement of the proximal aorta: comparison of techniques in 348 patients. Ann Thorac Surg 1992;54:427-39.
22. Svensson LG. Approach to the insertion of composite valve graft. Ann Thorac Surg 1992;54:376-8.
23. Svensson LG, Crawford ES. Aortic dissection and aortic aneurysm surgery: clinical observations, experimental investigations, and statistical analyses. Part I. Curr Probl Surg 1992;29:819-912.
24. Levy JH, Pifarre R, Schaff HV, et al. A multicenter, double-blind, placebo-controlled trial of aprotinin for reducing blood loss and the requirement for donor-blood transfusion in patients undergoing repeat coronary artery bypass grafting. Circulation 1995;92:2236-44.
25. Cosgrove DMI, Heric B, Lytle BW, et al. Aprotinin therapy for reoperative myocardial revascularization: a placebo-controlled study. Ann Thorac Surg 1992;54:1031-8.
26. Sundt TMI, Kouchoukos NT, Saffitz JE, et al. Renal dysfunction and intravascular coagulation with aprotinin and hypothermic circulatory arrest. Ann Thorac Surg 1993;55:1418-24.
27. Svensson LG, Sun J, Nadolny E, Kimmel WA. Prospective evaluation of minimal blood use for ascending aorta and aortic arch operations. Ann Thorac Surg 1995;59:1501-8.
28. Siegman MG, Anderson RV, Balaban RS, et al. Barbiturates impair cerebral metabolism during hypothermic circulatory arrest. Surg Forum 1991;42:272-4.

29. Guo J, White JA, Hunt Batjer H. The protective effects of thiopental on brain stem ischemia. Neurosurgery 1995;37:490-5.

30. Fei L, Statters DJ, Anderson MH, et al. Is there an abnormal QT interval in sudden cardiac death survivors with a "normal" QTc? Am Heart J 1994;128:73-6.

31. Elami A, Merin G, Flugelman MY, et al. Usefulness of late potentials on the immediate postoperative signal-averaged elctrocardiogram in predicting ventricular tachyarrhythmias early after isolated coronary artery bypass grafting. Am J Cardiol 1994;74:33-7.

32. Steinberg JS, Zelenkofske S, Wong S-C, et al. Value of the P-wave signal-averaged ECG for predicting atrial fibrillation after cardiac surgery. Circulation 1993;88:2618-22.

33. Seifert M, Josephson ME. P-wave signal averaging: high tech or an expensive alternative to the standard ECG? Circulation 1993;88:2980-2.

34. Suttorp MJ, Kingma JH, Peels HO, et al. Effectiveness of sotalol in preventing supraventricular tachyarrhythmias shortly after coronary artery bypass grafting. Am J Cardiol 1991;68:1163-9.

35. Barzilai B, Marshall WGJ, Saffitz JE, Kouchoukos N. Avoidance of embolic complications by ultrasonic characterization of the ascending aorta. Circulation 1989;80:i275-9.

36. Davila RVG, Barzilai B, Wareing TH, et al. Intraoperative ultrasonographic evaluation of the ascending aorta in 100 consecutive patients undergoing cardiac surgery. Circulation 1991;84(5 Supp):i1147-53.

37. Davis EA, Gillinov AM, Cameron DE, Reitz BA. Hypothermic circulatory arrest as a surgical adjunct: a 5-year experience with 60 adult patients. Ann Thorac Surg 1992;53:402-6.

38. Fisk GC, Wright JS, Hicks RG, et al. The influence of duration of circulatory arrest at 20° C on cerebral changes. Anaesth Intensive Care 1976;4:126-34.

39. Treasure T, Naftel DC, Conger KA, et al. The effect of hypothermic circulatory arrest time on cerebral function, morphology, and biochemistry. J Thorac Cardiovasc Surg 1983;86:761-70.

40. Loop FD, Szab J, Rowlinson RD. Events related to micro-embolism during extracorporeal perfusion in man: effectiveness of in-line filtration recorded by ultrasound. Ann Thorac Surg 1976;21:412-20.

41. Henriksen L, Hjelms E, Linderburgh T. Brain hyperperfusion during cardiac operations. J Thorac Cardiovasc Surg 1983;86:202-8.

42. Mills NL, Ochsner JL. Massive air embolism during cardiopulmonary bypass. J Thorac Cardiovasc Surg 1980;80:708-17.

43. Johnston WE, Vinten JJ, DeWitt DS, et al. Cerebral perfusion during canine hypothermic cardiopulmonary bypass: effect of arterial carbon dioxide tension. Ann Thorac Surg 1991;52:479-89.

44. Shaw PJ. Neurological complications of cardiovascular surgery. II. Procedures involving the heart and thoracic aorta. Internat Anesthesiol Clin 1986;24:159-200.

45. Shaw PJ, Bates D, Cartlidge NEF, et al. Neurologic and neuropsychological morbidity following major surgery: comparison of coronary artery bypass and peripheral vascular surgery. Stroke 1987;18:700-7.

46. Sotaniemi KA, Mononen MA, Hokkanen TE. Long-term cerebral outcome after open-heart surgery. Stroke 1986;17:410-6.

47. Engelman RM, Pleet AB, Rousou JA, et al. Does cardiopulmonary bypass temperature correlate with postoperative central nervous system dysfunction? J Card Surg 1995;10:493-7.

48. Guyton RA, Mellitt RJ, Weintraub WS. A critical assessment of neurological risk during warm heart surgery. J Cardiac Surg 1995;10:488-92.

49. Abe K, Aoki M, Kawagoe J, et al. Ischemic delayed neuronal death: a mitochondrial hypothesis. Stroke 1995;26:1478-89.

50. Chan PH. Editorial comment. Stroke 1995;26:1489.

51. Gerraty RP, Gates PC, Doyle JC. Carotid stenosis and perioperative stroke risk in symptomatic and asymptomatic patients undergoing vascular or coronary surgery. Stroke 1993;24:1115-8.

52. D'Agostino R, Svensson LG, et al. Evaluation of screening carotid ultrasonography and risk factors for stroke in coronary artery bypass surgery patients. Ann Thorac Surg, 1996. In press.

26

Complications of Distal Aorta Operations

ABDOMINAL AORTIC ANEURYSMS

The most frequent problems encountered after abdominal aortic aneurysm surgery are postoperative hemorrhage, peripheral arterial ischemia, hypothermia, and cardiac, renal, respiratory, neurological, and intestinal complications. Paraplegia after abdominal aorta surgery is rare (0.2% after elective repairs and 2.5% after ruptured abdominal aneurysm repairs)[1-4] and will be discussed in greater detail in the latter half of this chapter.[5-10]

Although peripheral ischemia after abdominal aortic aneurysm repair has a lower incidence than after bypasses for aortoiliac disease, it can be a serious problem, particularly if limb loss is a possibility. Many surgeons advocate the use of intraoperative heparin to prevent this complication. We consider this unnecessary if the procedure is a quick repair and the distal iliac arteries are not clamped. Furthermore, heparin will impair clotting at the anastomoses, and we deem it more important to ensure a safe operation without either the use of excessive blood products or the potential problem of postoperative bleeding complications. Despite our not having used heparin in the past in most of our patients, including those undergoing descending thoracic aorta and thoracoabdominal aorta operations, the need for a distal embolectomy for distal thrombosis has been rare. When a distal embolectomy is necessary in the postoperative period, we prefer to perform this through the distal popliteal artery so that a small embolectomy catheter can be passed into each artery of the leg, including the anterior tibial artery.[6] The condition called "trash foot," however, can sometimes be a difficult problem to deal with because it is often detected late and because the emboli are small and may be only platelet aggregates.[10] Deep venous thrombosis (DVT) may also be a problem after abdominal aortic aneurysm repairs, and Olin and colleagues[11] have reported that in a study of 50 of their patients, 18% had evidence of DVT formation.

Renal Complications

Renal failure after abdominal aorta surgery is usually due to either preexistent renal dysfunction with an elevated preoperative creatinine level or technical intraoperative problems.[6, 12-14] The technical problems include squeezing of

atheromatous material (*atheroma* means "porridge") by the aortic clamp into the renal arteries, with the potential problem of distal embolization; disruption of calcific plaques that can obstruct renal blood flow; failure to recognize accessory renal arteries arising from the infrarenal segment of the aorta; technical mishaps with endarterectomy or bypass of the renal arteries; inadvertent closure of a renal artery by a suture (particularly when the aorta has been clamped at the diaphragm and a juxtarenal aneurysm is being repaired); division of the left renal vein close to the left kidney; prolonged renal ischemia during repairs of the renal arteries; prolonged clamping of the aorta at the diaphragm[15]; ureteric obstruction (sutures inadvertently placed around or into the ureter, bypass grafts compressing the ureter, particularly at the iliac arteries, ureteric injury,[16] bleeding, inflammatory aneurysm wall); nephrotoxic agents such as radiographic dyes, aminoglycosides, ranitidine, or indomethacin; reduced cardiac preload; excessive use of diuretics; blood reactions; and postoperative bleeding. The increasing use of spiral computed tomography (CT) and magnetic resonance angiography (MRA)[17] should reduce the risk of renal failure due to preoperative administration of radiographic contrast material for evaluation of aortic anatomy. Although prolonged aortic cross-clamping will cause renal failure, a report by Breckwoldt and colleagues[18, 19] found that in 39 patients in whom the suprarenal aorta was clamped, the incidence of renal failure requiring dialysis was no different from that in patients undergoing infrarenal aortic cross-clamping alone (3% versus 2%). However, transient renal insufficiency was more frequent (28% versus 10%). We have noted that when both postoperative bleeding and increasing abdominal distention occur, then renal shutdown will often result, and if it is not immediately relieved, renal failure develops. This is probably the result of the increased intraabdominal pressure obstructing the renal veins by compression; if the intraabdominal pressure exceeds renal venous blood pressure, it will cause renal edema and reduced blood flow. Similarly, ureteric obstruction may also develop, leading to renal failure. When an "intraabdominal compartment syndrome" occurs, the procedure of secondary wound closure with a prosthetic mesh has been favored to relieve pressure and prevent complications.[20] Postoperative hypothermia may also be associated with an increased incidence of postoperative organ failure.[21, 22] It is difficult, however, to determine whether patients who return to the intensive care unit are hypothermic because of prolonged and complicated operations resulting in organ failure rather than because of hypothermia per se. For example, those of our patients who undergo thoracoabdominal aortic aneurysm repairs usually return to the intensive care unit in a hypothermic state, and how this influences the outcome is not clear, although most do well.[10]

Considerable research is being done on methods to reduce the incidence of renal failure and multiple organ failure after major surgery, such as increasing cardiac performance with the use of inotropes. Fluid loading before surgery and dopamine at a renal dose are probably effective in reducing the risk of renal failure.[23] In a recent study Gattinoni and colleagues[24] were unable to show that dopamine and dobutamine were beneficial in increasing cardiac output, although Boyd and colleagues[25] found the related compound, dopexamine, to be highly effective. Dopexamine is postulated not to increase oxygen consumption at the same time that it increases cardiac output, and this may partly account for its apparent efficacy. Unfortunately, the drug is not available in the United States, and its acquisition by a different company may further delay introduction to the United States market.[10]

Respiratory Complications

Respiratory complications after abdominal aorta surgery are not as frequent as those after thoracoabdominal aortic repairs.[26] However, with the increasing safety of infrarenal aortic repairs, older patients with more advanced respiratory disease (particularly chronic pulmonary disease) are being referred for surgery. Calligaro and colleagues[26] retrospectively reviewed 181 patients who underwent elective abdominal aorta surgery and found that 16% of the patients developed major respiratory complications, including pneumonia in 9%, prolonged ventilation in 5%, and reintubation in 2%. On univariate analysis, the risk factors were ($p < 0.05$) as follows: American Society of Anesthesiologists Class IV; age greater than 70 years; body weight greater than 150% of ideal; forced vital capacity less than 80% of predicted; FEF 25–75% less than 60% predicted; crystalloid fluid administration greater than 6 L; and total operative time more than 5 hours. Patients with ruptured abdominal aortic aneurysms undergoing surgery, however, are particularly prone to respiratory failure and multiple organ failure. A reason for this may be the combination of shock and supraceliac cross-clamping,[27] although many other factors clearly play a role, for example, the release of tumor necrosis factor (TNF∞) and various prostaglandins. In a prospective randomized study of transabdominal versus retroperitoneal incisions for abdominal aortic operations, Sicard and colleagues[28, 29] found that there was no difference in the incidence of pulmonary complications. One of the potential problems with retroperitoneal exposures that we have encountered is the postoperative occurrence of either chyloperitoneum or chylothorax; thus, if a retroperitoneal exposure is used, any potential chyle duct injuries or to the cisterna chyli must be ligated or oversewn. Chyloperitoneum, however, is rare after abdominal aorta surgery, and Pabst and colleagues[30] were able to find only 27 cases (including their own five) in the world literature. Abdominal distention, confirmed by paracentesis, was the most common presentation in 96% of the patients and occurred an average of 18.5 days after surgery. More than half of the patients (57%) were successfully treated with paracentesis and total parenteral nutrition, including medium-chain triglycerides. Peritoneovenous shunts were successful in four of five patients, as was operative ligation in five patients in whom previous conservative therapy had failed. Indeed, the latter procedure is recommended for cases in which conservative management has been unsuccessful.[10]

Intestinal Complications

Common to most major operations, particularly when either shock is present or excessive hemorrhaging occurs, is the increased risk of gastric stress ulceration and hemorrhages.[31-34] Brewster and colleagues,[35] in a retrospective review of 2137 patients who underwent abdominal aortic operations, showed that 1.1% developed signs of intestinal ischemia, with 0.9% related to colon ischemia and 0.2% related to small-bowel ischemia. There was no difference according to aneurysm or occlusive disease operations, although ruptured aneurysms and reoperations involved a greater risk. Half of those patients with colon ischemia required colon resections. The mortality rate was 25% but rose to 50% if a resection was required. Important factors that may account for this high mortality rate include failure to reattach the inferior mesenteric artery (74%); disease of the superior mesenteric artery, especially if occluded; retractor trauma; colon resection; and hypogastric perfusion exclusion. To reduce the risks of gastrointestinal complication, we recommend that the hemodynamics be optimized and that prophylactic agents be used both preoperatively and postoperatively. For example, our patients are routinely given Carafate, 1 g every 6 hours. In addition, the majority also receive an H2 blocker, such as ranitidine, even though this will reduce the action of Carafate and may increase the risk of gram-negative pneumonias caused by aspiration of gastric juice containing high counts of gram-negative bacteria.

Konno and colleagues[36] have found that in patients undergoing abdominal aortic aneurysm repairs, gastric mucosal blood flow is reduced before surgery and fibrin split products are also elevated and are associated with postoperative gastric and upper intestinal hemorrhage. Shenaq, in a study of our patients, also found that fibrin split products are elevated in patients having ascending arch repairs or thoracoabdominal aneurysm repairs. Konno and colleagues[36] also found that if patients with a reduced gastric mucosal blood flow were treated with H2 blockers, the incidence of upper gastrointestinal hemorrhage was reduced. Similarly, in patients with increased fibrin split products, postoperative bleeding was reduced if heparin was started before surgery.[10]

Research performed by Ernst and colleagues[37] has shown the importance of the inferior epigastric artery in the causation of left-sided colon and sigmoid ischemia. Techniques that have been used to establish whether the inferior mesenteric artery needs to be reanastomosed have included measurement of stump pressures, examination for retrograde blood flow, and detection of distal blood flow with a sterile Doppler probe or injection of fluorescein with examination for blood flow. To detect ischemia, intraluminal measurement of pH in the colon has also been proposed.[38, 39] Using this technique of pH monitoring, Soong and colleagues[40] have shown that a pH below 7 in patients who are undergoing abdominal aortic aneurysm repairs results in a higher level of blood endotoxin concentrations, which in turn, is associated with a higher postoperative aspartate transaminase level. The implication is that bowel ischemia results in endotoxemia and organ dysfunction. In those patients who have had previous colon resection and in whom the middle colic artery either has been sacrificed or has been damaged intraoperatively by a retractor (indicated by a mesenteric hematoma and loss of pulse), reimplantation of the inferior mesenteric artery is important for the viability of the colon.[6] Seeger and colleagues[41] have advocated routine reimplantation of patent inferior mesenteric arteries on the basis of the reduced incidence of colon ischemic complications and the lower mortality rate they observed in 151 patients in whom implantation was performed.[10]

Cardiac Complications

Cardiac complications after distal aorta surgery are the most common causes of death and have repeatedly been identified as independent predictors of death.[6, 42-51] In addition, patients with preoperative coronary artery disease have been recognized as being at greater risk of postoperative cardiac complications, and much research has been conducted to identify such patients.[42-45, 47, 48, 52-65] Kalra and colleagues[51] studied 555 patients who underwent elective abdominal aortic aneurysm repairs and found that 6.3% developed perioperative myocardial infarctions; one third of these died. On multivariate analysis, the risk factors were history of transient ischemic attacks (TIAs), raised serum creatinine level, age >60 years, and treatment for angina. Krupski and colleagues[60, 66] found that the risk was greater with infrainguinal repairs and that risk factors for all their patients were diabetes and definite coronary artery disease. The prospective study of 1000 patients by coronary angiography before peripheral vascular surgery at the Cleveland Clinic showed that 8% had normal coronary arteries, 32% had mild to moderate coronary artery disease, 29% had compensated for coronary artery disease by developing collateral vessels, 25% had disease that could be corrected by surgery, and 6% of patients were inoperable.[67] Severe bypassable coronary artery disease was found in 14% of patients who had no clinical evidence of coronary artery disease. The mortality rate for peripheral vascular operations was 0.8% in patients who had undergone previous myocardial

revascularization.[67] Whether a low left ventricular ejection fraction is still a risk factor with the advent of modern anesthesia techniques and invasive monitoring remains controversial.[33, 49, 61] The extent of preoperative tests and the cost benefits of such tests to detect coronary artery disease are much debated. Furthermore, screening by stress electrocardiography (ECG), Goldman criteria, Holter examination, MUGGA scans, echocardiography, dipyridamole-thallium 201 scans, high-speed CT, dobutamine echocardiography, and cardiac catheterization is not entirely reliable for detecting all at-risk patients. In high-risk patients with angina, coronary cardiac catheterization is the best alternative. We have found that in selected patients echocardiography combined with dobutamine infusion is highly satisfactory,[68, 69] for the screening of segmental wall-motion abnormalities during stressing. In addition, any valvular problems, calcification, or atheroma in the aorta, and ascending aortic size can be evaluated. Reports confirm that this may become a useful alternative for screening of patients[69, 70] and referral of those patients with positive dobutamine-echocardiograms for coronary angiography. Moreover, continuous transesophageal echocardiographic intraoperative monitoring is useful in high-risk patients. Our routine approach has been to perform the tests described previously[71] to detect asymptomatic coronary artery disease (namely, routine ECG, 24-hour Holter monitoring, and echocardiography). If significant coronary symptoms or ischemia are detected, then, when possible, the patients undergo coronary arteriography and balloon angioplasty. Patients with stable coronary artery disease and symptomatic abdominal aneurysms are monitored carefully during surgery, and appropriate agents such as nitroglycerin and dobutamine are used liberally. Increasingly, the use of transesophageal echocardiography (TEE) is also being espoused for these patients, and, when appropriate, the coronary artery disease is subsequently treated by invasive means. Clearly, because the aim of treatment should be to prolong long-term survival, the rare patients who have both symptomatic abdominal aortic aneurysms and unstable angina should undergo the combined operations of coronary artery bypass and abdominal aortic aneurysm repair. Patients with angina or significant coronary disease (more than 50% stenosis of the left main coronary artery, stenosis of the proximal left anterior descending coronary artery, and triple vessel disease) and asymptomatic aneurysms are best treated with preoperative coronary artery bypass. In our treatment of this subgroup of patients, we have found abdominal aortic aneurysm repair to be safe, with no postoperative deaths in 102 patients who underwent aortic procedures after coronary artery bypass operations.[43] However, in this group of patients there is a risk that the aneurysm will rupture in the postoperative period, and we favor performing the abdominal aortic repair 3 to 7 days after cardiac surgery, once the patient has recovered from the cardiac operation. Durham and colleagues[72] have reported that after cardiothoracic operations 11% of patients may have rupture of the aortic aneurysm an average of 39 days (range, 20 to 77 days) after surgery. Rupture is probably related foremost to the release of collagenases but possibly also to elastase (see Etiology of Degenerative Aneurysms).[73-80] Blackbourne and colleagues[81] reviewed their experience with 23 patients who had abdominal aortic aneurysms scheduled for repair and who also needed coronary artery bypass surgery. In the six patients who underwent simultaneous repair of abdominal aortic aneurysms and coronary artery bypass (five during bypass, one after discontinuing bypass) or the eight who underwent abdominal aortic repairs within 14 days of coronary artery bypass operations, there were no deaths (0/14). Of the nine patients who had repairs scheduled more than 14 days after coronary operations, however, three (33%) died ($p < 0.05$) of rupture with an average aneurysm size of 5.8 cm. The deaths occurred between 16 and 29 days after coronary surgery.

Recently, the issue of whether patients should even be studied extensively before vascular surgery has been raised. Mason and colleagues[82] compared three strategies of (1) immediate surgery, (2) coronary angiography with selective coronary revascularization before surgery and cancellation of surgery in patients with coronary disease who could not be revascularized, and (3) coronary angiography with selective coronary revascularization but without cancellation of surgery in patients with coronary artery disease who cannot be revascularized. They found that strategy 1 was the cheapest and had the lowest morbidity; strategy 3 (operating without revascularization) had a higher mortality rate; and strategy 2 (coronary revascularization and cancellation of surgery in patients with inoperable coronary disease) had a slightly lower mortality rate. They concluded that coronary angiography "leads to worse outcomes, even in patients at higher than average risk" and that only patients with "very high operative mortality due to vascular surgery" should have angiography. The problem with these recommendations is that they are premature in that they assess only the immediate mortality rate of surgery and fail to consider the long-term prognosis of the patient. For most patients undergoing vascular surgery, including most types of aortic operations, the 5-year survival rate is in the region of only 60% (Figs. 26–1 and 28–2) (see further discussion in Chapters 2 and 28). Since approximately half of the late deaths in patients having aortic surgery are due to cardiac causes, clearly, to improve long-term prognosis an aggressive perioperative search for and treatment of cardiac disease will improve both early and long-term prognosis. Thus controlled prospective studies are required to better elucidate the appropriate tests and strategies that should be instituted.[10]

DESCENDING THORACIC AND THORACOABDOMINAL AORTA OPERATIONS

Operative survival rate has improved over time, with recent reports documenting survival rates of 95% or better for descending thoracic or even, in some series (including our own and those of former associates, Drs. Coselli and Safi), for thoracoabdominal aneurysm repairs.[83-91] For both descending thoracic and thoracoabdominal aneurysm repairs at the Lahey Clinic (L.G.S.), the 30-day and in-hospital survival rate has been 96.2% (reported at the New England Society for Vascular Surgery, Sept. 30, 1995). Nevertheless, in a recent report on a series of 130 thoracoabdominal aneurysm repairs operated upon in Britain, the mortality rates for elective repairs varied from 42% for type II repairs, to 15% for type IV repairs, and to 73% for ruptured aneurysms.[92] The incidence of serious complications in recent reports by us and others indicates that with distal aortic perfusion, particularly with atriofemoral bypass (Fig. 26–2), the rate of renal failure and spinal cord injury has been reduced.[83-91]

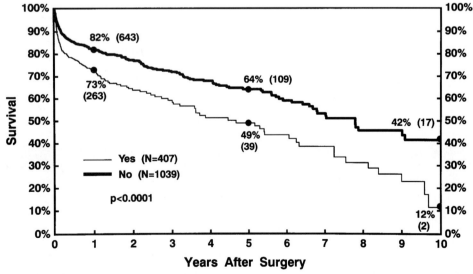

FIGURE 26–1 Effect of the preoperative presence of coronary artery disease on long-term survival of patients who had thoracoabdominal aneurysm repairs. (From Svensson LG, Crawford ES, Hess KR, et al. J Vasc Surg 1993;17:357–70.)

Nevertheless, the postoperative complications have assumed considerably more importance, not only to the patient, families, and the physician, but also to hospital administrators and health care underwriters who expect that patients will stay in the hospital no longer than a patient having a routine coronary artery bypass operation.[10]

Paraplegia/Paraparesis

In our series of 832 patients undergoing descending thoracic aortic repairs with a 98% (159/162) survival rate since 1988,[86] the independent predictors of spinal cord injury were ($p < 0.05$) extent of repair, aortic clamp time, postoperative renal complications, and gastrointestinal complications. When the clamp time exceeded 40 minutes, then the use of atriofemoral bypass was associated with a lower risk of spinal cord injury.[10]

The independent predictors of paraplegia/paraparesis in 1509 patients who underwent thoracoabdominal aorta operations, for 1494 of whom complete data were available ($p < 0.05$),[93] included extent of aneurysm resection, aortic cross-clamp time, presence of aortic rupture, increasing age, concurrent proximal aortic aneurysmal disease, and preoperative renal dysfunction. Figure 26–3 shows the relationship between total aortic cross-clamp time and the risk of paraplegia/paraparesis. Figures 26–4 and 26–5 show the effect of the extent of aneurysm repair according to clamp time by logistic regression and the effect by nonparametric

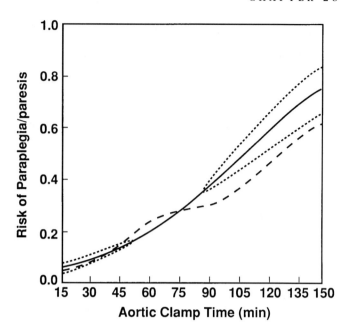

FIGURE 26–3 Relationship of aortic cross-clamp time to the risk of neurologic injury. The *solid curve* is from logistic regression analysis with the 95% confidence limits shown and the *dashed line* is for nonparametric analysis. (From Svensson LG, Crawford ES, Hess KR, et al. J Vasc Surg 1993;17:357-70.)

analysis. Figure 26–6 shows the influence of the visceral ischemia time on the risk of spinal cord injury. The incidence of paraplegia or paraparesis according to extent was 15% for type I, 31% for type II, 7% for type III, and 4% for type IV ($p < 0.0001$). The effect of postoperative spinal cord injury on long-term survival analyzed by Kaplan-Meier tables is shown in Figure 26–7.

FIGURE 26–2 Illustration of atriofemoral bypass. (From Svensson LG, Crawford ES, Hess KR, et al. J Vasc Surg 1992;16:378-90.)

FIGURE 26–4 Logistic regression analysis of the relationship of aortic cross-clamp time to risk of neurological injury according to Crawford type of aneurysm. (From Svensson LG, Crawford ES, Hess KR, et al. J Vasc Surg 1993;17:357-70.)

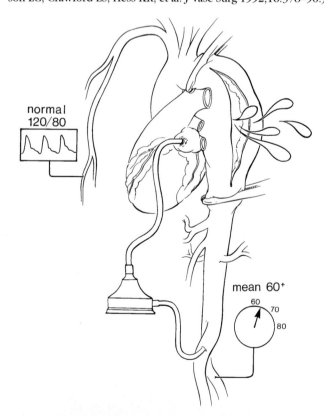

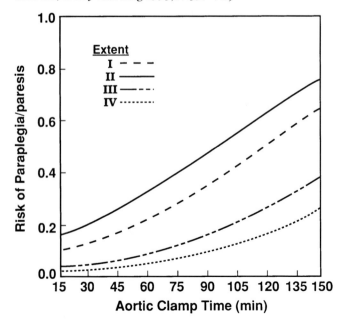

For acute dissection the incidence was 31%, for chronic dissection it was 24%, and for patients without aortic dissection it was 13% ($p < 0.0001$). Although aortic dissection was not found to be an independent determinant (on univariate analysis, this variable was highly significant), this was because the greater clamp time and more extensive resections in patients with aortic dissection displaced the variable aortic dissection from the stepwise logistic regression model. In a previous prospective study, with careful testing of the patients on a daily basis, including neurogenic bladder dysfunction, the incidence was 43% for type II aneurysms and reached 45% in patients with both aortic dissection and type II aneurysms.[94] Nevertheless, the incidence of paraplegia (excluding patients with paraparesis) in this subgroup was 13%. In the prospective study, 90 days after surgery, 7% of the survivors were still paraplegic and 7% were paraparetic, although two thirds of the latter were able to walk.[10, 94] On analysis of a total of 690 patients undergoing aortic dissection repairs, in that group of patients who had descending aorta repairs or thoracoabdominal aorta repairs, there was also a significant correlation with the aorta cross-clamp time and the risk of spinal cord injury as shown (Fig. 26–8).[95]

The cause of postoperative paraplegia/paraparesis, both at the cellular level and at a more gross pathophysiological level, is better understood as a result of extensive animal and clinical research, which has been reviewed previously.[50, 96–100] Etiological factors are discussed in other chapters, and more detailed discussions are beyond the scope of this chapter. The salient points in our understanding of the pathophysiological changes with aortic cross-clamping in humans are discussed below:

1. Cerebrospinal fluid pressure increases progressively with anesthetic maneuvers during aortic surgery, in addition to aortic cross-clamping, and this correlates with the central venous pressure.

2. Oxygenation of the spinal cord falls rapidly with aortic cross-clamping, even with deep hypothermia and circulatory arrest, and the longer the clamp time, the greater the risk of spinal-cord injury.

3. By gross inspection, segmental arteries supplying the spinal cord cannot be identified, as shown by hydrogen testing.

4. Perfusion of the vessels supplying the spinal cord by atriofemoral bypass does result in hydrogen reaching the spinal cord.

5. Identification of segmental arteries supplying the spinal cord, either by highly selective preoperative angiography or by intraoperative hydrogen testing, results in reestablishment of spinal cord blood flow.

6. Reattachment of segmental intercostal or lumbar arteries has to be successful since we have documented that a high proportion of the reattached arteries are not patent on postoperative highly selective angiographic examination.

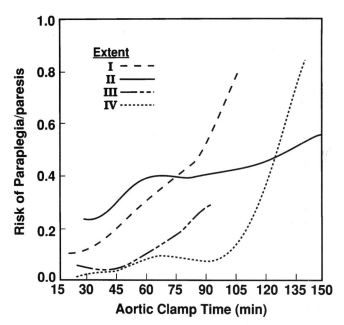

FIGURE 26–5 Non-parametric analysis of the relationship of aortic cross-clamp time to risk of neurologic injury according to Crawford type of aneurysm. (From Svensson LG, Crawford ES, Hess KR, et al. J Vasc Surg 1993;17:357–70.)

From our research, we conclude that the occurrence of immediate postoperative paraplegia or paraparesis is largely dependent on (1) the degree of spinal cord ischemia during aortic cross-clamping (the degree of ischemia is dependent on the diameter of available collateral arteries, including the anterior and posterolateral spinal arteries, and the extent of

FIGURE 26–6 Relationship of visceral ischemia time to the risk of neurological injury. The *solid curve* is from logistic regression analysis with the 95% confidence limits shown and the *dashed line* is for non-parametric analysis. (From Svensson LG, Crawford ES, Hess KR, et al. J Vasc Surg 1993;17:357–70.)

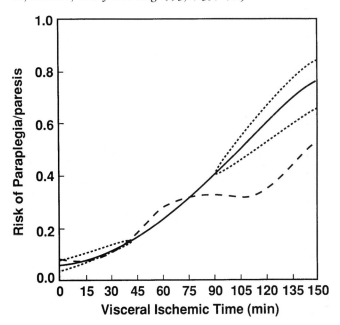

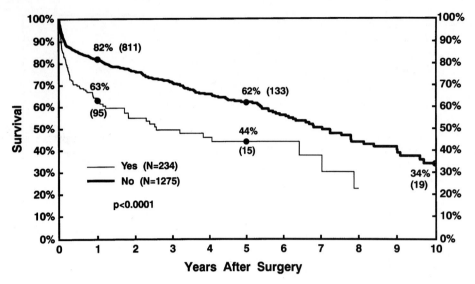

FIGURE 26–7 Effect of the postoperative neurological injury on long-term survival of patients who had thoracoabdominal aneurysm repairs. (From Svensson LG, Crawford ES, Hess KR, et al. J Vasc Surg 1993;17:357–70.)

the aneurysm); (2) the duration of the ischemia, particularly as the window of safety of approximately 30 minutes is exceeded; and (3) on the continuation of spinal cord ischemia after aortic unclamping due to failure of reattachment of critical segmental arteries.

After spinal cord ischemia there is marked hyperemia of the spinal cord with reperfusion. The reason for the hyperemia in the spinal cord is of interest insofar as the mechanism of injury is concerned. We[101, 102] have noted hyperemia in two previous nonhuman primate studies, particularly in those animals that were paralyzed, and we observed hyperoxygenation in our porcine experiments. Hyperemia has also been reported by others.[103, 104] This effect is possibly related to reperfusion injury and the generation of nitric oxide resulting in hyperperfusion (see Chapter 12). It is interesting to speculate that nitric oxide may play a role in the reported higher incidence of paraplegia in animals treated with nitroprusside during aortic cross-clamping because nitroprusside (and nitroglycerin to some extent) causes

arterial dilatation by releasing nitric oxide. Whether nitric oxide is protective or deleterious in the central nervous system is unclear at this stage (see Chapter 12). Rats fed nitric oxide synthetase inhibitor over a long term develop hypertension and spinal cord infarcts that result in leg paralysis.[105]

Delayed paraplegia/paraparesis, observed in about one third of the cases in our prospective randomized study of cerebrospinal fluid (CSF) drainage,[94] appears to be due to several factors, especially to decreased spinal cord oxygenation. This loss of spinal cord oxygenation is due either to hypotension with decreased blood supply through collaterals or to respiratory failure. In porcine experiments, we have shown that hypotension in animals dependent on the collateral blood supply to oxygenate the spinal cord resulted in paraplegia/paraparesis and that this could be reversed by immediately raising the blood pressure.[106] We have had similar experiences with humans by using dopamine and neosynephrine to raise the blood pressure and reverse delayed paraparesis. In addition, steroids and Narcan may

FIGURE 26–8 Logistic regression analysis of the relationship of aortic cross-clamp time to risk of neurological injury according to Crawford type of aneurysm and descending (DESC) aneurysm repair for aortic dissection. (From Svensson LG, Crawford ES, Hess KR, et al. Dissection of the aorta and dissecting aortic aneurysms. Improving early and long-term surgical results. Circulation 1990; 82(5 Suppl): IV2438. Reprinted with permission. Copyright 1990 American Heart Association.)

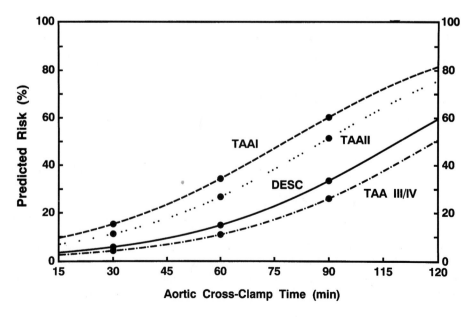

be of value. Other factors probably associated with delayed paraplegia/paraparesis include occlusion of critical segmental arteries, by either emboli or thrombosis; spinal cord edema; secondary spinal cord injury, which we have noted in porcine experiments and which was also noted by Moore and Hollier[104] in rabbit experiments; and a reperfusion injury, most likely related to white blood cells rather than to the de novo generation of oxygen radicals.[10] There is also some evidence that factors in the CSF after injury may inhibit recovery of the spinal cord, as shown by antibody studies against myelin-associated neurite growth-inhibitory proteins.[107] In patients with delayed spinal cord injury, CSF drainage with or without papaverine, in our experience and that of others[108] (personal communications from John Cunningham, M.D., George Letsakis, M.D.), has been demonstrated to reverse the transient injury. The mechanism for this is unknown, however, but may be related to removal of negative neurotrophic factors or decompression of the spinal cord with improved collateral blood flow. The factor could possibly be tissue plasminogen activator since tissue-type plasminogen activator (t-PA)-deficient mice are resistant to excitotoxin-induced neuronal loss.[109] It is interesting to speculate whether the higher incidence of stroke in patients given t-PA, as opposed to streptokinase, for acute myocardial infarction is also related to the negative neurotrophic effects of t-PA. It is of interest that research in rats has shown that segments of spinal cord can be replaced successfully with isotopic and isochronic grafts.[110] Neurotrophic factors apparently can result in sprouting of corticospinal tracts, even with long-distance regeneration of fibers.[107]

Although some of the origins of the multifactorial etiology of paraplegia/paraparesis have been established as a result of prospective studies, the means of fully preventing this dreaded complication in humans are still lacking, and no prospective randomized studies have proven any method to be particularly effective. In a prospective randomized study of CSF drainage, we were unable to show that drainage of 20 ml prior to aortic cross-clamping and a maximum of 50 ml during aortic cross-clamping (a median of 52.5 ml was withdrawn) prevented paraplegia or paraparesis; nor did CSF drainage significantly alter the severity of the neuromuscular deficits.[10, 94]

Nevertheless, several retrospective uncontrolled studies have reported a lower incidence of postoperative deficits based on the surgeon's preferred method of aortic repair.[83-91, 111] In nonhuman primate studies, we reported that vasodilatation of the anterior spinal artery with intrathecal papaverine increased spinal cord blood flow and prevented paraplegia after 60 minutes of normothermic aortic cross-clamping.[102] A subsequent prospective study in humans without reattachment of segmental intercostal or lumbar arteries was encouraging.[99, 106, 112-114] In a prospective randomized study that included preoperative localization of the spinal cord blood supply with reattachment of critical segmental arteries and femorofemoral cardiopulmonary bypass, Kieffer and colleagues[115] have shown that no per-

manent deficits and no paraplegia occurred in 29 patients selected at random to receive intrathecal papaverine whereas there were seven permanent deficits and three cases of paraplegia in the control group of 33 patients ($p < 0.05$). Four cases of reversible neurogenic bladder dysfunction or paraparesis occurred in the papaverine group. Furthermore, in Kieffer's continued use of intrathecal papaverine, paraplegia has occurred only in those patients whose spinal cord blood supply could not be identified or whose segmental arteries could not be successfully reattached.[115] Other preventive measures that may be important, according to animal studies or retrospective studies, are prevention of hyperglycemia; the use of steroids at a dosage of less than 2000 mg; prostaglandin E1 as used by Sandmann and his colleagues; the use of prostacyclin[116]; and the use of thiopental that has been shown to be effective in animal studies and is increasingly favored by some surgeons.[8, 10, 97, 111, 115, 117-129]

Distal aortic perfusion methods, particularly atriofemoral bypass, are increasingly being used, and our recent studies would suggest that distal perfusion protects both the kidneys and the spinal cord. Distal aortic perfusion was examined previously by Crawford and colleagues[8] and was found not to be effective. Nonetheless, in our more recent studies we have shown by hydrogen testing that if atriofemoral bypass is used in conjunction with sequential and segmental repairs of the aorta, blood supply to the spinal cord can be maintained while the proximal anastomosis is being performed.[93, 106] Our previous animal studies[101, 112] have demonstrated that distal aortic perfusion of only the arteria radicularis magna (ARM) results specifically in an increased blood flow to the lumbar spinal cord below the level of the ARM (artery of Adamkievicz) but not to the thoracic spinal cord. Moderate hypothermia, initially reported by DeBakey and colleagues,[130, 131] appears to be protective. We have shown that if we keep our patients normothermic, during aortic cross-clamping, with the atriofemoral bypass pump, then the incidence of neuromuscular dysfunction increases significantly.[93] Thus we now actively cool our patients before aortic clamping. Deep hypothermia is clearly also protective of the spinal cord in animal studies, and our experience with deep hypothermia and circulatory arrest has demonstrated the value of this technique in preventing paraplegia/paraparesis in the repair of both descending thoracic and thoracoabdominal aneurysms.[84, 88, 93, 128, 132, 133] Furthermore, Kouchoukos and colleagues[84, 88, 103, 133] favor this method.

In a previous report on 25 patients undergoing deep hypothermia with circulatory arrest for repair of descending thoracic or thoracoabdominal aortic aneurysms, mostly for technical indications, Crawford and colleagues[132] reported that four patients died and a further two developed postoperative paraplegia/paraparesis. Similarly, in our later report on the identification of the spinal cord blood supply with hydrogen testing,[106] one patient who did not have to have his segmental arteries reattached underwent deep hypothermia and circulatory arrest for technical indications but postoperatively had reversible paraparesis. In our study of the use of deep hypothermia with circulatory arrest,[134] 38 patients underwent resection of aneurysms distal to the left subclavian artery. Of these patients, 21% died and 15% had strokes. We (L.G.S.) have used deep hypothermic arrest for our replacements of the entire aorta during a single operation, and even though the spinal cord blood supply was arrested for as much as 90 minutes (considerably past the 30-minute window of "safety"), some patients have had no neurological deficits (see Chapter 24).[135]

Although the use of deep hypothermia may clearly reduce the incidence of lower limb neuromuscular deficits with prolonged aortic cross-clamp or spinal cord blood flow arrest times, complications still occasionally arise. However, it appears that these spinal cord injuries are related more often to technical problems with reattachment of the segmental intercostal or lumbar arteries, as we have previously noted (see Chapters 15 and 19). An important caveat is that application of this method on a strictly routine basis may sometimes be at the expense of an increased mortality rate, blood usage, and higher pulmonary complication rate.[134] Thus, when this method is used, great care must be taken not to injure the lung and also to obtain complete hemostasis before closure.[10]

Because spinal cord oxygenation falls during aortic cross-clamping, cooling of the spinal cord may slow the metabolic rate. In an attempt to cool the spinal cord locally, various means such as epidural cooling, continuous perfusion of the aneurysm, perfusion of the intrathecal space, and use of a single dosage of cold "spinoplegia" have been tried in animals, often with considerable success in preventing postoperative paraplegia or paraparesis.[117, 123, 128, 136, 137] As early as the 1960s, spinal cord cooling was used in both animals and patients in an effort to reduce the secondary injury of spinal cord trauma.[138-140] Thus, if such a technique can be developed for safe routine use in humans, it will undoubtedly be a useful adjunct. A recent report[125] has shown that perfusion of the intrathecal space with Fluosol, which also has a vasodilator action similar to that of papaverine, at a temperature of 32°C, prevented paraplegia in dogs. Of particular value would be the increased operative "window of safety"[99] period, allowing sufficient time for the successful reattachment of those identified segmental arteries that supply the spinal cord. In recent porcine experiments, we (L.G.S.) have been able to prevent paraplegia with 60 minutes of aortic cross-clamping ($p < 0.05$) using intrathecal papaverine combined with spinal cord perfusion with cold solution whereas spinal cord injury occurred in 100% of the control group of animals.[10]

The successful reattachment of segmental arteries that supply the spinal cord is clearly of great importance in reducing the incidence of postoperative neuromuscular deficits and is second only to the prevention of excessive ischemia during aortic cross-clamping. In our porcine experiments,[106] we demonstrated that division of the segmental arteries shown by hydrogen testing to supply the spinal cord largely resulted in either paraplegia or paraparesis, whereas preservation of only those identified vessels sup-

plying the spinal cord and division of the remainder significantly lowered the rate of deficits. Furthermore, perfusion of arteries supplying the spinal cord reduced the risk of spinal injury (see Chapter 15). Similarly, in our prospective randomized study of CSF drainage[33, 94, 106] we showed that if segmental arteries were present between T11 and L1 but were not reattached for technical or other reasons, then the postoperative paraplegia/paraparesis rate exceeded 60%, which was significantly higher than in patients in whom they were present and were reattached to the graft. When the intercostal arteries are sacrificed, sources of collateral blood supply, if adequate, become critical to spinal cord preservation.[98, 99] The potential sources of collateral blood supply that we[98, 99] have suggested possibly include the anterior and posterolateral spinal arteries, the scapular arteries, the internal mammary arteries, and other longitudinal arteries such as the lateral thoracic arteries. Giglia and colleagues[141] have shown that in the rat model the internal mammary arteries are essential to maintain the spinal cord blood supply and prevent paraplegia with short aortic cross-clamp times.

To deal with the problem of reattaching the segmental arteries, several approaches have been adopted: (1) simple expediency and reattachment of no arteries, thus shortening the aortic cross-clamp time[33, 94, 106, 142-144]; (2) reattachment of all segmental arteries from T8 to L1 (our standard approach[33, 95, 106, 145, 146] because these are more than 90% likely to supply the arteria radicularis magna[145]; (3) reattachment of all segmental arteries as practiced by Hollier and colleagues[121, 122]; (4) graft replacement of the proximal dissected descending aorta with tailoring of the distal third to the renal arteries and use of deep hypothermic circulatory arrest[147]; (5) selective reattachment of preoperatively identified arteries supplying the spinal cord with the use of highly selective angiography as espoused by Williams and associates[148] and Kieffer and colleagues[115, 149-150]; (6) intraoperative hydrogen identification of arteries supplying the spinal cord, as used by us experimentally,[106] which has been shown by postoperative highly selective angiography to be accurate (see Chapter 15).

There are significant problems, however, with all of these reattachment techniques. The arteries, because of either technical factors, calcification, or aortic dissection, cannot be reattached; the Carrel patch with the arteries may dissect and bleed; the vessels may thrombose or occlude, as we have noted on postoperative angiograms; and, with the preoperative localization techniques, correlation of the angiographic artery that supplies the spinal cord with the intraoperative determination of which artery supplies the spinal cord can be difficult. Intraoperative identification of those arteries that require reattachment avoids this latter problem. When no single artery supplies the spinal cord, because of occlusion of the ostia of the vessel by either atheroma or aortic dissection, then angiography may not identify the small collateral vessels supplying the spinal cord. We have shown in one patient, however, that hydrogen testing was able to identify the segmental artery that supplied the spinal cord as later diagnosed by postoperative angiography.[106] Using hydrogen to identify vessels supplying the spinal cord and postoperative highly selective angiography, we have noted five different patterns of spinal cord blood supply: (1) direct spinal cord perfusion via radicular arteries, (2) indirect perfusion via collaterals when the original intercostal arteries are occluded, (3) no identified arteries, (4) arteries arising from above or below the occluded segment, (5) atriofemoral bypass perfusion of vessels below the distal clamp.[10]

For our initial experiments on nonhuman primates, performed from 1983 to 1985 to study paraplegia after aortic cross-clamping, motor evoked responses were highly effective in documenting spinal cord injury.[102] In later porcine experiments, in which a stainless steel electrode was used alongside the spinal cord, we found that measurement of the amplitude of spinal motor evoked potentials (SMEPs) was similarly effective for studying spinal cord dysfunction, reversal with reperfusion, and the degree of permanent deficits.[106, 128] However, the monitoring of spinal cord electrical activity, either by somatosensory evoked potentials or motor evoked potentials, is of value only if something can be done to reverse signs of ischemia. Crawford and colleagues[8] have previously shown that somatosensory evoked potential monitoring may be inaccurate and influenced by many factors. Sandmann and colleagues,[119, 120, 123] however, have used epidural electrodes for the stimulation and recording of somatosensory evoked potentials and have found this to be a sound method. Our later research, based on porcine experiments,[106, 128] and the work of Allen and others[151] in canine experiments have shown that SMEPs elicited by stimulating the spinal cord directly and recording the potentials from lower limb muscle electrodes are highly accurate. Ellmore and colleagues,[152] however, found that at a higher level stimulation of the brain and recording over the thoracic spinal cord was not as accurate. This is probably because ischemia occurs in the more distal parts of the spinal cord.[101, 112, 128]

On the basis of our porcine experiments, we have used SMEP monitoring in humans, but the main problem we have encountered to date has been with measuring the potentials from muscles. The principal reason is that neuromuscular blockers cannot be used and the resultant twitching of the patient's legs during testing is disconcerting.[93] In our experience, if maximal uses are made of potential preventive measures, then monitoring is probably of little additional value, except perhaps for checking whether segmental arteries have been successfully reattached. Ongoing research by Shiiya and colleagues[153] has suggested that the technique may be of value in identifying the arteries that need to be reattached during aortic repairs, although in all of their cases the arteries were found each time to be in the T8 to L1 area, as expected. As stated earlier, this is also the segment that we recommend be routinely reattached to the new graft because we have demonstrated that these are more than 90% likely to supply the ARM.[145] Shiiya and associates have noted that controlling excessive back bleeding from intercostal

arteries will reverse adverse SMEP changes. This may be because of a "steal phenomenon" from the spinal cord to the opened aorta. Currently, Galla and colleagues[154] are studying the use of somatosensory evoked potentials for the selection and reimplantation of intercostal arteries. In a series of 26 descending thoracic or thoracoabdominal aneurysm repairs, nearly all the patients with uncorrected abnormal SMEP recordings developed deficits. The exceptions were one patient with an abnormal recording, who did not develop a deficit, and one patient with a normal recording, who developed postoperative paraplegia (4% false-negative rate).

When time permits, we use hydrogen testing to examine for patency of reattached segmental arteries. A notable caveat is that both intrathecal and hypothermic preventive measures interfere with the recording of SMEPs.[10]

Renal Failure

When we analyzed the 832 patients in whom descending aortic repairs had been performed, the independent predictors of renal failure (7%) were ($p < 0.005$) preoperative renal dysfunction (32% incidence of renal failure postoperatively), concurrent abdominal aortic aneurysm repair (18%), cardiopulmonary bypass (11%), or simple aortic cross-clamping alone (8%) compared with atriofemoral bypass (4%), cardiac complications (25%), sepsis (33%), and paraplegia/paraparesis (22%). These risk factors clearly show that the use of atriofemoral bypass for distal perfusion during repairs reduces the risk of renal failure and that the prevention of other complications is important for reducing the risk of renal failure.[10]

Of 1509 of our patients[93] who underwent thoracoabdominal aneurysm repairs, the data for 1396 were available to determine the independent predictors of renal failure ($p < 0.05$), which were increasing age, male gender, renal occlusive disease, preoperative renal dysfunction, history of cerebrovascular disease, preoperative serum creatinine level, and renal ischemic time. In a smaller study of 88 patients, Schepens and colleagues[155] also noted that age and preoperative serum creatinine level predicted the postoperative need for dialysis.

In our retrospective clinical study[156] of 1525 patients undergoing descending thoracic or thoracoabdominal repairs, the need for dialysis was not significantly reduced by the use of cold perfusion of the kidneys with Ringer's lactate solution or with atriofemoral bypass (Figs. 26–9 to 26–11). The risk factors for renal failure on multivariate analysis were preexistent renal dysfunction; diffuse atherosclerotic disease, including occlusive disease of branches of the aorta; use of pump bypass (largely because of cardiopulmonary bypass); and preoperative hemodynamic instability. The analysis also showed that renal artery endarterectomy and chronic aortic dissection were associated with a lower risk. Of 13 patients who were on hemodialysis preoperatively, eight were on chronic dialysis and four started dialysis immediately before surgery. Of the 68 patients who required postoperative dialysis, 63.2% died. However, in a

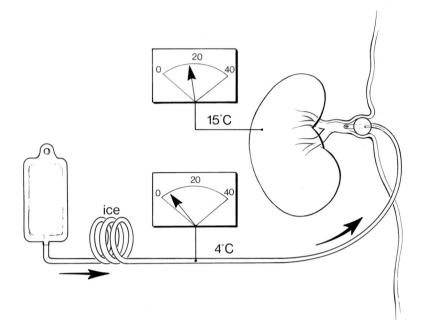

FIGURE 26–9 Protection of the kidney by perfusion of cold Ringer's lactate solution with monitoring of the renal temperature. (From Svensson LG, Crawford ES, Hess KR, et al. J Vasc Surg 1992;16: 378–90.)

more recent evaluation of patients who had visceral artery occlusive disease and who also had thoracoabdominal aortic repairs,[13] the patients appeared to benefit from cold perfusion of the renal arteries because of the high incidence of preoperative renal dysfunction.

From this, we conclude that most patients who have no preoperative renal dysfunction or renal artery occlusive disease or in whom a clamp time of less than 45 minutes is expected do not require cold perfusion.[93] If these adverse signs are present, however, then cold perfusion of the kidneys should be undertaken. Allen and colleagues[157] have also reported the benefit of cooling the kidneys during juxtarenal and suprarenal abdominal aortic aneurysm repairs, particularly if renal artery reconstruction is carried out at the same time. The addition of other medications, such as heparin, lidocaine, calcium channel blockers, and prostaglandins (PGE1 20 μg/L) to the solution may also be useful.[119, 120, 156, 158] Furthermore, prostacyclin may also reduce the risk of spinal cord injury, as reported in a rabbit model.[116] We have noted[93] that patients whose body temperature was allowed to drop during surgery to approximately 30° to 34° C had a significantly lower incidence of postoperative renal failure than patients in whom the temperature was kept normal in association with the use of atriofemoral bypass. Pelkey and colleagues[93, 159] have also reported that in animal experiments a lower body temperature is associated with a lower incidence of postoperative renal failure as measured by postoperative creatinine levels and renal histologic studies. Mannitol is used liberally because it has been reported to reduce the risk of renal failure.[160] Calcium channel blockers may also be protective when administered before and after the period of ischemia.[161] However, despite possible theoretical benefits, ACE inhibitors do not prevent postoperative renal failure.[12]

FIGURE 26–10 Perfusion of the renal arteries with side branches from the atriofemoral bypass pump. (From Svensson LG, Crawford ES, Hess KR, et al. J Vasc Surg 1992;16:378–90.)

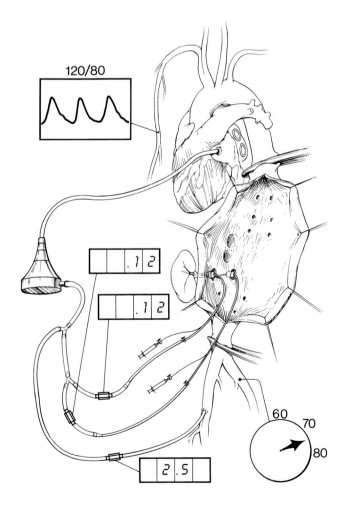

Postoperatively, we advocate the use of gentle diuresis with dopamine. We avoid the use of diuretics such as furosemide because of the risk that a precipitously reduced cardiac preload may result in hypotension and the development of delayed paraplegia or paraparesis, which has been reported to occur with excessively vigorous diuresis.[93] Although a higher preload may delay extubation of the patient, we deem this preferable to the risks of neuromuscular deficits and renal failure due to a reduced cardiac and renal preload.[10]

Postoperative renal dysfunction has a profound and significant influence on long-term survival after distal aortic surgery. Figure 26–12 shows the effect of renal dysfunction after descending thoracic or thoracoabdominal aortic repairs, as evidenced by an abnormally raised postoperative serum creatinine level, on long-term survival by Kaplan Meier analysis; it also shows the effect of postoperative dialysis. Note that the 5-year survival rate is only 7% for patients who require dialysis. Figure 26–13 shows the effect of postoperative renal failure, either a raised serum creatinine level or dialysis, on long-term survival in 1509 patients undergoing thoracoabdominal aneurysm repairs.

Respiratory Failure

In a prospective analysis of respiratory complications after 98 type I or type II thoracoabdominal aorta operations, the 30-day survival rate was 98%.[33] In this latter study, the incidence of respiratory failure was 43%. The independent predictors of respiratory failure were found to be chronic pulmonary disease, a smoking history, and cardiac and renal complications. In patients with chronic pulmonary disease (56%), the best independent predictor of

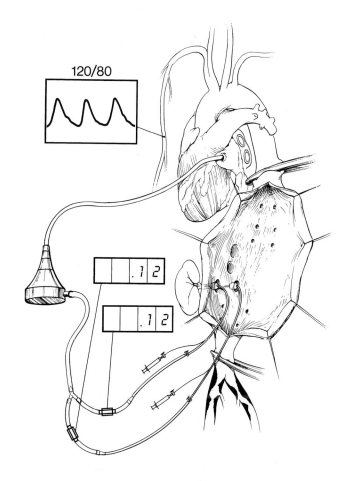

FIGURE 26–11 Perfusion of the renal arteries without atriofemoral bypass in patients with occlusive disease of the iliac arteries. (From Svensson LG, Crawford ES, Hess KR, et al. J Vasc Surg 1992;16:378–90.)

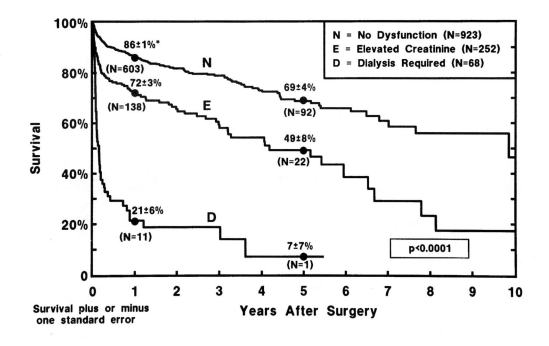

FIGURE 26–12 Effect of the postoperative renal dysfunction or dialysis on long-term survival of patients who had thoracoabdominal or descending thoracic aneurysm repairs. (From Svensson LG, Crawford ES, Hess KR, et al. J Vasc Surg 1992; 16:378–90.)

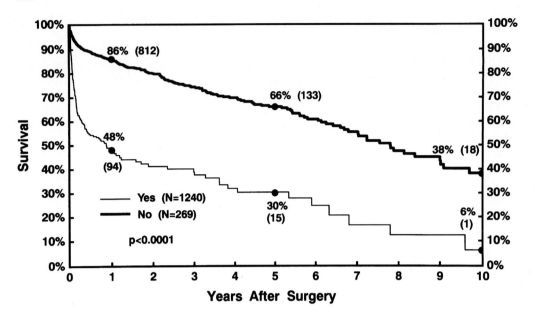

FIGURE 26–13 Effect of the postoperative renal failure on long-term survival of patients who had thoracoabdominal aneurysm repairs. (From Svensson LG, Crawford ES, Hess KR, et al. J Vasc Surg 1993;17:357–70.)

respiratory failure occurring was $FEF_{25\%}$, although this test also correlated closely with the FEV_1. (The chapter on preoperative assessment has dealt with this subject in more detail.) The presence of chronic pulmonary disease also significantly influences long-term survival after surgery (Fig. 26–14).

In summary, preoperative preparation of the patient is important in preventing respiratory failure. This includes cessation of smoking (preferably 2 weeks before surgery), use of bronchodilators for patients who are found to have reversible airway disease, coughing and breathing exercises, and control of productive secretions with appropriate antibiotics. Postoperative aminophylline (theophylline) may

be of value and has been shown to improve respiratory function after upper abdominal surgery.[10, 162-164]

Gastrointestinal Complications

We have documented the low incidence of gastrointestinal complications in patients with thoracoabdominal aneurysms in the entire series of 1509 patients.[93] The prospective studies of 98 patients undergoing high-risk surgery (Crawford types I and II),[33] and of patients undergoing visceral artery repairs[13] suggest that, with short aortic cross-clamp times and the liberal use of medications to prevent postoperative stress ulceration, gastrointestinal

FIGURE 26–14 Effect of the preparative chronic pulmonary disease on long-term survival of patients who had thoracoabdominal aneurysm repairs. (From Svensson LG, Crawford ES, Hess KR, et al. J Vasc Surg 1993;17:357–70.

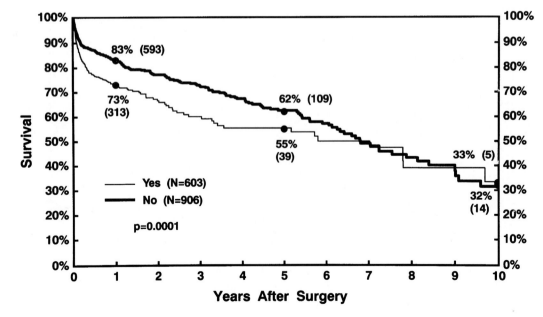

complications in patients should not be a frequent problem. Noteworthy, however, are the 13 patients who developed aortointestinal fistulae that resulted in their death.[93] The technique of transecting the aorta that was described earlier appears to reduce the risk of aortoesophageal fistulae developing at the proximal suture line.[10]

False Aneurysm Formation

As with the development of false aneurysms (pseudoaneurysms) at the coronary anastomoses and distal anastomoses in the ascending aorta or aortic arch, false aneurysms may occur in the distal aorta at the site of any anastomosis. For descending thoracic and thoracoabdominal aortic repairs, false aneurysms may occur at the proximal anastomoses, sites of intercostal artery reattachments, visceral artery anastomoses, and the distal anastomoses. In patients with Marfan syndrome, the intercostal and visceral anastomoses are particularly prone to the development of false aneurysms. In patients who have infrarenal aorta operations, the sites of false aneurysm development include the proximal anastomoses and distal anastomoses, particularly those at the femoral arteries.

With the current use of Prolene sutures for most anastomoses, suture failure is not the usual cause of false aneurysm formation unless the sutures were too small for the anastomosis or were held with a metal object such as forceps and frayed. In the past, the use of silk and other sutures that were not permanent often resulted in the formation of false aneurysms. The placement of sutures too close to the edge of either a Dacron or polytetrafluoroethylene (PTFE) graft may cause the sutures to pull loose, resulting in aneurysm formation. We have found that, even with the excision of ellipses out of grafts for the reattachment of intercostal or visceral arteries, as long as suture "bites" have been large, then fraying of the prostheses, later causing false aneurysms, has not been a problem. In most patients in whom false aneurysms develop, the cause is either poor aortic wall tissue or graft infection. An aortic wall with poor strength can be due to aneurysmal tissue (visceral and intercostal reimplantations), Marfan syndrome, medial wall degeneration, endarterectomy of the aorta, aortic dissection (particularly acute dissection), or residual infection of the aorta in the case of mycotic aneurysms or reoperation for graft infection.

Detection of false aneurysms may occur during clinical examination, ultrasound investigation, MRI or CAT scanning, or aortography. The natural course of false aneurysms is not clearly defined, although it is clear that many may rupture. Treatment is usually surgical, although femoral artery and some localized aortic false aneurysms can be treated with compression, embolization, or thrombosis. Craig Miller (personal communication) has also treated a false aneurysm after repair of a coarctation in the chest with a percutaneously placed stent excluding the aneurysm and resulting in its thrombosing. It should be noted, however, that the aorta wall that has been reimplanted for intercostal artery or visceral artery reattachments may appear to bulge after a successful repair of the aorta. This appearance should not be confused with a false aneurysm unless it is documented to expand with time and requires no further management other than close follow-up, particularly in patients with Marfan syndrome.

McCann and colleagues[165] reviewed a series of 61 patients who presented with either 25 false aneurysms or 41 graft infections late after abdominal aortic operations; 17 of the latter also had intestinal involvement. The 30-day mortality rates for operative repairs were 25%, 17% (excluding aortoenteric fistulae), and 35%, respectively. Only 47% of the patients with aortoenteric fistula, however, were discharged alive. Late aortic stump disruption after repair resulted in the death of five patients with aortoenteric fistulae, two with graft infections, and one with a false aneurysm. Allen and colleagues[166] reported on 31 aneurysms in 29 patients after abdominal aorta operations. In 19 patients the original operation was for an aneurysm and in 10 for occlusive disease. Six of the late aneurysms were true aneurysms (all after previous aneurysm repairs), and the remainder were false aneurysms. Twenty-seven of the para-anastomotic aneurysms were proximal to the previous graft insertions. Symptoms at presentation included abdominal pain, mass, claudication, and back pain. After surgical repair, 73% of the patients had serious morbidity and 21% died, whereas for elective repairs in symptom-free patients the morbidity rate was lower at 33%, as was the mortality rate at 17%. These results stress the importance of operating on these patients electively rather than on an emergency basis as has also been reported by Coselli.[167]

REFERENCES

1. Szilagyi DE, Hageman JH, Smith RF, et al. Spinal cord damage in surgery of the abdominal aorta. Surgery 1978;83:38–56.
2. Szilagyi DE. A second look at the etiology of spinal cord damage in surgery of the abdominal aorta. J Vasc Surg 1993;17:1111-3.
3. Salam AA, Sholkamy SM, Chaikof EL. Spinal cord ischemia after abdominal aortic procedures: is previous colectomy a risk factor? J Vasc Surg 1993;17:1108-10.
4. Picone AL, Green RM, Ricotta JR, et al. Spinal cord ischemia following operations on the abdominal aorta. J Vasc Surg 1986;3:94-103.
5. Crawford ES, Saleh SA, Babb JW, et al. Infrarenal abdominal aortic aneurysm; factors influencing survival after operation performed over a 25-year period. Ann Surg 1981;193:699-709.
6. Crawford ES. Symposium: prevention of complications of abdominal aortic reconstruction (introduction). Surgery 1983;93:91-6.
7. Crawford JL, Stowe CL, Safi HJ, et al. Inflammatory aneurysms of the aorta. J Vasc Surg 1985;2:113-24.
8. Crawford ES, Mizrahi EM, Hess KR, et al. The impact of distal aortic perfusion and somatosensory evoked potential monitoring on prevention of paraplegia after aortic aneurysm operation. (Published erratum appears in J Thorac Cardiovasc Surg 1989 May;97:665.) J Thorac Cardiovasc Surg 1988;95:357-67.
9. Crawford ES. Ruptured abdominal aortic aneurysm [editorial]. J Vasc Surg 1991;13:348-50.
10. Svensson LG, Crawford ES. Aortic dissection and aortic aneurysm surgery: clinical observations, experimental investigations, and statistical analyses. Part III. Curr Probl Surg 1993;30:1-172.
11. Olin JW, Graor RA, O'Hara P, Young JR. The incidence of deep venous thrombosis in patients undergoing abdominal aortic aneurysm resection. J Vasc Surg 1993;18:1037-41.
12. Svensson LG, Coselli JS, Safi HJ, et al. Appraisal of adjuncts to prevent acute renal failure after surgery on the thoracic or thoracoabdominal aorta. J Vasc Med 1989;10:230-9.

13. Svensson LG, Crawford ES, Hess KR, et al. Thoracoabdominal aortic aneurysms associated with celiac, superior mesenteric and renal artery occlusive disease: methods and analysis of results in 271 patients. J Vasc Surg 1992;16:378-90.

14. Svensson LG, Crawford ES. Aortic dissection and aortic aneurysm surgery: clinical observations, experimental investigations and statistical analyses. Part I. Curr Probl Surg 1992;29:819-912.

15. Nypaver TJ, Shepard AD, Reddy DJ, et al. Supraceliac aortic cross-clamping; determinants of outcome in elective abdominal aortic reconstruction. J Vasc Surg 1993;17:868-76.

16. Dalsing MC, Bihrle R, Lalka SG, et al. Vascular surgery-associated ureteral injury; zebras do exist. Ann Vasc Surg 1993;7:180-6.

17. Petersen MJ, Cambria RP, Kaufman JA, et al. Magnetic resonance angiography in the preoperative evaluation of abdominal aortic aneurysms. J Vasc Surg 1995;21:891-9.

18. Abbott ME. Coarctation of the aorta of the adult type. II. Am Heart J 1928;3:574-618.

19. Breckwoldt WL, Mackey WC, Belkin M, O'Donnell TF Jr. The effect of suprarenal cross-clamping on abdominal aortic aneurysm. Arch Surg 1992;127:520-4.

20. Rendl KH, Prenner K. Intra-abdominal compartment syndrome as a rare complication. Vasa 1992;21:81-4.

21. Bush HLJ, Hydo LJ, Fischer E, et al. Hypothermia during elective abdominal aortic aneurysm repair; the high price of avoidable morbidity. J Vasc Surg 1995;21:392-402.

22. Bush HL Jr, Huse JB, Johnson WC, et al. Prevention of renal insufficiency after abdominal aortic aneurysm resection by optimal volume loading. Arch Surg 1981;116:1517-24.

23. Bryan AG, Bolsin SN, Vianna PTG, Haloush H. Modification of the diuretic and natriuretic effects of a dopamine infusion by fluid loading in preoperative cardiac surgical patients. J Cardiothorac Vasc Anesth 1995;9:158-63.

24. Gattinoni L, Brazzi L, Pelosi P, et al. A trial of goal-oriented hemodynamic therapy in critically ill patients. N Engl J Med 1995;333:1025-32.

25. Boyd O, Grounds RM, Bennett ED. A randomized clinical trial of the effect of deliberate perioperative increase of oxygen delivery on mortality in high-risk surgical patients. JAMA 1993;270:2699-707.

26. Calligaro KD, Azurin DJ, Dougherty MJ, et al. Pulmonary risk factors of elective abdominal aortic surgery. J Vasc Surg 1993;18:914-21.

27. Lindsay TF, Walker PM, Romaschin A. Acute pulmonary injury in a model of ruptured abdominal aortic aneurysm. J Vasc Surg 1995;22:1-8.

28. Sicard GA, Reilly JM, Rubin BG, et al. Transabdominal versus retroperitoneal incision for abdominal aortic surgery; report of a prospective randomized trial. J Vasc Surg 1995;21:174-83.

29. Sicard GA, Freeman MB, VanderWoude JC, et al. Comparison between the transabdominal and retroperitoneal approach for reconstruction of the infrarenal abdominal aorta. J Vasc Surg 1987;5:19-27.

30. Pabst TS 3rd, McIntyre KEJ, Schilling JD, et al. Management of chyloperitoneum after abdominal aortic surgery. Am J Surg 1993;166:194-9.

31. Hinder RA, Fimmel CJ, Rickards E, et al. Stimulation of gastric acid secretion increases mucosal blood flow in immediate vicinity of parietal cells in baboons. Dig Dis Sci 1988;33:545-51.

32. Svensson LG, Von Ritter C, Oosthuizen MM, et al. Prevention of gastric mucosal lesions following aortic cross-clamping. Br J Surg 1987;74:282-5.

33. Svensson LG, Hess KR, Coselli JS, et al. A prospective study of respiratory failure after high-risk surgery on the thoracoabdominal aorta. J Vasc Surg 1991;14:271-82.

34. Von Ritter C, Hinder RA, Oosthuizen MM, et al. Gastric mucosal lesions induced by hemorrhagic shock in baboons: role of oxygen-derived free radicals. Dig Dis Sci 1988;33:857-64.

35. Brewster DC, Franklin DP, Cambria RP, et al. Intestinal ischemia complicating abdominal aortic surgery. Surgery 1991;109:447-54.

36. Konno H, Kaneko H, Maruo Y, et al. Prevention of gastric ulcer or acute gastric mucosal lesions accompanying bleeding after abdominal aortic aneurysm surgery. World J Surg 1994;18:944-7.

37. Tollefson DF, Ernst CB. Colon ischemia following aortic reconstruction. Ann Vasc Surg 1991;5:485-9.

38. Fiddian GRG, Gantz NM. Transient episodes of sigmoid ischemia and their relation to infection from intestinal organisms after abdominal aortic operations. Crit Care Med 1987;15:835-9.

39. Schiedler MG, Cutler BS, Fiddian GRG. Sigmoid intramural pH for prediction of ischemic colitis during aortic surgery: a comparison with risk factors and inferior mesenteric artery stump pressures. Arch Surg 1987;122:881-6.

40. Soong CV, Blain PHB, Halliday MI, et al. Bowel ischaemia and organ impairment in elective abdominal aortic aneurysm repair. Br J Surg 1994;81:965-8.

41. Seeger JM, Coe DA, Kaelin LD, Flynn TC. Routine reimplantation of patent inferior mesenteric arteries limits colon infarction after aortic reconstruction. J Vasc Surg 1992;15:635-41.

42. Cambria RP, Brewster DC, Abbott WM, et al. The impact of selective use of dipyridamole-thallium scans and surgical factors on the current morbidity of aortic surgery. J Vasc Surg 1992;15:43-50.

43. Crawford ES, Morris GC, Howell JF, et al. Operative risk in patients with previous coronary artery bypass. Ann Thorac Surg 1978;26:215-21.

44. Eagle KA, Singer DE, Brewster DC, et al. Dipyridamole-thallium scanning in patients undergoing vascular surgery: optimizing preoperative evaluation of cardiac risk. JAMA 1987;257:2185-9.

45. Hertzer NR, Beven EG, Young JR, et al. Coronary artery disease in peripheral vascular patients: a classification of 1000 coronary angiograms and results of surgical management. Ann Surg 1984;199:223-33.

46. Hertzer NR, Young JR, Beven EG, et al. Late results of coronary bypass in patients with infrarenal aortic aneurysms: the Cleveland Clinic Study. Ann Surg 1987;205:360-7.

47. Johnston KW, Scobie TK. Multicenter prospective study of nonruptured abdominal aortic aneurysms. I. Population and operative management. J Vasc Surg 1988;7:69-81.

48. Johnston KW. Multicenter prospective study of nonruptured abdominal aortic aneurysm. Part II. Variables predicting morbidity and mortality. J Vasc Surg 1989;9:437-47.

49. McCann RL, Wolfe WG. Resection of abdominal aortic aneurysm in patients with low ejection fractions. J Vasc Surg 1989;10:240-4.

50. Young JR, Hertzer NR, Beven EG, et al. Coronary artery disease in patients with aortic aneurysm: a classification of 302 coronary angiograms and results of surgical management. Ann Vasc Surg 1986;1:36-42.

51. Kalra M, Charlesworth D, Morris JA, Al-Khaffaf H. Myocardial infarction after reconstruction of the abdominal aorta. Br J Surg 1993;80:28-31.

52. Buckley MJ, Cheitlin MD, Goldman L, et al. Cardiac surgery and noncardiac surgery in elderly patients with heart disease. J Am Coll Cardiol 1987;10(2 Supp A):35A-37A.

53. Cutler BS, Leppo JA. Dipyridamole thallium 201 scintigraphy to detect coronary artery disease before abdominal aortic surgery. J Vasc Surg 1987;5:91-100.

54. Eagle KA, Coley CM, Newell JB, et al. Combining clinical and thalium data optimizes preoperative assessment of cardiac risk before major vascular surgery. Ann Intern Med 1989;110:859-66.

55. Golden MA, Whittemore AD, Donaldson MC, Mannick JA. Selective evaluation and management of coronary artery disease in patients undergoing repair of abdominal aortic aneurysm: a 16-year experience. Ann Surg 1990;212:415-20.

56. Golden MA, Donaldson MC, Whittemore AD, Mannick JA. Evolving experience with thoracoabdominal aortic aneurysm repair at a single institution. J Vasc Surg 1991;13:792-6.

57. Gouny P, Bertrand M, Coriat P, Kieffer E. Perioperative cardiac complications of surgical repair of infrarenal aortic aneurysms. Ann Vasc Surg 1989;3:328-34.

58. Grindlinger GA, Manny J, Weisel RD, et al. Volume loading and nitroprusside in abdominal aortic aneurysectomy. Surg Forum 1978;29:234-6.

59. Hertzer NR. Basic data concerning associated coronary disease in peripheral vascular patients. Ann Vasc Surg 1987;1:616-20.

60. Krupski WC, Layug EL, Reilly LM, et al. Comparison of cardiac morbidity between aortic and infrainguinal operations: study of Perioperative Ischemia (SPI) Research Group. J Vasc Surg 1992;15:354-63.

61. Mangano DT, London MJ, Tubau JF, et al. Dipyridamole-thallium 201 scintigraphy as a preoperative test: a re-examination of its predictive potential. Circulation 1991;84:493-502.

62. McEnroe CS, O'Donnell TF Jr, Yeager A, et al. Comparison of ejection fraction and Goldman risk factor analysis to dipyridamole-thallium 201 studies in the evaluation of cardiac morbidity after aortic aneurysm surgery. J Vasc Surg 1990;11:497-504.

63. Pairolero PC. Repair of abdominal aortic aneurysms in high-risk patients. Surg Clin North Am 1989;69:755-63.

64. Paterson IS, Klausner JM, Pugatch R, et al. Noncardiogenic pulmonary edema after abdominal aortic aneurysm surgery. Ann Surg 1989;209:231-6.

65. Yeager RA. Comparison of ejection fraction and Goldman risk factor analysis to dipyridamole–thallium 201 studies in the evaluation of cardiac morbidity after aortic aneurysm surgery [letter comment]. J Vasc Surg 1991;13:173.

66. Krupski WC, Layug EL, Reilly LM, et al. Comparison of cardiac morbidity rates between aortic and infrainguinal operations: two-year follow-up. J Vasc Surg 1993;18:609-17.

67. Beven EG. Routine coronary angiography in patients undergoing surgery for abdominal aortic aneurysm and lower extremity occlusive disease. J Vasc Surg 1986;3:682-4.

68. Berthe C, Pierard LA, Hiernaux M, et al. Predicting the extent and location of coronary artery disease in acute myocardial infarction by echocardiography during dobutamine infusion. Am J Cardiol 1986;58:1167-72.

69. Crawford MH. The preoperative cardiac evaluation of the patient with vascular disease: ejection fraction and stress echocardiography. Semin Vasc Surg 1991;4:77-82.

70. Lalka SG, Sawada SG, Dalsing MC, et al. Dobutamine stress echocardiography as a predictor of cardiac events associated with aortic surgery. J Vasc Surg 1992;15:831-42.

71. Svensson LG, Crawford ES. Aortic dissection and aortic aneurysm surgery: clinical observations, experimental investigations, and statistical analyses. Part II. Curr Probl Surg 1992;29:915-1057.

72. Durham SJ, Steed DL, Moosa HH, et al. Probability of rupture of an abdominal aortic aneurysm after an unrelated operative procedure: a prospective study. J Vasc Surg 1991;13:248-252.

73. Busuttil RW, Cardenas A. Collagenase activity of the human aorta. Arch Surg 1980;115:1373-8.

74. Tilson MD. Histochemistry of aortic elastin in patients with nonspecific abdominal aortic aneurysmal disease. Arch Surg 1988;123:503-5.

75. Zarins CK, Runyon HA, Zatina MA, et al. Increased collagenase activity in early aneurysmal dilatation. J Vasc Surg 1986;3:238-48.

76. Zarins CK, Glagov S, Vesselinovitch D, Wissler RW. Aneurysm formation in experimental atherosclerosis: relationship to plaque evolution. J Vasc Surg 1990;12:246-56.

77. Zarins CK, Xu CP, Glagov S. Aneurysmal enlargement of the aorta during regression of experimental atherosclerosis. J Vasc Surg 1992;15:90-8.

78. Menashi S, Campa JS, Greenhalgh RM, Powell JT. Collagen in abdominal aortic aneurysm: typing, content, and degradation. J Vasc Surg 1987;6:578-82.

79. Rizzo RJ, McCarthy WJ, Dixit SN, et al. Collagen types and matrix protein content in human abdominal aortic aneurysms. J Vasc Surg 1989;10:365-73.

80. Cohen JR, Mandell C, Margolis I, et al. Altered aortic protease and antiprotease activity in patients with ruptured abdominal aortic aneurysms. Surg Gynecol Obstet 1987;164:355-8.

81. Blackbourne LH, Tribble CG, Langenburg SE, et al. Optimal timing of abdominal aortic aneurysm repair after coronary artery revascularization. Ann Surg 1994;219:693-8.

82. Mason JJ, Owens DK, Harris RA, et al. The role of coronary angiography and coronary revascularization before noncardiac vascular surgery. JAMA 1995;273:1919-25.

83. Borst HG, Jurmann M, Buhner B, Laas J. Risk of replacement of descending aorta with a standardized left heart bypass technique. J Thorac Cardiovasc Surg 1994;107:126-33.

84. Kouchoukos NT, Wareing TH, Izumoto H, et al. Elective hypothermic cardiopulmonary bypass and circulatory arrest for spinal cord protection during operations on the thoracoabdominal aorta. J Thorac Cardiovasc Surg 1990;99:659-64.

85. Lawrie GM, Earle N, DeBakey ME. Evolution of surgical techniques for aneurysms of the descending thoracic aorta: twenty-nine years experience with 659 patients. J Cardiac Surg 1994;9:648-61.

86. Svensson LG, Crawford ES, Hess KR, et al. Variables predictive of outcome in 832 patients undergoing repairs of the descending thoracic aorta. Chest 1993;104:1248-53.

87. Svensson LG, Hess KR, Coselli JS, Safi HR. Influence of segmental arteries, extent, and atrio-femoral bypass on postoperative paraplegia after thoracoabdominal aortic aneurysm repairs. J Vasc Surg 1994;20:255-62.

88. Kouchoukos NT, Daily BD, Rokkas CK, et al. Hypothermic bypass and circulatory arrest for operations on the descending thoracic and thoracoabdominal aorta. Ann Thorac Surg 1995;60:67-77.

89. Najafi H. Descending aortic aneurysmectomy without adjuncts to avoid ischemia:1993 update. Ann Thorac Surg 1993;55:1042-5.

90. Coselli JS. Thoracoabdominal aortic aneurysms: experience with 372. J Cardiac Surg 1994;9:638-47.

91. Safi HJ. Neurologic deficit in patients at high risk with thoracoabdominal aortic aneurysms: the role of cerebral spinal fluid drainage and distal aortic perfusion. J Vasc Surg 1994;20:434-43.

92. Gilling-Smith GL, Worswick L, Knight PF, et al. Surgical repair of thoracoabdominal aortic aneurysm: 10 years' experience. Br J Surg 1995;82:624-9.

93. Svensson LG, Crawford ES, Hess KR, et al. Experience with 1509 patients undergoing thoracoabdominal aortic operations. J Vasc Surg 1993;17:357-70.

94. Crawford ES, Svensson LG, Hess KR, et al. A prospective randomized study of cerebrospinal fluid drainage to prevent paraplegia after high-risk surgery on the thoracoabdominal aorta. J Vasc Surg 1991;13:36-45.

95. Svensson LG, Crawford ES, Hess KR, et al. Dissection of the aorta and dissecting aortic aneurysms: improving early and long-term surgical results. Circulation 1990;82(5 Supp):IV 24-38.

96. Laschinger JC, Izumoto H, Kouchoukos NT. Evolving concepts in prevention of spinal cord injury during operations on the descending thoracic and thoracoabdominal aorta. Ann Thorac Surg 1987;44:667-74.

97. Shenaq SA, Svensson LG. Paraplegia following aortic surgery. J Thorac Cardiovasc Anesth 1993;7:81-94.

98. Svensson LG, Hinder RA. Hemodynamics of aortic cross-clamping: experimental observations and clinical applications. Surg Annu 1987;19:41-65.

99. Svensson LG, Loop FD. Prevention of spinal cord ischemia in aortic surgery. In: Bergan JJ, Yao JST, eds. Arterial Surgery: New Diagnostic and Operative Techniques. New York: Grune & Stratton, 1988:273-85.

100. Mauney MC, Blackbourne LH, Langenburg SE, et al. Prevention of spinal cord injury after repair of the thoracic or thoracoabdominal aorta. Ann Thorac Surg 1995;59:245-52.

101. Svensson LG, Richards E, Coull A, et al. Relationship of spinal cord blood flow to vascular anatomy during thoracic aortic cross-clamping and shunting. J Thorac Cardiovasc Surg 1986;91:71-8.

102. Svensson LG, Von Ritter CM, Groeneveld HT, et al. Cross-clamping of the thoracic aorta: influence of aortic shunts, laminectomy, papaverine, calcium channel blocker, allopurinol, and superoxide dismutase on spinal cord blood flow and paraplegia in baboons. Ann Surg 1986;204:38-47.

103. Rokkas CK, Sundaresan S, Shuman TA, et al. A primate model of spinal cord ischemia: evaluation of spinal cord blood flow and the protective effect of hypothermia. Surg Forum 1991;42:265-7.

104. Moore WM Jr, Hollier LH. The influence of severity of spinal cord ischemia in the etiology of delayed-onset paraplegia. Ann Surg 1991;213:427-31.

105. Blot S, Arnal J-F, Xu Y, et al. Spinal cord infarcts during long-term inhibition of nitric oxide synthase in rats. Stroke 1994;25:1666-73.

106. Svensson LG, Patel V, Robinson MF, et al. Influence of preservation or perfusion of intraoperatively identified spinal cord blood supply on spinal motor evoked potentials and paraplegia after aortic surgery. J Vasc Surg 1991;13:355-65.

107. Schnell L, Schneider R, Kolbeck R, Barde Y-A. Neurotrophin-3 enhances sprouting of corticospinal tract during development and after adult spinal cord lesion. Nature 1994;367:170-3.

108. Hill AB, Kalman PG, Johnston KW, Vosu HA. Reversal of delayed-onset paraplegia after thoracic aortic surgery with cerebrospinal fluid drainage. J Vasc Surg 1994;20:315-7.

109. Tsirka S, Gualandris A, Amaral DG, Strickland S. Excitotoxin-induced neuronal degeneration and seizure are mediated by tissue plasminogen acitivator. Nature 1995;377:340-1.

110. Iwashita Y, Kawaguchi S, Murata M. Restoration of function by replacement of spinal cord segments in the rat. Nature 1994;367:167-73.

111. Hollier LH, Money SR, Naslund TC, et al. Risk of spinal cord dysfunction in patients undergoing thoracoabdominal aortic replacement. Am J Surg 1992;164:210-4.

112. Svensson LG, Von Ritter CM, Groenveld HT, et al. Cross-clamping of the thoracic aorta: influence of aortic shunts, laminectomy,

papaverine, calcium channel blockers, allopurinol, and superoxide dismutase on spinal cord blood flow and paraplegia in baboons. Ann Surg 1986;204:38-47.

113. Svensson LG, Stewart RW, Cosgrove DM, et al. Preliminary results and rationale for the use of intrathecal papaverine for the prevention of paraplegia after aortic surgery. S Afr J Surg 1988;26:153-60.

114. Svensson LG, Stewart RW, Cosgrove DM 3rd, et al. Intrathecal papaverine for the prevention of paraplegia after operation on the thoracic or thoracoabdominal aorta. J Thorac Cardiovasc Surg 1988; 96:823-9.

115. The Marstrand workshop-group. Thoracoabdominal aortic aneurysms with special reference to technical problems and complications. Eur J Vasc Surg 1993;7:725-30.

116. Katircioglu SF, Kucukaksu DS, Kuplulu S, et al. Effects of postacyclin on spinal cord ischemia: an experimental study. Surgery 1993;114: 36-9.

117. Colon R, Frazier OH, Cooley DA, McAllister HA. Hypothermic regional perfusion for protection of the spinal cord during periods of ischemia. Ann Thorac Surg 1987;43:639-43.

118. Grabitz K, Freye E, Prior R, Braun M. Protection from spinal cord injury by intravenous prostaglandin E1 (PGE1) after one hour occlusion of the descending thoracic aorta. Prog Clin Biol Res 1989;301: 211-6.

119. Grabitz K, Freye E, Prior R, et al. The role of superoxide dismutase (SOD) in preventing postischemic spinal cord injury. Adv Exp Med Biol 1990;264:13-16.

120. Grabitz K, Freye E, Prior R, et al. Does prostaglandin E1 and superoxide dismutase prevent ischaemic spinal cord injury after thoracic aortic cross-clamping? Eur J Vasc Surg 1990;4:19-24.

121. Hollier LH, Symmonds JB, Pairolero PC, et al. Thoracoabdominal aortic aneurysm repair: analysis of postoperative morbidity. Arch Surg 1988;123:871-5.

122. Hollier LH, Moore WM. Avoidance of renal and neurologic complications following thoracoabdominal aortic aneurysm repair. Acta Chir Scand Supp 1990;555:129-35.

123. Kaschner AG, Sandmann W, Kniemeyer HW, et al. Evaluation of epidural perfusion cooling to protect the spinal cord during thoracic aortic cross-clamping: monitoring of spinal evoked electrogram. J Cardiovasc Surg 1985;26:97-8.

124. Kirshner DL, Kirshner RL, Heggeness LM, DeWeese JA. Spinal cord ischemia: an evaluation of pharmacologic agents in minimizing paraplegia after aortic occlusion. J Vasc Surg 1989;9:305-8.

125. Maughan RE, Mohan C, Nathan IM, et al. Intrathecal perfusion of an oxygenated perflurocarbon emulsion prevents paraplegia after extended normothermic aortic cross-clamping. Ann Thorac Surg 1992;54:818-24.

126. Nylander WA, Plunkett RJ, Hammon JW, et al. Thiopental modification of ischemic spinal cord injury in the dog. Ann Thoracic Surg 1982;33:64-8.

127. Shaw PJ, Bates D, Cartlidge NEF, et al. Neurologic and neuropsychological morbidity following major surgery: comparison of coronary artery bypass and peripheral vascular surgery. Stroke 1987;18:700-7.

128. Svensson LG, Crawford ES, Patel V, et al. Spinal cord oxygenation, intraoperative blood supply localization, cooling and function with aortic clamping. Ann Thorac Surg 1992;54:74-9.

129. Woloszyn TT, Marini CP, Coons MS, et al. Cerebrospinal fluid drainage and steroids provide better spinal cord protection during aortic cross-clamping than does either treatment alone. Ann Thorac Surg 1990;49:78-82.

130. DeBakey ME, Cooley DA, Creech O Jr. Resection of the aorta for aneurysms and occlusive disease with particular reference to the use of hypothermia; analysis of 240 cases. J Am Col Cardiol 1955; 5:153-7.

131. Pontius RG, Brockman HL, Hardy EG, et al. The use of hypothermia in the prevention of paraplegia following temporary aortic occlusion: experimental observations. Surgery 1954;36:33-8.

132. Crawford ES, Coselli JS, Safi HJ. Partial cardiopulmonary bypass, hypothermic circulatory arrest, and posterolateral exposure for thoracic aortic aneurysm operation. J Thorac Cardiovasc Surg 1987; 94:824-7.

133. Kouchoukos NT. Spinal cord ischemic injury: is it preventable? Semin Thorac Cardiovasc Surg 1991;3:323-8.

134. Svensson LG, Crawford ES, Hess KR, et al. Deep hypothermia with circulatory arrest: determinants of stroke and early mortality in 656 patients. J Thorac Cardiovasc Surg 1992;106:19-31.

135. Svensson LG, Shahian DM, Davis FG, et al. Replacement of entire aorta from aortic valve to bifurcation during one operation. Ann Thorac Surg 1994;58:1164-6.

136. Berguer R, Porto J, Fedoronko B, Dragovic L. Selective deep hypothermia of the spinal cord prevents paraplegia after aortic cross-clamping in the dog model. J Vasc Surg 1992;15:62-71.

137. Cambria RP, Brewster DC, Moncure AC, et al. Recent experience with thoracoabdominal aneurysm repair. Arch Surg 1989;124: 620-4.

138. Negrin JJ. Selective local hypothermia in neurosurgery. New York J Med 1961;1:2951-65.

139. Acosta-Rua GJ. Treatment of traumatic paraplegic patients by localized cooling of the spinal cord. J Iowa Med Soc 1970;LX:326-8.

140. Albin MS, White RJ, Acosta-Rua GJ, et al. Study of functional recovery produced by delayed localized cooling after spinal cord injury in primates. J Neurosurg 1968;29:113-20.

141. Giglia JS, Zelenock GB, D'Alecy L. Prevention of paraplegia during thoracic aortic cross-clamping; importance of patent internal mammary arteries. J Vasc Surg 1994;19:1044-51.

142. Svensson LG, Stewart RW, Cosgrove DM, et al. Intrathecal papaverine for the prevention of paraplegia after operation on the thoracic or thoracoabdominal aorta. J Thorac Cardiovasc Surg 1988;96: 823-9.

143. Svensson LG, Loop FD. Prevention of spinal cord ischemia in aortic surgery. In: Bergan JJ, Yao JST, eds. Arterial Surgery: New Diagnostic and Operative Techniques. New York: Grune & Stratton, 1988: 2273-85.

144. Cooley DA, Baldwin RT. Technique of open distal anastomosis for repair of descending thoracic aortic aneurysms. Ann Thorac Surg 1992;54:932-6.

145. Svensson LG, Klepp P, Hinder RA. Spinal cord anatomy of the baboon: comparison with man and implications on spinal cord blood flow during thoracic aortic cross-clamping. S Afr J Surg 1986; 24:32-4.

146. Svensson LG, Patel V, Coselli JS, Crawford ES. Preliminary report of localization of spinal cord blood supply by hydrogen during aortic operations. Ann Thorac Surg 1990;49:528-35.

147. Stone CD, Greene PS, Gott VL, et al. Single-stage repair of distal aortic arch and thoracoabdominal dissecting aneurysms using aortic taloring and circulatory arrest. Ann Thorac Surg 1994;57:580-7.

148. Williams GM, Perler BA, Burdick JF, et al. Angiographic localization of spinal cord blood supply and its relationship to postoperative paraplegia. J Vasc Surg 1991;13:23-33.

149. Kieffer E, Richard T, Chiras J, et al. Preoperative spinal cord arteriography in aneurysmal disease of the descending thoracic and thoracoabdominal aorta: preliminary results in 45 patients. Ann Vasc Surg 1989;3:34-46.

150. Kieffer E. Surgical treatment of aneurysms of the thoraco-abdominal aorta. Rev Prat 1991;41:1793-7.

151. Allen BT, Doblas M, Owen J, et al. Cerebrospinal fluid pressure, somatosensory and motor-evoked potentials in spinal cord ischemia after lumbar artery ligation. Surg Forum 1991;42:262-5.

152. Elmore JR, Gloviczki P, Harper CM, et al. Failure of motor evoked potentials to predict neurologic outcome in experimental thoracic aortic occlusion. J Vasc Surg 1991;14:131-9.

153. Shiiya N, Yasuda K, Matsui Y, et al. Spinal cord protection during thoracoabdominal aortic aneurysm repair: results of selective reconstruction of the critical segmental arteries guided by evoked spinal cord potential monitoring. J Vasc Surg 1995;21:970-5.

154. Galla JD, Ergin A, Sadeghi AM, et al. A new technique using somatosensory evoked potential guidance during descending and thoracoabdominal aortic repairs. J Cardiac Surg 1994;9:662-72.

155. Schepens MA, Defauw JJ, Hamerlijnck RP, Vermeulen FE. Risk assessment of acute renal failure after thoracoabdominal aortic aneurysm surgery. Ann Surg 1994;219:400-7.

156. Svensson LG, Coselli JS, Safi HJ, et al. Appraisal of adjuncts to prevent acute renal failure after surgery on the thoracic or thoracoabdominal aorta. J Vasc Surg 1989;10:230-9.

157. Allen BT, Anderson CB, Rubin BG, et al. Preservation of renal function in juxtarenal and suprarenal abdominal aortic aneurysm repair. J Vasc Surg 1993;17:948-59.

158. Torsello G, Schror K, Szabo Z, et al. Winner of the ESVS Prize 1988: effects of prostaglandin E1 (PGE1) on experimental renal ischaemia. Eur J Vasc Surg 1989;3:5-13.

159. Pelkey TJ, Frank RS, Stanley JJ, et al. Minimal physiologic

temperature variations during renal ischemia alter functional and morphologic outcome. J Vasc Surg 1992;15:619-25.

160. Schrier RW, Arnold PE, Gordon JA, Burke TJ. Protection of mitochondrial function by mannitol in ischemic acute renal failure. Am J Physiol 1984;247:F365-9.

161. Russell JD, Churchill DN. Calcium antagonists and acute renal failure. Am J Med 1989;87:306-15.

162. Siafakas NM, Stoubou A, Stathopoulou M, et al. Effect of aminophylline on respiratory muscle strength after upper abdominal surgery: a double blind study. Thorax 1993;48:693-7.

163. Jenne JW. What role for theophylline? Thorax 1994;49:97-100.

164. Banner AS. Theophylline: should we discard an old friend? Lancet 1994;343:618.

165. McCann RL, Schwartz LB, Georgiade GS. Management of abdominal aortic graft complications. Ann Surg 1993;217:729-34.

166. Allen RC, Schneider J, Longenecker L, et al. Paraanastomotic aneurysms of the abdominal aorta. J Vasc Surg 1993;18:424-32.

167. Coselli JS, LeMaire SA, Buket S, Berzin E. Subsequent proximal aortic operations in 123 patients with previous infrarenal abdominal aortic aneurysm surgery. J Vasc Surg 1995;22:59-67.

27

Statistical Analyses of Operative Results

This chapter is intended to help a physician decide whether a patient will survive an operation based on the independent risk factors for death, the best results that can be expected, and what the long-term prognosis will be for the patient. This chapter, therefore, contains statistical analyses of results according to the site of the operative procedure as well as analyses for aortic dissection. The early results of endovascular procedures are also discussed. The previous two chapters evaluate the risk factors and incidence of possible complications for proximal and distal operations.

ASCENDING AORTA OR AORTIC ARCH OPERATIONS

In our series of 717 patients who underwent ascending aorta or aortic arch operations,[1] we reported the following findings: 281 patients (39%) had composite valve graft replacements of the ascending aorta, the aortic arch, or both; 117 patients (16%) had separate valves and aortic tube grafts; 256 patients (36%) had grafts only; and 63 patients (9%) had other procedures such as aortoplasties. The cause was usually medial degenerative disease (384, 54%) but other etiologic factors included aortic dissection in 261 (36%) (of which 72 were acute), aortitis in 46 (6.4%), infection in 20, and trauma in 6. Of these 717 patients, 150 (21%) had undergone procedures done elsewhere and were having repeat operations because of recurrence of aneurysms, progression of disease, false aneurysms, rupture, valve regurgitation, aortocutaneous or aortoheart chamber fistulae, or infections, including mediastinitis (see Chapter 25). Concurrent aneurysmal disease distal to the left subclavian artery was present in 37% of the patients, and in patients with aortic arch involvement the incidence was 53%. The overall 30-day survival rate was 91%, although the associated risk factors of the patients strongly influenced survival. The independent predictors of 30-day deaths were increasing age, severity of aneurysm symptoms, diabetes, previous proximal aortic operations, need for postoperative cardiac support, postoperative tracheostomy for respiratory failure, cardiac complications, and stroke. In the 308 patients who had none of these preoperative risk factors, the survival rate was 97%. After a total of 1193 operations, 53 of the 717 patients (7.4%) had undergone total replacement of the entire aorta (see Chapter 24).

By Kaplan-Meier analysis, 66% of the initial 717 patients were alive 5 years after surgery. The independent predictors of long-term survival were severity of preoperative aneurysm symptoms, preoperative angina, extent of proximal aortic replacement, associated residual distal aneurysmal disease, use of a balloon pump, renal dysfunction, cardiac dysfunction, and stroke. The ameliorated results achieved in this study have been gained from numerous lessons learned over time, many of which were derived from retrospective research in consecutive series of patients who had undergone ascending aorta or aortic arch operations. The newer adjuncts, such as deep hypothermia with circulatory arrest and retrograde brain perfusion,[2] blood conservation,[3, 4] anesthetic techniques,[3] and operative techniques for aortic dissection, have been discussed in previous chapters and have further improved results, with up to a 98% survival rate now obtainable in our experience.[4]

Also, it is clearly important to resect all aneurysmal segments of the aorta to prevent later rupture and death,[1, 3, 5] particularly since there is a high incidence of aneurysmal disease in other segments of the aorta. In most patients, including those with aortic dissection, this involves tubular graft replacement of aneurysmal segments. For those patients with annuloaortic ectasia or Marfan syndrome, as discussed previously, the segment of aorta between the aortic valve and the ascending aorta must be replaced with either a composite graft of the valve, or a tube graft and reimplantation or remodeling of the aortic valve supported by an external tube graft. The latter procedure is described by David[6, 7] and others.[8-12] On late follow-up of patients in whom the sinuses of Valsalva are left and separate valve and tubular graft insertions are performed, we[4, 5, 13-15] and others[8, 16] have noted that quite a few patients go on to develop aneurysms in the unresected segment (see examples of reoperations in Chapter 18), although in carefully selected patients Lawrie and colleagues[17] have reported good long-term results. Lesser procedures, such as aortoplasties, will often fail.[15]

Aortic Arch Repairs

The increased use of deep hypothermia with circulatory arrest has made operations on the aortic arch considerably safer (Fig. 27-1), and the addition of retrograde brain

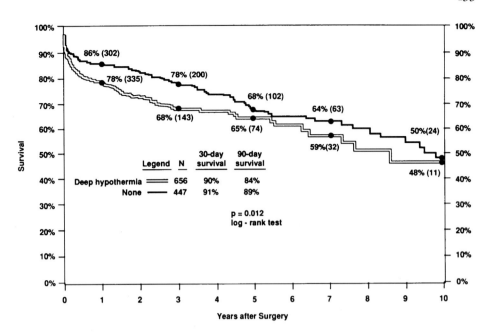

FIGURE 27-1 Long-term survival in 1103 patients who underwent ascending aorta or aortic arch repairs according to whether the operation was done with deep hypother- mic circulatory arrest *(double line)* or without. Although the long-term survival ($p = 0.012$) was significantly worse with circulatory arrest, it should be noted that these latter patients were undergoing more complex operations for more advanced or critical aortic disease (From Svensson LG, Crawford ES, Hess KR et al. J Thorac Cardiovasc Surg 1992;106:19–31.)

perfusion appears to have further improved results. In a study of 656 of our patients undergoing deep hypothermic arrest without retrograde brain perfusion,[2] the incidence of stroke was 7% and the predictors ($p < 0.05$) were a history of cerebrovascular disease, previous aortic surgery distal to the left subclavian artery, and cardiopulmonary bypass time (see Chapters 13 and 25). In this study the predictors of death (66/656, 10%) were ($p < 0.05$) increasing age, Marfan syndrome, concurrent distal aortic aneurysms, previous ascending aorta operations, cardiopulmonary bypass time, cardiac complications, renal complications, and stroke. The risk of stroke increased after 40 minutes, and the risk of death increased markedly after 65 minutes. In this study we also reported our initial experience with retrograde brain perfusion in 50 patients operated on by Coselli, Safi, and one of us (L.G.S.), with only one postoperative stroke due to an embolus from a thoracoabdominal aortic aneurysm. In this case the embolus probably broke off during retrograde perfusion through the femoral artery for cooling, since a change in the electroencephalogram (EEG) was noted and a passing embolus was detected by a Doppler flow probe over the middle cerebral artery.[18]

Coselli and associates[19] reported on a series of 227 patients who underwent aortic arch repairs and divided their patients into three groups according to acute dissection, chronic dissection, and medial degenerative aneurysms. They found that the respective mortality rates were 8.33% (4/48), 4.35% (3/69), and 6.36% (7/110), for an overall mortality rate of 6.17% (14/227). These results are particularly exemplary since the respective incidence of prior cardioaortic surgery was 21%, 70%, and 16%, for an overall reoperation rate of 33% (75/227). The postoperative incidence of stroke was excellent with only 3.1% of the patients having a stroke. It is noteworthy that, of the 111 patients who had retrograde brain perfusion, none had a postoperative stroke.

In a series of 60 consecutive patients undergoing ascending aorta or aortic arch repairs reported by one of us (L.G.S.),[4] 87% of the patients who had elective surgery required no operative blood transfusions and 69% left the hospital without having had a blood or blood product transfusion. The 30-day survival rate was 98%, with no patient sustaining a stroke or clinical neurocognitive deficit. On multivariate analysis, the predictors of in-hospital blood transfusion were ($p < 0.05$) increasing age, cardiopulmonary bypass time, and postoperative chest tube volume output. Preoperative blood donation was associated with a lower risk of blood transfusion. With adjustment for risk factors, patients who donated preoperative blood were ($p < 0.05$) less likely to have a homologous blood transfusion, required less intraoperative blood to be washed ("cell saver"), were extubated earlier, gained less weight postoperatively, had shorter hospital stays, and were discharged in a better functional state. The determinants for patients staying beyond the eighth postoperative day were ($p < 0.05$) preoperative valvular or aortic infection, in-hospital homologous blood transfusion, grade of aortic disease, lack of autologous fresh frozen plasma, increasing cardiopulmonary bypass time, delayed extubation, greater preoperative weight (obesity), and postoperative transfusion of homologous blood.

In a more recent update (L.G.S.) a total of 104 patients have undergone ascending aorta or aortic arch repairs. This series included 39 patients who had aortic dissection and 19 who had acute dissection. The ascending aorta alone was repaired in 54 and the aortic arch in 50; repair included replacement of the entire or nearly the entire aorta during one operation in four patients. The 30-day survival rate was 98% (102/104), and the in-hospital survival rate was 97% (101/104). The two early deaths occurred in patients with advanced atherosclerotic coronary artery disease, one with evolving myocardial infarction and heart failure and the other with an acute myocardial infarct with a 35% ejection fraction. The only patient who had a stroke or neurocognitive deficit had a transient expressive aphasia after repair of an extensive mycotic aneurysm of the aortic arch that was probably caused by eating a raw hamburger. In this patient retrograde brain perfusion could not be used. Also in this series, the findings for those patients who donated autologous blood versus those who did not were, respectively, homologous blood transfusion rates of 0.2 unit and 6.2 units; day of extubation, 1.2 days versus 5.4 days; and postoperative discharge at 10.1 days versus 16 days.

Clearly, patients who undergo urgent or emergency operations cannot donate autologous blood for surgery, and it is difficult to distinguish how much of the benefit of autologous blood is due to the blood per se and to the lack of use of homologous blood as opposed to the fact that the patients are having elective surgery. Nevertheless, we believe that, even in patients having elective surgery, those who have autologous blood available for surgery do better than those who do not.

COMPOSITE VALVE GRAFTS

In a review of 348 of our patients who underwent reattachment of the coronary ostia for composite valve grafts,[20] we found that the survival rate was no different between the Bentall, button, and Cabrol techniques (Fig. 27-2A). On late follow-up of these patients, however, the patients who had Bentall repairs, particularly those with Marfan syndrome,[14, 20, 21] were prone to the development of false aneurysms at the coronary ostia anastomoses because of tension on the suture lines (see Chapters 5 and 25). Furthermore, not infrequently patients who have been referred have required reoperation after failure of classic Bentall repairs. Patients with Cabrol repairs were prone to either early or late development of occlusion of the right graft limb to the right coronary artery,[20] whereas none of the patients who underwent the button technique required reoperation.[20] To circumvent the problems with these techniques and yet take advantage of the attributes, a newer procedure has been developed that is easy to perform, allows for control of bleeding from anastomoses, and offers the advantage of a button for the right coronary artery (see Chapters 17 and 18).[15, 20, 21]

Results of Operative Techniques

Many approaches have been proposed and successfully used for insertion of composite valve grafts and reattachment of the coronary artery ostia for repair of the ascending aorta.[1, 5, 14, 22-42] The Bentall, aortic button, and Cabrol techniques are the three most commonly used methods for insertion of composite valve grafts and reattachment of the coronary artery ostia.[1, 5, 14, 24, 27, 28, 31, 33-36, 38-40] With the Bentall technique, good results have been reported by Gott and colleagues[33] in patients undergoing elective repairs for Marfan syndrome, although more recently they have adopted the button technique without wrapping of the aortic prostheses (exclusion rather than inclusion technique). In previous reports[1, 5, 14] we have documented that, with the Bentall technique of direct reanastomosis of the coronary artery ostia, false aneurysms requiring later reoperation may form at the coronary ostial anastomoses, particularly at the left main coronary artery ostium in patients with Marfan syndrome[14] or in patients with aortic dissection.[5] Kouchoukos and colleagues[38] and other surgeons[35] have, in particular, stressed the importance of not wrapping the aneurysm wall around the aortic graft because of the increased incidence of false aneurysms associated with wrapping. The cause of the false aneurysms appears to be the tension exerted on those anastomoses when the gap between the aneurysmal wall and the tubular graft is excessive, especially when the collection of blood within the aneurysm wrap results in increased tension on the anastomoses. Tamponade of the aortic prosthesis by the accumulated blood within the wrap may also lead to an iatrogenic ascending coarctation. Moreover, bleeding from the anastomoses can be difficult to detect. To decompress the blood that accumulates around the wrapped graft, Cabrol[43] described creation of a shunt or fistula between the aneurysm wall and the right atrium to allow drainage of the blood. Although this technique can be used in cases where bleeding cannot be controlled after extensive searches for bleeding sites, there is the risk that the fistula may remain open, result in later heart failure, and have to be closed, as has been reported by Cooley in discussion of our paper on composite valve grafts[20] and by others.[44] To overcome the problem of late false aneurysm formation from wrapping of the graft, some surgeons have advocated the excision of coronary ostial buttons, mobilization of the proximal coronary arteries, and then reattachment of these ostia to the composite valve graft.[5, 37, 41, 42] This allows for an increased length of artery, which should usually bridge the gap between the aneurysm wall and the graft with minimal tension on the anastomoses. The drawback of this technique has been the time required to dissect out the ostia, particularly for the left coronary artery, and there is the risk of damage or stenosis of the left main coronary artery, the circumflex artery, or the first septal perforator because of tension or cutting the arteries. Furthermore, in patients with acute aortic dissection, mobilization of the coronary ostia may not be a feasible alternative. If bleeding should occur at the anastomosis between the left coronary ostium and the graft, as can also happen with the Bentall technique, then obtaining hemostasis by adding sutures to the anastomosis can be very difficult, since it is on the posterior aspect of the composite graft. Thus this technique has the potential for a higher operative mortality rate and increases the risk of uncontrolled bleeding at the anastomoses. On late follow-up, some surgeons report patients may develop left main coronary artery stenosis or calcification. Park and Maher[45] have described a technique of bringing the aortic button through the opening in the graft and then suturing the button in place so that it presses outward onto the composite graft from the pressure of arterial blood, thus decreasing the risk

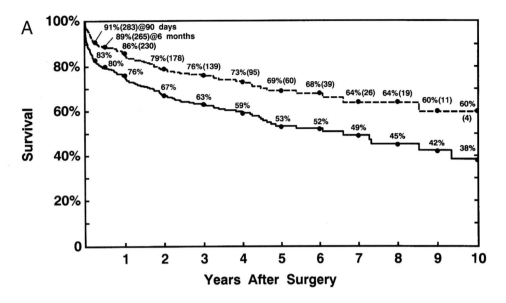

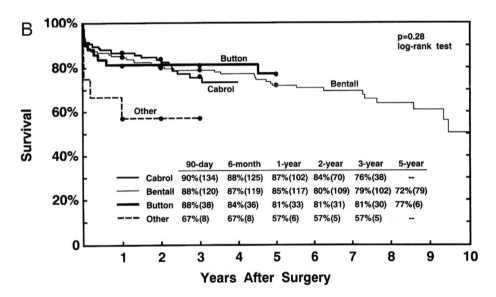

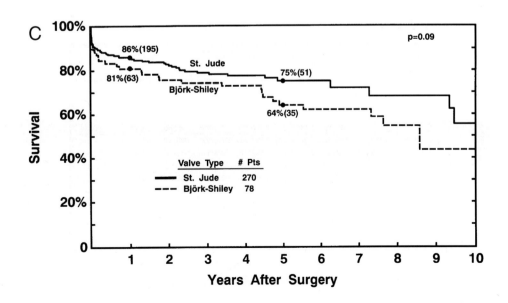

FIGURE 27-2 Kaplan-Meier analysis of late outcome after composite valve graft insertion in 348 patients. **A,** Overall survival *(broken line)* and event-free survival *(solid line)*: 30 fatal events, 50 nonfatal events, 59 nonevent deaths. **B,** 10-year survival by method of coronary ostia reattachment. **C,** 10-year survival by valve type used for the composite graft.

Illustration continued on following page

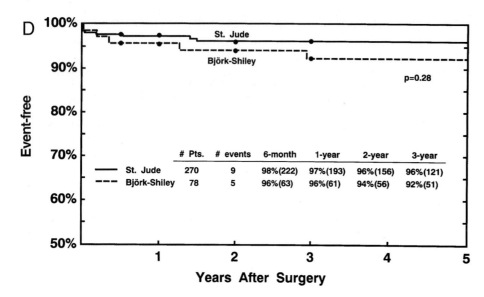

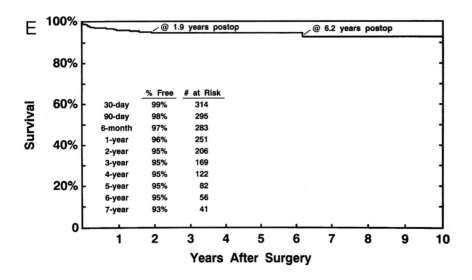

FIGURE 27-2 *Continued* Kaplan-Meier analysis of late outcome after composite valve graft insertion in 348 patients. **D,** 10-year freedom from permanent postoperative stroke by valve manufacturer. **E,** Overall 10-year freedom from reoperation: 15 reoperations in 348 patients. **F,** 10-year freedom from reoperation by method of coronary ostia reattachment. (Reprinted with permission from the Society of Thoracic Surgeons. From Svensson LG, Crawford ES, Hess KR, et al. Ann Thorac Surg;1992;54:427–39.)

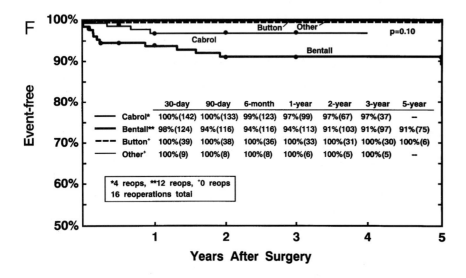

of bleeding. For the proximal anastomosis, Copeland and colleagues[46] have described placement of a second continuous row of sutures between the transected proximal aorta and the composite valve graft sewing ring to further improve hemostasis and reduce the risk of bleeding from around the aortic valve annulus. Nevertheless, the long-term results in patients who safely undergo repair by the button technique, whether for Marfan syndrome, aortic dissection, or medial degenerative disease, have been excellent,[1, 5, 14] with no patients in our experience requiring reoperation.[1, 5, 14, 20]

In an attempt to make the insertion of a composite graft easier, Cabrol and colleagues[23, 24] developed a technique whereby an interposition 10 mm tube graft was looped between the two coronary ostia and then the loop was attached to the ascending aortic composite valve graft by a side-to-side anastomosis. This approach also allowed easier access to the anastomoses for the purpose of obtaining hemostasis at the suture lines, including the aortic valve annulus and the coronary ostial anastomoses. The problem with this technique is that if the 10 mm intercoronary ostial tube graft loop is placed to the left of the ascending aortic graft, then the limb to the left coronary artery tends to kink. Similarly, with placement of the 10 mm tube graft to the right of the ascending aortic graft, the side-to-side anastomosis, which we prefer,[27] has to be placed high on the aortic graft and in a left anterolateral position so that the graft to the right coronary artery does not kink. Even when this is done, the left limb can kink from excessive tension over its long course at the tethered side-to-side anastomosis. Despite these modifications, the right limb can still be dysfunctional, or it can occlude because of both the angle at which the 10 mm tube graft to the right coronary artery ostium has to be performed or because the ostium has to be rotated through 90 degrees at the anastomosis. We have also noted on long-term follow-up that the limb to the right coronary artery can occlude.[14, 20]

Of 1108 patients who have undergone surgery on the ascending aorta or aortic arch, 348 had composite valve grafts inserted. We retrospectively analyzed our results with respect to the three techniques described above in 348 consecutive patients operated on between Sept. 17, 1979 and Jan. 29, 1991. Variables included aortic arch replacement in 88 (25%), necessity of deep hypothermia and circulatory arrest in 119 (34%), aortic dissection in 131 (38%), acute dissection in 34 (9.8%), reoperation in 79 (23%), and insertion of 270 (78%) St. Jude's prostheses. The 30-day survival rate was 91% (316/348), the in-hospital survival rate was 90% (312/348), and the 30-day postoperative incidence of new transient ($N = 6$) and permanent strokes ($N = 6$) was 3% (12/348). The respective 30-day survival rates for each method were Cabrol, 92% (144/157); Button, 91% (39/43); and Bentall, 91% (125/137). There was no difference in the operative mortality rate according to whether the aneurysmal sac was excised or wrapped around the composite valve graft to achieve hemostasis (excision 18/185 [10%] versus wrapping 14/163 [9%], $p = 0.71$). The mortality rate for the 112 patients who had Bentall repairs and wrapping was

10% (11/112) versus 4% (1/25) for those who did not have wrapping of the ascending aorta. None of the button repairs were performed with a wrap for obvious technical reasons. For the Cabrol repairs, the aneurysm sac was excised in 10% (11/106) and in the remaining patients it was loosely tacked or wrapped over the aortic prosthesis to protect it from the sternum, except in three patients in whom a Cabrol fistula to the right atrium was created.[20]

On univariate analysis, the following factors were associated with a higher mortality rate ($p < 0.05$): New York Heart Association (NYHA) classification for dyspnea symptoms, aneurysm symptom grade, presence of aortic dissection, atherosclerotic heart disease, aortic clamp time, cardiopulmonary bypass pump time, the need for concurrent coronary artery bypass, postoperative cardiac complications, renal complications, and stroke. On multivariate analysis, the independent predictors of death included ($p < 0.05$): NYHA classification for both dyspnea or angina, symptom grade severity, aortic dissection and acuity, concurrent distal aorta disease, atherosclerotic heart disease, aortic valve incompetence (reduced), pump time, cardioplegia (reduced), and postoperative cardiac complications or stroke. The causes of early (30-day) deaths are shown in Table 27–1. No significant difference in the cardiac causes of death, including myocardial infarction and ventricular arrhythmias, could be found between the different reattachment techniques.[20]

The incidence of new transient ($N = 6$) or permanent ($N = 6$) strokes within 30 days of surgery was 3% (12/348). On univariate analysis, the variables associated with stroke included ($p < 0.05$) heart failure, renal complications,

TABLE 27–1   CAUSES OF EARLY[32] AND LATE DEATH[57]: MORE THAN ONE CAUSE MAY APPLY

	Early	Late	Total
Arrhythmia	9	3	12
On cardiopulmonary bypass	7		7
Heart failure	9	6	15
Myocardial infarct	4	4	8
Sudden	1	3	4
Cardiac tamponade		1	1
Total cardiac	**30**	**17**	**47**
Stroke	4	6	10
Pulmonary	7	9	16
Renal	5	4	9
Rupture		7	7
Sepsis	2	5	7
Rupture anastomosis		6	6
Cancer		4	4
Hemorrhage	2	2	4
Hepatic	1	2	3
Unknown		3	3
Other	3	9	12

reoperation for bleeding, and the need for postoperative tracheostomy. The incidence of stroke decreased from 7% for the period from 1985 to 1986 to 1% for the period from 1989 to 1991 ($p = 0.18$, see multivariate model below). There was no significant difference according to the operative technique used to reattach the coronary ostia ($p = 0.44$). The independent predictors for the occurrence of postoperative stroke within 30 days of surgery were ($p < 0.05$) heart failure, history of cerebrovascular disease, concurrent mitral valve surgery, year of surgery, cardiac complications, renal complications, and reoperation because of bleeding. The use of cardioplegia was an independent predictor for a significantly reduced risk of stroke ($p = 0.0002$). Although the operative technique was not a predictor of the risk of stroke on multivariate analysis, on univariate analysis the risk was increased for patients undergoing Bentall repairs, button repairs, and other repairs when compared with Cabrol repairs ($p = 0.0001$). It is interesting to speculate whether the greater risk of loose atheromatous emboli may have been a factor. Nonetheless, when data were adjusted for the operation date, heart failure, presence of aortic valve incompetence and use of cardioplegia, there was no significant difference ($p = 0.44$) among the three repair methods.[20]

On late follow-up the Kaplan-Meier 5-year survival rate was 71% with no significant difference between the groups. Although the initial survival rate at 1 year was less for button repairs (81%, confidence interval [CI] 67%, 90%) than for Bentall repairs (85%, CI 78%, 90%) and for Cabrol repairs (87%, CI 80%, 92%), by 3 years after surgery, patients with button repairs had the best survival rate. At 3 years, 76% of patients undergoing Cabrol repairs were alive (95%, CI 63%, 86%), as were 79% with Bentall repairs (CI 71%, 85%), and 81% with button repairs (CI 66%, 90%). At 5 years, 72% of patients with Bentall repair and 77% of those with button repair were alive (Fig. 27–2B). The overall survival rate was 78% (175 patients) at 3 years, 71% (86) at 5 years, and 50% at 10 years; these figures include the 30-day operative deaths. The 5-year survival rate for patients in whom St. Jude's prostheses were inserted was 75% compared with 64% for those with Bjork-Shiley prostheses ($p = 0.09$); these figures also take into consideration operative deaths (Fig. 27–2C). The causes of the late deaths are shown in Table 27–1. Examination of the causes of death could not differentiate between the heart-associated causes of death according to type of operation. The incidence of myocardial infarction, ventricular arrhythmia, or sudden death for each repair type was as follows: Bentall, 11/125; button, 4/43; and Cabrol, 11/157. The Cabrol repairs, however, have the shortest follow-up.[20]

The 3-year freedom from reoperation was 95% (Cabrol, 97%; Bentall, 91%; button, 100%; $p = 0.1$). Reoperation was required in 12 patients with Bentall repairs, four patients with Cabrol repairs, and none with button repairs. The reasons for reoperation in the Cabrol repair group included occlusion of the right coronary artery in two patients and myocardial ischemia in one. The reasons for reoperations in

the Bentall group included six false aneurysms at the coronary anastomoses. Two of these six involved both the left and right coronary artery ostia; three involved the left and one the right coronary ostia. Four annular false aneurysms occurred, all in patients in whom the original operation was performed with a continuous 3-0 Prolene suture at the annulus. The predominant reasons for reoperation in three other patients included infection in one, right coronary occlusion in another, and false aneurysm arising from an unidentified source in the third. Of the Bentall reoperations, eight had involved wrapping of the aortic graft and four had not included wrapping of the aneurysmal wall around the composite graft. Of the latter four patients without wraps, three had some evidence of sepsis. One patient required a third operation to repair a recurrent false aneurysm of the proximal aorta. Comparison of the Kaplan-Meier curves by means of the log-rank test for the risk of reoperation revealed a tendency for the Bentall repairs to have a higher reoperation rate ($p = 0.1$, Fig. 27–2D), followed by Cabrol repairs. The comparison of the reoperation rate between button repairs and Bentall repairs yielded a value of $p = 0.069$ with the log-rank test. The overall freedom from reoperation was 95% (169 patients) at 3 years after surgery, 95% (82 patients) at 5 years, and 93% (4 patients) at 10 years (Fig. 27–2E).[20]

Late permanent strokes occurred in eight patients and transient strokes in six, for a total of 14 permanent strokes, including those strokes that occurred within 30 days of surgery. The Kaplan-Meier curves for permanent strokes according to type of valve inserted are shown in Figure 27–2F. At 5 years after surgery 96% of patients with St. Jude's valve prostheses were free of stroke events compared with 92% of those with the Bjork-Shiley prosthesis ($p = 0.28$). At 7 years after surgery, 95% of all patients were free of permanent strokes. The freedom from events (81 patients, 14 strokes, 43 hemorrhages, 16 reoperations, 3 emboli, 31 valve or prosthesis failures, including sepsis) and event-free survival at 5 years were 69% and 53%, respectively (Fig. 27–2A).[20]

In conclusion, despite the large sample size ($N = 348$) in this retrospective study, no strong statistical differences could be found. Nevertheless, we consider that the following important trends have occurred in our experience with the various techniques:

1. A continuous suture of the composite valve graft to the aortic annulus tends to disrupt.

2. The Bentall repair is prone to the development of false aneurysms at the coronary anastomoses.

3. Wrapping of the aortic graft after a Bentall procedure has a higher mortality rate and a greater risk of false aneurysm development, as has been reported by Kouchoukos et al.[38, 47] and others,[35] and by us in patients with Marfan syndrome or aortic dissection.[1, 5, 14] Nevertheless, complete excision of the aneurysm wall without loosely tacking it over the prostheses may increase the risk of late sepsis (valve endocarditis).

4. The button technique is more time consuming and difficult than a Bentall repair. It has a lower initial survival rate for the year after surgery, but thereafter has a better survival rate. No patients operated on by this technique required reoperation.

5. The Cabrol repairs are prone to intraoperative occlusion of the right coronary artery and, on late follow-up, to thrombosis of the right limb to the right coronary artery ostium. Nevertheless, this procedure has advantages over the other two in that no tension on the anastomoses occurs, all bleeding sites can be identified, the technique can be used for patients undergoing reoperation, complex repairs (including repair of aortic dissection involving the coronary ostia), and in our experience no patients required reoperation because of false aneurysms at the annulus or coronary ostia.

6. The St. Jude's prosthesis performs well as a composite valve graft prosthesis. Furthermore, with the collagen-impregnated tubular graft, baking the graft in albumin prior insertion is unnecessary and thus insertion is easier.

7. Patients in whom composite valve grafts are inserted, irrespective of operative technique, continue to be at risk of sepsis, late rupture developing beyond the repair, the onset of ventricular arrhythmias, and prosthetic valve-related events.[20]

On the basis of this retrospective study, we recommend that the button technique be used whenever feasible, with the Cabrol repair reserved for more complex lesions where tension on the ostial anastomoses may occur. If feasible, however, the button technique has better long-term results for both survival and rate of reoperation.[20]

An alternative to the above three methods involves the use of an interposition graft to reattach the left coronary artery and excision of an aortic button for reattachment of the right coronary artery. This latter technique has the advantage of technical ease in reattaching the left coronary artery, good results for reattachment of the right coronary artery, minimal tension on the anastomoses, and good visualization of all anastomoses.[21] In an ongoing prospective study we (L.G.S.) used this approach in operations on 46 patients. Thus far there have been no 30-day deaths or strokes, and only one patient (4%) of patients undergoing an elective repair has required an operative blood transfusion. None have required a reoperation on late follow-up. All patients had transesophageal echocardiography, transthoracic echocardiography, or angiography before discharge from the hospital; these showed no problems with the repairs, no false aneurysms, and preservation of myocardial function.

We also advise that after composite graft repairs all patients be evaluated every 6 months to 1 year by means of computerized tomography, magnetic resonance imaging, or transesophageal echocardiography to detect the development of any false aneurysms or progression of more distal disease; this is particularly important in patients with Marfan syndrome or aortic dissection.[5, 14] In addition to anticoagulation

with Coumadin, administration of beta-blockers on a long-term basis is recommended. Although selection bias and covariance may have influenced the results, we did find in a previous retrospective study that patients with aortic dissection, when placed on a regimen of beta-blockers, Coumadin, or aspirin, had a better long-term survival rate.[5] Similarly, DeBakey and colleagues[28] documented that the incidence of late aortic rupture in patients with aortic dissection was reduced when the patients' blood pressures were controlled. Patients should be aggressively treated with antibiotics for any infections or sites of sepsis, and prophylactic antibiotics should be prescribed before any invasive procedure. Unfortunately, despite the excellent valve performance of pulmonary autografts as reported by Ross and colleagues,[32] these repairs of the ascending aorta in young patients, like homograft repairs,[25, 26] are also still prone to the development of late sepsis, endocarditis, and calcification, although at a lower rate.[20, 25, 26, 32]

REPLACEMENT OF THE AORTA BY THE MODIFIED ELEPHANT TRUNK TECHNIQUE

The current technique of performing our modification of the elephant trunk procedure has made replacement of the aorta in patients with extensive aneurysmal disease considerably safer.[5, 13, 48] Among the 84 patients who underwent elephant trunk procedures, the survival rate for the first operation was 92% (76/84), with both of the two patients who had immediate repair of the descending aorta surviving.[2, 13, 48] Among the 56 patients who underwent second-stage operations, which were performed a median of 62 days later (range, 0 to 358 days), the survival rate was 96% for descending thoracic aorta repairs (20/21) and 97% (34/35) for thoracoabdominal repairs.[2, 5, 13, 48] Two of the initial deaths before 1988, when the technique was modified, were caused by rupture of the descending thoracic aorta at the distal suture line and two were the result of descending aortic aneurysm ruptures. The other deaths were due to stroke, multiple organ failure, and respiratory failure. The net result has been that nine patients have had staged repairs of the entire aorta, 27 of the entire thoracic aorta and upper abdominal aorta, and 22 of the entire thoracic aorta. One patient developed permanent paraplegia and two developed paraparesis after the initial operation; all of these had initially had very long elephant trunks inserted. Since a shorter elephant trunk (15 to 20 cm) came into use, however, this has not been a problem. The long-term survival analysis by Kaplan-Meier curves revealed an 82% 1-year and a 78% 2-year survival rate.[2, 5, 13, 15]

Heinemann and colleagues[49] reported on their experience with use of the elephant trunk technique at the aortic arch in 40 patients. Eight patients (20%) died in the early postoperative period, including all three who were operated on because of acute dissection; this supports our view that the elephant trunk technique should not be used for patients with acute dissection if possible. After a mean period of 9.6 months, 14 patients underwent second-stage repairs, with no operative deaths, and there were also no deaths in the three patients who had emergency second-stage repairs because of problems with distal perfusion related to the elephant trunk. The results are a tribute to the pioneering work of Borst and colleagues[50-52] for the safe repair of extensive aortic aneurysms, which continues to be the preferred technique for patients who can undergo staged repairs (see Chapters 17 and 18).

DESCENDING THORACIC AORTA

In an early report on 148 patients with descending thoracic aorta repairs for aneurysms between 1956 and 1980, the mortality rate had improved from 22% before 1967 to a 91% survival rate.[53] The improved survival rate was ascribed mainly to discontinuation of the use of either shunts or bypass for these operations. A more recent review of 832 patients revealed an overall survival rate of 92%, with an improvement to 98% after 1988. The mortality rate was significantly lower for patients who had atriofemoral bypass (4%) or none (9%) than for those who had cardiopulmonary bypass (11%, $p < 0.042$). Renal failure occurred in 7% (4% atriofemoral bypass, 8% none, and 11% with cardiopulmonary bypass, $p < 0.044$), paraplegia or paraparesis in 5% (2.3% were paraplegic), and strokes in 3%. On stepwise logistic regression analysis ($p < 0.05$), the predictors of death were increasing age, year of operation, extent repaired, cardiac complications, reoperation for bleeding, paraplegia or paraparesis, and postoperative dialysis. It should be noted that 5% ($N = 8$) of the patients died of acute postoperative dissection and 3% ($N = 2$) from ruptured anastomoses in the early period after surgery, and one early and three late deaths were due to aortoesophageal fistulae. The 5-year survival rate was 60% (Fig. 27-3).

Verdant,[54] in a 20-year experience, and Borst,[55] in a series of patients operated on between 1986 and 1992, have respectively reported 12% and 3% mortality rates with the use of passive shunts or atriofemoral bypass. Since the first report by DeBakey and Cooley[56] of a successful descending aortic repair with a prosthetic graft performed on Jan. 3, 1953, in the longest experience of 30 years reported by Lawrie and DeBakey[57] in 659 patients, the operative mortality rate was 24.2% and dropped to 14.3% after 1970. Lawrie and DeBakey[57] noted that the independent predictors of death during this study period were the aortic cross-clamp time, age, year of operation, acute dissection, concurrent ascending aortic aneurysm, rupture at presentation, and perioperative paraplegia. As discussed in Chapter 26, particularly noteworthy in this study was the increase in the incidence of paraparesis in the latter time period when distal aortic perfusion was not used, although the mortality rate was lower.

The operative techniques that we conclude have contributed to the improvement in the survival rate, particularly in those patients with aortic dissection, have been described earlier. We (L.G.S.) believe that atriofemoral bypass should be used whenever feasible, the intercostals should be reattached for repairs involving T7 to and including T12, and the proximal and distal anastomoses should be transected. Hypothermia is also of value while the aorta is cross-clamped. The postoperative complications of renal failure, respiratory failure, and paraplegia have been discussed in Chapter 26.[15]

THORACOABDOMINAL AORTA REPAIRS

Thoracoabdominal repairs continue to be challenging operations. In a series of 130 patients, Gilling-Smith et al.[58] reported a mortality rate of 42% for elective type II repairs, 73% for true ruptures, and 33% for contained or threatened ruptures.

Between 1960 and 1991 the senior author (E.S.C.) operated on 1509 patients who underwent 1679 thoracoabdominal aortic repairs.[59, 60] The extent of the repairs included 378

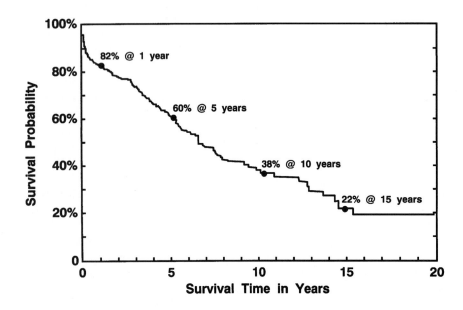

FIGURE 27-3 Kaplan-Meier curve of long-term survival after descending thoracic aortic repair. (From Svensson LG, Crawford ES, Hess, KR et al, Chest 1993;104:1248–53.).

(25%) for type I aneurysms (proximal descending to upper abdominal aorta); 442 (29%) type II (proximal descending thoracic aorta to below the renal arteries); 343 (23%) type III (distal descending thoracic aorta and abdominal aorta); and 346 (23%) type IV (most of the abdominal aorta). The median age was 66 years, aortic dissection was present in 276 (18%), and the median aortic cross-clamp time was 43 minutes. The 30-day survival rate over the 30-year period was 92% and the in-hospital survival rate was 90%. On stepwise logistic regression analysis, the significant predictors of death ($p < 0.05$) included increasing age, preoperative serum creatinine level, concurrent proximal aortic aneurysms, coronary artery disease, chronic pulmonary disease, and total aortic cross-clamp time. When postoperative events were also entered into the model, then cardiac complications, stroke, renal failure, and gastrointestinal complications also became significant factors. The incidence of paraplegia or paraparesis was 16% (234 patients). Renal failure occurred in 18% of the patients (creatinine > 3 mg/dl or dialysis), of whom 9% required dialysis. Gastrointestinal complications occurred in 7% of the patients. See Chapter 26 for

a further discussion of the complications. Figure 27–4 shows the Kaplan-Meier curves of cumulative survival.[60] In our presentation and discussion of this paper[60] in June, 1992, on thoracoabdominal aortic repairs, one of us (L.G.S.) reported improved results with cooling of the patient with atriofemoral bypass and sequential segmental repair of thoracoabdominal aortic aneurysms for lowering the risk of paraplegia and paraparesis. This was based on earlier animal research and studies in patients, particularly with the use of hydrogen testing, that showed improved spinal cord perfusion and a shorter period of spinal cord ischemia.[15, 61] Thus this is the technique that we currently advocate to improve results (see below and discussion in Chapters 12, 15, 19, 20, and 26).

In our prospective study regarding the influence of segmental arteries, the extent of repair, and the use of atriofemoral bypass on the risk of paraplegia after high-risk type I or II thoracoabdominal aneurysm repairs, the 30-day survival rate was 96%.[62] In this study the predictors on multivariate analysis of postoperative neurologic injury were ($p < 0.05$) increasing age and aortic cross-clamp time; however, the use of atriofemoral bypass was an independent

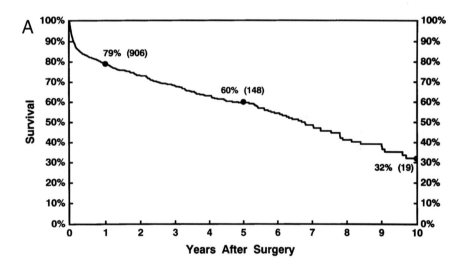

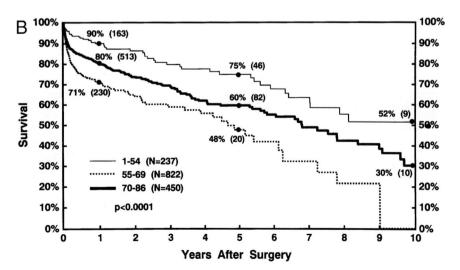

FIGURE 27-4   Survival in 1509 patients who underwent thoracoabdominal aortic repairs. **A,** Kaplan-Meier curve of long-term survival. **B,** Survival by age at the time of surgery.

Illustration continued on following page

predictor associated with a lower risk. Reattachment of arteries at T11 to L1 was associated with a lower risk. Our coauthors and former associates have also continued to report excellent results for thoracoabdominal aortic repairs. Coselli,[63] in a series of 372 patients undergoing thoracoabdominal aneurysm repairs, reported a 30-day survival rate of 95% and noted that the risk of neurological injury was reduced from 7.4% to 1.6% with the use of atriofemoral bypass. In a study of 45 patients with type I or II aneurysms, Safi et al.[64] reported a 96% survival rate and improved results when distal aortic perfusion was combined with cerebrospinal fluid drainage.

In the experience of one of us (L.G.S.) with 45 consecutive patients undergoing repairs of the descending aorta or the thoracoabdominal aorta, there have been two 30-day or in-hospital deaths (4.4%). In the last 2 years, including four patients undergoing replacement of the entire or nearly the entire aorta during one operation,[65] and nine with circulatory arrest, there was only one early death (3.3% mortality rate). The latter death was due to retrograde dissection and rupture of the ascending aorta on the third postoperative day. Two patients (7.7%) had permanent paraparesis after the operation. In one the paraparesis was due to intraoperative cardiopulmonary resuscitation for heart block and dysfunction for 15 minutes. The other patient had Marfan syndrome and underwent repair of a ruptured aortic arch dissection, which was done with deep hypothermic arrest; despite three attempts at reimplanting the intercostal arteries, the Carrel patch would tear each time and bleeding could not be controlled so that the arteries had to be oversewn.

Thoracoabdominal Aortic Aneurysms Associated With Visceral Artery Occlusive Disease

Of 1509 patients who underwent thoracoabdominal aortic repairs, we had 271 patients who had either celiac or superior mesenteric or renal artery occlusive disease.[59] These latter patients were treated with endarterectomy or bypass between June 20, 1960 and Jan. 10, 1991. After 1987 the 30-day survival rate was 93% (79/85) compared with 90% (245/271) before 1988. Multivariate predictors of death were ($p < 0.05$) age, postoperative reoperation because of

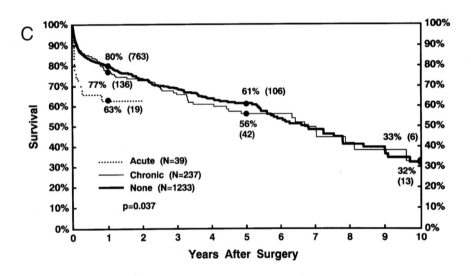

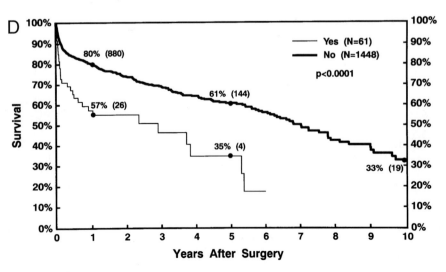

FIGURE 27-4 *Continued* Survival in 1509 patients who underwent thoracoabdominal aortic repairs. **C,** Survival by the presence or absence of aortic dissection and its acuity, if present. **D,** Survival by the presence or absence of preoperative aortic rupture. (From Svensson LG, Crawford ES, Hess KR, et al. J Vasc Surg 1993;17:357–70.)

bleeding, and cardiac complications. Renal complications (13% dialysis, 35/271) were associated with ($p < 0.05$) preoperative renal dysfunction, elevated preoperative serum creatinine level, urine clearance time of dye, extent of the aorta replaced, coagulopathy, and paraplegia or paraparesis. The incidence of postoperative renal dysfunction was reduced by ($p < 0.05$) renal artery endarterectomy. On univariate analysis ($p < 0.05$), the risk of renal failure was reduced by renal artery perfusion with cold Ringer's lactate solution. Gastrointestinal complications (9%, 25/271) were associated with ($p < 0.05$) a history of peptic ulcer disease on multivariate analysis. The Kaplan-Meier survival rates for patients with and without visceral occlusive disease were 53% and 60% at 5 years and 37% and 30%, respectively, at 10 years ($p = 0.08$).

We concluded from this study that (1) endarterectomy or bypass of occlusive visceral disease reduces the risk of renal failure after thoracoabdominal aortic aneurysm repairs, (2) it does not decrease early or late survival, (3) and it does not increase the risk of gastrointestinal complications. This study is also discussed in Chapter 9.[59]

ABDOMINAL AORTIC ANEURYSMS

In a previous review of our 920 consecutive patients undergoing infrarenal aortic repairs over a 25-year period, the operative mortality rate improved from 18% to 1.4%.[66] Risk factors for increased mortality included: atherosclerotic heart disease, heart failure, arrhythmias, peripheral vascular occlusive disease (including cerebrovascular disease), renal dysfunction, chronic lung disease, advanced age, hypertension, and morbid obesity.[66] At 5 years after surgery the survival rate by Kaplan-Meier analysis was 63%. Subsequent false aneurysms requiring reoperation occurred in 23 patients and graft erosion in 3 patients; 42 patients underwent subsequent coronary artery bypass. Sixty percent of the patients had tube grafts inserted without bifurcated limbs, and no patients subsequently needed surgery for iliac aneurysms. Reconstruction for distal occlusive disease was required, however, in 104 patients. Coselli and associates[67] have stressed the importance of long-term follow-up and surveillance of patients who have had abdominal aortic aneurysm repairs inasmuch as 3% to 8% will later develop a thoracic or thoracoabdominal aneurysm. In 123 patients with previous abdominal aortic aneurysm repairs (77 by the senior author [E.S.C.]), who required a subsequent repair at a mean interval of 8.2 years, 76.4% required a thoracoabdominal repair, 13.8% a juxtarenal repair, and 4.9% a descending thoracic aortic repair with 82% in continuity with the previously inserted graft. The operative mortality rate was 12.2%. Huber and colleagues,[68] in a study of elective abdominal aortic repairs, found that the predictors of death were age, history of myocardial infarction or heart failure, ejection fraction less than 50%, duration of operation, and additional operative procedures. O'Hara and colleagues[69] analyzed the results in 114 octogenarians who underwent abdominal

aortic aneurysm repairs. Bifurcation grafts were placed in 67%, and 25% had previously had coronary artery bypass operations. The overall 30-day mortality rate was 14% but declined to 8% during the last 5 years of the study. The 5-year survival rate was 48% compared with the 59% expected for the normal male population of the same age. However, it was 80% for patients who had previously undergone coronary artery bypass compared with 38% for those who had not ($p = 0.0077$). The predictors of a poorer long-term survival were perioperative homologous blood transfusion and a history of myocardial infarction. Symptomatic unruptured aneurysms have been reported by Sullivan and colleagues[70] to have a higher mortality rate (26%) and incidence of one or more of the following; myocardial infarction (21%), stroke (10%), respiratory failure (37%) and renal failure (31%). Bauer and colleagues,[71] in a series of 314 patients with ruptured abdominal aortic aneurysms, found a 29% mortality rate and reported that the predictors of death were duration of cross-clamp time, preoperative shock, suprarenal cross-clamping, history of coronary artery disease, as well as the postoperative complications of myocardial failure; renal failure; sepsis; and colon ischemia. Myocardial failure was associated with a history of coronary artery disease, volume of fluid given, suprarenal aorta clamping, and preoperative shock. The mortality rate for ruptured aortic aneurysms is reported to be as high as 70%.[72] In our own experience, the mortality rate has been 15% since 1980.[15, 73]

STATISTICAL ANALYSIS OF EARLY AND LATE SURVIVAL AFTER AORTIC DISSECTION REPAIR

The survival rate in patients following aortic dissection repair has improved to the extent that many centers have reported survival rates of greater than 90% for patients treated medically and surgically.[5, 19, 31, 38, 74–81] In fact, in our analysis of 690 patients, early survival was approximately 95% for patients undergoing aortic repairs irrespective of acuity or extent resected (Figs. 27–5 to 27–11).[5, 82] In our total experience of 844 patients with aortic dissection, the patients recently operated on continue to be operated on with a 95% survival rate. Nevertheless, acute dissection can be formidable and challenging to manage, particularly when the patients present in the emergency room with cardiac tamponade or shock, often comatose, and requiring emergency surgery.[5, 83]

In our series of 844 patients with aortic dissection, 188 had acute dissection; of these, 86 had type I, 20 had type II, and 82 had type III. Of the 656 patients with chronic dissection, 291 had type I, 77 had type II, and 288 had type III. Thus a total of 380 patients have had proximal repairs and 464 have had distal repairs, with an overall operative survival rate over a 33-year period of 91% and a 5-year survival rate of 57%, including operative deaths.[5, 83]

In a previous study of 690 patients, the independent determinants of early survival were obtained by stepwise logistic regression analysis.[5] The independent determinants of survival in all 690 patients who underwent surgery over a 33-year period ($p < 0.05$) were surgery before 1987, grade of aneurysm symptoms, history of atherosclerotic heart disease, diabetes mellitus, reoperation because of bleeding, cardiac complications, and postoperative stroke. Profound hypothermia with circulatory arrest has not been found to be a risk factor and, in fact, has contributed to a decline in the risk of postoperative stroke, which was permanent in only 1% of patients recently operated on. Notably, in those patients who have undergone surgery recently for both proximal aortic dissection (after 1985) and for distal aortic dissection (since 1983), the independent determinants included aneurysm symptom grade and cardiac complications. On examination of the risk factors according to extent and acuity over the entire 33-year period, the independent determinants for acute proximal dissection have been surgery before 1986, surgery within 1 day of dissection, repair of the ascending aorta and arch, postoperative balloon counterpulsation, and cardiac complications. In patients with distal acute dissection the independent risk factors were surgery before 1984, surgery within 1 day of dissection, and presence of chronic pulmonary disease. In patients with chronic proximal dissection the independent determinants were aneurysm symptom grade, atherosclerotic heart disease, previous aortic surgery, balloon pumping, cardiac complications, and postoperative stroke. Similarly, in patients undergoing chronic distal aortic dissection repairs the determinants were surgery before 1984, aneurysm symptom grade, and cardiac complications. These data suggest to us, as has also been shown by the Stanford group[77, 79] and reported by Rizzo and colleagues,[80] that the further reduction in operative mortality rate is dependent on both the earlier detection of aortic dissection by noninvasive measures and the referral of patients for surgery before the development of severe symptoms and complications related to aortic dissection.

Whether patients should have coronary artery arteriography before repair of acute aortic dissection of the proximal aorta is controversial,[80, 84] and we believe that it should be used selectively only in hemodynamically stable patients with no evidence of cardiac tamponade. The treatment of intraoperative hematoma is also controversial.[85-87] At the time of surgery, a tear is often found that has not been imaged by current techniques such as angiography, transesophageal cardiography (TEE), magnetic resonance imaging (MRI), and computed tomography (CT). The reason for this is that the clot in the false lumen ("intramural hematoma") has also sealed the entry site, and therefore flow outside the lumen is not seen, there is no oscillation of the septum, and the tear site is not seen. The other variant that we have noted (see illustrations in Chapters 4 and 18) is where the aortic intima and some of the media has torn but there is no undermining of the intima and, therefore, a septum is not seen. In two recent patients we have operated upon (L.G.S.) preoperative TEE, CT scan, and in one case angiography had failed to detect the limited dissection.

Our view is that many of the intramural hematomas will become classic dissections. We recommend surgery for proximal involvement and medical management initially for distal intramural hematomas unless a penetrating ulcer is present, in which case an emergency operation should be considered (see also Chapters 9, 18, and 20).[5, 83]

The Stanford group updated their results over a 30-year period in 360 patients.[81] Of the series, 174 had acute type A dissections (proximal dissections), 46 had acute type B dissections (distal dissections), 106 had chronic type A dissections, and 34 had chronic type B dissections. The respective operative mortality rates were 26%, 39%, 17%, and 15%. The respective mortality rates for the 1988 to 1992 time interval were 27%, 20%, 15%, and 17%. However, for acute dissection repairs during this time interval, if preoperative dissection complications (aortic rupture, cardiac tamponade, visceral ischemia, renal dysfunction, congestive heart failure, and shock) were not present, the mortality rate was 9%, emphasizing the effect of preoperative status on surgical outcome and results. The Stanford group also believes that a change in referral patterns may have resulted in their not maintaining the better result for all patients they had between 1977 and 1982, with a 7% mortality rate for acute proximal dissections and 13% for acute distal dissections. The stroke rates for acute and chronic proximal repairs were 4% and 3%, respectively. The aortic arch was replaced in only eight patients with acute proximal dissections, 10 with chronic proximal dissections, four with acute distal dissections, and one with chronic distal dissection. The paraplegia/paraparesis rate for acute and chronic distal repairs is not reported. The independent predictors of early death were earlier operative year, hypertension, cardiac tamponade, renal dysfunction, and older age. The respective 5-year survival rates were 55%, 48%, 65%, and 59% (p = ns). The independent predictors of late death were older age and previous operations. Freedom from reoperation in this updated series was 84% at 5 years.

Postoperative paraplegia (9%) or paraparesis (8%) in the 368 patients who underwent distal aorta surgery by us[5] was determined by the following independent factors ($p < 0.05$): aortic cross-clamp time, aneurysm grade of symptoms, hypertension, and extent replaced. The effect of cross-clamp time (Fig. 27-5B), and the influence of extent of replacement (Fig. 27-5B) probably are due to both the degree of ischemia and the loss of critical arteries that supply the spinal cord. Symptoms are likely due to perioperative hemodynamic instability, rupture, and insufficient time for adequate collaterals to develop. The effect of hypertension on the risk of spinal-cord injury is difficult to pinpoint but possibly may be similar to its effect on the brain, which is more prone to stroke in the presence of hypertension.[5, 83]

Preoperative and operative factors for both proximal and distal dissection were examined for their influence on late survival. Kaplan-Meier curves of patient survival are shown in Figure 27-5 C and D.[5] The independent determinants included the date of surgery, aneurysm symptoms, New York Heart Association grade of angina and dyspnea, the extent of aorta replacement, the type of operative procedure, postoperative complications, and residual aneurysms not removed from other segments. The latter point is stressed by the fact that the most important independent determinant for late rupture was the presence of residual aortic aneurysmal disease. Thus all aneurysmal segments of aortic dissection should be resected to reduce the risk of late death due to rupture. By aggressive surgical replacement, rupture as a cause of late death has been reduced from 30%[28] to 10% in the patients operated on since 1985.[5] At 5 years after surgery 9% of our patients required reoperation, and after 10 years 22% required reoperation. The corresponding results from Stanford[77, 78] were similar, namely, 13% at 5 years and 23% at 10 years. In the more recent, updated Stanford series the 5-year reoperation rate was 16%.[81] Once again, this stresses the importance of follow-up in these patients.[5, 83]

The influence of various factors on long-term survival can be seen in the illustrative Kaplan-Meier curves (Fig. 27–5 *C* and *D* and Fig. 27–8). For patients with proximal dissection, the 3-year survival rate, including operative deaths, is 87% for ascending aorta repairs and 72% for repairs that include the aortic arch. Similarly, for distal repairs, including operative deaths, the 5-year survival was 82% for the proximal part of the descending aorta repairs but was strongly influenced by extent replaced and associated risk factors. Approximately a 75% 5-year survival rate, including operative deaths, can be expected for patients who undergo surgery. Nevertheless, this is an oversimplification, as survival is affected by many factors.[5, 83]

Doroghazi and colleagues[88] from Massachusetts General Hospital reported a 76% 5-year survival rate for patients discharged from the hospital, irrespective of extent repaired. Similarly, Miller and colleagues[77, 78] reported a 72% 5-year

FIGURE 27-5 Analysis of outcomes for 690 patients undergoing aortic dissection repairs. **A,** 30-day survival by acuity and site of operation. ASC ± Arch = ascending aorta or aortic arch or both. DESC = descending thoracic. TAA = thoracoabdominal aorta. **B,** Risk of neurologic injury (paraplegia/paresis) by extent of repair and aortic cross-clamp time. I, II, III, IV = Crawford classification of extent of repair.

Illustration continued on following page

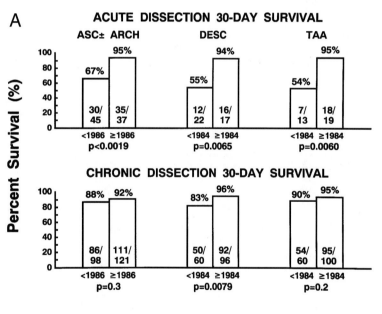

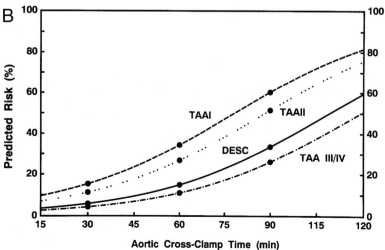

survival rate for patients discharged from the hospital. It can be expected that, with better techniques in postoperative care, these results will continue to improve. Thus, in a study by Glower and associates,[89] an 80% 5-year survival rate was noted for a selected group of patients undergoing surgical repair of uncomplicated descending aortic dissections. Nienaber and Kodolitsch[90] performed a meta-analysis of the world literature and came to the conclusion that, for a better long-term prognosis, both acute and chronic proximal dissections and chronic distal dissections should be treated surgically. The results tended to favor initial medical management, although the advantage was not as clear cut.[5, 83]

Of note, of our 22 patients who underwent elephant trunk repairs for aortic dissection, only one patient (5%) died.[5] Furthermore, of the entire series of 443 current survivors after aortic dissection repairs, 82% remain in either New York Heart Association functional class I or II.[5, 83]

In our more recent (L.G.S.) experience with aortic dissection repairs in 39 patients, with 19 for acute dissection, there have been no postoperative deaths or strokes, although the series is small in comparison with the series discussed above.

MARFAN SYNDROME

In patients with Marfan syndrome the results of surgery have continued to improve since our report on 151 patients.[14] However, as we and others have noted previously, the early and late survival rates are strongly influenced by whether preoperative aortic dissection is present (see Chapter 5).[14, 91, 92] The early survival rate has continued to improve and has been a large contributor to the better overall survival rate, so that in our experiences (L.G.S.) there

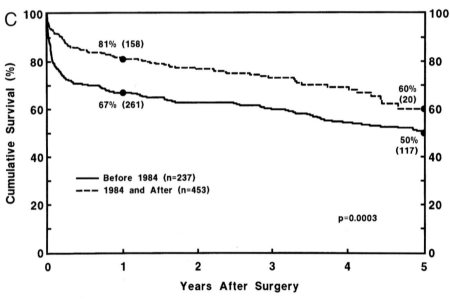

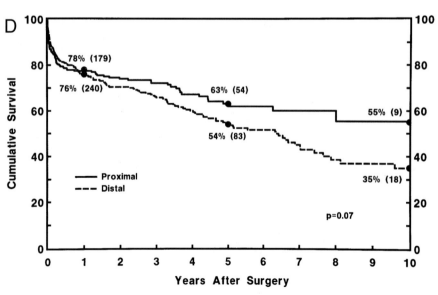

FIGURE 27-5 *Continued* Analysis of outcomes for 690 patients undergoing aortic dissection repairs. **C,** Overall survival by operative period. **D,** Survival by surgical approach (proximal [310] or distal [389]). (From Svensson LG, Crawford ES, Hess KR, et al. Dissection of the aorta and dissecting aortic aneurysms: improving early and long-term surgical results. Circulation 1990:82(5 supp): IV24–38. Reprinted with permission. Copyright 1990 American Heart Association.)

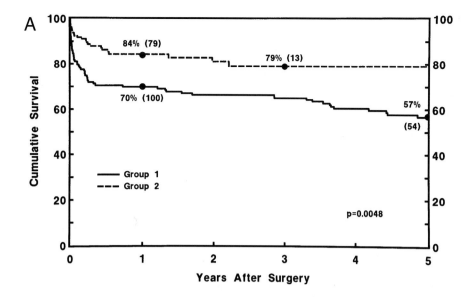

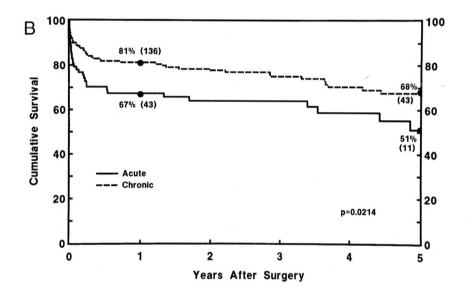

FIGURE 27-6 Survival for proximal aortic dissection. **A,** Survival by operative period (143 before 1986; 158 during 1986 and later). **B,** Survival by acuity for repairs (82 acute; 219 chronic). **C,** Survival by operative procedure (120 composite valve grafts [CVG], 46 separate valve grafts [SVG], 124 alone [GFT], 11 other procedures [OTH] such as aortoplasty).

Illustration continued on following page

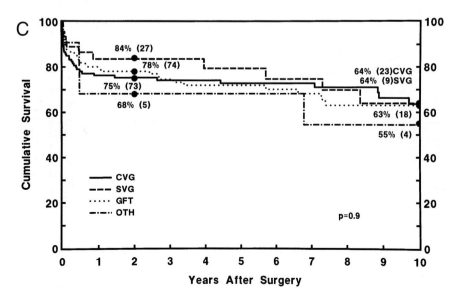

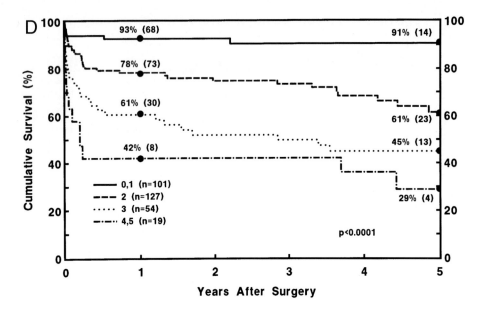

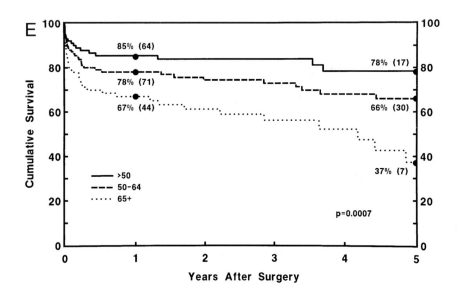

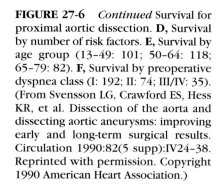

FIGURE 27-6 *Continued* Survival for proximal aortic dissection. **D,** Survival by number of risk factors. **E,** Survival by age group (13–49: 101; 50–64: 118; 65–79: 82). **F,** Survival by preoperative dyspnea class (I: 192; II: 74; III/IV: 35). (From Svensson LG, Crawford ES, Hess KR, et al. Dissection of the aorta and dissecting aortic aneurysms: improving early and long-term surgical results. Circulation 1990:82(5 supp):IV24–38. Reprinted with permission. Copyright 1990 American Heart Association.)

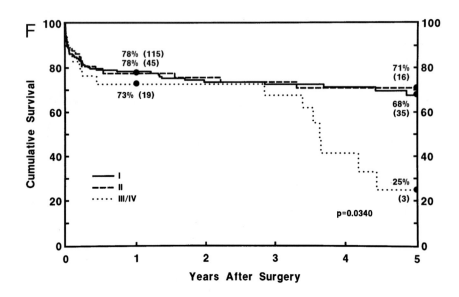

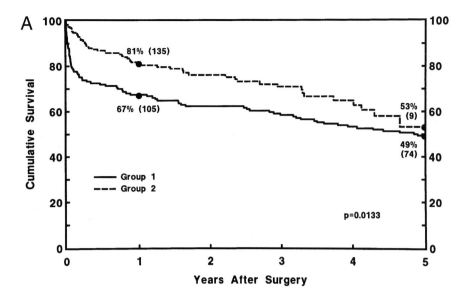

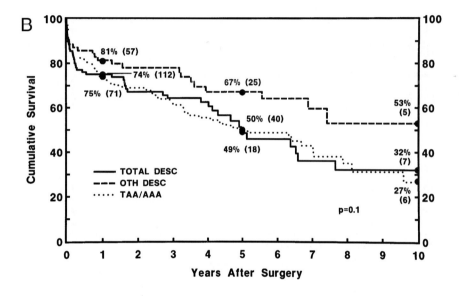

FIGURE 27-7 Survival for distal aortic dissection. **A,** Survival by operative period (157 before 1984; 232 during 1984 and later). **B,** Survival by operative procedure (117 total descending thoracic [DESC], 78 other descending aortic repairs less than total replacement [OTH DESC], 194 thoracoabdominal or abdominal aortic repairs [TAA/AAA]). **C,** Survival by number of risk factors.

Illustration continued on following page

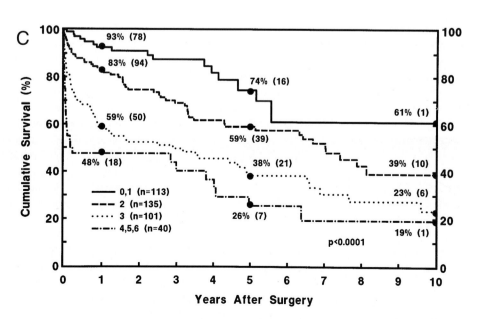

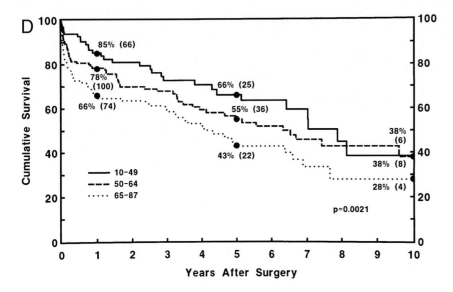

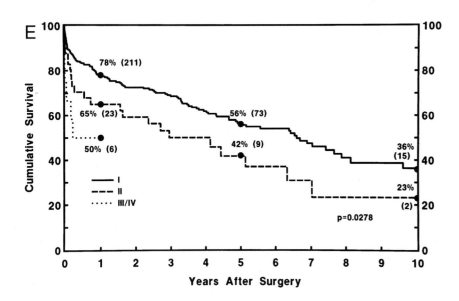

FIGURE 27-7 *Continued* Survival for distal aortic dissection. **D,** Survival by age group (10–49: 99; 50–64: 150; 65–87: 140). **E,** Survival by preoperative dyspnea class (I: 336; II: 41; III/IV: 12). (From Svensson LG, Crawford ES, Hess KR, et al. Dissection of the aorta and dissecting aortic aneurysms: improving early and long-term surgical results. Circulation 1990:82(5 supp):IV24–38. Reprinted with permission. Copyright 1990 American Heart Association.)

have been no early or late deaths after surgery. Coselli and colleagues[91] have reported a 98.7% 30-day survival rate and a 96.2% late survival rate. Currently, the average age at death has changed from 32 years to the eighth decade of life, with a median cumulative survival probability of 72 years.[93, 94] For surgically treated patients, a 70% or better 10-year survival can be expected, depending on whether aortic dissection is present or not.

PERCUTANEOUS AND ENDOVASCULAR METHODS OF MANAGEMENT

In 1964 Dotter and Judkins[95] and in 1969 Dotter[96] described treatment of atherosclerotic stenoses with balloon dilatation and also with tube endarterial grafts. Weibull and colleagues[97] reported a prospective randomized study of 58

patients in whom percutaneous transluminal renal angioplasty was successful in 83% of the patients with atherosclerotic renal artery stenosis and in 97% of the patients on whom operations were performed. Hypertension was cured or improved in 90% of the angioplasty patients and 86% of the patients who underwent operations. The respective incidence of improved or unchanged renal function was 83% and 72%. Seventeen percent of angioplasty patients required later operation. Weibull and colleagues concluded that initial angioplasty is acceptable therapy if combined with careful follow-up and aggressive reintervention. We have used percutaneous techniques to reperfuse the renal arteries after acute dissection or to reestablish blood flow to ischemic lower limbs, with either balloon angioplasty or stenting.[98] Since 1991 Parodi and colleagues[99, 100] have been placing endovascular stented grafts in patients. In a series of 57 patients (50 with abdominal or iliac aneurysms), this treatment was successful in 40 and secondary treatment was

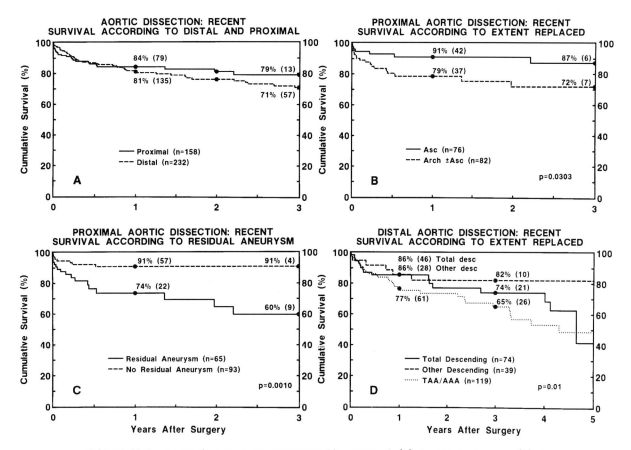

FIGURE 27-8 Aortic dissection. Recent survival by approach **(A)**, by proximal extent **(B)**, by proximal residual aneurysm **(C)**, and by distal extent **(D)**. (From Svensson LG, Crawford ES, Hess KR, et al. Dissection of the aorta and dissecting aortic aneurysms: improving early and long-term surgical results. Circulation 1990:82(5 supp):IV24–38. Reprinted with permission. Copyright 1990 American Heart Association.)

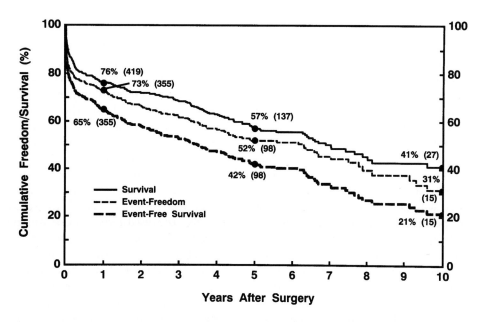

FIGURE 27-9 Aortic dissection. Overall survival and freedom from major postoperative events. (From Svensson LG, Crawford ES, Hess KR, et al. Dissection of the aorta and dissecting aortic aneurysms: improving early and long-term surgical results. Circulation 1990:82(5 supp):IV24–38. Reprinted with permission. Copyright 1990 American Heart Association.)

29. Donaldson RM, Ross DN. Composite graft replacement for the treatment of aneurysms of the ascending aorta associated with aortic valvular disease. Circulation 1982;66(Supp 1):116–21.

30. Edwards WS, Kerr AR. A safer technique for replacement of the entire ascending aorta and aortic valve. J Thorac Cardiovasc Surg 1970;59:837–9.

31. Galloway AC, Colvin SB, LaMendola CL, et al. Ten-year operative experience with 165 aneurysms of the ascending aorta and aortic arch. Circulation 1989;80(supp I):I-249–56.

32. Gerosa G, McKay R, Ross DN. Replacement of the aortic valve or root with a pulmonary autograft in children. Ann Thorac Surg 1991; 51:424–9.

33. Gott VL, Pyeritz RE, Cameron DE, et al. Composite graft repair of Marfan aneurysm of the ascending aorta: results in 100 patients. Ann Thorac Surg 1991;52:38–44.

34. Grey DP, Ott DA, Cooley DA. Surgical treatment of aneurysms of the ascending aorta with aortic insufficiency. J Thorac Cardiovasc Surg 1983;86:864–77.

35. Helseth HK, Haglin JJ, Monson BK, Wichstrom PH. Results of composite graft replacement for aortic root aneurysms. J Thorac Cardiovasc Surg 1980;80:754–9.

36. Jex RK, Schaff HG, Piehler JM, et al. Repair of ascending aortic dissection: influence of associated aortic valve insufficiency on early and late results. J Thorac Cardiovasc Surg 1987;93:375–84.

37. Kouchoukos NT, Karp RB, Blackstone EH, et al. Replacement of the ascending aorta and aortic valve with a composite graft: results in 86 patients. Ann Surg 1980;192:403–12.

38. Kouchoukos NT, Marshall WG Jr, Wedige STA. Eleven-year experience with composite graft replacement of the ascending aorta and aortic valve. J Thorac Cardiovasc Surg 1986;92:691–705.

39. Lewis CT, Cooley DA, Murphy MC, et al. Surgical repair of aortic root aneurysms in 280 patients. Ann Thorac Surg 1992;53:38–45.

40. Lytle BW, Mahfood SS, Cosgrove DM, Loop FD. Replacement of the ascending aorta: early and late results. J Thorac Cardiovasc Surg 1990;99:651–7.

41. Miller DC, Stinson EB, Oyer PE, et al. Concomitant resection of ascending aortic aneurysms and replacement of the ascending aortic valve: operative and long-term results with "conventional" techniques in ninety patients. J Thorac Cardiovasc Surg 1980;79:388–401.

42. Najafi H. Aneurysm of cystic medionecrotic root: a modified surgical approach. J Cardiovasc Surg 1973;66:71–4.

43. Cabrol C, Pavie A, Gandjbakhch I, et al. Complete replacement of the ascending aorta with reimplantation of the coronary arteries: new surgical approach. J Thorac Cardiovasc Surg 1981;81:309–15.

44. Rosero H, Nathan PE, Rodney E, et al. Aorta to right atrium fistula with congestive heart failure resulting from a patent Cabrol shunt after repair of aortic dissection. Am Heart J 1994;128:608–9.

45. Park SB, Maher TD Jr. Modification of the aortic composite graft using the button-in technique. Ann Thorac Surg 1994;57:1035–7.

46. Copeland JG III, Rosado LJ, Snyder SL. New technique for improving hemostasis in aortic root replacement with composite graft. Ann Thorac Surg 1993;55:1027–9.

47. Kouchoukos NT, Wareing TH, Murphy SF, Perrillo JB. Sixteen-year experience with aortic root replacement: results of 172 operations. Ann Surg 1991;214:308–18.

48. Svensson LG. Rationale and technique for replacement of the ascending aorta, arch, and distal aorta using a modified elephant trunk procedure. J Cardiac Surg 1992;7:301–12.

49. Heinemann MK, Buehner B, Jurmann MJ, Borst H-G. Use of the "elephant trunk technique" in aortic surgery. Ann Thorac Surg 1995; 60:2–7.

50. Borst HG, Schaudig A, Rudolph W. Arteriovenous fistula of the aortic arch: repair during deep hypothermia and circulatory arrest. J Thorac Cardiovasc Surg 1964;48:443–7.

51. Borst HG, Walterbusch G, Schaps D. Extensive aortic replacement using "elephant trunk" prosthesis. Thorac Cardiovasc Surg 1983; 31:37–40.

52. Borst HG, Frank G, Schaps D. Treatment of extensive aortic aneurysms by a new multiple-stage approach. J Thorac Cardiovasc Surg 1988;95:11–3.

53. Crawford ES, Walker HJ, Saleh SA, Normann NA. Graft replacement of aneurysm in descending thoracic aorta: results without bypass or shunting. Surgery 1981;89:73–85.

54. Verdant A, Cossette R, Page A, et al. Aneurysms of the descending thoracic aorta: three hundred sixty-six consecutive cases resected without paraplegia. J Vasc Surg 1995;21:385–91.

55. Borst HG, Jurmann M, Buhner B, Laas J. Risk of replacement of descending aorta with a standardized left heart bypass technique. J Thorac Cardiovasc Surg 1994;107:126–33.

56. DeBakey ME, Cooley DA. Successful resection of aneurysm of thoracic aorta and replacement by graft. JAMA 1953;152:673–6.

57. Lawrie GM, Earle N, DeBakey ME. Evolution of surgical techniques for aneurysms of the descending thoracic aorta: twenty-nine years experience with 659 patients. J Cardiac Surg 1994;9:648–61.

58. Gilling-Smith GL, Worswick L, Knight PF, et al. Surgical repair of thoracoabdominal aortic aneurysm: 10 years' experience. Br J Surg 1995;82:624–9.

59. Svensson LG, Crawford ES, Hess KR, et al. Thoracoabdominal aortic aneurysms associated with celiac, superior mesenteric and renal artery occlusive disease: methods and analysis of results in 271 patients. J Vasc Surg 1992;16:378–90.

60. Svensson LG, Crawford ES, Hess KR, et al. Experience with 1509 patients undergoing thoracoabdominal aortic operations. J Vasc Surg 1993;17:357–70.

61. Svensson LG, Patel V, Robinson MF, et al. Influence of preservation or perfusion of intraoperatively identified spinal cord blood supply on spinal motor evoked potentials and paraplegia after aortic surgery. J Vasc Surg 1991;13:355–65.

62. Svensson LG, Hess KR, Coselli JS, Safi HR. Influence of segmental arteries, extent, and atrio-femoral bypass on postoperative paraplegia after thoracoabdominal aortic aneurysm repairs. J Vasc Surg 1994;20:255–62.

63. Coselli JS. Thoracoabdominal aortic aneurysms: experience with 372. J Cardiac Surg 1994;9:638–47.

64. Safi HJ, Bartoli S, Hess KR, et al. Neurologic deficit in patients at high risk with thoracoabdominal aortic aneurysms: the role of cerebral spinal fluid drainage and distal aortic perfusion. J Vasc Surg 1994;20:434–43.

65. Svensson LG, Shahian DM, Davis FG, et al. Replacement of entire aorta from aortic valve to bifurcation during one operation. Ann Thorac Surg 1994;58:1164–6.

66. Crawford ES, Saleh SA, Babb JW, et al. Infrarenal abdominal aortic aneurysm: factors influencing survival after operation performed over a 25-year period. Ann Surg 1981;193:699–709.

67. Coselli JS, LeMaire SA, Buket S, Berzin E. Subsequent proximal aortic operations in 123 patients with previous infrarenal abdominal aortic aneurysm surgery. J Vasc Surg 1995;22:59–67.

68. Huber TS, Harward TRS, Flynn TC, et al. Operative mortality rates after elective infrarenal aortic reconstructions. J Vasc Surg 1995;22: 287–94.

69. O'Hara PJ, Hertzer NR, Krajewski LP, et al. Ten-year experience with abdominal aortic aneurysm repair in octogenarians: early results and late outcome. J Vasc Surg 1995;21:830–8.

70. Sullivan CA, Rohrer MJ, Cutler BS. Clinical management of the symptomatic but unruptured abdominal aortic aneurysm. J Vasc Surg 1990;11:799–803.

71. Bauer EP, Redaelli C, von Segresser LK, Turina MI. Ruptured abdominal aortic aneurysms: predictors for early complications and death. Surgery 1993;114:31–5.

72. Johansen K, Kohler TR, Nicholls SC, et al. Ruptured abdominal aortic aneurysm: the Harborview experience. J Vasc Surg 1991;13: 240–5.

73. Crawford ES. Ruptured abdominal aortic aneurysm [editorial]. J Vasc Surg 1991;13:348–50.

74. Crawford ES, Svensson LG, Coselli JS, et al. Aortic dissection and dissecting aortic aneurysms. Ann Surg 1988;108:254–73.

75. Ergin MA, Galla JD, Lansman S, et al. Acute dissection of the aorta: current surgical treatment. Surg Clin North Am 1985;65:721–41.

76. Gott VL, Pyeritz RE, Magovern GJ Jr, et al. Surgical treatment of aneurysms of the ascending aorta in the Marfan syndrome. N Engl J Med 1986;314:1070–4.

77. Haverich A, Miller DC, Scott WC, et al. Acute and chronic aortic dissections: determinants of long-term outcome for operative survivors. Circulation 1985;72(Supp II):II-22–34.

78. Miller DC. Surgical management of aortic dissections: indications, perioperative management, and long-term results. In: Doroghazi RM, Slater EE, eds. Aortic Dissection. New York: McGraw-Hill, 1983: 193–243.

79. Miller DC, Mitchell RS, Oyer PE, et al. Independent determinants of operative mortality for patients with aortic dissections. Circulation 1984;70(Supp I):I-153–64.

80. Rizzo RJ, Aranki SF, Aklog L, et al. Rapid noninvasive diagnosis and

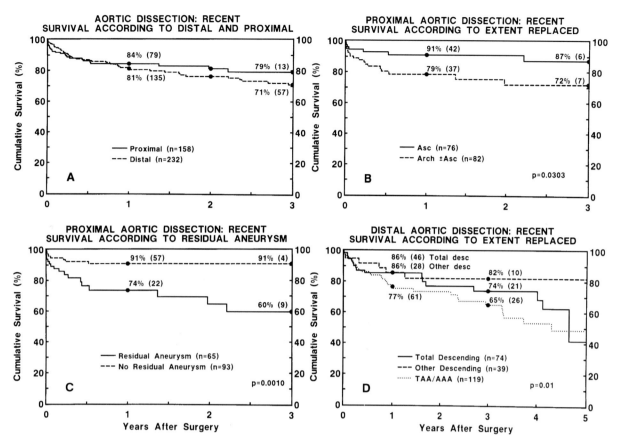

FIGURE 27-8   Aortic dissection. Recent survival by approach **(A)**, by proximal extent **(B)**, by proximal residual aneurysm **(C)**, and by distal extent **(D)**. (From Svensson LG, Crawford ES, Hess KR, et al. Dissection of the aorta and dissecting aortic aneurysms: improving early and long-term surgical results. Circulation 1990:82(5 supp):IV24–38. Reprinted with permission. Copyright 1990 American Heart Association.)

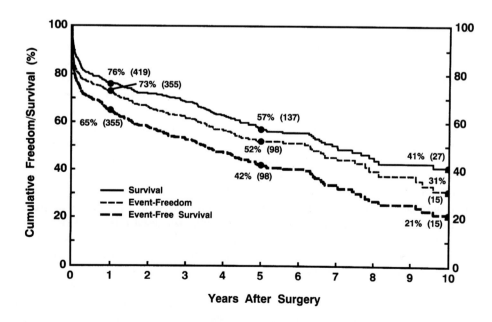

FIGURE 27-9   Aortic dissection. Overall survival and freedom from major postoperative events. (From Svensson LG, Crawford ES, Hess KR, et al. Dissection of the aorta and dissecting aortic aneurysms: improving early and long-term surgical results. Circulation 1990:82(5 supp):IV24–38. Reprinted with permission. Copyright 1990 American Heart Association.)

29. Donaldson RM, Ross DN. Composite graft replacement for the treatment of aneurysms of the ascending aorta associated with aortic valvular disease. Circulation 1982;66(Supp 1):116-21.

30. Edwards WS, Kerr AR. A safer technique for replacement of the entire ascending aorta and aortic valve. J Thorac Cardiovasc Surg 1970;59:837-9.

31. Galloway AC, Colvin SB, LaMendola CL, et al. Ten-year operative experience with 165 aneurysms of the ascending aorta and aortic arch. Circulation 1989;80(supp I):I-249-56.

32. Gerosa G, McKay R, Ross DN. Replacement of the aortic valve or root with a pulmonary autograft in children. Ann Thorac Surg 1991;51:424-9.

33. Gott VL, Pyeritz RE, Cameron DE, et al. Composite graft repair of Marfan aneurysm of the ascending aorta: results in 100 patients. Ann Thorac Surg 1991;52:38-44.

34. Grey DP, Ott DA, Cooley DA. Surgical treatment of aneurysms of the ascending aorta with aortic insufficiency. J Thorac Cardiovasc Surg 1983;86:864-77.

35. Helseth HK, Haglin JJ, Monson BK, Wichstrom PH. Results of composite graft replacement for aortic root aneurysms. J Thorac Cardiovasc Surg 1980;80:754-9.

36. Jex RK, Schaff HG, Piehler JM, et al. Repair of ascending aortic dissection: influence of associated aortic valve insufficiency on early and late results. J Thorac Cardiovasc Surg 1987;93:375-84.

37. Kouchoukos NT, Karp RB, Blackstone EH, et al. Replacement of the ascending aorta and aortic valve with a composite graft: results in 86 patients. Ann Surg 1980;192:403-12.

38. Kouchoukos NT, Marshall WG Jr, Wedige STA. Eleven-year experience with composite graft replacement of the ascending aorta and aortic valve. J Thorac Cardiovasc Surg 1986;92:691-705.

39. Lewis CT, Cooley DA, Murphy MC, et al. Surgical repair of aortic root aneurysms in 280 patients. Ann Thorac Surg 1992;53:38-45.

40. Lytle BW, Mahfood SS, Cosgrove DM, Loop FD. Replacement of the ascending aorta: early and late results. J Thorac Cardiovasc Surg 1990;99:651-7.

41. Miller DC, Stinson EB, Oyer PE, et al. Concomitant resection of ascending aortic aneurysms and replacement of the ascending aortic valve: operative and long-term results with "conventional" techniques in ninety patients. J Thorac Cardiovasc Surg 1980;79:388-401.

42. Najafi H. Aneurysm of cystic medionecrotic root: a modified surgical approach. J Cardiovasc Surg 1973;66:71-4.

43. Cabrol C, Pavie A, Gandjbakhch I, et al. Complete replacement of the ascending aorta with reimplantation of the coronary arteries: new surgical approach. J Thorac Cardiovasc Surg 1981;81:309-15.

44. Rosero H, Nathan PE, Rodney E, et al. Aorta to right atrium fistula with congestive heart failure resulting from a patent Cabrol shunt after repair of aortic dissection. Am Heart J 1994;128:608-9.

45. Park SB, Maher TD Jr. Modification of the aortic composite graft using the button-in technique. Ann Thorac Surg 1994;57:1035-7.

46. Copeland JG III, Rosado LJ, Snyder SL. New technique for improving hemostasis in aortic root replacement with composite graft. Ann Thorac Surg 1993;55:1027-9.

47. Kouchoukos NT, Wareing TH, Murphy SF, Perrillo JB. Sixteen-year experience with aortic root replacement: results of 172 operations. Ann Surg 1991;214:308-18.

48. Svensson LG. Rationale and technique for replacement of the ascending aorta, arch, and distal aorta using a modified elephant trunk procedure. J Cardiac Surg 1992;7:301-12.

49. Heinemann MK, Buehner B, Jurmann MJ, Borst H-G. Use of the "elephant trunk technique" in aortic surgery. Ann Thorac Surg 1995;60:2-7.

50. Borst HG, Schaudig A, Rudolph W. Arteriovenous fistula of the aortic arch: repair during deep hypothermia and circulatory arrest. J Thorac Cardiovasc Surg 1964;48:443-7.

51. Borst HG, Walterbusch G, Schaps D. Extensive aortic replacement using "elephant trunk" prosthesis. Thorac Cardiovasc Surg 1983;31:37-40.

52. Borst HG, Frank G, Schaps D. Treatment of extensive aortic aneurysms by a new multiple-stage approach. J Thorac Cardiovasc Surg 1988;95:11-3.

53. Crawford ES, Walker HJ, Saleh SA, Normann NA. Graft replacement of aneurysm in descending thoracic aorta: results without bypass or shunting. Surgery 1981;89:73-85.

54. Verdant A, Cossette R, Page A, et al. Aneurysms of the descending thoracic aorta: three hundred sixty-six consecutive cases resected without paraplegia. J Vasc Surg 1995;21:385-91.

55. Borst HG, Jurmann M, Buhner B, Laas J. Risk of replacement of descending aorta with a standardized left heart bypass technique. J Thorac Cardiovasc Surg 1994;107:126-33.

56. DeBakey ME, Cooley DA. Successful resection of aneurysm of thoracic aorta and replacement by graft. JAMA 1953;152:673-6.

57. Lawrie GM, Earle N, DeBakey ME. Evolution of surgical techniques for aneurysms of the descending thoracic aorta: twenty-nine years experience with 659 patients. J Cardiac Surg 1994;9:648-61.

58. Gilling-Smith GL, Worswick L, Knight PF, et al. Surgical repair of thoracoabdominal aortic aneurysm: 10 years' experience. Br J Surg 1995;82:624-9.

59. Svensson LG, Crawford ES, Hess KR, et al. Thoracoabdominal aortic aneurysms associated with celiac, superior mesenteric and renal artery occlusive disease: methods and analysis of results in 271 patients. J Vasc Surg 1992;16:378-90.

60. Svensson LG, Crawford ES, Hess KR, et al. Experience with 1509 patients undergoing thoracoabdominal aortic operations. J Vasc Surg 1993;17:357-70.

61. Svensson LG, Patel V, Robinson MF, et al. Influence of preservation or perfusion of intraoperatively identified spinal cord blood supply on spinal motor evoked potentials and paraplegia after aortic surgery. J Vasc Surg 1991;13:355-65.

62. Svensson LG, Hess KR, Coselli JS, Safi HR. Influence of segmental arteries, extent, and atrio-femoral bypass on postoperative paraplegia after thoracoabdominal aortic aneurysm repairs. J Vasc Surg 1994;20:255-62.

63. Coselli JS. Thoracoabdominal aortic aneurysms: experience with 372. J Cardiac Surg 1994;9:638-47.

64. Safi HJ, Bartoli S, Hess KR, et al. Neurologic deficit in patients at high risk with thoracoabdominal aortic aneurysms: the role of cerebral spinal fluid drainage and distal aortic perfusion. J Vasc Surg 1994;20:434-43.

65. Svensson LG, Shahian DM, Davis FG, et al. Replacement of entire aorta from aortic valve to bifurcation during one operation. Ann Thorac Surg 1994;58:1164-6.

66. Crawford ES, Saleh SA, Babb JW, et al. Infrarenal abdominal aortic aneurysm: factors influencing survival after operation performed over a 25-year period. Ann Surg 1981;193:699-709.

67. Coselli JS, LeMaire SA, Buket S, Berzin E. Subsequent proximal aortic operations in 123 patients with previous infrarenal abdominal aortic aneurysm surgery. J Vasc Surg 1995;22:59-67.

68. Huber TS, Harward TRS, Flynn TC, et al. Operative mortality rates after elective infrarenal aortic reconstructions. J Vasc Surg 1995;22:287-94.

69. O'Hara PJ, Hertzer NR, Krajewski LP, et al. Ten-year experience with abdominal aortic aneurysm repair in octogenarians: early results and late outcome. J Vasc Surg 1995;21:830-8.

70. Sullivan CA, Rohrer MJ, Cutler BS. Clinical management of the symptomatic but unruptured abdominal aortic aneurysm. J Vasc Surg 1990;11:799-803.

71. Bauer EP, Redaelli C, von Segresser LK, Turina MI. Ruptured abdominal aortic aneurysms: predictors for early complications and death. Surgery 1993;114:31-5.

72. Johansen K, Kohler TR, Nicholls SC, et al. Ruptured abdominal aortic aneurysm: the Harborview experience. J Vasc Surg 1991;13:240-5.

73. Crawford ES. Ruptured abdominal aortic aneurysm [editorial]. J Vasc Surg 1991;13:348-50.

74. Crawford ES, Svensson LG, Coselli JS, et al. Aortic dissection and dissecting aortic aneurysms. Ann Surg 1988;108:254-73.

75. Ergin MA, Galla JD, Lansman S, et al. Acute dissection of the aorta: current surgical treatment. Surg Clin North Am 1985;65:721-41.

76. Gott VL, Pyeritz RE, Magovern GJ Jr, et al. Surgical treatment of aneurysms of the ascending aorta in the Marfan syndrome. N Engl J Med 1986;314:1070-4.

77. Haverich A, Miller DC, Scott WC, et al. Acute and chronic aortic dissections: determinants of long-term outcome for operative survivors. Circulation 1985;72(Supp II):II-22-34.

78. Miller DC. Surgical management of aortic dissections: indications, perioperative management, and long-term results. In: Doroghazi RM, Slater EE, eds. Aortic Dissection. New York: McGraw-Hill, 1983:193-243.

79. Miller DC, Mitchell RS, Oyer PE, et al. Independent determinants of operative mortality for patients with aortic dissections. Circulation 1984;70(Supp I):I-153-64.

80. Rizzo RJ, Aranki SF, Aklog L, et al. Rapid noninvasive diagnosis and

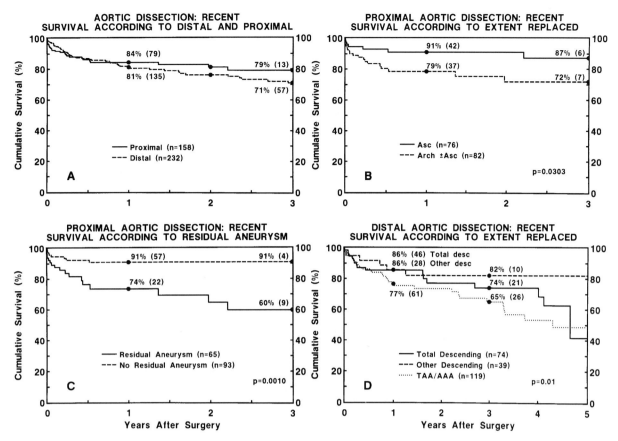

FIGURE 27-8 Aortic dissection. Recent survival by approach **(A)**, by proximal extent **(B)**, by proximal residual aneurysm **(C)**, and by distal extent **(D)**. (From Svensson LG, Crawford ES, Hess KR, et al. Dissection of the aorta and dissecting aortic aneurysms: improving early and long-term surgical results. Circulation 1990:82(5 supp):IV24-38. Reprinted with permission. Copyright 1990 American Heart Association.)

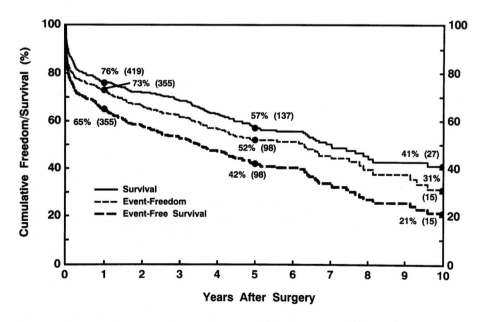

FIGURE 27-9 Aortic dissection. Overall survival and freedom from major postoperative events. (From Svensson LG, Crawford ES, Hess KR, et al. Dissection of the aorta and dissecting aortic aneurysms: improving early and long-term surgical results. Circulation 1990:82(5 supp):IV24-38. Reprinted with permission. Copyright 1990 American Heart Association.)

29. Donaldson RM, Ross DN. Composite graft replacement for the treatment of aneurysms of the ascending aorta associated with aortic valvular disease. Circulation 1982;66(Supp 1):116-21.

30. Edwards WS, Kerr AR. A safer technique for replacement of the entire ascending aorta and aortic valve. J Thorac Cardiovasc Surg 1970;59:837-9.

31. Galloway AC, Colvin SB, LaMendola CL, et al. Ten-year operative experience with 165 aneurysms of the ascending aorta and aortic arch. Circulation 1989;80(supp I):I-249-56.

32. Gerosa G, McKay R, Ross DN. Replacement of the aortic valve or root with a pulmonary autograft in children. Ann Thorac Surg 1991; 51:424-9.

33. Gott VL, Pyeritz RE, Cameron DE, et al. Composite graft repair of Marfan aneurysm of the ascending aorta: results in 100 patients. Ann Thorac Surg 1991;52:38-44.

34. Grey DP, Ott DA, Cooley DA. Surgical treatment of aneurysms of the ascending aorta with aortic insufficiency. J Thorac Cardiovasc Surg 1983;86:864-77.

35. Helseth HK, Haglin JJ, Monson BK, Wichstrom PH. Results of composite graft replacement for aortic root aneurysms. J Thorac Cardiovasc Surg 1980;80:754-9.

36. Jex RK, Schaff HG, Piehler JM, et al. Repair of ascending aortic dissection: influence of associated aortic valve insufficiency on early and late results. J Thorac Cardiovasc Surg 1987;93:375-84.

37. Kouchoukos NT, Karp RB, Blackstone EH, et al. Replacement of the ascending aorta and aortic valve with a composite graft: results in 86 patients. Ann Surg 1980;192:403-12.

38. Kouchoukos NT, Marshall WG Jr, Wedige STA. Eleven-year experience with composite graft replacement of the ascending aorta and aortic valve. J Thorac Cardiovasc Surg 1986;92:691-705.

39. Lewis CT, Cooley DA, Murphy MC, et al. Surgical repair of aortic root aneurysms in 280 patients. Ann Thorac Surg 1992;53:38-45.

40. Lytle BW, Mahfood SS, Cosgrove DM, Loop FD. Replacement of the ascending aorta: early and late results. J Thorac Cardiovasc Surg 1990;99:651-7.

41. Miller DC, Stinson EB, Oyer PE, et al. Concomitant resection of ascending aortic aneurysms and replacement of the ascending aortic valve: operative and long-term results with "conventional" techniques in ninety patients. J Thorac Cardiovasc Surg 1980;79:388-401.

42. Najafi H. Aneurysm of cystic medionecrotic root: a modified surgical approach. J Cardiovasc Surg 1973;66:71-4.

43. Cabrol C, Pavie A, Gandjbakhch I, et al. Complete replacement of the ascending aorta with reimplantation of the coronary arteries: new surgical approach. J Thorac Cardiovasc Surg 1981;81:309-15.

44. Rosero H, Nathan PE, Rodney E, et al. Aorta to right atrium fistula with congestive heart failure resulting from a patent Cabrol shunt after repair of aortic dissection. Am Heart J 1994;128:608-9.

45. Park SB, Maher TD Jr. Modification of the aortic composite graft using the button-in technique. Ann Thorac Surg 1994;57:1035-7.

46. Copeland JG III, Rosado LJ, Snyder SL. New technique for improving hemostasis in aortic root replacement with composite graft. Ann Thorac Surg 1993;55:1027-9.

47. Kouchoukos NT, Wareing TH, Murphy SF, Perrillo JB. Sixteen-year experience with aortic root replacement: results of 172 operations. Ann Surg 1991;214:308-18.

48. Svensson LG. Rationale and technique for replacement of the ascending aorta, arch, and distal aorta using a modified elephant trunk procedure. J Cardiac Surg 1992;7:301-12.

49. Heinemann MK, Buehner B, Jurmann MJ, Borst H-G. Use of the "elephant trunk technique" in aortic surgery. Ann Thorac Surg 1995; 60:2-7.

50. Borst HG, Schaudig A, Rudolph W. Arteriovenous fistula of the aortic arch: repair during deep hypothermia and circulatory arrest. J Thorac Cardiovasc Surg 1964;48:443-7.

51. Borst HG, Walterbusch G, Schaps D. Extensive aortic replacement using "elephant trunk" prosthesis. Thorac Cardiovasc Surg 1983; 31:37-40.

52. Borst HG, Frank G, Schaps D. Treatment of extensive aortic aneurysms by a new multiple-stage approach. J Thorac Cardiovasc Surg 1988;95:11-3.

53. Crawford ES, Walker HJ, Saleh SA, Normann NA. Graft replacement of aneurysm in descending thoracic aorta: results without bypass or shunting. Surgery 1981;89:73-85.

54. Verdant A, Cossette R, Page A, et al. Aneurysms of the descending thoracic aorta: three hundred sixty-six consecutive cases resected without paraplegia. J Vasc Surg 1995;21:385-91.

55. Borst HG, Jurmann M, Buhner B, Laas J. Risk of replacement of descending aorta with a standardized left heart bypass technique. J Thorac Cardiovasc Surg 1994;107:126-33.

56. DeBakey ME, Cooley DA. Successful resection of aneurysm of thoracic aorta and replacement by graft. JAMA 1953;152:673-6.

57. Lawrie GM, Earle N, DeBakey ME. Evolution of surgical techniques for aneurysms of the descending thoracic aorta: twenty-nine years experience with 659 patients. J Cardiac Surg 1994;9:648-61.

58. Gilling-Smith GL, Worswick L, Knight PF, et al. Surgical repair of thoracoabdominal aortic aneurysm: 10 years' experience. Br J Surg 1995;82:624-9.

59. Svensson LG, Crawford ES, Hess KR, et al. Thoracoabdominal aortic aneurysms associated with celiac, superior mesenteric and renal artery occlusive disease: methods and analysis of results in 271 patients. J Vasc Surg 1992;16:378-90.

60. Svensson LG, Crawford ES, Hess KR, et al. Experience with 1509 patients undergoing thoracoabdominal aortic operations. J Vasc Surg 1993;17:357-70.

61. Svensson LG, Patel V, Robinson MF, et al. Influence of preservation or perfusion of intraoperatively identified spinal cord blood supply on spinal motor evoked potentials and paraplegia after aortic surgery. J Vasc Surg 1991;13:355-65.

62. Svensson LG, Hess KR, Coselli JS, Safi HR. Influence of segmental arteries, extent, and atrio-femoral bypass on postoperative paraplegia after thoracoabdominal aortic aneurysm repairs. J Vasc Surg 1994;20:255-62.

63. Coselli JS. Thoracoabdominal aortic aneurysms: experience with 372. J Cardiac Surg 1994;9:638-47.

64. Safi HJ, Bartoli S, Hess KR, et al. Neurologic deficit in patients at high risk with thoracoabdominal aortic aneurysms: the role of cerebral spinal fluid drainage and distal aortic perfusion. J Vasc Surg 1994;20:434-43.

65. Svensson LG, Shahian DM, Davis FG, et al. Replacement of entire aorta from aortic valve to bifurcation during one operation. Ann Thorac Surg 1994;58:1164-6.

66. Crawford ES, Saleh SA, Babb JW, et al. Infrarenal abdominal aortic aneurysm: factors influencing survival after operation performed over a 25-year period. Ann Surg 1981;193:699-709.

67. Coselli JS, LeMaire SA, Buket S, Berzin E. Subsequent proximal aortic operations in 123 patients with previous infrarenal abdominal aortic aneurysm surgery. J Vasc Surg 1995;22:59-67.

68. Huber TS, Harward TRS, Flynn TC, et al. Operative mortality rates after elective infrarenal aortic reconstructions. J Vasc Surg 1995;22: 287-94.

69. O'Hara PJ, Hertzer NR, Krajewski LP, et al. Ten-year experience with abdominal aortic aneurysm repair in octogenarians: early results and late outcome. J Vasc Surg 1995;21:830-8.

70. Sullivan CA, Rohrer MJ, Cutler BS. Clinical management of the symptomatic but unruptured abdominal aortic aneurysm. J Vasc Surg 1990;11:799-803.

71. Bauer EP, Redaelli C, von Segresser LK, Turina MI. Ruptured abdominal aortic aneurysms: predictors for early complications and death. Surgery 1993;114:31-5.

72. Johansen K, Kohler TR, Nicholls SC, et al. Ruptured abdominal aortic aneurysm: the Harborview experience. J Vasc Surg 1991;13: 240-5.

73. Crawford ES. Ruptured abdominal aortic aneurysm [editorial]. J Vasc Surg 1991;13:348-50.

74. Crawford ES, Svensson LG, Coselli JS, et al. Aortic dissection and dissecting aortic aneurysms. Ann Surg 1988;108:254-73.

75. Ergin MA, Galla JD, Lansman S, et al. Acute dissection of the aorta: current surgical treatment. Surg Clin North Am 1985;65:721-41.

76. Gott VL, Pyeritz RE, Magovern GJ Jr, et al. Surgical treatment of aneurysms of the ascending aorta in the Marfan syndrome. N Engl J Med 1986;314:1070-4.

77. Haverich A, Miller DC, Scott WC, et al. Acute and chronic aortic dissections: determinants of long-term outcome for operative survivors. Circulation 1985;72(Supp II):II-22-34.

78. Miller DC. Surgical management of aortic dissections: indications, perioperative management, and long-term results. In: Doroghazi RM, Slater EE, eds. Aortic Dissection. New York: McGraw-Hill, 1983: 193-243.

79. Miller DC, Mitchell RS, Oyer PE, et al. Independent determinants of operative mortality for patients with aortic dissections. Circulation 1984;70(Supp I):I-153-64.

80. Rizzo RJ, Aranki SF, Aklog L, et al. Rapid noninvasive diagnosis and

surgical repair of acute ascending aortic dissection: improved survival with less angiography. J Thorac Cardiovasc Surg 1994;108: 567-75.

81. Fann JI, Smith JA, Miller CD, et al. Surgical management of aortic dissection during a 30-year period. Circulation 1995;92(Supp II): 113-21.

82. Crawford ES, Kirklin JW, Naftel DC, et al. Surgery for acute dissection of ascending aorta: should the arch be included? "See comments." J Thorac Cardiovasc Surg 1992;104:46-59.

83. Svensson LG, Crawford ES. Aortic dissection and aortic aneurysm surgery: clinical observations, experimental investigations, and statistical analyses. Part II Curr Probl Surg 1992;29:915-1057.

84. Creswell LL, Kouchoukos NT, Cox JL, Rosenbloom M. Coronary artery disease in patients with type A aortic dissection. Ann Thorac Surg 1995;59:585-90.

85. Robbins RC, McManus RP, Mitchell RS, et al. Management of patients with intramural hematoma of the thoracic aorta. Circulation 1993;88(5 Pt 2):II1-10.

86. Nienaber CA, von Kodolitsch Y, Petersen B, et al. Intramural hemorrhage of the thoracic aorta: diagnostic and therapeutic implications. Circulation 1995;92:1465-72.

87. O'Gara PT, DeSanctis W. Acute aortic dissection and its variants: toward a common diagnostic and therapeutic approach. Circulation 1995;92:1376-78.

88. Doroghazi RM, Slater EE, DeSanctis RW, et al. Long-term survival of patients with treated aortic dissection. J Am Coll Cardiol 1984;3: 1026-34.

89. Glower DD, Fann FJI, Speier RH, et al. Comparison of medical and surgical therapy for uncomplicated descending aortic dissection [abstract]. Circulation 1990;80(supp IV):IV-39-46.

90. Nienaber CA, Kodolitsch YV. Metaanalyse zur Prognose der thorakalen Aortendissektion: Letalität im Wandel der letzten vier Jahrzehnte. Herz 1992;17:398-416.

91. Coselli JS, LeMaire SA, Buket S. Marfan syndrome: the variability and outcome of operative managment. J Vasc Surg 1995;21:432-43.

92. Smith JA, Fann JI, Miller C, et al. Surgical management of aortic dissection in patients with the Marfan syndrome. Circulation 1994;90: II-235-242.

93. Silverman DI, Burton KJ, Gray J, et al. Life expectancy in the Marfan syndrome. Am J Cardiol 1995;75:157-60.

94. Finkbohner R, Johnston D, Crawford ES, et al. Marfan syndrome: long-term survival and complications after aortic aneurysm repair. Circulation 1995;91:728-33.

95. Dotter CT, Judkins MP. Transluminal treatment of arteriosclerotic obstruction: description of a new technic and a preliminary report of its application. Circulation 1964;30:654-70.

96. Dotter CT. Transluminally-placed coilspring endarterial tube grafts: long-term patency in canine popliteal artery. Invest Radiol 1969;4: 329-32.

97. Weibull H, Bergqvist D, Bergentz S-E, et al. Percutaneous transluminal renal angioplasty versus surgical reconstruction of atherosclerotic renal artery stenosis: a prospective randomized study. J Vasc Surg 1993;18:841-52.

98. Svensson LG, Labib S. Aortic dissection and aneurysm surgery. Curr Opin Cardiol 1994;9:191-9.

99. Parodi JC, Palmaz JC, Barone HD. Transfemoral intraluminal graft implantation for abdominal aortic aneurysms. Ann Vasc Surg 1991; 5:491-9.

100. Parodi JC. Endovascular repair of abdominal aortic aneurysms and other arterial lesions. J Vasc Surg 1995;21:549-57.

101. Marin ML, Veith FJ, Cynamon J, et al. Initial experience with transluminally placed endovascular grafts for the treatment of complex vascular lesions. Ann Surg 1995;222:449-69.

102. Moore WS, Vescera CL. Repair of abdominal aortic aneurysm by transfemoral endovascular graft placement. Ann Surg 1994;220: 331-41.

103. White RA, Verbin C, Kopchok G, et al. The role of cinefluoroscopy and intravascular ultrasonography in evaluating the deployment of experimental endovascular prostheses. J Vasc Surg 1995;21:365-74.

104. Buckmaster MJ, Hyde GL, Arden WA, et al. An angioscopic method for intraluminal aortic evaluation and stent placement. J Vasc Surg 1995;21:818-22.

105. Brock RC. The life and work of Sir Astley Cooper. Ann R Coll Surg Engl 1969;44:1-18.

106. Matas R. An operation for the radical cure of aneurysms based on arteriography. Ann Surg 1903;37:161.

107. Matas R. Aneurysm of the abdominal aorta at its bifurcation into the common iliac arteries. Ann Surg 1960;112:909.

108. Carpentier A, Fabiani JN. La thrombo-exclusion dans les dissections et les aneurysmes de l'aorte thoracique descendante. In: Kieffer E, ed. Chirugie de l'aorte throracique descendante et thoraco-abdominale. Paris: Expansion Scientifique Française, 1986:245-51.

109. Criado E, Marston WA, Woosley JT, et al. An aortic aneurysm model for the evaluation of endovascular exclusion prostheses. J Vasc Surg 1995;22:306-15.

110. Sayers RD, Thompson MM, Nasim A, Bell PRF. Endovascular repair of abdominal aortic aneurysm: limitations of the single proximal stent technique. Br J Surg 1994;81:1107-10.

111. Chuter T, Green RM, Ouriel K, et al. Transfemoral endovascular aortic graft replacement. J Vasc Surg 1993;18:185-97.

112. Chuter TAM, Green RM, Ouriel K, DeWeese JA. Infrarenal aortic aneurysm structure: implications for transfemoral repair. J Vasc Surg 1994;20:44-50.

113. Quinones-Baldrich WJ, Deaton DH, Mitchell RS, et al. Preliminary experience with the endovascular technologies bifurcated endovascular prosthesis in a calf model. J Vasc Surg 1995;22:370-81.

114. Marin ML, Veith FJ, Cynamon J, et al. Human transluminally placed endovascular stented grafts: preliminary histopathologic analysis of healing grafts in aortoiliac and femoral artery occlusive disease. J Vasc Surg 1995;21:595-604.

115. Piquet P, Rolland P-H, Bartoli J-M, et al. Tantalum-Dacron coknit stent for endovascular treatment of aortic aneurysms: a preliminary experimental study. J Vasc Surg 1994;19:698-706.

116. Marin ML, Veith FJ, Panetta TF, et al. Transluminally placed endovascular stented graft repair for arterial trauma. J Vasc Surg 1994;20:466-73.

117. Rosenthal E, Qureshi SA, Tynan M. Stent implantation for aortic recoarctation. Am Heart J 1995;129:1220-1.

118. Kato M, Matsuda T, Kaneko M, et al. Experimental assessment of newly devised transcatheter stent-graft for aortic dissection. Ann Thorac Surg 1995;59:908-15.

119. Moon MR, Dake MD, Pelc LR, et al. Intravascular stenting of acute experimental type B dissections. J Surg Res 1993;54:381-8.

120. Walker PJ, Dake MD, Mitchell RS, Miller DC. The use of endovascular techniques for the treatment of complications of aortic dissection. J Vasc Surg 1993;18:1042-51.

121. Marin ML, Veith FJ, Sanchez LA, et al. Endovascular aortoiliac grafts in combination with standard infrainguinal arterial bypasses in the management of limb-threatening ischemia: preliminary report. J Vasc Surg 1995;22:316-25.

122. van de Ven PJG, Beutler JJ, Kaatee R, et al. Transluminal vascular stent for ostial atherosclerotic renal artery stenosis. Lancet 1995; 346:672-4.

123. Dake MD, Miller DC, Semba CP, et al. Transluminal placement of endovascular stent-grafts for the treatment of descending thoracic aortic aneurysms. N Engl J Med 1994;331:1729-34.

28

Late Follow-up and Management

To improve the long-term quality and quantity of life after aortic surgery, patients require careful long-term management.

POSTOPERATIVE STUDIES

Before patients who have had an aortic dissection repair, particularly if acute, are discharged from the hospital, we routinely obtain a postoperative imaging study, whereas for patients with type I dissection we order a computed tomography (CT) scan (with contrast) of the chest and abdomen. In patients who have had acute repairs it is not infrequent to see that the distal aortic false lumen and aorta have enlarged since the preoperative study. If the distal aorta, typically the proximal descending or the abdominal aorta, is larger than 6 cm we will also repair this segment. If a composite valve graft was inserted, a transesophogeal echocardiogram (TEE) is performed. Alternatively, some patients will undergo angiography. For type II proximal dissections, TEE studies are usually performed before discharge, particularly if a composite valve graft was inserted. Distal dissection repairs are checked with CT scans with contrast before discharge. For those patients who do not have aortic dissection repairs but only degenerative aneurysm repairs, no special studies are obtained before discharge other than routine chest radiographs or the occasional angiograph. For these patients, as for those with aortic dissection repairs, however, routine CT scans are obtained at 6 months, then at 1 year, and thenceforth at 2-year intervals. If warranted for other reasons (for example valve replacement) some patients will also have TEE studies.

FOLLOW-UP

All patients should be considered as having ongoing disease that requires long-term management and follow-up. Acute emergency surgery for aortic dissection is often only palliative, whereas surgery for chronic dissection is prophylactic against later rupture. Rarely is surgery curative for aortic dissection, as in the case of type II dissections or traumatic injuries. Enlargement of the unresected but dissected aorta can be expected in 20% to 40% of patients.[1-5] Some 5% to

10% of patients who have degenerative aneurysm repairs, depending on the site and other factors, may later require another operation.

After operative repair, patients require careful follow-up to control blood pressure and to check for the development of complications such as false aneurysms or further aneurysmal formation. Coselli has reviewed the course of patients who have abdominal aortic aneurysms repaired and who subsequently require the most thoracoabdominal aneurysm repairs. The late development of false aneurysms and aneurysms is discussed in previous chapters.[6, 7]

DeBakey and colleagues[1] reported that in patients who had undergone aortic dissection repairs, the risk of aneurysm development in the remaining aorta was 45.5% if the blood pressure was uncontrolled but only 17% if the patients were normotensive postoperatively. This result was confirmed by Neya and colleagues,[8] who reported a rupture-free survival rate of 96% at 5 years for normotensive patients and a 61% survival rate for patients with uncontrolled blood pressure ($p < 0.05$).

Continuous monitoring of aneurysm size is important because of the dismal prognosis for those patients in whom rupture from a subsequent aneurysm occurs and is a frequent cause of death on late follow-up.[7, 9-13] Furthermore, the poor long-term survival of patients with aneurysms has previously been reviewed in Chapter 3.[14-26]

We found that if there was residual dilatation of the aorta after repair of the ascending aorta, the ascending aorta plus arch, or the descending aorta, then the dilatation was a significant risk factor on long-term follow-up for aortic rupture and death (see Chapter 27). Clearly, patients with dilated aortas after aortic dissection repair still have double lumina, usually without thrombosis. Our data, however, did not show that the risk of rupture was greater when a double lumen was present and the aorta was not dilated or aneurysmal. Thus, it would appear to us that the risk of subsequent rupture is mostly influenced by the diameter of the residual aorta and probably a growth rate of more than 0.5 to 1 cm per year, rather than the presence of a double lumen. Erbel and colleagues[27] performed a multicenter prospective study of 168 patients who had undergone operations and followed them up with TEE. They found that 80% of patients with type I repairs had some thrombosis of the false lumen, with only 6.6% showing complete thrombosis; 93% of the patients had a residual patent false lumen; and 11% of those with type II repairs had a residual lumen. After medical therapy for type III dissections, 81% of type III dissection repairs showed evidence of some thrombosis in the false lumen. After operation for type III dissection, however, only 17% (2/12) had complete thrombosis of the false lumen. For both type II and type III dissections, 4% healed spontaneously.

These data emphasize that after either medical treatment or operation, complete obliteration of the remaining dissected aorta is rare, which warrants meticulous follow-up of the aorta for possible aneurysm formation. The risk of reoperation or rupture may be higher in patients with communication between the true and false lumina or with no thrombus formation in the false lumen.[28] Nonetheless, with their careful follow-up, Erbel and colleagues[27] were unable to prove conclusively that this was the case. Dinsmore and colleagues[29] also have argued that the long-term results are better if the false channel is thrombosed. Whether either the size of the aorta or the presence of thrombus is the critical factor is unknown because the two factors are directly interrelated. Parenthetically, the history of vascular surgery is replete with early reports of induction of thrombosis in aneurysms that still ruptured later despite the thrombus formation. Roudaut and colleagues[30] used CT, transthoracic echocardiography (TTE), or TEE, to follow up 32 patients who had ascending aorta (25) or ascending aorta plus arch (7) repairs for type A proximal aortic dissection. Of the patients, 31% developed dilatation of the ascending aorta. Persistence of flow in the distal false lumen was significantly ($p < 0.05$) more frequent in patients with a dilated (> 4 cm) distal aorta (77%, 7/9) than in those with nondilated aortas (14%, 3/21). It made no apparent difference whether the aortic arch was repaired, although the numbers were small. Roudaut found that, in comparison with CT, TEE consistently underestimated the size of the aortic root (0.6 cm), ascending aorta (0.6 cm), aortic arch (1.1 cm), upper descending aorta (0.5 cm), and lower descending aorta (0.3 cm). However, it is not clear from the study whether the internal diameter of the aorta was measured with TEE, whereas the external diameter is usually measured with CT. Of interest, all of the six patients (19%) in whom late false aneurysms developed at the suture lines had been operated on with the use of glue to reapproximate the layers of the aorta. By contrast, none of those whose repairs were done without glue, developed false aneurysms. Ergin and colleagues[31] followed up 58 patients who had proximal dissection repairs and for whom 38 late postoperative studies were available. All the distal repairs had been performed by the open method with circulatory arrest. Patent distal false lumina were found in 47.3%, with 45.8 % (11/24) being antegrade for sutured anastomoses versus none for intraluminal grafts ($p < 0.01$). The 5-year survival and event-free survival rates were no different between groups with or without a patent distal lumen, although patients without a patent distal lumen tended to do better. With longer follow-up and a larger series, this study may later show better survival results for those patients with an obliterated false lumen.

With the Bentall technique, development of false aneurysms is not uncommon,[13] particularly in patients with Marfan syndrome.[32] We have found that false aneurysms can be detected by echocardiography.[33] Currently, our (L.G.S.) patients routinely undergo TEE after insertion of a composite valve graft. No false aneurysms have been detected at any of the anastomoses in those patients in whom both the left main ostium was reanastomosed by a separate tube graft and the right coronary artery was reattached as an aortic button with a Teflon doughnut.[34] We perform TTE on all patients who have undergone a tube graft replacement of the ascending aorta or arch.

Peigh and colleagues,[35] in a series of 27 patients who had composite valve graft repairs, of whom 20 (74%) were survivors, noted that 10 patients (50%) had episodes of neurological or visual signs, including scotomata in seven, transient ischemic attacks in two, amaurosis fugax in four, and attention lapses in one. In none of a group of patients who had separate aortic valve and graft insertions was this noted. The reasons for these episodes in patients with composite valve grafts in this series are unclear. In our own study of 348 patients with composite valve grafts, the risk of late neurological deficits (see Chapter 27) was rare and no different from the results to be expected with an aortic valve replacement alone, but we found that the risk was slightly higher with the Bjork-Shiley valve. We have inserted a separate tube graft to the left main coronary artery and reattached the right coronary artery as a button in 34 patients and have observed them with careful yearly follow-up, and to date none has presented with a new transient or permanent neurological deficit.

Rofsky and colleagues[36] examined the aorta with MRI or CT after repair by the graft inclusion technique for either aortic dissection or aneurysms of the ascending aorta. The two methods were found to be equivalent in detecting flow outside the graft (15% versus 17%), mass effect on the graft (12% and 13%), and persistence of the false lumen after dissection repair (50% and 40%). For late follow-up, we tend to favor CT because of the greater accuracy in measuring aorta diameter and because CT is possibly also better for detecting false aneurysms.[30] Furthermore, evidence of calcification of the aortic neointima and aortic wall may indicate a lower risk of rupture.

For patients who have had ascending aorta or aortic arch repairs, we prescribe aspirin to reduce both the risk of cardiac events and the risk of stroke. Late results of aortic dissection and factors influencing results are shown in the Chapter 27. Although we did not perform a prospective randomized study and there were undoubtedly selection factor biases, it is of interest how postoperative medications were associated with improved long-term survival in patients who had aortic dissection repairs (see Chapter 4, Fig. 4-29). In an unpublished analysis of postoperative factors that influenced long-term survival, we noted that survival was decreased by uncontrolled blood pressure

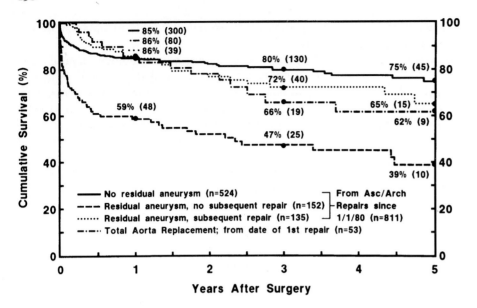

FIGURE 28–1 Kaplan-Meier survival curve of long-term survival according to resection of all aneurysmal disease or failure to resect all aneurysmal disease.

and improved by the use of aspirin, anticoagulation with Coumadin, and beta-blockers. These data should be interpreted with caution, since the correlation with other factors in the retrospective analysis may have influenced the result. Thus patients who were not given beta-blockers may have had severe heart or respiratory disease, favoring the long-term results in the patients treated with beta-blockers. We prefer to use beta-blockers for blood pressure control to reduce the risk of the *dP/dt* max of cardiac contraction and the possibility of further dissection requiring a repeat operation. There is also evidence that beta-blockers will reduce the rate of growth of aneurysms, including abdominal aortic aneurysms[37, 38] and in patients with Marfan syndrome.[39-41] Furthermore, there are reports that beta-blockers may increase collagen and elastic cross-linking, possibly resulting in a stronger aorta to resist dilatation and aneurysm formation.[42-44] Beta-blockers may further reduce cardiac causes of late death from the current rate of 25% in

our patients.[9-13, 44-46] All patients who can tolerate beta-blockers should be maintained on them for life.[2, 9, 39, 45-47]

If the long-term survival rate after aortic repairs is to be improved, other than by monitoring of the aorta and resecting all aneurysmal disease (Fig. 28-1), further attention will have to be focused on the evaluation of coronary artery disease, depending on the planned operation, either before or on late follow-up after surgery. It is noteworthy that, irrespective of the site of aortic repair, we have reported a 5-year survival rate of approximately 60% for all types of aneurysm (see discussion of preoperative evaluation and complications after distal aortic operations) (Fig. 28-2). Clearly, the results for young patients with Marfan syndrome who undergo elective operations are considerably better. Nevertheless, data from the Cleveland Clinic Foundation have shown that, even in octogenarians, if a preoperative coronary artery bypass is performed, the survival rate is 80% at 5 years versus 38% if it is not performed

FIGURE 28–2 Kaplan-Meier survival curve of long-term survival according to segment of aortic repair.

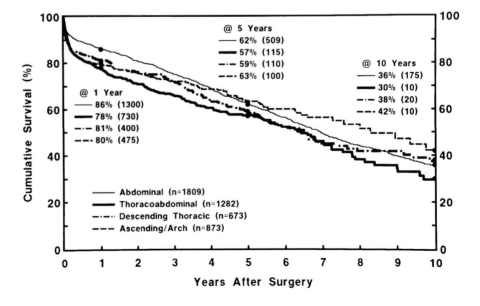

(p = 0.0077). The issue of cost containment will also have to be addressed and is beyond the scope of this review of aortic surgery.

REFERENCES

1. DeBakey ME, McCollum CH, Crawford ES, et al. Dissection and dissecting aneurysms of the aorta: twenty-year follow-up of five hundred twenty-seven patients treated surgically. Surgery 1982;92: 1118-34.
2. DeSanctis RW, Doroghazi RM, Austen WG, et al. Aortic dissection. N Engl J Med 1987;317:1060-7.
3. Doroghazi RM, Slater EE, DeSanctis RW, et al. Long-term survival of patients with treated aortic dissection. J Am Coll Cardiol 1984;3: 1026-34.
4. Haverich A, Miller DC, Scott WC, et al. Acute and chronic aortic dissections: determinants of long-term outcome for operative survivors. Circulation 1985;72(Supp II):II-22-34.
5. Heinemann M, Laas J, Karck M, Borst HG. Thoracic aortic aneurysms after acute type A aortic dissection: necessity for follow-up. Ann Thorac Surg 1990;49:580-4.
6. McCann RL, Schwartz LB, Georgiade GS. Management of abdominal aortic graft complications. Ann Surg 1993;217:729-34.
7. Coselli JS, LeMaire SA, Buket S, Berzin E. Subsequent proximal aortic operations in 123 patients with previous infrarenal abdominal aortic aneurysm surgery. J Vasc Surg 1995;22:59-67.
8. Neya K, Omoto R, Kyo S, et al. Outcome of Stanford type B acute aortic dissection. Circulation 1992;86(Supp II):II-1-7.
9. Svensson LG, Crawford ES, Hess KR, et al. Dissection of the aorta and dissecting aortic aneurysms: improving early and long-term surgical results. Circulation 1990;82(5 Supp):IV 24-38.
10. Svensson LG, Crawford ES, Hess KR, et al. Variables predictive of outcome in 832 patients undergoing repairs of the descending thoracic aorta. Chest 1993;104:1248-53.
11. Svensson LG, Crawford ES, Hess KR, et al. Experience with 1509 patients undergoing thoracoabdominal aortic operations. J Vasc Surg 1993;17:357-70.
12. Svensson LG, Crawford ES. Aortic dissection and aortic aneurysm surgery: clinical observations, experimental investigations, and statistical analyses. Part III. Curr Probl Surg 1993;30:1-172.
13. Svensson LG, Crawford ES, Hess KR, et al. Composite valve graft replacement of the proximal aorta: comparison of techniques in 348 patients. Ann Thorac Surg 1992;54:427-39.
14. Nevitt MP, Ballard DJ, Hallett JW Jr. Prognosis of abdominal aortic aneurysms: a population-based study. N Engl J Med 1989;321:1009-14.
15. Johansson G, Markstrom U, Swedenborg J. Ruptured thoracic aortic aneurysms: a study of incidence and mortality rates. J Vasc Surg 1995;21:985-8.
16. Perko MJ, Norgaard M, Herzog TM, et al. Unoperated aortic aneurysm: a survey of 170 patients. Ann Thorac Surg 1995;59:1204-9.
17. Agnagnostopoulos CE, Prabhakar MJS, Vittle CF. Aortic dissections and dissecting aneurysms. Am J Cardiol 1972;30:263-73.
18. Darling RC, Messina CR, Brewster DC, Ottinger LW. Autopsy study of unoperated abdominal aortic aneurysm: the case for early resection. Circulation 1976;56(2 Supp):161.
19. Szilagyi DE, Elliot JP, Smith RF. Clinical fate of the patient with asymptomatic abdominal aortic aneurysm and unfit for surgical treatment. Arch Surg 1972;104:600-6.
20. Pressler V, McNamara JJ. Thoracic aortic aneurysm: natural history and treatment. J Thorac Cardiovasc Surg 1980;79:489-98.
21. Pressler V, McNamara JJ. Aneurysm of the thoracic aorta: Review of 260 cases. J Thorac Cardiovasc Surg 1985;89:50-4.
22. Bickerstaff LK, Pairolero PC, Hollier LH, et al. Thoracic aortic aneurysms: a population-based study. Surgery 1982;92:1103-8.
23. Bickerstaff LK, Hollier LH, Van Peenen H, et al. Abdominal aortic aneurysms: the changing natural history. J Vasc Surg 1984;1:6-12.
24. Dapunt OE, Galla JD, Sadeghi AM, et al. The natural history of thoracic aortic aneurysms. J Thorac Cardiovasc Surg 1994;107:1323-32.
25. Cronenwett JL, Murphy TF, Zelenock GB, et al. Actuarial analysis of variables associated with rupture of small abdominal aortic aneurysms. Surgery 1985;98:472-83.
26. Cronenwett JL, Sargent SK, Wall MH, et al. Variables that affect the expansion rate and outcome of small abdominal aortic aneurysms. J Vasc Surg 1990;11:260-8.
27. Erbel R, Oelert H, Meyer J, et al. Effect of medical and surgical therapy on aortic dissection evaluated by transesophageal echocardiography: implications for prognosis and therapy. Circulation 1993; 87:1604-15.
28. Khandheria B. Aortic dissection: the last frontier. Circulation 1993; 87:1765-8.
29. Dinsmore RE, Rourke JA, DeSanctis RD, et al. Angiographic findings in dissecting aortic aneurysm. N Engl J Med 1966;275:1152-7.
30. Roudaut RP, Marcaggi XL, Deville C, et al. Value of transesophageal echocardiography combined with computed tomography for assessing repaired type A aortic dissection. Am J Cardiol 1992;70: 1468-76.
31. Ergin MA, Phillips RA, Galla JD, et al. Significance of distal false lumen after type A dissection repair. Ann Thorac Surg 1994;57: 820-4.
32. Svensson LG, Crawford ES, Coselli JS, et al. Impact of cardiovascular operation on survival in the Marfan patient. Circulation 1989;80(3 Pt 1):i233-42.
33. Barbetseas J, Crawford S, Safi HJ, et al. Doppler echocardiographic evaluation of pseudoaneurysms complicating composite grafts of the ascending aorta. Circulation 1992;85:212-22.
34. Svensson LG. Approach to the insertion of composite valve graft. Ann Thorac Surg 1992;54:376-8.
35. Peigh PS, DiSesa VJ, Cohn LH, Collins JJ Jr. Neurological and ophthalmological phenomena after aortic conduit surgery. Circulation 1990;82(supp IV):IV-47-50.
36. Rofsky NM, Weinreb JC, Grossi EA, et al. Aortic aneurysm and dissection: normal MR imaging and CT findings after surgical repair with the continuous-suture graft-inclusion technique. Radiology 1993;186:195-201.
37. Leach SD, Toole AL, Stern H, et al. Effect of beta-adrenergic blockade on the growth rate of abdominal aortic aneurysms. Arch Surg 1988;123:606-9.
38. Gadowski GR, Pilcher DB, Ricci MA. Abdominal aortic aneurysm expansion rate: effect of size and beta-adrenergic blockade. J Vasc Surg 1994;19:727-31.
39. Pyeritz RE. Propranolol retards aortic root dilatation in the Marfan syndrome. Circulation 1983;68(Supp II):II-356.
40. Shores J, Berger KR, Murphy EA, Pyeritz RE. Progression of aortic dilatation and the benefit of long-term β-adrenergic blockade in Marfan's syndrome. N Engl J Med 1994;330:1335-41.
41. Taherina AC. Cardiovascular anomalies in Marfan's syndrome: the role of echocardiography and beta-blockers. South Med J 1993;86: 305-10.
42. Brophy C, Tilson JE, Tilson MD. Propranolol delays the formation of aneurysms in the male blotchy mouse. J Surg Res 1988;44:687-9.
43. Brophy CM, Tilson JE, Tilson MD. Propranolol stimulates the crosslinking of matrix components in skin from the aneurysm-prone blotchy mouse. J Surg Res 1989;46:330-2.
44. Boucek RJ, Gunja-Smith Z, Noble NL, Simpson CF. Modulation by propranolol of the lysyl cross-links in aortic elastin and collagen of the aneurysm-prone turkey. Biochem Pharmacol 1983;32:275-80.
45. Yusuf S, Wittes J, Friedman L. Overview of results of randomized clinical trials in heart disease. I. Treatments following myocardial infarction. JAMA 1988;260:2088-93.
46. Yusuf S, Wittes J, Friedman L. Overview of results of randomized clinical trials in heart disease. II. Unstable angina, heart failure, primary prevention with aspirin, and risk factor modification. JAMA 1988;260:2259-63.
47. Eagle KA, DeSanctis RW. Aortic dissection. Curr Probl Cardiol 1989; 14:225-78.

Index

Note: Page numbers in *italics* refer to illustrations; page numbers followed by t refer to tables.

A

Abdominal aorta, acute occlusion of, 183
    aneurysm of. See *Aortic aneurysm, abdominal.*
    aortography of, 13–14, *13*
    definition of, 29
    juxtarenal segment of, definition of, 29
    occlusive disease of, *180,* 182–183, *182, 373*
    rupture of, *304*
    supraceliac segment of, definition of, 29
    suprarenal segment of, definition of, 29
Aberrant right subclavian artery, 161, 163–164, *165–169*
Adenosine, in ischemia, 201–202, *202*
Adenosine deaminase, in ischemia, 201–202, *202*
Afterload, intraoperative, 252, 253
Allopurinol, in reperfusion injury prevention, 205
Amino acids, excitatory, in ischemia, 198–201
Amlodipine, in neuronal ischemia, 198
AMPA (α-amino-3-hydroxy-5-methyl-4-isoxazole propionate) receptor, 199, 200
Anastomoses, in cardiopulmonary bypass discontinuation, 255–256
Angioplasty, 19
    in coarctation of aorta, 155, 159–160
    results of, 450, 452–453
Anion transport inhibitor, in neuronal ischemia, 210
Ankylosing spondylitis, aortitis in, 118
Annuloaortic ectasia, 29
Anterior spinal artery, anatomy of, 232, 233, 234
Antibiotics, prophylactic, for prosthesis placement, 133
Antioxidants, 205–206
alpha₁-Antitrypsin, in degenerative aortic aneurysm, 34
Aorta, congenital abnormalities of, 153–173. See also *Aortic arch; Coarctation of aorta.*
    diameter of, calculation of, 95
        in Marfan syndrome, 95, 97
    normal histology of, 30–31
    occlusive disease of. See *Occlusive disease.*
    segments of, 29
    traumatic rupture of, 184–190

Aorta *(Continued)*
    diagnosis of, 185, *186–188*
    management of, 185–190, *188–190*
   tumors of, 192
Aortic aneurysm(s), 29–40
    abdominal, coronary artery disease and, 16–17
        expansion rate of, 37
        genetic factors in, 33–34
        iliac artery stenosis with, *384*
        incidence of, 36
        monitoring of, 37
        mortality from, 38
        repair of, 39, *357*
        rupture of, 38, *357*
        ultrasound in, 36
        with horseshoe kidney, *395, 395–399, 396, 398*
    aortic arch, *12,* 281–283, *281–285,* 286
        distal, *338–342*
    aortocaval fistulae with, 391, *392*
    atherosclerosis in, 29, *30*
    autoimmune disease and, 35
    bacterial infection in, 34–35
    biochemical factors in, 34–35
    clinical presentation of, 38–39
    collagenase in, 34
    definition of, 29
    distal, repair of, 335–358
        abdominal aortic repair for, *357*
        descending thoracic aorta replacement for, 343–345, *343, 344*
        infrarenal aortic repair for, 350, *351, 352, 356*
        juxtarenal aortic repair for, 350, *353, 354*
        proximal aorta repair with, 335, *336–342*
        suprarenal aortic repair for, 350, *355*
        thoracoabdominal aortic repair for, 345–350, *345, 347–349*
    elastase in, 34
    etiology of, 33–35

Aortic aneurysm(s) *(Continued)*
   false, 29, *268, 329, 330-331,* 427
   fusiform, aortic dissection and, 45
   genetic factors in, 33-34
   histology of, 31-33, *31-33*
   in Kawasaki disease, 35
   in Marfan syndrome, 93, *94, 96*
   in syphilis, 126
   incidence of, 35-36
   inflammatory, 32-33, *33.* See also *Aortitis.*
      of infrarenal aorta, 119-124, *120-123*
   infrarenal, 119-124, *120-123*
      computed tomography of, *11*
      inflammatory, 119-124, *120-123*
      renal artery stenosis with, *388, 389*
      repair of, 350, *351, 352, 356*
      ultrasound in, 36-37
      with horseshoe kidney, 395-399, *397*
   juxtarenal, aortography of, 14
      repair of, 350, *353-354*
   medial atherosclerosis in, *30,* 32
   medial degeneration in, 31, *31*
   medial necrosis in, 31, *32*
   mortality from, 35
   mycotic, 126-133. See also *Mycotic aneurysm.*
   noninflammatory fibroplasia and, 33
   postcoarctation, *154,* 156, *156*
   proximal, repair of, 263-294, *264*
         aortic arch replacement for, 281-283, *281-285,*
            286
         aortic valve insertion for, 264-265, *265, 266*
         ascending aortic tubular graft insertion for,
            263-264, *264*
         composite valve graft insertion for, 265-273,
            266-272, 274
            Bentall technique of, *266, 268*
            button technique of, *267*
            Cabrol technique of, *269-271*
         distal aortic arch replacement for, *292,* 293-294,
            293
         elephant trunk procedure for, 286-295,
            287-290
            results of, 291-293
         homograft insertion for, 273-281, *275-280*
         patient preparation for, 283-286
         pulmonary autograft insertion for, 278-279,
            278-280
   rupture of, clinical presentation of, 39
      expansion rate and, 37
      incidence of, 35
   saccular, acute dissection and, *300-301*
      aortography of, *12*
      chest radiography of, *11*
      computed tomography of, *12*
      magnetic resonance imaging of, *16*
   suprarenal, repair of, 350, *355*

Aortic aneurysm(s) *(Continued)*
   surgical treatment of, 39-40, 263-294, 335-358. See
      also *Aortic aneurysm(s), distal; Aortic
      aneurysm(s), proximal.*
      evaluation for, 39-40
      incidence of, 36
      prophylactic, 38
   syndromes with, 35
   thoracic, coronary artery disease and, 17
      incidence of, 35-36
      monitoring of, 37-38
      mortality from, 38
      repair of, 343-345, *343, 344*
      rupture of, 38
   thoracoabdominal, celiac artery stenosis with, *374, 376,
      379,* 380-382, 381t, 382t
      classification of, 29, *30*
      iliac artery stenosis with, *375*
      in Marfan syndrome, *94, 361*
      mortality from, 38
      renal artery stenosis with, *375,* 380-382, 381t, 382t
      repair of, 345-350, *345, 347-349*
      rupture of, 38
      superior mesenteric artery stenosis with, *374, 376,
         379,* 380-382, 381t, 382t
      umbilical artery catheter infection and, *129-131,*
         132, 132t
      with horseshoe kidney, 395-399, *397*
   ultrasound in, 36-37
   with horseshoe kidney, 395-399, *395-398*
Aortic arch, 29
   cervical, 165
   distal, repair of, 335, *338-342*
   double, 161
   embryology of, 160-161
   interrupted, 161
   replacement of, 72-74
   right-sided, 164-165, *170-172*
Aortic arch arteries, occlusive disease of, 175-178, *177*
Aortic cross-clamping, 226-245
   cardiovascular alterations with, 226
   central venous pressure during, *228,* 230-231
   cerebrospinal fluid pressure changes during, 230-232
   hemodynamic alterations with, 226
   hyperemic unclamping response after, 228-229, *229*
   motor evoked potentials after, 245, *245*
   renal blood flow with, 226-227, *228*
   spinal cord blood flow and, 227-230, *228-230*
   spinal cord blood supply during, 232-245, *232, 233,
      235-245*
   spinal cord injury and, 257, *257,* 419-420, *419*
Aortic disease, diagnosis of, 6-25
   aortography in, 10-15
      abdominal views for, 13-14, *13*
      advantages of, 14
      anterior abdominal view for, 13, *13*

Aortic disease *(Continued)*
    catheter-induced complications of, 14-15
    disadvantages of, 14-15
    indications for, 10-11, *11, 12*
    lateral abdominal view for, 13-14, *13*
    renal failure with, 14
    standard thoracic views for, 11-13, *13*
  carotid artery screening during, 21-22
  comorbid disease detection during, 21-25
  computed tomography in, 6, 8-10, *8, 9*
    advantages of, 6, 9
    disadvantages of, *8,* 9-10
    indications for, 6, 9
  magnetic resonance imaging in, 15-16, *16*
    advantages of, 15-16
    disadvantages of, 15-16
    history of, 15
    indications for, 15
  pulmonary function tests during, 22-25, *22, 23, 24*
  strategies for, 21
Aortic dissection, 42-80
  acute, 42
    clinical manifestations of, 55-56
    diagnosis of, 57-67
      aortography in, 62-66, *64-66*
      chest radiography in, 57
      computed tomography in, 57-59, *58*
      magnetic resonance imaging in, 59, 63-64
      tranesophageal echocardiography in, 59-62, *61, 62, 63-64*
    prognosis for, 67
    signs of, 55-56
    symptoms of, 55
    treatment of, 67-70
      beta-blockers in, 67
      results of, 443-446
      surgical, 296, 298-307, *299-309,* 359, *360*
        indications for, 68
        results of, 443-446
      vasodilators in, 67-68
  aortic regurgitation in, 55-56
  aortic rupture in, 53, 55
  aortic valve defects in, 45
  aortography of, 7, 62-66, *64-66*
  atherosclerosis in, 46-47
  atherosclerotic ulcer in, 178, *181*
  auscultation in, 55, 56
  cardiac tamponade in, 55, 56
  chronic, 42
    clinical presentation of, 56-57, *57*
    prognosis for, 67
    surgical treatment of, 68, 311-319, 359-370. See also
      Aortic dissection, distal, chronic; Aortic dissection, proximal, chronic.
  classification of, 42-43, *43, 44*
    management and, 43

Aortic dissection *(Continued)*
  claudication in, 56
  clinical manifestations of, 55-57
  coarctation of aorta and, 45
  computed tomography in, 10, 80
  congenital factors in, 45
  Crawford classification of, 43, *44*
  DeBakey classification of, 43, *43*
  definitions of, 42
  diagnosis of, 57-67
    aortography in, *7,* 62-66, *64-66*
    chest radiography in, 57, *65*
    computed tomography in, *8,* 57-59, *58, 59,* 63-64
    echocardiography in, 20, 59-64, *59-62*
    magnetic resonance imaging in, 59, 63-64, *65*
  distal, 43
    acute, medical management of, 69-70
      repair of, 359, *360*
        indications for, 68
        results of, 443-446
    chronic, repair of, 68, 359-370
      descending thoracic aorta repair for, 359, *360, 361*
      indications for, 68
      peripheral vascular procedures for, 68, 362-363, *368-369,* 370
      results of, 443-446
      second-stage elephant trunk procedure for, 362
      thoracoabdominal aortic repair for, 360, *361,* 362, *363-367*
  echocardiography in, 20, 59-64, *59-62,* 80
  etiology of, 46-48, *47-53*
  experimental, 48
  extent of, 43, *43, 44*
  false lumen of, 42, 50-51, 53, *54, 75*
  fusiform aortic aneurysm and, 45
  genetic factors in, 44-45
  healing of, 46
  histology of, 46
  historical note on, 42
  hormonal abnormalities and, 45-46
  hypertension in, 47, 55
  iatrogenic factors in, 47-48, *47, 48, 51-53*
  in animals, 48
  in Marfan syndrome. See *Marfan syndrome.*
  incidence of, 44
  infection and, 45-46
  inflammatory disease and, 45-46
  intimal intussusception in, 53, *54*
  ischemia in, 56
  magnetic resonance imaging in, 59, 63-64, *65,* 80
  medial degenerative disease in, 46
  medical management of, 67-70
    beta-blockers in, 67
    vasodilators in, 67-68
  mortality from, 35

Aortic dissection *(Continued)*
  pain in, 55, 56
  pathophysiology of, 48, 50-51, 53
  pregnancy and, 45
  prognosis for, 67
  proximal, 43
    acute, medical management of, 69-70
      repair of, 68, 296, 298-307
        aortic arch management for, 296, *300-303*
        aortic valve management for, 303-307, *303-309*
        elephant trunk procedure for, 296, *302, 303*
        indications for, 68
        proximal aortic arch anastomosis for, 296, *298, 299*
    chronic, repair of, 68, 74-75, *75-77*, 307, *310, 311-319*
        aortic arch repair for, 307, *310*, 311
        aortic valve management for, 311-315, *311-315*
        ascending aorta reconstruction for, 307
        elephant trunk technique for, 316, *316-317*
        indications for, 68
        reoperation for, 316-319, *318-333*
        results of, 319, 334
  septal disappearance in, 46
  Stanford classification of, 43, *43*
  surgical treatment of, 43, *64*, 70-80, 298-319, 359-370
    See also *Aortic dissection, distal; Aortic dissection, proximal.*
    aortic arch repair in, 72-74
    aortic dilatation after, 79-80
    composite valve graft in, 75, *75-77*
    echocardiography after, 80
    indications for, 68
    interventional cardiovascular procedures in, 70
    intraluminal grafts in, 70, *71-74*
    principles of, 70, *71-73*
    reoperation risk after, 79-80
    rupture risk after, 79-80
    survival after, 56, *57, 66*, 75, *77-79, 79-80*
  syncope in, 55
  syphilitic aortitis and, 46
  transesophageal echocardiography in, 59-62, *61, 62*, 63-64, 80
  traumatic factors in, 47-48, *47*
Aortic fistulae, repair of, 391-393, *392, 393*
Aortic incompetence, in chronic aortic dissection, 57
Aortic isthmus, saccular aneurysm of, magnetic resonance imaging of, *16*
Aortic pressure, in spinal cord perfusion, 230
Aortic prosthesis, infection of, 133-149
    clinical presentation of, 134
    definition of, 134
    diagnosis of, 134
    incidence of, 134
    management of, 134-149

Aortic prosthesis *(Continued)*
      conservative, 134-136, *135*
      dead space obliteration in, 139
      extraanatomic bypass for, 139-140
      homografts for, 136, 138
      in situ repair for, 136-139, *137-150*
      long-term, 140
      operative strategy for, 140, 147
    prevention of, 133-134
Aortic replacement, entire, 400-405
    elephant trunk procedure for, 286-295, *287-291*, 400, 404-405 *402-405*
      results of, 291-293, 439-440
    in Marfan syndrome, *99*
    in planned stages, 400, *401*
    in unplanned stages, 400, *401*
Aortic rupture, in aortic dissection, 53, 55, *304*
  traumatic, 184-190
    diagnosis of, 185, *186-188*
    management of, 185-190, *188-190*
Aortic stenosis. See *Occlusive disease.*
Aortic surgery, distal, complications of, 414-427
      cardiac, 416-417
      gastrointestinal, 426-427
      intestinal, 415-416
      renal, 414-415, 423-425, *424, 425*
      respiratory, 415, 425-426, *426*
      spinal, 418-423, *418-420*
    for aneurysms, 335-358. See also *Aortic aneurysm(s).*
    for dissection, 359-370. See also *Aortic dissection.*
  follow-up after, 456-459
  history of, 2-3
  monitoring during, 248-260
      cardiac, 248, 251-253
      fluid, 252-253
      intrathecal, 248-251, *249-251*
      intravenous, 251
      transfusion, 258-260, *259*
  proximal, complications of, 407-412
      cardiac, 407-408
      neurological, 408-412, *409-411*
    for aneurysms, 263-294. See also *Aortic aneurysm(s).*
    for dissection, 296-334. See also *Aortic dissection.*
  results of, for abdominal aortic repair, 443
      for angioplasty, 450, 452-453
      for aortic arch repairs, 432-434, *433*
      for aortic dissection repair, 443-446, *445-453*
      for balloon dilatation, 450, 452-453
      for composite valve grafts, 434-439, *435-436*, 437t
      for descending thoracic aorta repairs, 440, *440*
      for elephant trunk procedure, 439-440
      for thoracoabdominal aorta repairs, 440-443, *441-442*
Aortic valve defect, congenital, aortic dissection and, 45
Aortic valve disease, 19

Aortic valve regurgitation, aortic aneurysm and, *321, 333*
  aortic dissection and, 55-56, *332*
  in Marfan syndrome, *89, 92, 94*
Aortic valve replacement, aortic dissection after, 45
  in Marfan syndrome, 87, *96,* 97
  in proximal aortic aneurysm repair, 264-265, *265, 266*
  in proximal aortic dissection repair, 303-307, *303-309,* 311-315, *311-315*
Aortitis, 32-33, *33,* 105-119
  autoimmune disease and, 35
  in aortic dissection, 46
  noninfective, 105-116. See also *Takayasu's disease.*
    etiology of, 118-119
    in ankylosing spondylitis, 118
    in Beçhet's disease, 118
    in cocaine abuse, 118
    in giant cell arteritis, 116-117, *117,* 119
    in polymyalgia rheumatica, 118
    in relapsing polychondritis, 118
    in rheumatoid arthritis, 117-118
    in systemic lupus erythematosus, 118
  syphilitic, 126
    aortic dissection and, 46
  tuberculous bacilli in, 32-33
Aortocaval fistulae, aortography of, 14
  repair of, 391, *392*
Aortoduodenal fistulae, repair of, 391, 393, *393*
Aortography, 10-15
  abdominal views for, 13-14, *13*
  advantages of, 14
  anterior abdominal view for, 13, *13*
  catheter-induced complications with, 14-15
  disadvantages of, 14-15
  in aortic dissection, *7,* 62-66, *64-66*
  in traumatic aortic rupture, 185
  indications for, 10-11, *11, 12*
  lateral abdominal view for, 13-14, *13*
  postoperative, in ascending aorta replacement, *8*
  renal failure after, 14
  Seldinger technique for, 10
  standard thoracic views for, 11-13, *13*
Aortoiliac segment, occlusive disease of, 382-389, *384-389*
  aortobifemoral bypass graft in, 382-383, *384-389*
  endarterectomy in, 382, 383
Aortointestinal fistulae, repair of, 391, 393, *393*
Apoptosis, 202
Aprotonin, postoperative, 260
Arachidonic acid, in neuronal ischemia, 210
  in reperfusion injury, 204
Arfonad (trimetaphan camsylate), in aortic dissection, 67-68
Arrhythmias, ventricular, postoperative, 407-408
Arteria radicularis magna (ARM, artery of Adamkiewicz), anatomy of, 232, *233,* 234, 235, *235*
Arterial pressure, during aortic surgery, 228, *228*
  spinal cord blood flow and, 226

Arteriography, in giant cell arteritis, 117
Arteritis, giant cell, 116-117, *117,* 119
  temporal, 116-117, *117*
Arthritis, rheumatoid, noninfective aortitis in, 117-118
Ascending aorta, definition of, 29
Aspartate, in ischemia, 198
Atheroma, echocardiography of, 20
Atherosclerosis. See also *Occlusive disease.*
  echocardiography of, 20
  in aortic dissection, 46-47
  in degenerative aortic aneurysm, 29, *30*
  of ascending aorta, 175
  of descending aorta, 178
  of thoracoabdominal aorta, 178
Atriofemoral bypass, 256-258, *257*
  in intraoperative spinal cord protection, 230
Auscultation, in aortic dissection, 55, 56
Autotransfusion, 258-260, *259*
Avitene, postoperative, 260

B

Balloon angioplasty, in coarctation of aorta, 155, 159-160
Beçhet's disease, aortitis in, 118
Beta-blockers, in aortic dissection, 67, 69
  in Marfan syndrome, 93
Blood gases, in cardiopulmonary bypass discontinuation, 256
Blood transfusion, intraoperative, 258-260, *259*
Blue toe syndrome, 178, *179, 180*
Brachiocephalic artery, occlusive disease of, 178
Brain, ischemic injury to, 195-212, *209*
  adenosine in, 201-202, *202*
  anion transport inhibitor in, 210
  arachidonic acid in, 210
  calcium in, 196-197, 197t
  dizocilpine in, 211
  DNA damage in, 202-203
  doxycycline prevention of, 211
  excitatory amino acids in, 198-201, *200*
  free fatty acids in, 201
  gangliosides in, 210
  hypothermia in, 210
  leukocytes in, 211
  neurotransmitters in, 198
  nitric oxide in, 207-209, *209*
  pentoxifylline in, 210
  polyamines in, 210-211
  prostaglandins in, 201

C

Calcification, after aortic rupture repair, 189, *190*
  of ascending aorta, 175
Calcium, in ischemia, 195, 196-197, 197t, 200-201

Calcium channel, voltage-gated, 196–197, 197t

Calcium channel blockers, in neuronal ischemia, 197–198

Calpain, in neuronal ischemia, 198

Cannulation, for cardiopulmonary bypass, 253–255, *254, 255*

Cardiac arrest, 223–225. See also *Deep hypothermia with circulatory arrest.*

Cardiac catheterization, 18–19
  complications of, 19
  disadvantages of, 19

Cardiac failure, intraoperative, 407

Cardiac index, during aortic surgery, 228, *228*
  in cardiopulmonary bypass discontinuation, 256

Cardiac output, intraoperative, 248, 252

Cardiac surgery, iatrogenic aortic dissection with, 47–48, *47–53*

Cardiac tamponade, echocardiography of, 20
  in aortic dissection, 55, 56

Cardiac valves, evaluation of, 19

Cardioplegia, 223, 224–225. See also *Deep hypothermia with circulatory arrest.*
  solutions for, 224

Cardiopulmonary bypass, 253–256
  cannulation for, 253–255, *254, 255*
  cardiac fibrillation during, 223–224
  cardioplegia during, 223, 224–225
  discontinuation of, 255–256

Carotid artery disease, hsp65 autoantibody and, 34
  postoperative stroke and, 412
  screening for, 21–22

Carotid endarterectomy, 21

Catheter, intrathecal, insertion of, 249–250, *250, 251*
    intraoperative, 248–251, *249–251*
  intravenous, intraoperative, 251

Cbz-Val-Phe-H (MDL-28170), in neuronal ischemia, 198

Cefamandole, prophylactic, for prosthesis placement, 133

Cefazolin, prophylactic, for prosthesis placement, 133

Celiac artery, occlusive disease of, *373, 374, 376, 379,* 380–382, *380,* 381t, 382t

Cell-saver blood, respiratory failure risk and, *24*

Central venous pressure, intraoperative, 228, *228,* 230–231

Cerebrospinal fluid (CSF), drainage of, 231–232

Cerebrospinal fluid (CSF) pressure, intraoperative, 228, *228,* 230–232
  measurement of, 231
  spinal cord blood flow and, 226

Chacma baboons, spinal cord blood flow in, 227–330, *227, 229, 230*

Chest pain, in aortic dissection, 55

Chest radiography, in aortic dissection, 57
  in traumatic aortic rupture, 185, *186, 190*
  reversed 3 sign on, 7

Children, coarctation of aorta repair in, 153, 155
  mycotic aneurysm in, *129–131,* 132, 132t

Chronic obstructive pulmonary disease, 22, *22*
  in aortic dissection, 69
  postoperative respiratory failure and, 415, 425–426, *426*
  pulmonary function tests in, 22–25, *23, 24*

Circulatory arrest, deep hypothermia with, 219–222. See also *Deep hypothermia with circulatory arrest.*

Claudication, in aortic dissection, 56

Coagulation, postoperative, 259–260

Coarctation of aorta, 153–160, *154*
  abdominal, 157, 159, *164*
  aortic dissection and, 45
  magnetic resonance imaging of, 7
  operative repair of, in adults, 155–157, *155–164,* 159–160
    in children, 153, 155
    results of, 159–160
  with Von Recklinghausen's neurofibromatosis, 157, 159

Cocaine abuse, aortitis in, 118

COL3A1 gene, in aortic dissection, 45

Collagen, in aortic aneurysm, 34

Collagenase, in aortic aneurysm, 34

Compartment syndrome, with aortography, 14

Computed tomography, 6, 8–10
  advantages of, 6, 9
  disadvantages of, 9–10
  in aortic dissection, *8,* 10, 57–59, *58, 59,* 63–64, 80
  in infrarenal aortic aneurysm, *11,* 119, *120, 122*
  in Marfan syndrome, *9*
  in mycotic aneurysm, 132
  in traumatic aortic rupture, 185, *187, 188*
  indications for, 6, 9

Connective tissue disorders, 44–45, 84–102. See also *Marfan syndrome.*

Cooper, Astley, 2

Coronary artery (arteries), photographic positive substraction angiography of, 12, *13*

Coronary artery disease, abdominal aortic disease and, 16–17
  evaluation of, 16–21
    cardiac catheterization in, 18–19
    echocardiography in, 19–21
    24-hour Holter electrocardiography in, 18
    preoperative, 416–417, *417*
  preoperative, 416–417, *417*
  prognostic implications of, 17–18
  thoracic aortic disease and, 17

Creatinine, respiratory failure risk and, *24*

Cross-clamping, aortic, 226–245. See also *Aortic cross-clamping.*

Crystalloid volume, respiratory failure risk and, *24*

Cyclophosphamide, in Takayasu's disease, 110

Cytokines, in aortitis, 118–119

Cytomegalovirus, in infrarenal aortic aneurysm, 119

D

Dacron graft, fibrous histiocytoma and, 192
DDAVP (1-deamino- (8-D-arginine)- vasopressin, desmopressin), postoperative, 259-260
Deep hypothermia with circulatory arrest, 219-222
    ancillary measures during, 221
    barbiturates during, 221
    blood transfusion during, 259
    cannula arrangement for, *220*
    duration of, 408, 411
    electroencephalogram monitoring during, 220-221
    history of, 219
    membrane stabilizers during, 221
    neurological dysfunction after, 411-412
    pH during, 219-220, 219t
    results with, 221-222, 408-412, *409-411*
    retrograde brain perfusion during, 221
    temperature measurement during, 220-221
Deoxyribonucleic acid (DNA), damage to, in ischemia, 202-203
Descending aorta, definition of, 29
Disseminated intravascular coagulation, postoperative, 260
Dizocilpine (MK-801), in neuronal ischemia, 211
Double aortic arch, 161
Doxycycline, in neuronal ischemia, 211
Duplex sonography, 21
Dural ectasia, in Marfan syndrome, 87, *88*

E

Echocardiography, 19-21. See also *Tranesophageal echocardiography (TEE).*
    dobutamine, 19
    Doppler, 21, 60
    for long-term follow-up, 20-21
    in aortic dissection, 20, 59-64, *61, 62*
    in atherosclerosis, 20
    in cardiac tamponade, 20
    in mycotic aneurysm, 132
    in traumatic aortic rupture, 185
    intraoperative, 20, 60
    of atheroma, 20
Ectopia lentis, of Marfan syndrome, 86, *87*
Ehlers-Danlos syndrome, 100, 102
    management of, 102
    pathology of, 102
    type I, 100
    type IV, 100, 102
Ejection fraction, calculation of, 18-19
Elastase, in degenerative aortic aneurysm, 34
Elastin, in degenerative aortic aneurysm, 34
Electrocardiography, after coronary artery bypass surgery, 408

Electrolytes, in cardiopulmonary bypass discontinuation, 256
Elephant trunk procedure, for distal aortic dissection, 362
    for entire aortic replacement, 286-295, *287-291,* 400, 404-405 *402-405,* 439-440
    for proximal aortic aneurysm, 286-295, *287-290*
    for proximal aortic dissection, 296, *302, 303,* 316, *316-317*
    in Marfan syndrome, *94, 96, 99*
(S)-Emopamil, in ischemia, 201
Encephalopathy, respiratory failure risk and, 24-25
Endocarditis, bacterial, mycotic aneurysms and, 126-127
Epigastric artery, inferior, in postoperative gastrointestinal tract ischemia, 416
Esmolol, in aortic dissection, 67
Eye, abnormalities of, in Marfan syndrome, 86, *87,* 90

F

False aneurysm, 29, *268, 329, 330-331,* 427
Fatty acids, free, in ischemia, 201
$FEF_{25\%}$, in chronic pulmonary disease, 23, *23*
$FEF_{25\%-75\%}$, in chronic pulmonary disease, 23-24, *23*
FEV_1, in chronic pulmonary disease, 23-24, *23*
FEV_1/FVC, in chronic pulmonary disease, 23-24, *23*
Fibrillation, cardiac, 223-224
Fibrillin, gene for, in Marfan syndrome, 85-86
Fibroplasia, arterial, noninflammatory, 33
Fibrous histiocytoma, Dacron graft and, 192
Fistulae, aortic, repair of, 391-393, *392, 393*
Fluid loading, during aortic surgery, 252-253
    guidelines for, 253
Flunarizine, in neuronal ischemia, 197
Follow-up, 456-459
Free fatty acids, in ischemia, 201
Free radicals, in reperfusion injury, 203-205, *203,* 205
    protection against, 205-206

G

Galen, 1
Gangliosides, in neuronal ischemia, 210
Gastric stress ulceration, postoperative, 415-416
Genetic factors, in Marfan syndrome, 85-86
    in Takayasu's arteritis, 107
Giant cell arteritis, 116-117, *117,* 119
Glutamate, in ischemia, 198-199, *199*
Glutamate receptors, in neuronal ischemia, 199-201, *200*
    inotropic, 199-200, *200*
    metabotropic, 199
Glutathione peroxidase, in reperfusion injury, *203,* 204
Graft. See *Aortic prosthesis.*

H

Haplotype-segregation analysis, in Marfan syndrome, 86
Harvey, William, 1
Heart, arrest of, 223-225. See also *Deep hypothermia with circulatory arrest.*
    contractility of, in cardiopulmonary bypass discontinuation, 256
    evaluation of, 16-21
        cardiac catheterization in, 18-19
        echocardiography in, 19-21
        24-hour Holter electrocardiography in, 18
        preoperative, 416-417, *417*
    fibrillation of, 223-224
    intraoperative function of, 223-225
    oxygen requirements of, 224
    preoperative preparation of, 223
Heart beat, in cardiopulmonary bypass discontinuation, 256
Heart failure, intraoperative, 407
Heat-shock protein 65, carotid artery plaques and, 34
    in aortitis, 119
Hematocrit, in cardiopulmonary bypass discontinuation, 256
    postoperative, 259-260
Hemoglobin, postoperative, 259-260
Hemorrhage, gastric, 415-416
    postoperative, 259-260
Hippocampus, CA1 sector of, ischemic injury to, 202-203
    long-term potentiation of, 210
Histiocytoma, fibrous, Dacron graft and, 192
Holter electrocardiography, 18
Horseshoe kidney, aortic aneurysm with, 395-399, *395-398*
    blood supply of, 398
    cooling of, 398
    renal artery anatomy in, 14
Hunter, John, 2
Hydration, preoperative, 252
Hydrogen peroxide, in reperfusion injury, 203, *203,* 204
Hydrogen testing, intraoperative, of spinal cord blood supply, 235-245, *236-244*
Hydroxyl ion, in reperfusion injury, *203,* 204
Hyperemia, after aortic cross-clamping, 228-229, *229*
Hypertension, in aortic dissection, 47, 55
    postoperative, after coarctation repair, 156
        after traumatic aortic rupture repair, 188
Hypoplastic aorta syndrome, 175
Hypotension, in cardiopulmonary bypass discontinuation, 256
Hypothermia. See also *Deep hypothermia with circulatory arrest.*
    neuroprotective effects of, 210

I

Iliac artery, occlusive disease of, *375, 384, 386*
Iliac vein fistula, repair of, *392*
Infant, coarctation of aorta in, operative repair of, 153, 155
Infection, 126-149
    bacterial, aortic dissection and, 45-46
        chronic, 126
    in aortitis, 119
    in degenerative aortic aneurysm, 34-35
    mycotic, 126-133. See also *Mycotic aneurysm.*
    of aortic prosthesis, 133-149. See also *Aortic prosthesis, infection of.*
    syphilitic, 126
Inflammatory aortic aneurysm, 32-33, *33.* See also *Aortitis.*
    of infrarenal aorta, 119-124, *120-123*
Inflammatory disease, aortic dissection and, 45-46
Infrarenal aorta, aneurysm of, computed tomography of, *11*
        inflammatory, 119-124, *120-123*
        renal artery stenosis with, *388, 389*
        repair of, 350, *351, 352, 356*
        ultrasonography of, 36-37
        with horseshoe kidney, 395-399, *397*
    diameter of, 36
    occlusive disease of, *377-378, 387*
Innominate artery, occlusive disease of, 371, *372*
Intercostal arteries, anatomy of, *232,* 233-234
Interferon-J, in aortitis, 119
Interleukins, in aortitis, 119
Internal mammary artery bypass graft, in descending thoracic aortic operation, 17
Interrupted aortic arch, 161
Intestinal fistulae, repair of, 391, 393, *393*
Intraoperative monitoring, 248-260
    cardiac, 248, 251-253
    fluid, 252-253
    intrathecal, 248-251, *249-251*
    intravenous, 251
    transfusion, 258-260, *259*
Iron, in reperfusion injury, 205
Ischemia, 195-203, 209-211, *209.* See also *Reperfusion injury.*
    adenosine in, 201-202, *202*
    anion transport inhibitor treatment in, 210
    arachidonic acid metabolites in, 210
    calcium in, 196-197, 197t, 200-201
    definition of, 194
    dizocilpine treatment in, 211
    DNA damage in, 202-203
    doxycycline treatment in, 211
    excitatory amino acids in, 198-201, *199, 200*
    free fatty acids in, 201
    ganglioside treatment in, 210

Ischemia *(Continued)*
  glutamate in, 198-199, *199*
  glutamate receptors in, 199-201, *200*
  hypothermia prevention of, 210
  in aortic dissection, 55, 56
  lactic acidosis in, 195-196
  leukocytes in, 211
  neural injury from, 195
  neurotransmitters in, 198
  nitric oxide in, 211, *211*
  pentoxifylline treatment in, 210
  polyamines in, 210-211
  prevention of, 210-211
Isradipine (PN200-220), in neuronal ischemia, 197

J

Juxtarenal aorta, 29
  aneurysm of, 14, 350, *353-354*

K

Kainate receptor, 199, 200
Kawasaki disease, aneurysms in, 35
Ketanserin, in ischemia, 201
Kidneys, blood flow of, aortic cross-clamping and, 226-227, *228*
  cold perfusion of, 424, *424*
  failure of, contrast-induced, 9, 14
    postoperative, 415-415, 423-425, *424, 425, 426*
  function of, in cardiopulmonary bypass discontinuation, 256
  horseshoe, aortic aneurysm with, 395-399, *395-398*
    blood supply of, 398
    cooling of, 398
    renal artery anatomy in, 14
  ischemia of, aortic cross-clamping and, 226-227, *228*

L

Labetalol, in aortic dissection, 67
Lactic acid, in ischemia, 195-196
Left subclavian artery steal syndrome, 175-176, *177*
Left ventricular distention, intraoperative, 223
Lens, displacement of, in Marfan syndrome, 86, *87*
Leukocytes, in reperfusion injury, 211
Leukotrienes, in neuronal ischemia, 210
  in reperfusion injury, 204
Lipids, peroxidation of, in reperfusion injury, 204
Long-term management, 456-459
Long-term potentiation, of CA1 hippocampal synapses, 210

M

Magnetic resonance imaging, 15-16, *16*
  advantages of, 15-16
  disadvantages of, 16
  history of, 15
  in aortic dissection, 59, 63-64, 80
  in infrarenal aortic aneurysm, 119, *120*
  in mycotic aneurysm, 132
  indications for, 15
  technique of, 15
  vs. transesophageal echocardiography, 15
Marfan syndrome, 84-100
  aortic aneurysm in, 93, *94, 96*
  aortic diameter in, 95, 97
  aortic dissection in, *9*, 45, *49, 50, 76*, 87, 90, 93
    aortic arch extension of, *90*
    aortic replacement for, 400, *401*
    during pregnancy, 93
    operative repair of, *89-91*, 92-100, *94-96, 98-101*
      history of, 84-85
      indications for, 95, 97
      infection after, *135*
      results of, 446, 450
      technique for, 97-100, *98-101*
    type II, *89, 95*
    type III, *91, 92*
  aortic valve regurgitation in, *89, 92, 94*
  beta-blockers in, 93
  cardiovascular abnormalities in, 87, *89*, 90, *90-92*
  clinical manifestations of, 86
  computed tomography in, *9*
  death in, 92-93
  diagnosis of, 92
  dural ectasia in, 87, *88*
  ectopia lentis of, 86, *87*
  family history of, 87
  fibrillin gene in, 85-86
  genetic counseling in, 93
  genetic findings in, 85-86
  histology of, 86
  historical perspective on, 84-85
  incidence of, 86
  major criteria for, 86-90, *87-92*
  medical management of, 93
  minor criteria for, 90, 92
  mitral valve disease in, 93
  palate in, *89*
  sinus of Valsalva aneurysm in, *95*
  Steinberg thumb sign in, 86-87, *88*
  thoracoabdominal aortic aneurysm in, *94, 361*
Mechanical ventilation, duration of, respiratory failure risk and, 25
Media, atherosclerosis of, *30, 32*
  degeneration of, 31, *31*. See also *Aortic aneurysm(s).*
    in aortic dissection, 46

Media *(Continued)*
  necrosis of, 31, *32*
Medionecrosis aortae idiopathica cystica, 46
Mega-aorta, aortic replacement in, 335, *336-337, 402-404*
Menkes' syndrome, 102
Mesenteric artery, superior, occlusive disease of, *373, 374, 376, 379,* 380-382, *380,* 381t, 382t
Metals, transition, in reperfusion injury, 205
Methotrexate, in Takayasu's disease, 110
Metoprolol (Lopressor), in aortic dissection, 67, 69
Middle aortic syndrome, 105, 108. See also *Takayasu's arteritis.*
Mitral valve disease, in Marfan syndrome, 93
Monckeberg's sclerosis, *vs.* pseudoxanthoma elasticum, 102
Motor vehicle accident, aortic rupture with, 184-190
    diagnosis of, 185, *186-188*
    management of, 185-190, *188-190*
Mycotic aneurysm, 126-133
  aortography of, 14
  bacterial endocarditis and, 126-127
  clinical presentation of, 132
  definition of, 126-127
  diagnosis of, 132
  etiology of, 128-132, *129-131*
  historical perspective on, 126-127
  in child, *129-131,* 132, 132t
  management of, 132-133, 132t
  organisms in, 127-128, *128*
  pathology of, 127-128, *127, 128*
  predisposing factors in, 132
Myocardial ischemia, silent, Holter monitoring for, 18

N

Necrosis, 202
Neurological dysfunction, deep hypothermia with circulatory arrest and, 411-412
  in traumatic aortic rupture, 188
Neurotransmitters, in ischemia, 198
Nimodipline, in neuronal ischemia, 198
Nitric oxide, functions of, 207-209
  in neuronal ischemia, 207-209, *209*
  in no-reflow phenomenon, 206-209, *209, 211*
  NMDA receptor effect of, 209-210
Nitric oxide synthase, 207, 207t, 208
  inhibitors of, 208
Nitroglycerin, intraoperative, 252, 253
  preoperative, 252
Nitroprusside, in aortic dissection, 67-68
  in spinal cord injury, 230
  intraoperative, 253
NMDA receptor, 199-200
  nitric oxide effect on, 209-210
No-reflow phenomenon, 206-209
  definition of, 194-195

No-reflow phenomenon *(Continued)*
  nitric oxide in, 206-209, 207t
  nitric oxide synthase in, 207, 207t

O

Occlusive disease, 175-183
  of abdominal aorta, *180,* 182-183, *182, 373*
  of aortic arch arteries, 175-178, *177*
  of aortoiliac segment, 382-389, *384-389*
  of ascending aorta, 175, 371, *372*
  of celiac artery, *373, 374, 376, 379,* 380-382, *380,* 381t, 382t
  of iliac artery, *375, 384, 386*
  of infrarenal aorta, *377-378, 387*
  of innominate artery, 371, *372*
  of left subclavian artery, 175-178, *177*
  of renal artery, *373, 375,* 380-382, 381t, 382t, *388, 389*
  of right subclavian artery, 371, *372*
  of superior mesenteric artery, *373, 374, 376, 379,* 380-382, *380,* 381t, 382t
  of thoracoabdominal aorta, 178, *179, 180*
  of visceral arteries, 371-380, *373-380*
Ornithine decarboxylase, in neuronal ischemia, 211
Oxygen, cardiac requirements for, 224

P

Pain, in aortic dissection, 55, 56
PaO$_2$, respiratory failure risk and, *24*
Paralysis, respiratory failure risk and, 24-25
Paraparesis, postoperative, 418-423, *418-420*
    delayed, 420-421
    prevention of, 421-423
Paraplegia, postoperative, 233-245, *235-245,* 418-423, *418-420*
    delayed, 420-421
    prevention of, 421-423
Par, Ambrose, 1
Pectus carinatum, in Marfan syndrome, 86, *87*
Pectus excavatum, in Marfan syndrome, 86
Pentoxifylline, in neuronal ischemia, 210
Percutaneous transluminal coronary angioplasty (PTCA), 19
pH, in deep hypothermia with circulatory arrest, 219-220, 219t
Photographic positive substraction angiography, 12, *13*
Polychondritis, relapsing, aortitis in, 118
Polymyalgia rheumatica, aortitis in, 118
Porcelain aorta, 175, *176*
Posterior spinal artery, anatomy of, 233
Potassium, in cardiopulmonary bypass discontinuation, 256
  in ischemia, 195
Pregnancy, aortic dissection during, 45
  with Ehlers-Danlos syndrome, 102

Preload, intraoperative, 252, 253

Procollagen gene, in aortic dissection, 45
    in degenerative aortic aneurysm, 34

Propranolol (Inderal), in aortic dissection, 67, 69

Prostacyclin (PGI$_2$), in neuronal ischemia, 210
    in reperfusion injury, 204

Prostaglandins, in ischemia, 201
    in reperfusion injury, 204

Prosthesis, aortic, infection of, 133-139. See also *Aortic prosthesis, infection of.*

Pseudocoarctation, 156, *157*

Pseudoxanthoma elasticum, 102

Pulmonary arterial pressure, in cardiopulmonary bypass discontinuation, 256

Pulmonary autograft, for proximal aortic aneurysm repair, 278-279, *278-280*

Pulmonary disease, 22, *22*
    postoperative respiratory failure and, 415, 425-426, *426*
    pulmonary function tests in, 22-25, *23, 24*

Pulmonary function tests, in pulmonary disease, 22-25, *23, 24*

R

Relapsing polychondritis, aortitis in, 118

Renal artery (arteries), anatomy of, in horseshoe kidney, 14
    occlusive disease of, *373, 375, 379,* 380-382, *380,* 381t, 382t, *388, 389*

Renal failure, contrast-induced, 9, 14
    postoperative, 414-415, 423-425, *424, 425, 426*

Reperfusion, definition of, 194

Reperfusion injury, 203-206. See also *Ischemia.*
    allopurinol prevention of, 205
    antioxidant prevention of, 205-206
    leukocytes in, 211
    lipid peroxidation in, 204
    oxygen-derived free radicals in, 203-205, *203*
    prevention of, 205-206
    superoxide dismutase prevention of, 206
    transition metals in, 205

Respiratory failure, postoperative, 415, 425-426, *426*
    risk for, 22-25, *22, 23, 24*

Rheumatoid arthritis, noninfective aortitis in, 117-118

Right-sided aortic arch, 164-165, *170-172*

Riluzole, in neuronal ischemia, 199

S

Segmental arteries, reattachment of, 422-423

Sepsis, nitric oxide in, 208

Serotonin, in ischemia, 201

Sinus of Valsalva, 29
    aneurysm of, in Marfan syndrome, *95*
    dilatation of, *270*

Solutions, cardioplegic, 224

Spinal arteriography, 12-13

Spinal cord, blood flow of, aortic pressure in, 230
        arterial pressure and, 226
        CSF pressure and, 226
            during aortic cross-clamping, 234-245, *235-245*
            in chacma baboons, 227-330, *227, 229, 230*
        blood supply of, aortic cross-clamping and, 232-234, *232, 233*
            hydrogen testing of, 235-245, *236-244*
            intraoperative identification of, 235-245, *236-244*
        cooling of, 422
        operative injury to, 418-423, *418-420*
            aortic cross-clamping and, 233-245, *235-245,* 257, *257*
            prevention of, 421-423

Spinal motor evoked potentials, 423

Spirometry, in chronic pulmonary disease, 23-24, *23*

Steinberg thumb sign, in Marfan syndrome, 86-87, *88*

Stenosis. See also *Occlusive disease.*
    aortic, supravalvular, 165, 170-173, *173*

Steroids, in giant cell arteritis, 117
    in Takayasu's disease, 110

Stroke, postoperative, 408-412, *409-411*
        carotid artery stenosis and, 412
        risk for, carotid artery screening for, 21-22
        with aortography, 15

Subclavian artery, right, aberrant, 161, 163-164, *165-169*
        occlusive disease of, 371, *372*

Subclavian artery steal syndrome, left, 175-176, *177*

Superoxide, in reperfusion injury, *203, 204*

Superoxide dismutase, in reperfusion injury prevention, 206

Suprarenal aorta, 29

Supravalvular aortic stenosis, 165, 170-173, *173*

Surgicel, postoperative, 260

Syncope, in aortic dissection, 55

Syphilitic aortitis, 126

Systemic lupus erythematosus (SLE), aortitis in, 118

T

Takayasu's disease, 105-116
    anatomic site of, 107
    angiography in, 107
    classification of, 105-106, *106*
    clinical presentation of, 107
    cyclophosphamide in, 110
    demography of, 107
    diagnosis of, 107-110
    genetic factors in, 107
    histology of, 106-107
    historical perspective on, 105-106
    medical treatment of, 110
    methotrexate in, 110
    prognosis for, 110, 116

Takayasu's disease *(Continued)*
   steroids in, 110
   surgical treatment of, *108-109,* 110, *111-115*
Temperature, body. See also *Deep hypothermia with circulatory arrest.*
     in cardiopulmonary bypass discontinuation, 256
Temporal arteritis, 116-117, *117*
Thoracic aorta, aneurysm of. See *Aortic aneurysm, thoracic.*
   aortography of, 11-13, *13*
   definition of, 29
   descending, cross-clamping of, 226-245. See also *Aortic cross-clamping.*
Thoracoabdominal aorta, aneurysm of. See *Aortic aneurysm, thoracoabdominal.*
   dissection of, 360, *361, 362, 363-367*
   occlusive disease of, 178, *179, 180*
Three-dimensional spiral computed tomographic angiography, 9
Thromboxane, in neuronal ischemia, 210
   in reperfusion injury, 204
Transesophageal echocardiography (TEE), 19-21
   in aortic dissection, 59-64, *61, 62,* 80
   in mycotic aneurysm, 132
   in traumatic aortic rupture, 185
   intraoperative, 60
   limitations of, 60-62, *61, 62*
   vs. magnetic resonance imaging, 15
Transgenic mice, superoxide dismutase activity in, 206
Transition metals, in reperfusion injury, 205
Transthoracic echocardiography (TTE), 19-21
   in aortic dissection, 59, 80
Trauma, 184-190
   blunt, 184-190
     diagnosis of, 185, *186-188*
     management of, 185-190, *188-190*
   in aortic dissection, 47-48, *47-53*
   penetrating, 184
Trimetaphan camsylate (Arfonad), in aortic dissection, 67-68
Tuberculosis, aortitis in, 32-33
Tumors, 192

U

Ulcer, atherosclerotic, 178, *181*
Ultrasonography, for aortic aneurysm screening, 36-37
Umbilical artery catheter, infection of, thoracoabdominal aortic aneurysm with, *129-131,* 132, 132t
Urine output, in cardiopulmonary bypass discontinuation, 256

V

Vancomycin, prophylactic, for prosthesis placement, 133
Vascular resistance, systemic, during aortic surgery, 228, *228*
Vasodilators, in aortic dissection, 67-68
Ventricular arrhythmia, postoperative, 407-408
Ventriculography, segmental wall motion on, 18
Vesalius, Andreas, 1
Visceral arteries, occlusive disease of, 371-380, *373-380*
Von Recklinghausen's neurofibromatosis, abdominal coarctation with, 157, 159

W

Wheat procedure, 264-265, *265, 266, 303, 305*
Williams syndrome, supravalvular aortic stenosis and, 165, 170-173, *173*

X

Xanthine oxidase, in ischemia, 201-202, *202*
   in reperfusion injury, 205

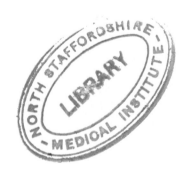

ISBN 0-7216-5426-6